Textbook of International Health
SECOND EDITION

Textbook of International Health

SECOND EDITION

PAUL F. BASCH

To David Pyle
With fond recollections of
our wanderings
Paul

New York   Oxford
OXFORD UNIVERSITY PRESS
1999

Oxford University Press

Oxford   New York
Athens   Auckland   Bangkok   Bogotá   Buenos Aires   Calcutta
Cape Town   Chennai   Dar es Salaam   Delhi   Florence   Hong Kong   Istanbul
Karachi   Kuala Lumpur   Madrid   Melbourne   Mexico City   Mumbai
Nairobi   Paris   São Paulo   Singapore   Taipei   Tokyo   Toronto   Warsaw

and associated companies in
Berlin   Ibadan

Published by Oxford University Press, Inc.
198 Madison Avenue, New York, New York 10016

Oxford is a registered trademark of Oxford University Press

Library of Congress Cataloging-in-Publication Data
Basch, Paul F., 1933–
Textbook of international health / Paul F. Basch. - - 2nd ed.
p. cm. Includes bibliographical references and index.
ISBN 0-19-513204-1
1. World health.   I. Title.
RA441.B38   1999
362.1- -dc21   98-50118

9 8 7 6 5 4 3 2 1
Printed in the United States of America
on acid-free paper

Preface

Like a distant, exotic place, international health is strangely alluring but difficult to reach, replete with unfamiliar tribal customs, and perhaps a bit dangerous, but with the prospect that the journey there would be immensely worthwhile. This book is intended as a travelers' guide. But what is *international health*? I see it broadly as *a systematic comparison of the factors that affect the health of all human populations*. Please feel free to write your own definition. It is a big subject that can accommodate many interpretations.

This book is a complete rewriting of the first edition, which was published in 1990. In the intervening decade the field has grown more than I or anyone else expected. Technology and world events have affected the health scene in many ways. The Soviet Union has collapsed, to be replaced by diverse new sovereign states, Germany has been reunified, and health reform has burgeoned in those places and throughout the world. Accordingly, chapters have been added on management information systems and health sector reform. The network of organizations involved in this field has expanded in number and broadened in outlook. These groups and their policies and programs are reviewed and updated. Trends in development assistance "(foreign aid,")" such as sector-wide approaches, are highlighted. A list of useful Internet sites is included as an appendix to Chapter 5 to facilitate direct access to these groups, and to their documents and records. There are new discussions of structural adjustment; the global burden of disease; application of the disability-adjusted life year (DALY); poverty, equity, and health; disaster and refugee relief programs; aging populations; and development, resource use, and the environment. The sections on child health, women's and reproductive health, maternal mortality, and emerging infectious diseases, including AIDS have been updated. There is expanded coverage of the basic models of health and medical care systems and their variants.

In an increasingly interconnected world every element is linked to all others, so it is a daunting challenge to depict the multidimensional nature of international health in a linear text. It is equally demanding to depict the world with accuracy. People tend to buy into one or another consensus reality, based on their affiliations, attitudes, experiences, and presumed knowledge, and all interpretation is colored by inevitable biases. We concede that there is a real world out there, but have access only to limited information about it, of variable and often unrecognized quality. A certain number of children died in West Africa in 1998, but we can only estimate the exact tally. Of those children, a number were reported to have died from malaria, but with better nutrition or less diarrheal disease or pneumonia many of those children might have recovered. It becomes very difficult, then, to specify how many deaths were in fact attributable specifically to malaria. Much of international health is that way. We must function with a level of uncertainty somewhere between unlimited acceptance and universal skepticism.

This book is an attempt to frame some of the larger issues in international health in ways that serve the needs of students, scholars, and workers in this and related fields and to provide a base from which to expand knowledge wherever interest and opportunity may lead. Each major topic contains enough complexity to consume a lifelong career. I have sought a balance between principles and specifics to satisfy both planners and technicians; between the past and the present to build an appreciation of why we are where we are; and between advocates and critics of various approaches to highlight the challenges of fulfilling the best of intentions. I have tried to maintain the attitude of an observer who is both passionately interested and earnestly disinterested—that is, impartial, unbiased, having no personal stake in one outcome or another.

In a work intended to be comprehensive without being encyclopedic, and comprehensible without being simplistic, my decision to include this or omit that will inevitably differ from the choices that would have been made by others. As interpretation and rebuttal have no logical end, my tendency to write on has been restrained by pleas from the editor to keep the page count within reason. I have tried to comply and trust that clarity has grown along with brevity. A multiauthor anthology would be superior in expertise and authenticity, but consistency may be better served when a single, admittedly fallible, mind confronts the subject.

My job has been made easier by the information and assistance given by many people. Among these are Valery Abramov, Howard Barnum, David Brandling-Bennett, Robert Bergquist, Neil Boyer, Guy Carrin, James Cheyne, Alice Clague, Andrew Creese, Bob Emrey, Tore Godal, Jeffrey Hammer, Robert Hata, Robert Hecht, Peter Heywood, Chris Howson, Michel Jancloes, Katia Janovsky, Jayakaran Job, Etsuko Kita, Chris Lovelace, Halfdan Mahler, Sara Newman, Armen Panossian, David Peters, Alexander Preker, Richard Saynor, Helen Saxenian, Alfredo Solari, Lane Smith, Gill Walt, Roy Widdus, Ronald Wilson, and Ken Yamashita. All of these colleagues, and many others, have improved this book immeasurably. I am sincerely grateful for the generous loan of their time and knowledge, which I have tried to repay through these pages. Many students over the years have focused my attention on their concerns. I have had them in mind while writing, and much of the discussion is aimed at questions they would be likely to ask. Jeffrey House, Susan Hannan and Nancy Wolitzer of Oxford University Press have eased the transition from textfile to textbook with patience and professionalism.

Despite my best efforts, there must be statements in this book that are not true: simple factual mistakes, lapses of judgment, failures of comprehension, and explanations overrun by the passage of time. The responsibility for these errors of commission, omission, opacity, and interpretation is mine alone. I wish I knew what and where they are.

Stanford, California   P.F.B.
October 1998

Contents

Some Abbreviations and Acronyms Used in International Health

ACMR   Advisory Committee on Medical Research (WHO)

ADB   Asian Development Bank

AfDB   African Development Bank

AID   See USAID

AIDS   Acquired Immunodeficiency Syndrome

AKF   Aga Khan Foundation

ALRI   Acute Lower Rerpiratory Infection

ARI   Acute Respiratory Infection

AURI   Acute Upper Respiratory Infection

BCG   Bacille Calmette-Guèrin (TB vaccine)

CBA   Cost–Benefit Analysis

CBR   Crude Birth Rate

CCCD   Combatting Childhood Communicable Diseases

CDC   Centers for Disease Control and Prevention, US Public Health Service

CDR   Division of Diarrheal and Acute Respiratory Disease Control (WHO)

CEA   Cost-Effectiveness Analysis

CEE   Central and Eastern Europe

CGAP   Consultative Group to Assist the Poorest

CHE   Complex Humanitarian Emergency

CHW	Community Health Worker
CIDA	Canadian International Development Agency
CIOMS	Council for International Organizations of Medical Sciences
CIS	Commonwealth of Independent States
CMR	Child Mortality Rate; Crude Mortality Rate
CPHC	Comprehensive Primary Health Care
CVI	Children's Vaccine Initiative
DAC	Development Assistance Committee (OECD)
DALY	Disability-Adjusted Life Year
DDT	Dichlorodiphenyltrichloroethane
DPT	Diphtheria, Pertussis, Tetanus (immunization)
ECA	East Europe and Central Asia
EPI	Expanded Programme of Immunization (WHO)
ES	Epidemiological Surveillance
FAO	Food and Agriculture Organization (UN)
FHW	Family Health Worker
FP	Family Planning
FSE	Formerly Socialist Economy
FSU	Former Soviet Union
GBD	Global Burden of Disease
GDP	Gross Domestic Product
GHC	Global Health Council (formerly National Council for International Health)
GIS	Geographic Information System
GNP	Gross National Product
GPS	Global Positioning System
GOBI	Growth Monitoring, Oral Rehydration, Breastfeeding, Immunization (UNICEF)
GOBI/FFF	GOBI plus Family Planning, Food Production, Female Education
HFA	Health for All (WHO)
HFA2000	Health for All by the Year 2000
HIS	Health Information System
HIV	Human Immunodeficiency Virus
H/MIS	Health (and) Management Information System

HMO	Health Maintenance Organization
HNP	Health, Nutrition and Population (World Bank)
HPI	Human Poverty Index
HPN	Health, Population and Nutrition (USAID)
HYE	Health Years Equivalent
IBRD	International Bank for Reconstruction and Development (World Bank)
ICD	International Classification of Diseases
ICDDR,B	International Centre for Diarrhoeal Disease Research, Bangladesh
IDA	International Development Association
IDB	Inter-American Development Bank
IFPMA	International Federation of Pharmaceutical Manufacturers Associations
IGO	Intergovernmental Organization
IHD	International Health Division of the Rockefeller Foundation
ILO	International Labor Organization
IMCI	Integrated Management of Childhood Illness
IMF	International Monetary Fund
IMR	Infant Mortality Rate; Institute for Medical Research
INCLEN	International Clinical Epidemiology Network
IPPF	International Planned Parenthood Federation
IPV	Inactivated Poliomyelitis Vaccine
IRB	Institutional Review Board
IRH/FP	Integrated Rural Health and Family Planning
IT	Information Technology
LDC	Less Developed Country; sometimes Least Developed Country
LEB	Life Expectancy at Birth
LLDC	Least Developed Country (sometimes)
LNHO	League of Nations Health Office
MCH	Maternal and Child Health
MCO	Managed Care Organization
MIS	Management Information System
MMR	Maternal Mortality Rate
MOH	Ministry of Health

MSA	Medical Savings Account; Most Seriously Affected (Countries)
NCIH	National Council for International Health (U.S.) (renamed Global Health Council)
NGHA	Non-governmental Humanitarian Agency
NGO	Non-governmental Organization
NHS	National Health Service (Great Britain)
NIH	National Institutes of Health (US)
NIS	Newly Independent States
NNMR	Neonatal Mortality Rate
OC	Oral Contraceptive
ODA	Official Development Assistance
OECD	Organization for Economic Cooperation and Development
ODM	Overseas Development Ministry (UK)
OIH	Office of International and Refugee Health (US)
OIHP	Office Internationale d'Hygiène Publique
OPV	Oral Poliomyelitis Vaccine
ORS	Oral Rehydration Solution
ORT	Oral Rehydration Therapy
OTA	Office of Technology Assessment, U.S. Congress (Closed in 1995)
PAHO	Pan American Health Organization
PASB	Pan American Sanitary Bureau
PEM	Protein-Energy Malnutrition
PHC	Primary Health Care
PNN	Postneonatal
PNNMR	Postneonatal Mortality Rate
PPO	Preferred Provider Organization
PRC	People's Republic of China
PRICOR	Primary Health Care Operations Research
PVD	Program for Vaccine Development
PVO	Private Voluntary Organization
QALY	Quality-Adjusted Life-Year(s)
SAL	Structural Adjustment Loan
SAP	Structural Adjustment Policy (or Program)

SEP	Sector Expenditure Program
SIP	Sector Investment Program
SPHC	Selective Primary Health Care
STD	Sexually Transmitted Disease
SWAP	Sector-Wide Approach
TB	Tuberculosis
TBA	Traditional Birth Attendant
TDR	UNDP/World Bank/WHO Special Programme for Research and Training in Tropical Diseases
TFBSSA	Task Force on Basic Social Services for All (UN)
TFR	Total Fertility Rate
UN	United Nations
UNCTAD	United Nations Conference on Trade and Development
UNFPA	United Nations Population Fund
UNICEF	United Nations Children's Fund
UNDP	United Nations Development Programme
UNHCR	United Nations High Commissioner for Refugees
UNRRA	United Nations Relief and Rehabilitation Agency
USAID	United States Agency for International Development
WDR93	The World Bank's World Development Report 1993, Investing in Health
VHW	Village Health Worker
WHA	World Health Assembly (WHO)
WHO	World Health Organization
WHOQOL	World Health Organization Quality of Life Index
YPLL	Years of Productive (or Potential) Life Lost

Textbook of International Health

SECOND EDITION

1

Introduction

We will invert the usual order of things and start this book with a quiz. Simply decide whether you agree or disagree with each of the 20 following statements. Don't worry: You cannot fail because there are no right answers.

International Health: First Quiz

1. All people have a right to health care provided by their government.
2. People's indigenous cultural traditions should be respected even if known to be harmful to their health.
3. In wealthy countries most health problems are caused by people's inappropriate behavior.
4. The most urgent health need in poor countries is for more doctors and hospitals.
5. The best medicine is the least medicine.
6. Most health problems originate in the environment and can be combated only in the environment.
7. Population control in the developing countries is the world's most urgent health priority.
8. Most of the major endemic communicable diseases will disappear by themselves with economic development.
9. Providing medical care to people in poor countries is a good way to promote religious or political viewpoints.
10. A person's genes basically determine his or her health and not much can be done about it.
11. If we eradicated smallpox we can do the same for any disease if we really want to.

12. People in the wealthy countries have a moral obligation to help people in the poor countries.
13. Saving lives from disease and starvation may produce more problems than it solves.
14. Governments in most poor countries are corrupt, so foreign aid is generally a waste of money and effort.
15. The main health problems in developing countries are caused simply by lack of water and sanitation.
16. To help reduce the burden of illness in the world one must first become a physician.
17. Most people in developing countries really do not want modern biomedical science.
18. The world is running out of many important resources so we must all learn to get by with less.
19. The best argument to a government official for financing health services is that it is a good economic investment.
20. As soon as we learn to control one disease another comes up: look at AIDS. The whole effort is basically useless.

How did you do? Why did you answer as you did? Was it easy to say yes or no, or did you have to stop and hesitate? If so, about which statements? Have you compared your answers with those of others? It should be clear by now that each person's interpretation of issues in international health depends on preexisting attitudes that color how he or she views the world. Although we are all born equally naked and ignorant, the unique personal combination of heredity plus life experience defines capabilities, attitudes, and interests, and influences receptivity to new ideas. While clearly idiosyncratic and highly variable, these global outlooks fall naturally within a fairly small number of internally consistent packages.

Herman Kahn and colleagues[1] defined four views of *the earth-centered perspective* which capture the main characteristics of four different attitudes toward the future of the world. The original descriptions, which were not concerned with health issues, cover many pages, but they are summarized in the paragraphs below. I have also added to each a description of views on world health likely to be held by people who hold each of the four basic attitudes. Look at these statements with some care and find the one with which you feel most comfortable. This selection is likely to color your interpretation of everything that is to follow in this book.

FOUR BASIC OUTLOOKS ON WORLD AND HEALTH FUTURES

Convinced Neo-Malthusian

Mankind is steadily depleting the earth's resources for food, fuel, and minerals. The world may run out of many critical nonrenewable resources in the next 50 years, and whatever remains must be shared more equitably among the nations. We have also created an increasingly serious pollution problem. Population and economic growth are almost cancerous and have passed the earth's long-term capacity to sustain. The domination of the world's resources by the rich countries must lead to increased and prolonged poverty in less developed countries. The rich may benefit temporarily but the gap between rich and poor is growing. Industrialization is a major culprit. Bigness must be discouraged, and more emphasis must be placed on local action. Proposed technological solutions to pollution and resource problems are short-term at best and will eventually make things worse. The 21st century will see environmental catastrophe; billions will die from hunger, pollution, and wars over shrinking resources. A completely new approach is needed now, with severe restraints, cutbacks, and a basic change in values and objectives. However, firmly held ideological differences among nations and groups make any effective action highly unlikely. Therefore the future is extremely gloomy.

The world's really serious health problems are caused by misuse of the environment, by pollution, by overpopulation, and by unequal distribution of wealth. The poor are kept ignorant and forced to cope with inadequate food, water, sanitation, and social services. These chronic problems are bound to get worse with increasing industrialization and soaring population, leading to the starvation of billions of people. As pandemics sweep the world, medical care will be increasingly scarce for most people in the world. So-called medical research is irrelevant to the health needs of the vast majority, whose problems are of little interest to developed-country researchers. In any case, there will be no logistical way to apply the results of sophisticated research, and most people will be too poor for it to be economically reasonable. As environmental and population pressures mount, governments will devote ever more attention to military issues and less to the welfare of their citizens. No real improvement in health can come about until the underlying causes are corrected, which will require no less than a radical restructuring of societal attitudes and governmental priorities, both of which are extremely unlikely ever to happen.

Guarded Pessimist

Efforts to obtain more minerals and food will accelerate pollution and exhaustion of resources, making some sort of disaster probable. As no practical solutions to resource and pollution problems are at hand, the best prudent strategy is immediate conservation of the remaining resources. Although the supply of materials is truly uncertain, it should be said that past projections have usually been underestimates. Nevertheless, ceaseless demands for growth, coupled with political turmoil, poor management, and inept planning, compound the problems. Demand must be limited. The rapidly increasing complexity of life makes effective management of these issues, and resolution of conflicts, very difficult. People in less developed countries should not seek big industry but should instead remain at a modest, appropriate scale that preserves their culture as well as their resources. Marginal returns from new investments will decline, so technology and investment should be discouraged. The time bought by technological advances must be used constructively to find ways to reduce expansion. We must reduce the growth of overcrowded cities, inhibit suburban sprawl, and slow demand for material things to avoid unwanted painful political and economic changes. Conditions in poor countries are becoming more desperate and may lead to extended warfare. A more equitable distribution of income and opportunities is urgently needed. Care and good planning are needed but may not prevent some disasters related to environmental degradation, population growth, and excessive demand.

Most of the world's health problems are caused by abuse of the environment, by excessive population, by social inequities, and by inappropriate health behavior. To minimize these to the extent possible, it is urgently important to augment educational, family planning, and environmental programs such as water supply and sanitation. In general, economic development merely substitutes one set of diseases for another. There are growing problems of environmental degradation, pesticide resistance in agricultural pests and vector mosquitoes, and drug resistance of disease-causing organisms. Epidemics of new diseases such as acquired immunodeficiency syndrome (AIDS) may appear from time to time, with substantial loss of life. To overcome such problems will require ever more effort, knowledge, and innovation. Large-scale world transfers of food may be needed to avert starvation in certain areas, but it is not clear who will pay for this. Medical care, although not an ultimate answer, can help people to live better lives. Great efforts will be needed to improve human knowledge and behavior and establish better health services. These are difficult problems with no easy solution, but concerted action can bring about gradual improvement.

Guarded Optimist

Despite some dangers, only new technology and investment can increase production; protect and improve the environment; hold down the costs of energy, minerals and food; and provide surpluses to improve living standards in less developed countries (LDCs). Even if world population approaches 20 billion, economic and technologic progress can yield living standards markedly better than present ones. However, it seems likely that internal societal forces will limit world population to about twice the current level, or about 12 billion. The progress made in developed countries suggests that increasing production is likely to increase further the potential for future production. We must push ahead, with caution. Higher consumption in developed countries benefits everyone; progress in one region leads to progress elsewhere, so the poor will also benefit. Absolute poverty is likely to vanish as economic development—the only hope of poor countries—is accelerated. Because reserves of energy, resources, and space are adequate for most populations, average per capita world production can reach two or three times the current U.S. level.

Overall, the best bet is for continued technological and economic development. Then, given good management, reasonable environmental protection, and attention to health and safety, outstanding progress is possible. In fact, most misery in the future will come from the anxieties of relative wealth, not poverty. As to corporations, some public regulation may be needed, but economic mechanisms can make most private organizations responsive to environmental problems. But it is possible that cartels and politial conflicts may lead to occasional problems in maintaining adequate supplies at reasonable prices.

The increased longevity typical of developed countries will be achieved in the currently less developed countries. Through carefully planned, patiently executed public health programs most serious diseases will be controlled, if not eradicated. Of course, education, family planning, and so on will need to be maintained, and will become increasingly effective through improvements in data processing and communication technology. Research in environmental and vector control, plus new vaccines, will lead to great reductions in diseases formerly considered intractable. The "green revolution" will have an increasingly positive impact on nutrition in poorer countries. Some hunger may be inevitable in local areas, but with adequate planning this will not be a major worldwide problem. Medical research will continue to provide new information to alleviate chronic diseases and enable people to live longer and in better physical condition. Better administrative and management techniques will lead to more efficient and cost-effective health services. These will be paid for by improved economies resulting from industrial development in poorer countries. Although some problems will remain formidable, the combination of improved knowledge, more efficient medical care, and better health services will lead to general and substantial improvement.

Technology-and-Growth Enthusiast

Sufficient land and resources exist for continued progress on a bountiful earth. Most current problems result from too little technology and capital, not too much. Greater growth means greater potential. Fantastic economic and technological progress lies ahead in fields such as agronomics, electronics, biotechnology, information processing, and power generation. The important resources are capital, technology, and educated people. Although there have been some problems from careless uses of technology, any dangers can be remedied by proper application of additional technology. Modern communications and information systems make rapid adjustments more feasible provided that governments do not interfere. The currently industrialized countries were once poor, and the currently poor countries will someday be rich. All those who wish to can share in the benefits of modern civilization. No imposed limits are needed except for population growth in some LDCs. Mankind has always faced problems, has always found a way to solve them, and will continue to do so despite gloomy predictions from some. Those doomsayers are probably disgruntled or unhappy people who oppose progress for ideological reasons. In any case there is always the likelihood of expansion into extraterrestrial habitats.

Medical researchers have made and will continue to make incredible strides in understanding basic biomedical science. Diseases such as polio that formerly caused panic are now a thing of the past in most developed countries. Other diseases such as malaria and even cancer are likely to lose their place as major killers of mankind. Organ transplants will be commonplace and will be able to maintain almost everybody in peak condition. The problem of excessive population in some countries will be solved by technology such as contraceptive vaccinations. Other advances in biotechnology will lead to improved strains of food crops and animals that will solve the world's problems of hunger forever. Even today a major problem of agriculture is persistent surpluses of food and fiber. Means of redistribution can readily be worked out to bring these surplus materials to people in need, whose industrialization will pay for the food imports, as has long been the case in Japan. Dams will redistribute water for irrigation and domestic purposes and at the same time provide abundant hydroelectric power for industrialization and full employment. Any new diseases that may appear can be conquered by application of ever more powerful research and technology. Advances in communications will bring health education to the whole world. Medical care will be generally available so that all people can live long, comfortable, and productive lives.

WHAT INTERNATIONAL HEALTH IS ALL ABOUT

So there you have it: an attempt to characterize people's attitudes about the future of health in the world. Now that we have established, or at least groped for, an individual philosophical underpinning, it seems reasonable to consider more concretely what "international health" is all about:

- Is it actually a distinct, definable discipline, or merely a collection of exotic health-related related data, anecdotes, and experiences?
- Is there a special body of concerns, knowledge, and practice shared uniquely by those persons who claim professional status within the field?
- Are there any special axioms, precepts, or guiding principles according to which we may order our observations and base our interpretations?

By way of analogy, look at the field of pathology and search for unique characteristics. Pathology is based on the findings of students of gross and microscopic anatomy, microbiology, immunology, physiology, endocrinology, and so on, many of whom might be surprised to be called a pathologist. It might be difficult even to define a subset of concerns, knowledge, and practice that is truly *unique* to pathology. Nevertheless, few would argue that pathology is not a distinct academic discipline. It follows that exclusivity is not a criterion for the legitimacy of any discipline. In fact, all disciplines, with the exception perhaps of pure mathematics, are made up of contributions from many others. Preexisting fields may always be reshaped through discovery and novel methodologies into a newly coherent body of knowledge, such as molecular biology.

Some persons are reductionist by temperament. They seek to understand the intimate workings of nature by probing more and more closely into mechanisms. The same kinds of intellectual processes drive those who probe into the cell nucleus or the atomic nucleus; indeed, a molecular biologist who happens to work in a medical school may have more in common intellectually with an atomic physicist than with a public health specialist. Alternatively, some persons are integrators by nature. They like to assemble observations and facts into big, interrelated constructs, and anything in the world, or the universe, for that matter, is fair game. International health offers plenty of scope for people with either outlook. But a subject that pretends to cover everything covers nothing, or at least nothing very well.

What then is included in international health?

- An understanding of the principles of epidemiology and public health. The general orientation is toward alleviating the burden of ill health in populations, while acknowledging that all populations are made up of individuals.
- An appreciation of the root causes of ill health in the world in general and in defined populations in particular; a certain level of technical understanding of the biology of pathogens causing infectious diseases, and their vectors or reservoirs where present; and of risk factors relevant to nutritional, environmental, and chronic diseases.
- A degree of sympathetic understanding of the emotional and psychological consequences which illness causes individuals, families, and communities, and of the means adopted within various cultures to diminish its burden
- Some understanding of the economic significance of illness to the individual, family, and community; and of the economic aspects of preventive, curative, and rehabilitative services, including their value to society and the flow of money and resources through the system.
- A recognition of the social and environmental consequences of human population growth and a knowledge of the methods of noncoercive family planning.
- Special consideration of similarities and differences among people in different countries, and among population segments within individual countries differentiated by age, sex, ethnicity, genetic makeup, residence, educational, occupation, culture, behavior, or other characteristics that affect health status.
- Familiarity with the structure and functioning of governments, especially ministries of health and other sectors responsible for public well-being. These may include ministries or agencies dealing with education; social security; planning,

finance, and evaluation. Knowledge of national, international, and intergovernmental donor and development agencies and their programs; and of nongovernmental and private voluntary organizations
- Understanding the variety of healing professions and their relation to the health of individuals and groups; including not only licensed physicians, nurses, and other practitioners of scientific western medicine but also midwives, community and village health workers, and traditional and folk healers of all sorts.
- Sensitivity to the ethical aspects of research and practice in poor and marginalized populations, and to the drive toward equity in the design and delivery of services.
- Humanitarian response to disasters and emergencies, especially those involving large numbers of people whose lives are disrupted by natural or civil calamity.

To the extent that international health (small letters) is considered by the general public at all, it is likely that threats of Ebola virus, AIDS and cholera, and images of relief workers feeding emaciated children will predominate over issues of economics and policy. The popular view, shaped by the media, is understandably skewed toward immediate and dramatic themes such as epidemics and disasters rather than the unsensational struggle for rational and equitable development.

The professional constituency for International Health (capital letters) consists of a smallish network of scholars, bureaucrats, consultants, and activists whose work and training are described further in Chapter 15. Many other individuals have greater or lesser involvement (Table 1-1). Their interests may be influenced by the underlying attitudes described earlier; by current news reporting of a famine or disaster; by concepts of equity, morality, and social conscience; by personal experience abroad; and even by a certain sense of adventure. The wisdom bought by experience is always expensive in time and effort, and competent professionals are both rare and valuable. Less experienced people may expect rapid resolution of problems that have evolved over years or decades, or perhaps have always existed. They may believe, in concert with some of the world views described earlier, that every problem is amenable to a technical solution—perhaps a new vaccine, or laptop microcomputers in health centers, or a novel form of contraceptive. Others will be convinced that some particular social scheme or political change is bound to achieve a rapid and permanent resolution. Advocates of either view may not appreciate the true complexity of issues and may denigrate the very solution so obvious to the other, while both may overlook other crucial aspects such as the economic dimensions. Hence the importance of the broad overview.

Throughout this text, we speak of "industrialized (or developed) countries" and "developing countries" as if these were real, and mutually exclusive, categories. Development cannot be measured solely by per capita Gross National Product (GNP), because some countries with high per capita GNPs have not undergone balanced

Table 1-1. What Different People Want From International Health

Academician	Study and publish about health problems and their solutions
Administrator	Organize and operate health services
Advocate	Promote a viewpoint
Anthropologist	Study human customs and behaviors related to health
Biotechnologist	Evaluate a new vaccine
Businessman	Obtain raw materials and market drugs and devices
Clinician	Practice medicine in a remote area
Development banker	Finance various investment projects
Economist	Study health resource allocation and financing
Epidemiologist	Study distribution and control of diseases
Escapist	Go to romantic places as far away as possible
Environmentalist	Protect habitats from human exploitation
Historian	See effects of past epidemics and policies
Humanitarian	Help suffering people
Militarist	Protect troops from exotic illnesses
Missionary	Gain converts through healing
Pharmacologist	Find new medicines
Politician	Control spheres of influence
Public health worker	Protect populations from illnesses
Scholar	Observe, analyze, and write books like this one

social and industrial growth. Countries that have experienced the demographic and epidemiologic transitions (Chapter 8) are generally thought of as "developed," but the per capita GNP of Mexico, a mid–transitional country, is 50% higher than that of Poland, a post–transitional country. In another viewpoint, the former colonialist powers must be considered developed, in contrast to the undeniably less developed tropical countries that were once their possessions. However, there is great variation within the ex-colonialist group; for example, France has four times the per capita GNP of Portugal, and some former colonies are doing very well indeed.

For our purpose, "industrialized" nations are, in general, those having specialized agencies to provide Official Development Assistance (ODA) in the form of financial flows and technical cooperation intended for the sociocultural and economic advancement of poorer countries. These are the 18 member countries of the Development Assistance Committee (DAC) of the Organization for Economic Cooperation and Development (OECD) (Chapter 3) and their economic peers. The member countries of the Organization of Petroleum Exporting Countries (OPEC) also provide some development assistance, as do other individual countries, such as Israel. Some countries, such as Israel and some OPEC members, receive and provide aid at the same time. Some donors, such as the Scandinavian countries, the Netherlands, and Canada, are often considered to have more altruistic policies, while others such as the United States and Japan are viewed as tending more toward self-interest. In fact, the situation is everywhere quite fluid, in response to a variety of ever-shifting domestic and global pressures and needs.

NOTES
   1. Kahn *et al.* (1976).

2

International Health Before 1900

PREHISTORY

Persons recognizable as fellow humans are thought to have evolved during the middle to late Pleistocene (250,000 to 100,000 BC), perhaps earlier, and most likely in East Africa. Existence at that time, in the words of Thomas Hobbes,[1] was marked by, "no arts; no letters; no society; and which is worst of all, continual fear and danger of violent death; and the life of man, solitary, poor, nasty, brutish, and short." Although there have been minimal physical changes since that era, every human population movement, war, and technological development has in some way left its mark on the current state of world health. That is why a knowledge of history is important.

Being as restless as we ourselves, our distant ancestors wandererd into the Middle East about 120,000 years ago, and throughout the habitable earth, even to Australia, by about 40,000 years ago. We are happy to believe that our ancient forebears lived a gentle and idyllic life, taking only what they needed and leaving little but footprints, but it has never been so. From the very beginning, humans have been hard on their environment. The tasty pigmy hippopotamus became extinct on Cyprus from overhunting in prehistoric times, as did the mammoths, sloths, giant tapirs, and camels in the Americas. Craftsmen on Crete stopped making ivory jewelry around 950 BC because elephants in Syria had been hunted to extinction. On Pacific islands, even quite remote ones, approximately 20% of all bird species were exterminated by the actions of ancient humans.[2]

By 10,000 to 30,000 years ago, Hobbes notwithstanding, some humans had developed substantial cultures with a sophisticated artistic sense, reflected in the many Neolithic cave paintings from this era found particularly in Spain and France. Estimates vary as to the number of humans in those early days. Most observers believe that around 10,000 years ago there were four to ten million humans on earth. Most lived in small groups or bands and over a lifetime were unlikely to see more than a few hundred different people, or any with gray hair.

The size of early human tribes was critical to the state of health of their descendants, because the genetic makeup of small populations can change quite rapidly. A small number of individuals in an isolated population is the classic material for genetic diversification through the process of *genetic drift*. Some characteristics are conserved and others are lost by chance or in relation to their survival value in the local setting. The isolation of populations need not be geographic, but must be reproductive. Subgroups of people can drift genetically even when they live side by side with others, so long as they do not interbreed.

Some early human health problems were not very different from those we know today. Although most of our information about ancient diseases comes from bones, careful sifting through the earth beneath skeletal remains has yielded recognizable eggs of intestinal parasites. Gallstones and bladderstones have remained in place in some prehistoric burials. Mummies found in Egypt, China, and elsewhere have been rich sources of medical information and have shown that schistosomiasis, arteriosclerosis, emphysema, syphilis, silicosis, and anthracosis, among others, are long-standing maladies of man. A study of 500 skulls of aristocrats from the Old Kingdom of Egypt showed that tartar formation, dental caries, and alveolar abscesses were no less common than in modern Europeans; by contrast, the teeth of persons from the poorer classes of that era, accustomed to a coarse and uncooked diet, were in much better condition.[3] Disturbances in development such as dwarfism and clubfoot are demonstrated in early remains, and osteomyelitis, gout, and spondylitis all register their presence in ancient bones. Rickets occurred in neolithic bones in Denmark, but, as may be expected, it has not been recorded from the then-tropical areas which had abundant sunlight. (Rickets usually requires an absence of sunlight or vitamin D.) Levels of lead and other elements can be determined directly in bones and teeth. Little is known of metabolic diseases such as diabetes, nor of cancers of blood or soft tissues that have left no permanent trace, but there seems no reason to doubt their presence. Some bones have shown signs of what is interpreted to be metastatic carcinoma thought to derive from primary sites in prostate, breast, and other organs. It is possible that with improved molecular techniques DNA from more recent or better-preserved specimens may provide direct testimony of ancient illnesses.

In the hunting–gathering stage of human development the small size of social groups and low degree of contact among them would probably have limited epidemics. The number of new susceptible people available in such bands was probably not enough to maintain an infective agent once an immunity-producing disease had run its course. Afflictions such as head and body lice, pinworms, yaws, and malaria most likely evolved along with humans from their primate ancestors. Hunter–gatherers must have confronted infectious viruses and bacteria carried by biting insects and the tissues of animals that they killed, skinned, and ate. They faced tetanus and fungal spores in the soil, parasites in the water, and other living hazards directly from the environment that did not depend on person-to-person transmission. Our Cro-Magnon ancestors hunted animals for a thousand years but seem never to have domesticated them. At some point nomadic hunters got control over herd animals, which they used for food (meat, milk, blood), wool, fur, and leather. They were now pastoralists with mobile, low-density populations living in close relations with their livestock and subject to diseases of animals such as plague, anthrax, Q fever, brucellosis, tuberculosis, hydatid cysts, and toxoplasmosis.

Because of their continual wanderings, migratory herdsmen faced starvation in lean times and certainly suffered from seasonal and regional nutritional deficiencies, but little is known about these. Although these nomads probably did not plant crops, others did. Agriculture began perhaps 10,000 years ago around fields of grasses such as wheat, barley, rye, and emmer and spread rapidly around the world in the succeeding six or eight millennia. Although it may seem easier to live off the land as a nomadic hunter–gatherer than to be a fixed farmer or villager, the benefits from animal husbandry and agriculture made settlements and villages viable. Health risks were both increased and decreased in the process. The accumulation of human feces around homesteads led to buildups of intestinal parasites and bacteria, causing diarrheal diseases. The need to store seeds and harvests, and the inevitable garbage and refuse heaps near habitations, brought molds, insects, and rodents. Eventually crowding, deficient hygiene, and unprotected water sources must have led to transmission of respiratory and intestinal infections with a huge toll, particularly among the young. Epidemics of measles, smallpox, and other infectious diseases with person-to-person transmission would also have occurred with migrations and trade whenever populations became large enough to maintain them.

In addition to a more predictable food supply, settling down may have reduced the hardships of pregnancy in nomadic life and helped in the survival of infants. Fixed communities also promoted occupational specialization leading to food production, weaving, refining metals, and making pottery for trade. Perhaps the need for a reliable source of fuel, ores, clays, and fibers, or the construction of permanent ovens or workshops helped convince people to stay put, at least for extended periods each year. Occupational diseases undoubtedly began around this time. One can imagine smoky environments from firing pots or smelting ores and toxicity from working unprotected with natural minerals. Cooking fires in caves and huts were also a source of respiratory illnesses and eye irritation, and remain so to this day in many countries of the world.

Indirect evidence of illness is seen in representations on artifacts, burial items, paintings, bas-reliefs, and statuettes found in Egyptian, Assyrian, Greek, Roman, and pre-Columbian digs. Among other afflictions these clearly depict dwarfism, rickets, polio, goiter, spinal tuberculosis, and leishmaniasis. Writings, stories, and legends are less certain sources of information. A condition mentioned in Indian texts from the sixth century BC and Chinese texts from the third century BC was probably leprosy. This disease may have been brought to Europe by soldiers of Alexander the Great returning from India in the fourth century BC. The famous Plague of Athens, which raged between 430 and 425 BC, killed a third of the inhabitants of the city-state, or about 300,000 people, who died rapidly in terrible agony. Many historians have suggested causes ranging from measles to influenza, but none seems reasonable for an epidemic of such virulence. Only recently has a tantalizing suggestion come forth: Could the plague of Athens have been caused by Ebola virus? Many aspects of the epidemic match those of recent outbreaks of Ebola fever in Zaire, even including a characteristic hiccoughing by infected people.[4]

In a remarkable discovery, a well-preserved complete body 5300 years old has been found recently in the Alps.[5] The deep-frozen "ice man" was only 25 to 40 years old when he died, but he had arthritis; calcium deposits in the blood vessels of his chest, pelvis, and neck; heart disease; atherosclerosis; healing broken ribs; and fairly severe osteoarthritis in the neck, lower back, and hip; and lacked one toe, possibly from frostbite. His lungs were very black, probably from cave fires. Finally, his bones showed growth retardation at ages 9, 15, and 16, most likely from repeated starvation. It was no Garden of Eden. Atherosclerotic heart disease has also been found in Egyptian mummies 3000 years old.[6]

Health hazards associated with the development of settlements have not been limited to ancient times. There have been analogous situations down through the millennia. In the decades following the Russian Revolution in 1917, for example, outbreaks of severe disease occurred among road builders, woodcutters, and settlers in new communities being developed in the taiga and steppe regions. Many persons died, and others were permanently paralyzed. The dramatic nature of these outbreaks stimulated investigation and led to the discovery of tick-borne encephalitis, spirochetosis, relapsing fever, and other diseases in these remote, formerly uninhabited regions. These diseases had several common elements: association with particular habitats or even specific locations, animal reservoirs, and, often, arthropod vectors. Outbreaks among humans resulted from intrusion into natural disease cycles occurring in the local fauna, particularly rodents, around whose burrows the agents and vectors were concentrated. Pioneering development in new areas—for instance, in the Brazilian Amazon or the Indonesian rain forest—results in similar disease outbreaks to the present day.

Humans did not kill only hippos, camels, and birds, but have themselves always been at risk from other humans. In early times infanticide was practiced, presumably to limit population size in times of stress, and may have accounted for 15% to 20% of births, as judged by skeletal remains.[7] The existence of cannibalism is shown by the cracked and isolated human bones in domestic waste piles. These bones may have been those of slaves or captives from tribal and territorial conflicts, a result of the sacrifice of older or weaker individuals, or the consequence of ritual consumption of the deceased. Such practices have continued until modern times in some parts of the world, and were responsible quite recently for transmission of *kuru* among the Fore people of Papua New Guinea.[8]

Ancient Medical Care

The first traces of medical lore appeared perhaps 10 to 12 thousand years ago,[9] in a period when agriculture and animal husbandry had their beginnings, tools were used to build huts and clear forests, and baskets and pottery were made. Lacking direct evidence, we presume that in ancient times healers attended to trauma, set broken bones, assisted at childbirth, and conducted healing rituals. They must have used medicinal plants including hallucinogens and narcotics, and processed plant products such as alcohol. We know that surgery was done even in very early times. In many regions, including Europe and the Pacific, trephining of the skull was practiced, a surgical procedure that reached its peak of perfection in the mountains of Peru. These daring operations in which a hole was cut through the skull may have been undertaken for ritual purposes, possibly for treatment of epilepsy, spirit possession, or some other disorder. The level of surgical skill is reflected in hundreds of neatly healed skulls with new bone growing around the aperture. The process has been depicted in colorful terms:

> There he squats, his back braced against a tree trunk, the patient's head firmly held between his knees. He selects a sharp-edged stone or fleam and makes an incision in the scalp, then bores into and through the bone. Such a stone, if expertly used, can penetrate the human skull in five minutes. He exchanges the dull stone for a new sharp one and bores another hole adjacent to the first, and so on until a complete circle of holes is made. These holes are joined and the disk of bone is lifted out ... What a glorious enterprise was his! Alone, beneath the open sky, no team of consultants, assistants, and nurses milling about ... Only his crafty hands, sharp stones, and compassion for his injured tribesman. One thrills at his performance.[10]

EARLY HISTORICAL TIMES

The development of civilizations with urban commercial and ceremonial centers surrounded by agricultural lands marked an enormous turning point in human history. Improved survival led to perhaps 100 million people by ancient historic times, around 500 BC. At the beginning of the Christian era the world population was probably about 250 million, a figure that did not change appreciably for a thousand years. Human communities became concentrated in such numbers that water supply and sanitation became critically important. Engineering works such as reservoirs and water distribution systems were built by Aztecs, Mayas, and Incas in the Western Hemisphere; by the peoples of the eastern Mediterranean; and by the Khmers, Aryans, Chinese, and others in Asia. Existing ponds or lakes were incorporated into the systems, or artificial ones were constructed. Custom, ritual, and political power must have regulated the use of water for domestic and agricultural purposes. Epidemics of waterborne diseases such as cholera and typhoid fever may have occurred wherever the proper microorganisms, environmental conditions, and susceptible populations coexisted. Mosquito breeding sites and, in some areas, snail habitats created by those developments undoubtedly led to outbreaks or permanent establishment of malaria, yellow fever, and schistosomiasis where conditions were favorable. As populations grew, the disposal of sewage and waste became more of a problem. Urban dwellers became vulnerable to food shortages as artisan, priest, and trader depended for their nutrition upon the labor of others, and all were subject to the vagaries of weather, microorganisms, insects, and other natural hazards.

The Dispersal of Humans

Three types of human movements should be distinguished. The first, and probably oldest, is the cyclical or irregular travel of a small group or band in a limited area, following the seasons and availability of plant and game foods. Hunter–gatherer groups must have moved in such orbits, which are still followed by some nomadic populations to this day.

The second is actual geographic migration from one area to another, with establishment of permanent residence in the new locality. Planned or unintentional ocean voyages have carried individuals or groups to distant shores. Thor Heyerdahl demonstrated this on the Kon-Tiki expedition, in which he and his companions drifted 3700 miles from Peru to the island of Raroia in Polynesia. Persons from Malaya, Sumatra, and Java migrated to Madagascar in ancient times, and the most remote piece of land on earth, Easter Island, was settled by the fourth century BC by peoples of the Pacific skilled in navigation. Continual, slow extension of range overland resulted in the occupancy of North and South America by emigrants from Asia probably between 20,000 and 10,000 years ago, and other continental areas were being colonized in the same general time period.

The third kind of human travel falls under the very general heading of "visiting," or movement from one place to another with the intention of returning. Invaders or marauders seized slaves, wives, cattle, or goods from near or far. Establishment of permanent settlements was followed by roads or tracks between them, and by the time of the Bronze Age in Europe, for instance, paths had been established from the Atlantic to the Caspian and from Scandinavia to Italy. Trading followed raiding.

Records of travels and voyages are available from early classical times onward, although some may be questionable. Phoenecian navigators reached Spain and Britain, and may have circumnavigated Africa about 600 BC to trade for spices in the area of India now known as Kerala. Carthaginians had commerce with West Africa (Guinea?) in the following century. By Greek and Roman times travel was well established, and even elephants from India were seen in Italy in the third and fourth centuries BC. Three ancient "silk roads" linked China, India, and Rome, and an alternate overland route passed from China through Yunnan and Burma to India. In the time of the emperor Trajan (AD 98–117) the Roman Empire extended from Scotland to the Sahara and from the Atlantic Ocean to the Persian Gulf, but goods of Mediterranean origin found their way to more remote places. Phoenecian beads have been discovered in Sarawak, on the island of Borneo, and Roman beads in the southern Malay Peninsula.[11] Articles originating in China about the ninth century AD have been unearthed in Zimbabwe, showing that a thousand years ago there was commerce between the African interior and the eastern seacoast, and from there with the great empires of Asia. "The world is infinitely more permeable than one would believe."[12]

Since the earliest days, genes, infectious agents, and ideas have been distributed, along with articles of booty or commerce, within and between human populations. Concepts relating to the body, to maintenance of health, and to avoidance or cure of disease were disseminated along the paths of human movements. Charms, amulets, herbs, and drugs have always been items of trade and exchange, and some early travels were undertaken specifically for purposes of medical learning. For example, a Chinese scholar traveled to Baghdad about AD 400, learned Arabic, and copied the works of Galen; later Arab scholars in turn collected writings on Indian, Chinese, Persian, Greek, and Roman medicine.[13]

GREECE AND ROME

An abundance of writings and artifacts from the Mediterranean classical periods has survived to modern times, and there is no lack of description and commentary upon medical practice at that time. It is clear that the Greek tradition did not spring fully formed from the pen of Hippocrates but developed from the collection and elaboration of previous ideas. From the Minoans came ideas of hygiene, healing temples, and the association with serpents (both as a source of illness and for treatment of mental illness) still seen today in the caduceus, symbol of medicine. Egypt contributed its pharmaceutical lore and surgical techniques; Mesopotamia (present-day Iraq and Iran), various drugs and some patterns of medical practice. These sources were blended with magical and mystical ideas. Later contributions, particularly from Sicily, brought the rudiments of anatomical dissection. Persian and Indian elements were also incorporated into the Greek medical lore around 300 BC.

An essential part of Greek thinking was the early idea of balance of the four basic elements: fire, water, air, and earth. To each of these elements there was later associated one of the four bodily *humors*—blood, black bile, yellow bile, and phlegm, respectively—with behavioral characteristics assigned to persons according to their predominant humor. Those favoring the blood–fire combination were *sanguine*—fat, with hot blood, and prone to laughter. Excess of black bile produced a *melancholy* disposition—peevish, depressed, and passive, while yellow bile made people *choleric*—violent and fierce. *Phlegmatic* persons, slow and plodding, made up the last of four primary categories. These terms remain in common usage today, even though the underlying associations have long since been discarded. The basic idea of bodily humors, with illness ascribed to their imbalance, is a recurrent theme in many philosophic systems, not only in India and China but throughout the world (see also Chapter 6).

A strong rational element existed in Greek medical thought and writings, including clear descriptions of diseases such as tuberculosis, malaria, epilepsy, and puerperal fever. Signs and symptoms were carefully observed and reasonable prognoses were made as to the outcome of episodes of illness. Many medicinal plants were known, collected, used, and recorded. The importance of hygiene, sport, good diet, and clean water was recognized, and individual and social well-being was emphasized. Yet despite the superb natural history of Aristotle, Greek medicine was deficient in practical knowledge of anatomy and physiology, failings that were to hinder European medicine for well over a millennium.

The aqueducts, baths, and public conveniences of Rome are too well known to require description here, but the state of medical knowledge can be briefly mentioned. The hard lot of workers and slaves gave rise to studies of occupational diseases. Martial wrote on sulfur workers, Juvenal on blacksmiths, and Lucretius on gold miners. Around AD 30, Celsus compiled current knowledge in his treatise *De Re Medica,* preceding by a century the writings of Galen, which were to form the basis of European medical practice for the following 1500 years. The Romans, like the Greeks some 400 years earlier, suffered from lack of good anatomical and, especially, physiological observations. Galen had himself examined a human skeleton and done dissections of animals, but anatomical study of human remains was uncommon, even though Celsus had noted that "criminals were procured from prison by royal permission, and dissected alive."

The actual practice of medicine in Roman times was carried out in large part by public physicians (*archiatri*) employed by the state, who were sent to towns and institutions to provide care for the poor. These men also engaged in private consultation for paying patients in a pattern familiar today in many countries. The Justinian Code near the end of the Roman Empire (AD 533) reminded these public officers that it was their duty "to choose to do honest service for the poorest rather than be disgracefully subservient to the rich."[14] Some physicians had private practices, and some were salaried employees of the gladiators, baths, the courts, or other organizations. Although medical knowledge was scant, the needs of the military and the gladiators stimulated a substantial surgical practice, and many different instruments, such as scalpels, forceps and syringes (some of Egyptian or Babylonian origin) were described by Celsus. In the ruins of Pompeii hundreds of such instruments have been found, some of which, such as vaginal specula, barely differ from those used in modern practice.

Finally, public health measures and hospitals in Roman times were closely regulated by the legal and administrative systems. Control over the baths and aqueducts, the sanitation and maintenance of streets, and the wholesomeness of food and marketplaces was placed in the hands of public officials in an organization that functioned until the decay of the empire about AD 400 to 500. Military hospitals were built all over the empire, and institutions (*valetudinaria*) originally intended for care of sick and aged slaves were in later years made available to the general poor.

NON-MEDITERRANEAN MEDICINE

Indigenous ideas about the body, the maintenance of health, and the cure of disease must have developed wherever human civilization flourished. Of the Aztec, Maya, Inca, Khmer, and other high cultures not a great deal is known, and their influence upon other and succeeding peoples has been limited. Two major systems of medical thought should, however, be mentioned because of their antiquity, extent, and importance. These are the Indian and the Chinese.

Traditional Indian Medicine and Surgery

Earliest Indian medical writings date from the second millennium BC, when the so-called Vedic practice consisted largely of charms and magical practices for control of demons. From about 800 BC to AD 1000 Brahmanistic medicine predominated and several large technical treatises have survived from this period. Among the conditions described in such detail that they are recognizable today were tuberculosis, cancer, diabetes, leprosy, and smallpox. The practice of physicians was well described, with ample warnings against quacks who, failing to obtain a cure, blame the patient for disobeying directions. Healers should direct full attention toward curing the patient and under no circumstances cause him harm; the patient should be treated as if he were the physician's own son. Diagnoses were made by listening to the sounds of the breath and entrails; observing color of the eyes, tongue, and skin; feeling the pulse and even tasting the urine for the characteristic sweetness of diabetes. A careful history was taken including the patient's origin and travel, diet, duration of illness, etc. Early prognosis was important because the clever physician did not wish to risk his reputation by treating an incurable patient.[15]

Stress was placed upon diet, hygiene, and mental preparation of both physician and patient, and foods were endowed with mystical properties. Specific remedies, based primarily upon herbs, were prescribed for fevers, cough, diarrhea, abscesses, and other common maladies. Among the hundreds of medicinal plants known was the snakeroot, *Rauwolfia serpentina,* a source of "pacifying remedies" whose active principle of reserpine is still in use as a tranquilizer and hypotensive agent. Opium, introduced later from Arabia, was used especially as a cure for diarrhea, an application widely employed today in tincture of paregoric, an opium derivative. Drugs were classified by taste (sour, sweet, salt, pungent, bitter, astringent), power (hot or cold), and elemental properties (vacuum, wind, fire, water, and earth). They were given by mouth or enema, as drops in the eye, nose, or ear; by inhalation or as sneezing powders; as suppositories; or applied to the body in poultices and oint-ments. Steam and sweat baths were used, as were cupping and bleeding. Certain drugs were burned and the smoke was inhaled through pipes. Mineral-based medi-cines used mercury, arsenic, sulfur, and antimony.

Surgical operations were classified under eight headings: excision, incision, scar-ification, puncturing, probing, extraction, drainage, and suturing. Cauterization was also practiced. Patients were anesthetized with wine in order not to faint or feel the knife so sharply. A wide variety of procedures was undertaken, including laparo-tomy, removal of bladderstones, repair of fistulas, caesarian section, and even re-moval of cataracts and other ophthalmic maneuvers. More than one hundred dif-ferent surgical instruments were in use.

A pervasive theme of Ayurvedic medicine is the triad of wind, bile, and phlegm. Diseases arise from derangement of the balance among these three entities and may be treated with substances having opposite qualities in order to neutralize excesses. There are also seven basic elements of the body: chyle, blood, flesh, fat, bone, mar-row, and sperm. Their increase or decrease induces the whole range of diseases. A large and complex body of commentary has naturally developed over the centuries, but basic principles of Ayurveda remain today as they were developed thousands of years ago. Many of the themes of Indian theory and practice sound familiar to students of early European medicine, with which there was considerable transfer of knowledge. Alexander the Great employed Indian physicians in his armies, and other contacts have already been mentioned.

Traditional Chinese Medicine

Europe and America are currently passing through the latest of many cycles of fas-cination with the world's oldest and largest sustained cultural system. Medical texts from early dynastic times have been reprinted, often for the first time in many cen-turies, and have been widely distributed around the world. More recent innovations, such as the barefoot doctors of the 1960s and 1970s (Chapter 8) have inspired wide-spread imitation, and the Chinese mandate to merge traditional and western prac-tices has led to a resurgence of interest in herbal drugs and acupuncture.

Lendings and borrowings between Chinese and other traditions have gone on for millennia, but China has retained its distinctive system of medical and health lore. Chinese medicine can be traced back at least to the time of Fu Hsi, an extraordi-nary personage who about 3322 BC "taught his people how to keep domestic ani-mals, how to fish, how to cook, and how to get married. He also invented musical instruments and needles of nine different shapes. The needles were made of stone and used, in many instances, for the treatment of diseases."[16]

Writers on classical Chinese medicine of the "great tradition" (as opposed to rus-tic folk remedies) invariably relate concepts of the body to those referring to the universe in general: "The basic idea behind these may be seen as a homeostatic concept of health and disease related to the cosmological ideas of Han philosophers. Just as equilibrium, or harmony, within an endless cycle of fluctuating changes is the basic principle of the natural order and of human society, so man (the microcosm of the universe) is healthy when his basic life forces are in harmony and unhealthy when the harmony is disturbed."[17]

The Chinese concept of *ch'i* or life essence represents an abstraction unrelated to the anatomy of the body or to scientific physiology. It is the function, the essence, that is important. Born of chaos, ch'i gives rise to *yin* and *yang*, whose relative amounts and proportions help determine health and disease and many other things besides. Yin forces represent night, dark, cold, negative, passive, and female and are inherent in solid organs of the body; yang forces represent day, light, warm, positive, and male, and inhere in hollow organs. Balances must be properly maintained through careful observance of outside forces and attention to activities and diet. Because of the unity of all nature, there is no sharp distinction between food and medicines, although certain concentrated substances, usually powdered, ashed, or extracted, may provide the essence of one or another force.

As early as 2700 BC Shen-Nung published a book listing 365 kinds of medicines— 46 from minerals, 67 from animals, and 252 from plants. Many of these, and the thousands of other natural products in the Chinese traditional pharmacopeia, are empirical remedies containing specific active ingredients. Other aspects of classical Chinese medicine, including the 12 meridians of the body bearing 132 acupuncture points, and certain organs such as the "triple warmer," are more difficult to interpret but retain a firm position within a coherent system of medicine.

In comparison with the medical tradition of India, the Chinese system is often characterized as having a poor morphologic sense and little or no knowledge of surgery. The traditional Chinese ignorance of anatomy may be explained by the enormous importance attached in classical times to the symbolic aspects of health, which was viewed in theoretical and cosmologic terms and not as structural and functional constructs.

Traditional Practices in Other Cultures

There are of course a great many traditions in all parts of the world developed in harmony with local religious thought. As shrewd observers with finely developed powers of perception and deduction, native peoples in Africa, Asia, and the Americas long ago discovered many practical and useful substances—along with much that, to our eyes, is of little value. North American Indians knew laxative, diuretic, emetic, and antipyretic drugs and were familiar with the use of foxglove (digitalis) as a heart stimulant. South American Indians developed the use of cocaine, cinchona (quinine), curare, ipecac (emetine), and numerous other drugs. The Aztecs, Mayas, and other Middle American groups made use of a wide variety of substances, including tobacco, which have not been without influence in the course of later world developments.

THE MIDDLE AGES IN EUROPE

With the decline of the Roman Empire in the fifth century AD, western Europe passed into a millennium of scientific somnolence, but several developments relevant to international health may be described. Knowledge, including medical knowledge, passed into the hands of the Catholic Church, and such of the Greek and Roman writings as were preserved in the west survived in the monasteries of Europe. Galen continued as the primary authority during this time and little of value was added to his writings. Especially in the earlier part of the long decline, the Byzantine Eastern Church in Constantinople (modern Istanbul) surpassed the European church in preserving and copying classical texts, and it was here that exchange continued with cultures to the east.

In the ninth century a medical school was founded in Salerno, near Naples, where during the next few hundred years Arabian, Byzantine, and Jewish scholars came to translate their texts and carry medical writings to Europe. Here was written the *Regimen Sanitatis Salernitanum*, a series of aphorisms on hygiene and healthful living which became immensely popular. With the invention of printing in the 15th century these jingles were translated into all known western languages and enjoyed the widest distribution of any book of the time with the exception of the Bible.[18]

Plague and the Beginnings of International Health Regulation

The crowded cities of medieval Europe, far below Greek and Roman standards in water supply, sanitation, personal hygiene, and enlightenment, were excellent candidates for outbreaks of epidemic disease, and it may be said that the Middle Ages were bracketed by two great outbreaks of plague. The first pandemic, also known as the *Plague of Justinian*,[19] struck in AD 542 and decimated the known world from Asia to Ireland, but the great *Black Death* of the 14th century is known as the most destructive epidemic in the history of mankind. AIDS pales by comparison, at least to date. Starting from wild rodents in the plains of Central Asia, the plague reached the Black Sea in 1346, spreading by 1348 to the British Isles and all over the then known world. The entire social, economic, agricultural, and ecclesiastical structure of Europe was shaken to its foundations. Europe alone lost perhaps 25 million people, and through the Middle East, India, and China similar devastation resulted in the deaths of additional tens of millions. Physicians had no conception of the cause of the disease, ascribing it to a conjunction of the planets or to other cosmic and divine causes. Scapegoats were sought and many blamed Jews, who a suffered greatly as a result.

Despite ignorance of its true cause, recognition of the contagious nature of plague led to the earliest attempts at international disease control. In the belief that plague was introduced by ships, the city-state of Venice in 1348 adopted a 40-day detention period for entering vessels, soon copied by Genoa, Marseilles, and other major ports. This period of *quarantine* (from the Italian word for forty, possibly representing the period during which Moses wandered alone in the desert), although only partially effective in stopping plague, established a concept, the *cordon sanitaire*, that was to be used frequently in succeeding centuries.

Subsequent visitations of the Black Death were no less kind. In 1630–1631 plague in Bologna killed 24% of the population; in Venice, 33%; in Milan, 46%, and in Verona, 61%. A scant generation later 19% of the inhabitants of Rome succumbed to the plague of 1656–1657, as did 50% of Naples and 60% of Genoa. In the current epidemic HIV has infected 30% to 50% of the population in some limited areas of sub-Saharan Africa. The visitation of disease was considered by some the wrath of God in punishment for intemperate behavior, but it was clear to others at the time that plague was transmitted from person to person. Daniel Defoe, writing a half century after the great 1665 plague of London, described the contagion vividly:

the calamity was spread by infection; that is to say, by some certain steams or fumes, which the physicians call effluvia, by the breath or by the sweat or by the stench of the sores of the sick persons or some other way, . . . which effluvia affected the sound, who came within certain distances of the sick, immediately penetrating the vital parts of the said sound persons, putting their blood into an immediate ferment, and agitating their spirits to that degree which it was found they were agitated; and so the newly infected persons communicated it in the same way to others.[20]

Plague was not the only great epidemic disease of the Middle Ages. Smallpox, diphtheria, measles, influenza, tuberculosis, scabies, erysipelas, anthrax, and trachoma were also rife.[21] Mass hysteria in the climate of superstition and ignorance led to outbreaks of dancing mania. Ergotism, arising from fungal contamination of rye, killed or crippled large numbers of people in dozens of epidemics between the 9th and 15th centuries. It is possible that leprosy, present in Europe for centuries, became epidemic in the 13th and 14th centuries, moving Voltaire to say that of all things gained in the Crusades, leprosy was the only thing that Europe kept. After the Black Death, which carried off numerous inhabitants of leprosaria, the disease was never again important in Europe. The causative bacillus, however, was not eradicated and cases continued to occur. It was not until 1868 that *Mycobacterium leprae* was identified, not in the tropics but in a leprosarium near Bergen, Norway. This discovery by the Norwegian investigator Gerhard Hansen resulted in the modern term of *Hansen's disease* or *Hansenosis* as the preferred designation for leprosy. To this day many leading investigators of this disease come from Norway.

The Sanitary Awakening

It was during the Middle Ages that hospitals became established in Europe. Stimulated in part by ideas of contagion, these institutions were at the time the only places that specialized in the care of the sick. Religious orders dedicated to charity and healing were chartered in this period, partly to meet the needs of returning crusaders. Some institutions, such as St. Bartholemew's (St. Bart's) and St. Thomas's in London, founded in 1123 and 1215 respectively, still function today. From about the 13th century on, secular hospitals were founded in many municipalities, staffed primarily by monks and nuns.

Concepts of cleanliness and sanitation took hold slowly in Europe's cities. Through public awareness and legislation, urban centers began to approach the hygienic standards of the Roman Empire a thousand years before as towns controlled the cleaning of streets, disposal of dead animals, and pollution of streams. Bathing became popular and the printing press brought enlightenment to the popular mind. The stage was being set for the Renaissance.

THE PERIOD OF EUROPEAN COLONIAL EXPANSION

During the Middle Ages in Europe, classical scientific and medical knowledge was retained by the Arabs, who established learned settlements in Spain, Portugal, and Sicily. Much of European medieval thought was expended on the rivalry with Islam, and although the Crusades had by and large failed, contacts with the Muslim world opened new vistas to European eyes. Commodities of high value, mostly from the East, were in great demand, but the traditional routes of passage for such goods went through the Mediterranean and the Italian city-states. Partly as a continuation of the Christian–Muslim rivalry, partly for riches and adventure, and partly because of technical improvements in navigation and seamanship, western Europeans of the early 15th century embarked on a series of conquests by sea. The Iberian countries were early entrants, and Portugal, by virtue of its maritime traditions, large fleet, and well-established coastal trade, was first.

Beginning in 1415, the Portuguese attacked Muslim settlements in nearby North Africa, and instead of plundering and retreating, they established permanent garrisons. In some ways the early 15th-century voyages may be considered extensions of the Crusades. The influence of Islam had expanded rapidly during the preceding few centuries—to the Balkan States, western Asia, Egypt, East Africa, India, and the East Indies (now, Indonesia), and the opportunity to spread Christianity was a powerful stimulus to the conquistadores of Portugal and Spain. Final success in the long struggle for eradication of the Moorish Kingdom of Granada coincided with the arrival of Colombus in the Caribbean in the year 1492. The excitement generated by discoveries of islands in the western Atlantic, thought to be a gateway to China, can only be imagined. The writings of men such as Bernal Diaz about the civilizations of the New World, disseminated by the recently developed but already widespread printing presses, fired the imagination, and the booty of gold and precious objects stimulated baser emotions.

The Portuguese arrived in India in 1498 and loaded the first of many cargoes of spices for the return voyage to Lisbon, challenging Italy for this trade; the English and Dutch in the 17th century finally ended Mediterranean dominance and extended European influence to the farthest corners of the world. The colonial period thus begun lasted essentially until the 1950s and 1960s, with very few colonies remaining, in a *de jure* sense, beyond 1970 (see next chapter).

The period of exploration and colonization had extremely important effects upon international health. Consider the "fatal impact" of early European ships on the natives of the South Pacific. The *Dolphin*, under Captain Wallis, arrived in Matavi Bay, Tahiti, in 1697, and the exhausted sailors, long at sea, found to their delight that "the girls were prepared to make love at any time for the most trifling gifts; most of all they preferred ordinary carpenter's nails which they seemed to value as the Europeans value gold. There had been a commotion aboard the Dolphin when it was discovered that the sailors were not only withdrawing nails from the ship's planks but had even filched the nails from which their hammocks were suspended so that most of them were sleeping on the deck."[22] By 1769, Captain James Cook noted that within a few weeks of going ashore in Tahiti, a third of his crew was ill with sexually transmitted diseases, which he felt "may in time spread itself over all the islands in the South Seas to the eternal reproach of those who first brought it among them." Later, in the same vein, "we debauch their morals already prone to vice and we introduce among them wants and perhaps diseases which they never before knew and which serve only to disturb that happy tranquility they and their forefathers had enjoyed. If any one denies the truth of this assertion let him tell what the natives of the whole extent of America have gained by the commerce they had had with Europeans."[23] Destruction of the fragile cultures of the South Seas was accomplished within a few years, sometimes just months, after the first landfall by Europeans and their introduction of rum, gunpowder, and disease. Although still a matter of controversy, some investigators believe that syphilis itself may have been introduced to Europe by early Iberian explorers who acquired it in the Western Hemisphere. The worldwide spread of AIDS is a bicentennial echo demonstrating once again that, as in ancient times, genes and germs follow the trade routes of humans.

In other parts of the world, destruction of aboriginal cultures and peoples was even more dramatic than in the South Pacific. It is commonly believed, for example, that the first footfall of Columbus in the New World was on San Salvador (Watling's Island) in the Bahamas group, an archipelago from which the entire native population was quickly carried off to slavery and death on nearby Cuba and Hispaniola. The Spanish bishop Bartolomé de las Casas reported that the native population of the Antilles when Columbus arrived in 1492 was 3,770,000; by 1518 the number had declined to 15,600.[24] Although these numbers may not be accurate, similar scenarios were then in progress, or were soon to occur, in other parts of the Western Hemisphere.

Many authors[25] have considered the interchange of infectious agents between Europe and the Americas arising from the early explorations, and their consequences for New World populations.

> At present, the following three facts are widely accepted: a) in the 15th century the American population was not numerically very far from the European, which was estimated around 50 to 80 million; b) in the 16th century, Europe experienced demographic growth, in part because of the import of goods from the conquered lands; and c) America by contrast experienced a sudden decline in its population (followed by the massive import of slaves from Africa), and this is considered to be the greatest demographic tragedy in history.[26]

The exchange of specific diseases is a subject of continual review and argument. Many imported diseases have been implicated by different authors. Those that probably accompanied the Europeans were influenza, typhus, smallpox, measles, cholera, and yellow fever. Some believe that certain kinds of malaria parasites[27] were present in pre-Columbian times but that the deadly malignant tertian (*falciparum*) malaria came from Africa in European ships. The microbial unification of the world has been in progress in a major way for the past 500 years or so and is now complete as shown by the almost instantaneous and universal dissemination of HIV.

The fatal impact was to prove two-edged, and European adventurers and settlers were often cruelly treated by the many endemic diseases to which they had scant resistance. Nowhere was this more true than in West Africa, the "White Man's Grave." The Portuguese had established slaving stations along the coast as early as the 15th century, but the small disease-ridden outposts did not develop into colonial settlements. Dysentery (then known as the *bloody flux* and by many other names) and malaria were rampant. Many European attempts at colonization were decimated by disease. Similar events occurred in the New World. Of ten thousand French colonists who landed in Guiana in 1765, eight thousand were dead within a few months, and the colony failed to develop despite the fact that France sent more persons there than to Canada.[28]

Mungo Park, the English botanist and explorer, entered the Gambia on his second reconnaissance expedition in May 1805. A few months later he was to write to Lord Camden:

> Your lordship will recollect that I always spoke of the rainy season with horror, as being extremely fatal to Europeans; and our journey from the Gambia to the Niger will furnish a melancholy proof of it. We had not contact with the natives, nor was any one of us killed by wild animals or any other accidents; and yet I am sorry to say that of forty-four Europeans who left the Gambia in perfect health five only are at the present alive—viz., three soldiers (one deranged in his mind), Lieutenant Maclyn and myself.[29]

Shortly thereafter, Park himself and the last few stragglers were drowned in an accident. Of the original 44 Europeans, 35 had died of malaria, 3 of dysentery, 1 of epilepsy, and 5 of drowning. James Tuckey's expedition to the Congo, July–September 1816, was scarcely more fortunate—in just $2^1/_2$ months 21 of the original 44 Europeans died of malaria. In the 1832 Niger expedition, 32 of 41 died of fever. The extreme susceptibility of Caucasians vis-à-vis Africans was illustrated in the Niger expedition of 1841, which carried 145 Europeans and 158 Africans. Not one African, but 42 Europeans died of malaria, and only 15 failed to become ill.[30]

The Slave Trade

The hope of obtaining quick riches in West Africa apparently outweighed the fear of sickness and death in many European minds. Gold from the Gold Coast, ivory from the Ivory Coast—to say nothing of palm oil and, above all, slaves—provided the stimulus for frequent expeditions to the coasts of Africa.

Slavery was, of course, not a new phenomenon, having been common in antiquity. The early African slave trade went to North Africa and Europe, but with the discovery of America and the "unsuitability" of its natives for plantation labor, by far the greatest number of West African slaves made the dismal passage across the Atlantic. The total number captured has been estimated at some 11 million, of whom some 9.6 million were landed in North or South America or the Caribbean region.[31]

The slave trade was a source of enormous profit for those who invested in it, including (it is said) Queen Elizabeth I of England. By the middle of the 18th century, the city of Liverpool alone had 87 ships engaged in transport of slaves from West Africa to the Caribbean and southern United States. An Englishman named Lovett Cameron observed:

> a gang of fifty-two women tied together in three lots; some had children in their arms, others were far advanced in pregnancy, and all were laden. They were covered with weals and scars. To obtain these fifty-two women, at least ten villages had been destroyed, each with a population of one to two hundred, or about 1500 in all ... In chained gangs the unfortunate slaves are driven by the lash from the interior to the barracoons on the beach; there the sea-air, insufficient diet and dread of their approaching fate, produce the most fatal diseases; dysentery and fever release them from their sufferings ... On a short march, of six hundred slaves intended for the Emma Lincoln one hundred and twenty-five expired on the road. The mortality on these rapid marches is seldom less than twenty per cent.[32]

The eons needed for humanoid dispersal from their African origins to the Americas in prehistoric times is in contrast to the rapid carriage of individuals to the New World via the slave trade. As these dismal journeys were fairly brief, weeks or perhaps months at the most, infectious microorganisms and parasites were certainly carried across the Atlantic. During the centuries in which this appalling commerce continued, millions of Africans were transported to tropical America where climatic conditions were relatively similar to their homelands. Brazil alone received three times as many slaves as the United States, and millions more went to the islands of the Caribbean. Some pathogens, such as African hookworms, found fertile ground and became part of the tropical American landscape. Others did not become established because the needed insect vector wasn't there.

Several helminth parasites were probably introduced with the slave trade. Schistosomiasis due to *Schistosoma mansoni* was almost certainly such a legacy, since it has been known in Africa for a very long time. Another form of the disease, that caused by *S. haematobium*, was also introduced to the Americas but did not become established for want of a suitable snail host. Similarly, some people with African sleeping sickness must have been brought to America, but without tsetse flies there was no way to maintain the infection and the disease quickly died out. The filarial worm *Wuchereria bancrofti*, a causative agent of elephantiasis, was endemic in the region of Charleston, South Carolina, from some time before 1808 until about 1920. This mosquito-transmitted parasite of humans was probably introduced to the Charleston area from Barbados in the West Indies, which in turn had had the filaria brought to it from Africa through the slave trade. The peculiar ecological conditions in the Charleston area, together with its close commercial ties to the West Indies during the colonial period, led to conditions ideal for the introduction and maintenance of the filarial parasite.[33]

Europe and the Tropical World

European intervention in the tropics has gone on for many centuries. The Romans sent expeditions to Africa to collect wild animals for popular amusement and ships to the Malabar coast of India (the present-day state of Kerala) for spices. From the 13th to the 18th century European traders, plunderers, explorers, missionaries, and scholars crisscrossed the seas to carry out their own plans and dreams.

It is important to understand the tropics as a conceptual, and not merely a physical, space. There is, of course, a vast body of geographical, ecological and medical literature which finds little difficulty with the idea that the tropics actually exist, nestling in the middle latitudes of the globe or spilling over into the adjacent "sub-tropical" regions. A further distinction is sometimes made between the hot, wet tropics, the dry savannas and the alpine zones, but in the medical literature as elsewhere it is mainly the hot, wet regions that are taken to represent the tropics in their most essential form. Calling a part of the globe 'the tropics' became a way of defining something culturally alien to, as well as environmentally distinct from, Europe and the other parts of the temperate world ... The idea of the tropics was in origin and essence the perception and the experience of white men and women venturing into an unfamiliar world in which climate, vegetation, disease and people all appeared to be different, and in which the familiar forms of temperate life were threatened, overturned, or inverted.[34]

Early travelers carried cultivated plants from one continent to another. Rice, bananas, yams, taro, and sugar from Asia; coffee and oil palm from Africa; maize, cassava, peanuts, tomatoes, papayas, pineapples, and potatoes from the New World have all become generally distributed and form common articles of diet throughout the world. European tastes for some of these products and needs for others stimulated development of estates or plantations in tropical areas, and the need for labor was met either by the importation of slaves or large-scale hiring of contract workers. A good example of the latter is in the rubber estates of Malaya.

The rubber tree (*Hevea brasiliensis*) is native to the rain forests of South America. Some seedlings, smuggled out of Brazil and grown in London hothouses, served as the basis of commerical plantings of natural rubber trees in several countries of the British Empire in the late 19th century. Conditions on the Malay Peninsula were close to ideal for this tree, and the development of motor transport and other industrial uses for rubber generated an enormous demand for latex. Large numbers of Tamil-speaking people were brought from the Madras region of southeastern India. Almost immediately severe health problems were encountered on the rubber estates, particularly with regard to malaria:

> Between the years 1892 and 1898 there were on an average fifty Tamil women upon the check-roll each year. Yet in the whole period no living child was born. Several women became pregnant, but only in one case did the child become quick, and even in this case the woman eventually had a miscarriage. The estate was so riddled with malaria that the coolies were all miserably anemic and lacking in strength and the estate had eventually to be abandoned.[35]

Quinine

The severity of malaria in many parts of the world and the enormous impediment that it places in the way of economic development have put this disease in a special category at least since the time of Hippocrates. The recognition, in the early 1600s, of a cure for malaria is a milestone in human history. The cure consisted of quinine, an alkaloid that occurs in the bark of *Cinchona officinalis*, a tree native to the forests of Peru. By the middle of the 17th century the fame of this "Jesuit Bark" or "lignum febrium" had spread throughout Europe, where it rapidly gained favor as a specific for agues and fevers. The great demand for cinchona bark almost led to the destruction of the trees in Peru, Bolivia, and Ecuador. Growing wild in the forests, they were searched out and killed by bark collectors without regard to the future. Several attempts at estate cultivation of the trees met with indifferent success until the Dutch finally established profitable plantations in Java. Careful se-

lection, grafting, and cultivation resulted in growth of high-quality trees rich in quinine, and the Dutch had a virtual monopoly of quinine production until the Second
World War. The Japanese occupation of the East Indies cut off the world supply of
quinine and created an additional incentive to the development of synthetic antimalarial drugs such as chloroquine. The spread of chloroquine-resistant malaria in
recent years has renewed demand for the natural product and quinine has enjoyed
a resurgence.

Sleeping sickness

One further example may be cited here of the pervasive importance of disease as a
determinant of economic development: the case of trypanosomiasis in Africa, mentioned earlier in connection with the slave trade. The parasite, transmitted by biting
tsetse flies, has prevented introduction of large domesticated animals for food, labor, or transportation in many areas of the continent. Many attempts have been made
to introduce ox-drawn carts or ploughs, horses, and livestock. All fell victim to *na-
gana*, the animal version of African sleeping sickness. Pictures of early European
travelers in Africa usually show long lines of porters, each carrying a box or bale
on his head as the safari meanders through the bush. One may wonder why the conquistadores in Latin America or early European travelers in India or East Asia are
not depicted in this way. The reason, of course, is that their animals survived to
carry the burdens. Domestic animals are used for much more than power and
transport—the meat and milk provided by cattle are major sources of protein, still
greatly deficient in tropical Africa, and hides and wool are important items of commerce.

The toll of trypanosomes on humans, both natives and expatriates, has also been
great. It seems certain that the commerical and agricultural activities of Europeans
have acted to spread these pathogens to new areas of Africa. Until late in the last
century sleeping sickness was not recorded in East Africa. Its probable introduction
by the Stanley expedition from the Congo area to the East African lake region resulted in an enormous outbreak among residents of Uganda from about 1900 to
1908. In Busoga, on the north shore of Lake Victoria, the government tried to estimate the severity of sleeping sickness and "instructed the local chiefs to report to
headquarters and to carry with them a twig to represent the death of each individual they thought died of sleeping sickness within their chiefdoms. A solemn pro-
cession of chiefs came to headquarters on the first day and the twigs numbered
eleven thousand." The chiefs were too modest. In fact, the toll along the fertile
lakeshore of Uganda had exceeded 200,000 people.[36]

Panama

Unfamiliar diseases encountered by Europeans abroad were of crucial importance
to empire builders. The threats to colonizers, to labor forces, and to resident populations have already been mentioned, but disease was also a potent inhibitor of con-

struction projects and other commercial ventures. The Panama Canal is perhaps the most compelling example. After eight years of effort, 300 million dollars in expenditure, and almost 20,000 deaths from malaria and yellow fever, the Compagnie Universelle du Canal Interoceanique de Panama went bankrupt and abandoned its efforts in 1888. Almost no planning or funds had been allocated by the company for hygiene and sanitation; indeed, at the start of the French effort, the cause and means of transmission of the two great diseases that killed their canal had not yet become known. The successful completion of the Panama Canal by the Americans was accomplished in the years 1906 to 1914. In the interim between the French and American attempts, mosquito transmission of both malaria (by *Anopheles)* and of yellow fever (by *Aedes)* had been proven.

To understand the events in Panama we must turn to Havana, where, from 1881 onward, Carlos Finlay had been proclaiming that yellow fever was transmitted only by the bite of a mosquito. Few people believed him, and it would be well over a decade before Ronald Ross would demonstrate the mosquito transmission of malaria. After an outbreak of yellow fever at the U.S. military garrison in Havana, the American Yellow Fever Commission, headed by Walter Reed, conducted experiments using mosquitoes fed on patients and then on uninfected volunteers. The commission fully confirmed Finlay's observation and announced at the Pan American Medical Congress in Havana in 1901 that the mosquito *Stegomyia fasciata* (now called *Aedes aegypti)* is the sole vector of yellow fever. William C. Gorgas, in charge of sanitation in Havana since 1898, established a series of ordinances that resulted, within a few years, in a dramatic decline in yellow fever prevalence within the city. These rules included the abolition, or protection by screening, of all collection of domestic water likely to breed mosquitoes; daily inspection of houses and yards by an army of sanitarians; the imposition of a stiff fine on property owners found to have mosquito larvae on their premises; and the reporting and isolation of every suspected case of yellow fever.

In 1904 when the United States took over the Canal Zone, Gorgas was appointed to head the medical department of what may have been the most fever-ridden place on earth. By 1905 more than 4000 men were employed in mosquito extermination alone. Two brigades were formed: the *Stegomyia* brigade to work primarily around houses and settlements, and the *Anopheles* brigade to clear jungles, drain and oil swamps, and work to reduce the recently confirmed vector of malaria. Piped water supplies were constructed to eliminate the barrels that had formerly produced clouds of mosquitoes. Houses were screened and bed-nets provided to the canal workers. Quinine was issued both as a prophylactic against malaria and as a cure, and persons with fevers were isolated behind mosquito-proof screening. As the engineers blasted and dredged, the war waged against *Aedes* and *Anopheles* by the sanitarians gradually brought yellow fever and malaria under control and marked a high point in the history of applied epidemiology in international health.

The few examples cited here can do no more than hint at the multitude of health-related effects set in motion by worldwide exploration, colonization, and commerce since the 15th century. Very significant demographic changes have occurred. Massive emigration from Europe has changed the character of populations most dramatically in North America, Australia, New Zealand, South Africa, and parts of Latin America. The establishment of colonial governments resulted in the inevitable introduction of the cultures and social institutions of the ruling country, which blended with preexisting local norms. This is true of languages, legal systems, and medicine, including concepts of causality and treatment and patterns of medical organization and practice.

PRELUDE TO THE PRESENT

The period from 1750 to the beginning of the 20th century was characterized by a complex web of interlocking developments in technology and science and in social and political thought. The great impact of the industrial revolution reverberated throughout this period and continues to the present day. Advances in science and technology both contributed to industrialization and in large part were stimulated by it. Revolutionary movements in France, North America, and elsewhere generated and disseminated ideas of the innate rights of man to political freedom while, paradoxically, the largest colonial empires in history were being assembled. Between 1750 and 1900 the world's population doubled, from about 800 million to 1.7 billion, fueled by a tenfold increase in the rate of population growth.

The Industrial Revolution in England

The term "industrial revolution" is now commonly used to denote the period from about 1750 to 1830 during which power-driven machinery was first employed in factories for mass production of articles of commerce. A constellation of basic social and economic changes of considerable significance to health accompanied the development of the factory system, which was itself made possible by the rapid advances in technology during the 18th century. The textile industry played the leading role in early industrialization in England, with the flying shuttle, spinning machines, and, above all, intricate powered looms making possible the production of vast amounts of cotton cloth. Early textile machinery was operated by water power, limiting the placement of the mills, but after James Watt's invention of the rotary steam engine in 1781, factories could be located at almost any site, limited only by supplies of labor, coal, and materials.

The requirement for factory workers produced a whole new category of specialized wage laborers derived largely from impoverished rural folk, apprentices, and destitute women and children. Some owners of these early factories displayed an indifference to the welfare of the workers comparable to the attitudes of their colleagues in the West African slave trade. Safety devices were unheard of and small children, sometimes literally chained to the machines, toiled from dawn to dusk in dusty, noisy, unventilated workrooms. Many who fell asleep at their work paid with fingers, hands, or worse. The exploitation of women and children in Midlands factories was exceeded by dreadful conditions in the coal mines.

Many people were outraged at the shocking conditions in factory and mine. A rising tide of humanitarianism and social concern was gaining momentum in England, on the Continent, and in America. Wesleyan Methodism gained great influence in the industrial and mining towns of England in the middle of the eighteenth century. The writings of the French intellectual and social philosophers—Rousseau, Voltaire, and Diderot—of John Locke, and of the Americans Thomas Paine, Thomas Jefferson, and many others served to disseminate concepts of the perfectability of humanity, inalienable human rights, and the essential dignity of the person.

> the question of health serves as a focal point around which the doctrines of economic freedom and political liberalism can be seen in various stages of modification. This transformation did not occur simply because of the growth of humanitarian sentiment or of a social conscience. Legislation on health and sanitation resulted from a variety of forces within the social and economic order.[37]

Legislation in England to control abuses of the Industrial Revolution began with the Health and Morals of Apprentices Act of 1802, limiting the work of children in textile factories to 12 hours per day, but setting no lower age limit for employment. The Factory Act of 1833 finally set a minimum age of nine years for work in textile factories, limited the work day of children from 9 to 13 years old to 9 hours daily and that of children from 13 to 16 years old to 12 hours. Certain other reforms, such as two hours of compulsory schooling each day, were instituted. The Mines and Collieries Act of 1842 set 10 years as the minimum age for boys to work underground and forbade the employment of women and girls within the pits, but it was not until 1874 that employment of children under 10 in factories was prohibited in England. The writings of William Blake (*Songs of Innocence*) in the 18th century, and of Dickens, Elizabeth Barrett Browning, and other social reformers in the 19th were influential in inducing these changes, which were instituted over the vigorous opposition of the leaders of the industries concerned.

The cities of England and of other industrializing nations grew enormously in the first half of the 19th century. Between 1800 and 1841 the population of London doubled, and that of Leeds almost tripled. Birmingham grew tenfold in 50 years, and the populations of towns such as Bradford and Oldham increased a hundred times. Birmingham, Manchester, and other cities had instituted cleanup campaigns in the 1760s, correcting centuries of decay by installation of paving, sewerage, and piped water, but these civic improvements were swamped by the rapid growth of population. As wageworkers came in from the countryside and Irish emigrant laborers flocked to the factory towns, housing was constructed as quickly and cheaply as possible. City planning was nonexistent and sanitation neglected. Neighborhood standpipes provided water of poor quality to numerous residences. The smoke from innumerable coal fires filled the air and blackened buildings and lungs alike. The lack of recreational facilities combined with general illiteracy and cheap alcohol from the colonies to produce the conditions immortalized in Hogarth's famous "Gin Lane" etchings. Despite improvements in agricultural production, nutrition was poor. Rickets became common in children rarely exposed to sunshine, and contagious diseases such as tuberculosis, diphtheria, and louse-borne typhus took a great toll. The first cholera pandemic to strike England and western Europe took thousands of lives in the early 1830s and quickly extended to North America via shipping. Occupational accidents were common, as were diseases arising from unrestricted use of lead, mercury, phosphorus, and other toxic substances in industrial processes and even in household "cottage industries."

Sanitary Reform in England

Widespread and more or less coordinated efforts to alleviate many unhealthful conditions began around 1830. In England this can be seen as consisting of four principal movements.[38] First, the aftermath of the cholera epidemic of 1831–1833 saw the formation of more than 1200 locally elected boards of health, which functioned mainly in the area of environmental hygiene and proposed to prevent future epidemics by early detection of cases, isolation, quarantine, and similar measures. The true cause of cholera was still unknown, but the association of that and other diseases with crowded and insanitary conditions had become clear. Second, the increase in wage dependency and altered socioeconomic conditions had placed intolerable burdens upon the parish-based relief mechanisms contained in the Elizabethan Poor Laws of 1601. A royal commission, appointed in 1832 to look into these matters, was eventually responsible for the Poor Laws of 1834. This legislation provided for a centralized Poor Law Commission with a medical officer and medical inspectors, and it acknowledged the need for some sort of generalized health services for the poor. Third, the Factory Act of 1833 incorporated provision for enforcement inspectors in the field under the supervision of the Home Office. Increasing interest in industrial health problems was reflected in the publication in 1831 of Charles Thackrah's monograph, *The Effects of the Principal Arts, Trades and Professions, and of Civic States and Habits of Living, on Health and Longevity, With Suggestions for the Removal of Many of the Agents Which Produce Disease and Shorten the Duration of Life*. Finally, the establishment of the Registrar General's Office and the division of the country into districts for registration of births, marriages, and deaths made possible the orderly accumulation of basic demographic data as a basis for further legislation and action.

The situation in American hospitals was so dismal that Thomas Jefferson was provoked to write:

> And I will ask how many families . . . would send their husbands, wives or children to a hospital, in sickness to be attended by nurses hardened by habit against the feelings of pity, to lie in public rooms harassed by the cries and sufferings of disease under every form, alarmed by the groans of the dying, exposed as a corpse, to be lectured over by a clinical professor, to be crowded and handled by his students, to hear their case learnedly explained to them, its threatening symptoms developed, and its probable termination foreboded?[39]

Edwin Chadwick

The movement for reform in Britain culminated in the activities of Edwin Chadwick, a towering figure in the history of public health. Chadwick had headed a royal commission in 1832 to suggest revision of the Poor Laws which dated from Elizabethan times. The investigations of the Poor Law Commission emphasized the importance of collecting accurate data about health and sanitation and resulted in the new Poor Law of 1834. A few years later, the Commission was asked to extend its work beyond the indigent poor to the health of the working classes of England, Wales, and Scotland. Chadwick's 1842 *Report . . . on an Inquiry Into the Sanitary Condition of the Labouring Population of Great Britain* was a fundamental document in the development of modern public health. Chadwick pointed out that the majority of children of the working classes died before their fifth birthday and showed how mortality varied among social and economic classes. He also made a key point about public health measures:

> The great preventives, drainage, street and house cleansing by means of supplies of water and improved sewerage, and especially the introduction of cheaper and more efficient modes of removing all noxious refuse from the towns, are operations for which aid must be sought from the science of the Civil Engineer, not from the physician, who has done his work when he has pointed out the disease that results from the neglect of proper administrative measures, and has alleviated the sufferings of the victims.

Chadwick's report was based on an extensive survey and analysis of conditions in various parts of England and stimulated the appointment of a royal commision in 1843 charged with investigating sanitary conditions in the larger towns. The findings of this commission, which surveyed 50 towns, eventually formed the basis of the Public Health Act of 1848 that established the General Board of Health and authorized the post of Medical Officer of Health to local boards. As it happened, that very year there was a major epidemic of cholera in London.

Cholera had been endemic for centuries in the Ganges River basin, but in 1818 it spread to Southeast Asia, China, Japan, East Africa, the eastern Mediterranean (Syria and Palestine), and southern Russia. Less than a decade later another wave, originating in India in 1826, swept Russia, where hundreds of thousands died, and into the major cities of Europe, from which it reached the British Isles in 1831. Within a year, transatlantic ships brought cholera to New York, New Orleans, Montreal, and other seaports. It spread to the American interior, reaching the Pacific Coast and Mexico in 1833. The Middle East was not spared, and Muslim pilgrims returning from the Haj in Mecca carried cholera to Egypt and the countries of northern Africa.[40] In 1882 the Ottoman Empire set up a quarantine station in the Red Sea specifically to prevent spread of infectious diseases through the Haj. The station persisted until 1956.[41]

The first Medical Officer of Health of London, John Simon, was imbued with the spirit of the environmental reformer and fully recognized the economic implications of ill health. He wrote that, "Sanitary neglect is mistaken parsimony. Fever and cholera are costly items to count against the cheapness of filthy residences and ditch-drawn drinking water: widowhood and orphanage make it expensive to sanction unventilated work places and needlessly fatal occupations . . . The physical strength of a nation is among the chief factors of national prosperity." Simon knew very well the cost of cholera; he had assumed his office the year before the great cholera epidemic of 1848, of which William Farr was to write:

> If a foreign army had landed on the coast of England, seized all the seaports, sent detachments over the surrounding districts, ravaged the population through the summer, after having destroyed more than a thousand lives a day, for several days in succession, and in the year it held possession of the country, slain 53,293 men, women and children, the task of registering the dead would be inexpressibly painful; and the pain is not greatly diminished by the circumstance, that in the calamity to be described, the minister of destruction was a pestilence that spread over the face of the island, and found on so many cities quick poisonous matters ready at hand to destroy the inhabitants.[42]

The year 1849 also marked the publication of a slender pamphlet, *On the Mode of Communication of Cholera*, by John Snow, a work expanded and augmented in 1854 and destined to become one of the great classics of epidemiological reasoning. Although ignorant of the still-undiscovered world of microbiology, Snow correctly deduced the mode of transmission of cholera through contaminated drinking water. He showed how water drawn from the lower Thames, after passage through London, was far more likely to transmit cholera than was water taken from localities upstream of the city. These developments, so briefly reviewed here, helped to build the foundations of modern public health practice.

Sanitary Reform in Other Countries

The appalling conditions in England at the turn of the nineteenth century were not unique to that country but occurred also on the Continent wherever industrial centers developed. In many areas they prompted a similar response. France occupied the premier position in social and political thought at the time but did not adopt legislation limiting child labor until 1841. Seven years later, when the British General Board of Health was created, laws were also passed in Paris to establish a national public health advisory committee and a network of local public health councils. In Germany agitation for similar legislation was led largely by the famous pathologist Rudolf Virchow and a small reformist group. The year 1848 was marked by revolution and political turmoil in Germany, and it was not until 1873 that a Reich Health Office was set up. In that year Max von Pettenkofer delivered his well-known orations on *The Value of Health to a City*, in which he reiterated the necessity of sanitation and added observations on nutrition, housing, bathing, customs and habits, and political and social conditions. Pettenkofer showed that the crude mortality rate in London had fallen from 35 per thousand around 1750 to 22 per thousand in 1873 while the population had increased fivefold to more than three million. He compared available mortality data from cities around the world with his own Munich, where the death rate was 50% higher than that of contemporary London or Paris, and exemplified the growing mood toward social responsibility in these words:

> In every large community there are always many people who have not the means to procure for themselves the things that are absolutely necessary to a healthy life. Those who have more than they need, must contribute to supply these wants, in their own interest. It is not a matter of indifference if, in a city, the dwellings of the poor become infested with typhoid and cholera but is a threat to the health of the richest people also. This is true for all contagious or communicable diseases. Whenever causes of disease cannot be removed or kept away from the individual, the citizens must stand together and accept taxation according to their ability. When a city provides good sewerage, good water supplies, good and clean streets, good institutions for food control, slaughter houses and other indispensable and vital necessities, it creates institutions from which all benefit, both rich and poor. The rich have to pay the bill and the poor cannot contribute anything; yet the rich draw considerable advantages from the fact that such institutions benefit the poor also. A city must consider itself a family, so to say. Care must be taken of everybody in the house, also of those who do not or cannot contribute toward its support.[43]

A decade later the paternalistic German state under Otto von Bismarck was to undercut the growing power of the Social Democrats and introduce a comprehensive scheme of social security legislation providing insurance for workers against the hazards of accident, sickness, and old age (see Chapter 12). The Sickness and Maternity Law (1883); the Work-Injury Law (1884); and the Old Age, Invalidity, and Death Law (1889) soon became models for similar legislation in every other country of Europe, and eventually throughout the world.

The cities of North America had the advantage of relative newness, but by the middle of the 19th century the crush of immigration had rendered the larger urban centers of the East Coast fully as noxious as their European counterparts. New York City, for instance, increased in population from about 75,000 in 1800 to more than half a million by 1850. Local boards of health had been established in some of the larger eastern cities even before 1800, but these were ineffective in stemming the tide of disease. From early colonial times North America had been swept by epidemics of smallpox, yellow fever, typhoid, and typhus; and tuberculosis, malaria, and other communicable diseases were firmly entrentched. The cholera pandemics of the 1830s and 1840s struck America with full force, the latter coming to California along with the gold fever of the '49ers.

Using Chadwick's 1842 report as a model, John Griscom in 1845 published *The Sanitary Condition of the Laboring Population of New York*, followed five years later by Lemuel Shattuck's *Report of the Sanitary Commission of Massachusetts*. The gradual awakening of interest in such matters resulted in the National Quarantine Conventions of the late 1850s, and a National Board of Health was established by Act of Congress in 1879.

The Internationalization of Health

The 19th century in the western countries opened on a technological upbeat: ingenious mechanical devices were transforming the pattern and quality of life in city and farm. Industrial processes, based on advances in engineeering and chemistry, were flourishing. Agriculture was becoming more efficient and less labor-intensive. Unprecedented volumes of raw materials and consumer goods crisscrossed the world. A philosophical outlook of realism and pragmatism was becoming firmly established. However, rational understanding of health and disease were hardly better than in Roman times.

The repeated pandemics of cholera forced the European powers to develop feasible steps to control transmission.[44] The idea of the *cordon sanitaire*, enforced by quarantine regulations and sometimes by military force, had been prevalent since the 14th century, but as international commerce grew these blockades were increasingly seen by the maritime nations as obstacles to trade. By the mid-1800s the pressure had become intense for some sort of international agreement. Accordingly, an International Sanitary Conference was organized to be held in in Paris in 1851.[45] International health was not the only topic for such conferences at the time. During the same year of 1851 the "Great Exhibition" in London, actually the first World's Fair, celebrated trade and manufacturing, while the First International Congress on Statistics was held in Brussels. "The congress on statistics was only the first in a vast series of subjects which became the bases of international congresses during the period. Demography and hygiene followed in 1852, ophthalmology in 1857, and veterinary medicine in 1863."[46] During the same era, in 1864, the first international nongovernmental agency, the International Red Cross, was founded by Jean-Henri Dunant, a Swiss national inspired by the terrible suffering of soldiers. The founding document of the Red Cross, which promoted neutral humanitarian assistance to wounded combatants, has come to be known as the original *Geneva Convention.*[47]

Despite the classic studies of John Snow just a few years earlier, the most learned men of Europe, debating for six months at the First International Sanitary Conference, could not agree whether cholera was or was not contagious. The marathon 1851 conference eventually produced a lengthy convention dealing mainly with the quarantine of ships against plague, cholera, and yellow fever, but it came to naught as only France, Portugal, and Sardinia ratified the document, whereupon the latter two then revoked their acceptance. At least that was better than a similar convention generated by the second (1859) conference, which was never ratified by anyone. Among the reasons that these very early conferences ended in frustration was that they were attended by waistcoated and top-hatted diplomats representing national interests rather than by scientists. In any event the state of scientific ignorance concerning the causes and transmission of the diseases in question would have hindered any rational measures for control. A third conference, held in Constantinople in 1866, was the first one to invite participation of the United States, which declined to attend. The 1866 delegates reviewed voluminous evidence regarding the cause of cholera, including the works of Snow and Pettenkofer, and concluded that the disease is transmitted through what we would today call the "fecal-oral" route:

> . . . cholera dejections being incontestably the principal receptacle of the morbific agent, it follows that everything that is contaminated by these dejections becomes also a receptacle from which the generative principle may be disengaged, under the influence of favorable conditions; it follows also that the production of the cholera germ takes place very probably in the alimentary canal, to the exclusion, perhaps, of all other parts of the system.

In 1854 the Italian researcher Filippo Pacini had discovered (and named) the cholera vibrio in the stools and intestines of cholera patients and cited it as the cause of the illness. Exactly 30 years later, a year after Pacini's death, Robert Koch showed that cholera in Calcutta was caused by the same organism.[48]

From such a shaky foundation, through a remarkably concerted achievement of the human intellect, a flood of discoveries poured from the world's laboratories in the latter half of the 19th century, identifying the causal agent and basic means of transmission of almost every major bacterial and parasitic disease of man and domestic animals. Within the span of one human lifetime, from about 1850 to 1910, vague theories of miasma and divine displeasure gave way to experimentally based laboratory data regarding the genesis of infectious disease and its effects upon the body. Repeated epidemics of cholera in Europe and continuing havoc from other communicable diseases were intense stimuli for investigators. The extreme intellectual ferment provoked by Darwin's theories provided a further incentive to biological studies after about 1860. Knowledge of physiology, nutrition, and many other aspects of biomedical science also advanced during this period with the dawn of an understanding of endocrine and metabolic conditions.

Although some important work on disease control had been done in the 18th century (for instance, James Lind's demonstration of the prevention of scurvy and Edward Jenner's work on vaccination with cowpox to prevent smallpox), the rise of microbiology awaited the chemical and technological underpinning provided by the Industrial Revolution. Refinements in microscope design produced the lenses of the 1880s, close forerunners to those in use today. The chemistry of dye manufacture, developed for the textile industry, was incorporated into histology and bacteriology. Little by little the basis of modern medical laboratory and clinical practice was hammered together.

In this chapter we have touched lightly upon a range of human conditions, attitudes, interactions, and developments over a span of millennia, all of which have left their imprint upon world health as we find it today. But more than this—the hunter, farmer, city dweller, exploiter, humanitarian, and scientist are all still here, and so are the basic problems of health that mankind has encountered from the beginning. That is why the study of history has the same relevance for students of international health as does the study of embryology for students of medicine. As William Faulkner said, "History is not dead. It is not even past."

NOTES

1. Hobbes (1651).
2. Steadman (1995).
3. Sigerist (1951).
4. This suggestion has been made by Patrick Olson, who has pointed out the similarities with modern Ebola outbreaks, even showing that green monkeys, a known host of Ebola virus, lived on the island of Santorini in ancient Greek times.
5. Fowler (1995); Holden (1995).
6. Zimmerman (1993).
7. Life was risky for paleolithic infants, who were also at risk of death from malnutrition, infection, predation, and trauma (Goldsmith, 1993; McKeown, 1988).
8. A discovery for which Carleton Gajducek received a Nobel Prize.
9. Sigerist (1951).
10. Selzer (1975).
11. Hoeppli (1959).
12. Siegfried (1965).
13. Hoeppli (1959).
14. Leff and Leff (1957).
15. Jolly (1951).
16. Li (1974).
17. Crozier (1972).
18. Wain (1970).
19. Some authorities believe that the Plague of Justinian was toxic shock syndrome and not bubonic plague.
20. Defoe (1722).

21. Rosen (1958).
22. Moorehead (1966).
23. Quoted by Moorehead (1966).
24. de las Casas (1552). Cited by Guerra (1993).
25. See for example Berlinguer (1993), Guerra (1993), and Merbs (1992).
26. Berlinguer (1993). The claim of "greatest demographic tragedy" is a contentious one, having been made also for the great epidemics of plague, the destruction of the peoples of central Africa, the Nazi holocaust or the deaths of millions of Russians in World War II, the Cambodian genocide, and for other large-scale human tragedies.
27. Specifically, *Plasmodium vivax* and *Plasmodium malariae*. See Chapter 14.
28. Gourou (1980).
29. Quoted by Scott (1939).
30. Gelfand (1964).
31. Curtin (1968).
32. Scott (1939).
33. Savitt (1977).
34. Arnold (1997).
35. Sandosham (1959).
36. McKelvey (1973).
37. Rosen (1958).
38. Brockington (1966). For a description of the wretched health conditions in 19th-century English cities see Wohl (1983).
39. Thomas Jefferson, 1824, in a letter to James Cabell, quoted by Savitt (1978).
40. Many historians have traced the paths of these and subsequent cholera pandemics. See, for example, Pollitzer (1959) and Marks and Beatty (1976).
41. Weindling (1995).
42. Quoted by Pollitzer (1959).
43. Pettenkofer (1873).
44. The early history of international cooperation in health work has been well documented—for example by the World Health Organization (1958) and in Goodman (1971), Brockington (1975), Howard-Jones (1975), Cooper (1986), Bynum (1993), and World Health Forum (1995).
45. Representing 12 states: Austria, France, Great Britain, Greece, the Papal States, Portugal, Russia, Sardinia, Spain, Tuscany, and the Two Sicilies.
46. Bynum (1993).
47. Convention for the Amelioration of the Condition of the Wounded in Armies in the Field, entered into force June 22, 1865. Many more Geneva conventions have been signed, covering topics such as maritime warfare, asphyxiating gases, expanding bullets, the dropping of explosives from balloons, treatment of noncombatants, and similar topics. The full texts of these international humanitarian conventions and agreements can be found at the website of the University of Minnesota Human Rights Library, <www.umn.edu/humanarts/>.
48. Koch never mentioned the various papers on the cholera vibrio published by Pacini between 1854 to 1879.

3

The Organization of International Health Since 1900

The legal profession distinguishes neatly between comparative law and international law, the latter dealing specifically with issues between and among different countries. We can make a similar distinction. The essence of things international lies in the crossing of borders, those imaginary lines on which so much of the world's emotion, energy, and treasure are spent. With regard to health, what functions are served, and what sorts of events occur, at national borders? Retained within these limits is the legal jurisdiction of governments, both central and regional, with their regulations, policies, currency, and other apparatus of sovereign states. Concentrated, but often not restricted inside these wiggly lines are the culture(s) of a people, their languages and customs, and, to some extent, their gene pools. More or less constrained by authority are ideas, materials and merchandise of all sorts, and people. Other things are oblivious to goverment decrees: air and water, migratory birds, and other organisms. If we need reminders, the chemical spill on the Rhine, the disaster at Chernobyl, and the spread of the AIDS virus have shown that pollution, radioactivity, and viruses do not respect national borders.

For centuries the wealthier countries have had an influence on the well-being and health of populations outside their borders. Their people have reached over national borders to become involved in international health through thousands of voluntary, religious, charitable, professional, and commercial organizations. Motivations for both private and official programs have varied widely in their blend of self-interest and altruism. On the government side, motives include:

- National protection and defense against introduced diseases
- Desire for goodwill, influence, and prestige

- Support or protection of private investments
- Humanitarianism
- Furtherance of knowledge, research, and learning in medical sciences
- A response to specific requests or pressure from other governments or international organizations

The early history of international cooperation in health was discussed briefly in the previous chapter, which closed at about the end of the 19th century. The 20th century can be divided into three blocks by the major landmarks of the world wars: before the first, between the first and second, and since the Second World War. The year 1900 saw a symbolic opening of the new century's scientific internationalism with the awarding of the first Nobel prizes. From that point on the nations of the world have become enmeshed in a great variety of regional and global organizations established for every conceivable purpose. International health activities have grown steadily in breadth and complexity as more and more actors are involved in a process that continues to accelerate. Official agreements between sovereign states in the field of health exist in many forms. Some are developed through membership in multilateral agencies. Others derive from bilateral cooperative contracts between pairs of countries, often developed and developing. Here we will describe the evolution and structure of some of these organizations from about 1900 to the present. Their activities will be reviewed in Chapter 9.

OFFICIAL AGENCIES

Intergovernmental Organizations

At the fourth International Sanitary Conference in Vienna (1874) a proposal was made to establish a permanent International Commission on Epidemics, but the world was not yet ready. The idea was finally accepted in 1903, barely two years after the earliest Nobel Prize for medicine and one year after the First Pan American Sanitary Conference in Washington established the International Sanitary Bureau[1] among the nations of the Western Hemisphere. Over the three decades from 1874 to 1903 biomedical science advanced far more than it had in the previous three millennia. The acceptance of Darwin's concept of evolution, the application of quantitative reasoning, and developments in chemistry and microscopy led to an unprecedented accumulation of new knowledge. This knowledge, combined with field-based research all over the world,[2] revealed for the first time the means of transmission and causative agent[3] of almost every infectious disease important to human and veterinary medicine.

One product of the 1903 agreement was a conference four years later in Rome that set up *L'Office Internationale d'Hygiène Publique* (OIHP), known informally to English speakers as the "Paris Office." The Paris Office opened its doors in 1909, and was charged "To collect and bring to the knowledge of the participating states the facts and documents of a general character which relate to public health and especially as regards infectious diseases, notably cholera, plague, and yellow fever, as well as the measures to combat these diseases." A formal internationalism in health had now become firmly established within the first decade of the new century.

The Paris Office, with a permanent staff of barely half a dozen people, worked diligently but could hardly keep up with its stated mission. Nevertheless, progress was made; for example, studies on water pollution and the deratting of ships, an international agreement to control sexually transmitted diseases among seamen, standardization of some biological products, and a study of hospital organization. The permanent committee of directors, representing each of the member states, did not meet at all in the wartime years of 1914–1919, as conditions in Europe continued to deteriorate. During this period the great influenza epidemic of 1918–1919 killed 20 million people worldwide, and the deprivations of World War I led to outbreaks of diseases such as typhus that infected millions of people in war-torn Europe.

A conference in London in 1920 recommended the establishment of a health section of the newly minted League of Nations, to include the Paris Office, but this plan was aborted by the United States. Since the US had declined to join the League of Nations, it refused to permit the OIHP (of which it was a member) to be absorbed by the League. Nevertheless the Health Section of the League of Nations was formed without American participation. Where there had been none a scant 20 years before, now three official international health organizations functioned more or less separately: the International Sanitary Bureau in Washington, the OIHP (Paris Office), and the League of Nations Health Office (LNHO) in Geneva.[4] Further international networking was provided by the League of Red Cross Societies and the *Comité Internationale de la Croix Rouge* (which competed and feuded with each other), and other organizations of worldwide scope.

Operations of the OIHP and the LNHO in the 1930s were marked by international bickering and the chaos of the worldwide economic depression, with resultant wavering support and a chronic shortage of funds. Communication was carried out by (sea) mail, telegrams, and, where possible, by telephone or two-way radio. Obtaining timely information about disease outbreaks in remote areas was a continuing problem.

The principles governing the work of the LNHO were "to inform national health authorities on matters of fact, to document them on methods of solving their technical problems and to afford them such direct assistance as they may require."[5]

The LNHO became involved in many health-related activities, far broader than the quarantine mandate of previous decades. In matters of epidemics and outbreaks and gathering epidemiological information, the office collaborated closely with the OIHP. It pioneered in the collection, standardization, and dissemination of vital and health statistics from around the world. In 1926 the LNHO started publication of the *Weekly Epidemiological Record*, which has been continued to the present time by the World Health Organization. Considering itself a worldwide organization, the LNHO established a branch in Singapore in 1925 to gather information on health conditions in Asia, and it held conferences in South Africa. It established many scientific and technical commissions to set standards for drugs and vaccines; to study general subjects such as medical education, housing, and the operations of medical facilities; and to report not only on major infectious diseases (syphilis, tuberculosis) but also on nutrition, cancer, and heart disease. Health personnel were sent to other countries for training and consultation and to establish international networks of professionals.

> Expert opinion was provided, for instance, on measures against malaria in Albania, syphilis in Bulgaria and dengue in Greece. Ireland was helped in reorganizing its hospitals and Chile in solving nutritional problems. Advice was given on reorganization of the entire public health administration in countries such as Bolivia, China, Greece, Liberia, and Romania. In addition, courses and study tours were conducted, covering many aspects of disease control and public health. The experience of the Health Organisation showed for the first time the full value of international collaboration in health, and much of its scientific work has been recognized as being of the highest standard.[6]

The OIHP was the agency with official jurisdiction over international agreements in the health field, and served, in principle, as an advisory council to the LNHO. This arrangement permitted the United States, as a nonmember of the League of Nations, to keep a small window open into the LNHO.[7] The period between the wars saw for the first time the interactions of official governmental and intergovernmental agencies with private and voluntary organizations. An important American connection was through the Rockefeller Foundation, which exerted considerable influence by providing advice and funding for many LNHO activities. Both the Paris and Geneva offices ceased operation with the advent of the Second World War.

A "semiofficial" organization, the Pasteur Institutes

It is sometimes difficult to tell whether an organization is private or public. A good example of this in the health field is the *Institut Pasteur*, headquartered in Paris. This institute was founded in the flush of the new microbiological era in the 1880s with an outpouring of funds donated by a citizenry anxious to help in the development of Pasteur's antirabies vaccine. The institute flourished, attracted many outstanding researchers, and set up a teaching program of high quality. Our interest in this organization arises from the remarkable network of Instituts Pasteur that began to appear throughout the Francophone world within a very few years after the Paris Institut was founded. Pasteur's dictum to "Go and teach all nations" was quickly implemented. Starting in Saigon (now Ho Chi Minh City) in 1891, Pasteur Institutes were established in many parts of the world,[8] all tracing their *raison d'etre* back to the hopes and financial support of thousands of private citizens. The institutes are mostly government laboratories producing sera and vaccines, offering diagnostic services, and conducting research on a wide range of infectious and parasitic diseases. In these outlying laboratories pioneering work was done on plague by Yersin, on malaria by Laveran, and on the bacille Calmette-Guérin (BCG) by Albert Calmette. Between the world wars the institutes "could be envisioned as organs of the LNHO."[9] Although the institutes and the Rockefeller Foundation were active competitors in development of yellow fever vaccine, they worked together in the first demonstration of the value of DDT for delousing against typhus at the Institut Pasteur (Algiers) in 1943. This procedure was used extensively among civilian populations in immediate postwar Europe, saving many lives in a fine example of international cooperation.

> The network of Pastorian researchers illustrates the far-reaching influence of a flamboyant community united by strong ideological links . . . the doctors working in the domain of public health, tended to adopt a more internationalist style of practice, due to the scientific necessities of addressing epidemiological issues across national borders and elaborating common guidelines . . . the success of the overseas institutes, compared to the relative stagnation of the mother house, illustrated the shift in the scientific drive away from the centre and raised the issue of the integration of biological research into the economic development of what we now call the third world.[10]

The Rockefeller Foundation

Of all the private foundations in international health work, the best known and most significant has been the Rockefeller Foundation (RF). Arising from the earlier Rockefeller Institute for Medical Research (1901) and the General Education Board (1903), the foundation began in 1909 with some 72,000 shares of stock in Standard Oil of New Jersey. Its ambitious purposes were: "To promote the well-being and to advance the civilization of the peoples of the United States and its territories and possessions and of foreign lands in the acquisition and dissemination of knowledge, in the prevention and relief of suffering and in the promotion of any and all of the elements of human progress." The International Health Commission was set up within the RF in 1913, changed to a board in 1916, and finally designated a division. In its 38 years of operation, the IHD cooperated with 75 governments in campaigns on 21 separate diseases or health problems, including tuberculosis, yaws, rabies, influenza, schistosomiasis, and malnutrition, but it is best known for its work with hookworm, malaria, and yellow fever. These campaigns have been well chronicled.[11] The RF played a major part in ridding the southern United States of hookworm and malaria, which were both widespread in the early decades of this century. The 17D yellow fever vaccine (often considered the best vaccine ever made) was developed in RF laboratories in 1936, resulting in a Nobel Prize for Max Theiler and the saving of millions of lives. In the late 1930s the introduced African mosquito *Anopheles gambiae* was responsible for an immense outbreak of malignant tertian malaria in Brazil, with more than 100,000 cases and 14,000 deaths in 1938 alone. Rockefeller Foundation money and workers, together with the Brazilian government, eventually eradicated *A. gambiae* from that country after years of effort, demonstrating the effectiveness of vector control. In Egypt, Nigeria, India, Trinidad, and many other countries, the International Health Division of the Rockefeller Foundation established laboratories and trained local workers in methods of investigating and combating endemic diseases.

The Rockefeller Foundation was involved in aspects of international health work other than disease control. In medical education the foundation contributed to reorganization of American medical schools following Abraham Flexner's famous report of 1910 (which had been supported by the Carnegie Foundation for the Advancement of Teaching). Overseas, RF support was given to medical schools in Bangkok, Beirut, Brussels, and elsewhere, but none became so well known as the Peking Union Medical College (PUMC). The PUMC was the only medical school created and operated by the Rockefeller Foundation.[12] From establishment of the China Medical Board in 1914 to the opening of the PUMC in 1917 to its takeover by the Japanese during World War II and then by the new government of the People's Republic of China in 1951, the RF spent some $47 million (under a budget separate from the IHD) on this experiment in international medical education. In 1951 the people's government took over PUMC and renamed it as the Union Medical College of China (UMCC). The UMCC stopped enrolling new students in 1953 and in 1957 was amalgamated into the Chinese Academy of Medical Sciences. The medical school was reestabished in 1959 under the name of the Medical College of China, which closed in 1970. In 1979 it was reopened as the the Capital Medical University of China, which came full circle in 1985 by restoring the name of the Peking Union Medical College. The emphasis at PUMC was on high quality: In its first 18 years it produced only 166 graduates, which included a large proportion of the leaders of modern medicine in China. Many of the "patriotic health campaigns" in the early years of the People's Republic of China were based on knowledge derived from investigations carried out by the old PUMC, which has had a profound long-term effect upon the health of the Chinese people.

The Rockefeller Foundation also financed and supported many schools of Public Health, first at Johns Hopkins University, which became a major center for international health, and extending to many sites overseas. Their role in launching the International Clinical Epidemiology Network (INCLEN) is discussed elsewhere.

TWENTIETH CENTURY: SECOND HALF

International health since the Second World War can be viewed as a series of consecutive and overlapping eras (Table 3-1). On the table, each era is designated by

Table 3-1. Trends in International Health, 1945–2000

1940s–1950s
Era of organization and integration

Model:	Intergovernmental; reconstructionist
Focus:	Peace; economic and political stability
Theme:	International cooperation
Agents:	American and European National governments
Events:	Bretton Woods, United Nations, World Health Organization

1950s–1970s
Era of consolidation

Model:	Medical
Focus:	Diseases
Themes:	Health and development; institution building
Agents:	United Nations, World Health Organization, National governments
Events:	Decolonization; Cold War; international voting blocs; world conferences

1970s–1980s
Era of programs and projects

Model:	Community
Focus:	Clients
Themes:	Primary Health Care, Child Survival, Health for All by the Year 2000, Community empowerment, women's Issues
Agents:	WHO, UNICEF, UNDP, governments, donors, NGOs
Events:	Alma Ata, Smallpox eradication

1980s–1990s
Era of health sector reform

Model:	Economic
Focus:	Providers
Themes:	Resources, Investment, Cost-effectiveness, Efficiency, Equity, Privatization; Environment; Structural Adjustment
Agents:	World Bank, IMF, WHO; governments; private sector
Events:	Debt crisis; Child Summit; Earth Summit; World Development Report 1993

a few key words and phrases that summarize the general spirit of the time in a multidimensional reality that occupies much of the remainder of this book.

Planning the Postwar World

The first half of the twentieth century had been a miserable time for most the world's people. The First World War had left much of Europe devastated. The economic turmoil, hyperinflation, depression, and unemployment of the 1930s were both a product of that war and precursors of the one to come. By the 1940s many leaders within and outside the United States had learned a painful lesson from America's isolationism during the interwar years and realized that such a policy of by any major power was ultimately self-defeating. The intense collaboration needed to defeat the axis powers and rebuild after the war helped American and Western European planners to envision a future of international economic cooperation and political stability. The closely interconnected issues demanding immediate attention were: paying for the reconstruction of industries and economies ravaged by the war and assuring monetary stability, realistic exchange rates, and convertibility of currencies to promote orderly international trade and commerce. To do these things, new postwar institutions were envisaged to deal with official intergovernmental issues such as currency stabilization and the like and commercial trade and investment policies. The emphasis of these planners was clearly on Europe, and globalization was not yet on the (brand new) radar screens.

In addition to such pressing economic problems, some minds had already turned to larger concerns of world peace and security. Forward-looking thinkers with a worldwide vision foresaw that the war would mark the end of the colonial era, but few would dare to predict the torrent of newly independent nations that were soon to appear (Table 3-2). The idea that every bit of land on earth should be part of a distinct sovereign state arose only after the war. Decolonization came first in Asia, where Japanese armies had occupied French Indo-China, British Singapore and Malaya and parts of Greater India, and the Dutch East Indies. Indeed, Indonesian rebels proclaimed independence from the Netherlands in August 1945 just after the Japanese surrender. By 1950 the British rule over India, Pakistan, Burma, and Sri Lanka and the French colonization of Laos and Cambodia were essentially gone. The unification of an independent Vietnam 25 years later and the return of Hong Kong to China in 1997 marked the last major events of the colonial era and a distant echo of the avalanche started by World War Two. In the interim, dozens of African colonies had also achieved independence. Created in the rush of imperial divestment, these newly minted countries were generally superimposed on the borders of former colonies which had been created with little regard for the ethnic composition of the population.

From the start, many of the nascent nation-states were tugged at from above by

Table 3-2. Major Former European Colonies Since World War II: Month of Independence[a] and of Membership in the World Health Organization

Independence Year	Month	Nation	Former colony of	WHO Membership, Month and Year
1947	August	India	England	January 1948
	August	Pakistan	England	June 1948
1948	January	Myanmar (Burma)	England	July 1948
	February	Sri Lanka	England	July 1948
1949	July	Laos	France	May 1950
	November	Cambodia	France	May 1950
	December	Indonesia	Netherlands	May 1950
1954	July	Vietnam[b]	France	May 1950
1956	January	Sudan	England and Egypt	May 1956
	March	Morocco	France	May 1956
	March	Tunisia	France	May 1956
1957	March	Ghana	England	April 1957
	August	Malaysia	England	April 1958
1958	October	Guinea	France	May 1959
1960	January	Cameroon	United Nations Trust, administered by France	May 1960
	April	Togo	United Nations Trust, administered by France	May 1960
	June	Madagascar	France	January 1961
	June	Republic of Congo (Zaire)	Belgium	February 1961
	July	Somalia	England and Italy	January 1961
	August	Benin	France	September 1960
	August	Niger	France	October 1960
	August	Burkina Faso	France	October 1960
	August	Cote d'Ivoire	France	October 1960
	August	Gabon	France	November 1960
	August	Chad	France	January 1961
	August	Central African Republic	France	September 1960
	August	Congo (Brazzaville)	France	October 1960
	August	Senegal	France	October 1960
	September	Mali	France	October 1960
	October	Nigeria	England	November 1960
	November	Mauritania	France	March 1961
1961	April	Sierra Leone	England	October 1961
1962	July	Burundi	United Nations Trust, administered by Belgium	October 1962
	July	Rwanda	United Nations Trust, administered by Belgium	November 1962

(*continued*)

Table 3-2. Major Former European Colonies Since World War II: Month of Independence[a] and of Membership in the World Health Organization *(continued)*

Independence Year	Month	Nation	Former colony of	WHO Membership, Month and Year
	July	Algeria	France	November 1962
	October	Uganda	England	March 1963
1963	December	Kenya	England	January 1964
1964	April	Tanzania	England	March 1962
	(December 1961	Tanganyika	United Nations Trust Administered by England)	
	(December 1963	Zanzibar	England)	
	July	Malawi	England	April 1965
	October	Zambia	England	February 1965
1965	February	The Gambia	England	April 1971
	July	Maldives	England	November 65
	August	Singapore	(Separated from Malaysia)	February 1966
1966	September	Botswana	England	February 1975
	October	Lesotho	England	July 1967
1968	March	Mauritius	England	December 1968
	September	Swaziland	England	April 1973
	October	Equatorial Guinea	Spain	May 1980
1971	December	Bangladesh	(Separated from Pakistan)	May 1972
1974	September	Guinea-Bissau	Portugal	July 1974
1975	June	Mozambique	Portugal	September 1975
	July	Cape Verde	Portugal	January 1976
	July	Comoros	France	December 1975
	July	São Tome & Principe	Portugal	March 1976
	September	Papua New Guinea	United Nations Trust, administered by Australia	April 1976
	November	Angola	Portugal	May 1976
1976	June	Seychelles	England	September 1979
1977	June	Djibouti	France	March 1978
1980	April	Zimbabwe	England	May 1980
1990	March	Namibia	South African Mandate	April 1990

Source: Modified from Central Intelligence Agency Internet database (independence) and WHO reports (membership).

[a]Dates of proclamation and achievement of independence may differ. Some national entities have merged, separated, changed names, or transformed in other ways.

[b]The Geneva Accords of May 20 and 21, 1954, established a provisional boundary between North and South Vietnam at the 17th parallel. The nation was reunited at the end of the Vietnam War on April 30, 1975, with the surrender of the government of South Vietnam.

their old colonial regimes and by the demands of intergovernmental organizations and competing big powers; from below by their own citizens with varying ethnic, religious, political, linguistic, or separatist allegiances; and from the side by possibly belligerent, corrupt, or ineffectual neighbors. The new nations lacked almost everything except problems. With no tradition of self-government, a skeletal civil service, a shortage of trained staff in all fields, and few resources, they assumed the responsibility of operating viable administrations that could provide essential services to their populations. Any functioning public health and medical services were inherited from the former colonial power. "It was very soon apparent that these imposed health service systems simply could not work in countries where there was virtually no formal medical treatment, other than by mission clinics or traditional healers, outside the big cities; where there were far too few doctors and nurses for the fast-growing population; and where a large proportion of that population would never be able to make regular cash contributions to support a national health service."[13]

The decade of the 1950s marked the beginning of the Cold War and early collaboration among countries in the process of decolonization. As early as 1955 a conference of Asian and African states in Bandung, Indonesia, established the "non-aligned" movement of countries that resisted allegiance to either the United States or the USSR.

The Bretton Woods Institutions

In 1944, a year before the end of the war, the U.S. government organized the *United Nations Monetary and Financial Conference* in Bretton Woods, New Hampshire, and invited representatives from 43 countries to attend.

> It goes without saying that the influence of the underdeveloped countries on these negotiations and on the institutions that emerged was nil or negligible. Of the 43 countries invited to attend the Bretton Woods Conference, 27 were from the underdeveloped regions of Africa, Asia and Latin America, with the overwhelming majority being Latin American countries. Indeed there were only three African countries present (Egypt, Ethiopia and Liberia) and five countries from Asia (India, Iran, Iraq, the Philippines, and China). The bulk of Africa was still under European colonial rule, as was a large part of Asia. Given the complexity of the issues involved, the late stage at which they were brought in to the picture, and the minimal real bargaining power that they could in any event exert, it is not surprising that the influence of these countries on the conference and its outcome was minimal.[14]

The relative weakness of what is now often called the Third World[15] is certainly to be expected; nevertheless, it seems remarkable that more than half the countries invited to participate in Bretton Woods were non-European. The Latin American countries had already been independent for a very long time, and most of the others had never been colonies. The participation of India, then still a part of the British Empire, foreshadowed its independence in 1949.

The main outcome of the conference was the establishment of the International Monetary Fund (IMF) and the International Bank for Reconstruction and Development (IBRD), more commonly called the World Bank. An International Trade Organization was also planned but failed to achieve ratification at the time.[16]

The International Monetary Fund

The IMF was relatively inactive during the early postwar years, as the various countries sorted out their liquidity and convertibility issues. The international financial experts at the fund exhorted countries to adopt responsible monetary and fiscal policies, but some countries considered this to be unattainable. After vigorous negotiations, access to IMF support was made conditional on adoption of certain anti-inflationary and international payments policies, particularly so for the developing countries.[17] In more recent years, such conditionalities, under the name of *Structural Adjustment Programs* (SAPs), have generated an enormous amount of comment in the international health literature. More information on SAPs is found in Chapter 9.

The World Bank

The charter of the *International Bank for Reconstruction and Development* (IBRD)—the World Bank—limits its operations to lending for specific types of projects. During its first decades of operation the bank concentrated its development lending on transportation, public utilities, and certain other infrastructure projects. More recently the bank has provided support to more human welfare-oriented sectors such as education and health. World Bank project loans are made at prevailing market interest rates.[18] Many modifications and "add-ons" have expanded the bank's scope and functions. In 1955 the *International Finance Corporation* (IFC) was set up as a bank affiliate to help promote private (i.e., nongovernmental) investment in developing countries. While cooperating closely, the IFC is legally and financially independent of the IBRD and has its own shareholders and staff. It raises most of the money for its lending activities through the sale of bonds in international financial markets. As the private investment arm of the bank, the IFC has not been involved in the health sector until recently, but in line with the growing trend to privatization of health services in some countries, the IFC is likely to play a larger role in health. The inherent uncertainties that interfere with the flow of private investment to developing countries have stimulated the founding of the latest member of the World Bank Group, the *Multilateral Investment Guarantee Agency* (MIGA). Started in early 1988, MIGA provides investment guarantees against the risks of currency transfer, expropriation of property, war, and civil disturbance.

In the mid-1950s it became evident that the poorer countries were unable to repay standard World Bank (IBRD) loans. The demand for money on easier terms ("soft" loans) led in 1960 to the establishment of the *International Development Association* (IDA) as a separate member of the World Bank Group.[19] Although the procedures and staff are the same for IBRD and IDA, eligible countries receive IDA assistance at much lower interest rates and far better terms. Typically there is a ten-year grace period; then, several decades are allowed for repayment. Considering the future value of today's money we can calculate that IDA funding is really more grant than loan. For this and other reasons the bank speaks of IBRD loans and IDA credits.

To be eligible for World Bank loans a country must fall below a certain level of income per capita. The establishment of the IDA recognized a second, lower threshold. The actual income levels (based on purchasing power parities) have changed over the years. In the mid-1990s the IDA threshold was roughly equal to US$1000 per year and the IBRD limit was about $6000. Recipient governments naturally prefer to get money at lower rates, and those whose incomes are near the IDA limit argue for the best terms when a loan is negotiated. In practice, many countries receive IBRD loans in some sectors and, at the same time, IDA credits in others. Many projects are co-financed; that is, bank loans are linked with funds from other donors to gain additional leverage, as described in the latter part of this chapter.

In the late 1980s the bank formed the *Division of Population, Health and Nutrition*, since transformed into *Health, Nutrition, and Population (HNP)*. Following a reorganization in the late 1990s HNP became a sector of the *Human Development Network* of the Bank, the other two sectors being Education and Social Protection. Besides HDN, the three other networks are: the Poverty Reduction and Economic Management Network; the Environment and Socially Sustainable Network; and the Finance, Private Sector and Infrastructure Network. Bank personnel are grouped into these networks, and into six regional vice presidencies: for Africa, East Asia and Pacific, Europe and Central Asia, Latin America and Caribbean, Middle East and North Africa, and South Asia.

An increasing number of bank programs impinge in some way on international health. One example is the *Consultative Group to Assist the Poorest* (CGAP), set up within the bank in 1995. Although formally constituted, the CGAP is not a separate entity such as the IMF, IFC, IDA, or MIGA. It was inspired by the success of the Grameen Bank in Bangladesh, which provides small cash loans primarily to help women become economically self-sufficient. The CGAP, supported by international donors,[20] is an effort to reduce poverty by devoting resources to the field of "microfinance." A sum of more than $200 million contributed by the bank and the donors is made available in small increments to enable very poor men and women to become more productive by channeling funds to help build sustainable local institutions to support micro-enterprise development. These 'retail institutions' include non-governmental organizations (NGOs), specialized banks, credit unions and cooperatives, and microfinance projects, which then provide the loans to individuals.

Other Development Banks

In addition to the World Bank Group itself, lending on a regional level is conducted by the Inter-American Development Bank, also based in Washington; the Asian Development Bank in Manila, Philippines; the African Development Bank in Abijan, Côte d'Ivoire; the Caribbean Development Bank in Barbados; and the East African Development Bank in Kampala, Uganda. The newest such bank, the European Bank for Reconstruction and Development, was set up in 1991 mainly to support the advancement of market economies in the countries of central and eastern Europe and the former Soviet Union. All provide loans in various fields, including health-related projects.

The United Nations Family of Organizations

For the origins of the United Nations we return to the Second World War and the "Declaration by United Nations" of January 1, 1942, when representatives of 26 nations pledged to continue fighting against the Axis Powers. Then representatives of China, the Soviet Union, the United Kingdom, and the United States met at Dumbarton Oaks, an estate in Washington, DC, in 1944 to make further plans. The actual charter of the UN was drawn up by representatives of 50 countries in San Francisco from April to June 1945. The United Nations officially came into existence on October 24, 1945, when the charter had been ratified by the major powers and a majority of other signatories. Since then, the UN has developed many programs directly under the General Assembly which promote UN activities in development and health, including:

- *The UN Development Programme* (UNDP), the UN's largest source of grants for sustainable human development, works to facilitate technical cooperation in 174 countries and territories
- *The UN Children's Fund* (UNICEF), the lead UN organization working for survival, protection and development of children. Founded in 1946 as the UN Children's Emergency Fund as a temporary agency for war relief, its charter was extended indefinitely by the UN General Assembly in 1953. Working in some 150 countries, UNICEF's programs focus on immunization, primary health care, nutrition, maternal health, and basic education
- *The UN Environment Programme* (UNEP) works to encourage sound environmental practices everywhere
- *The UN High Commission for Refugees* (UNHCR), which replaced the International Refugee Organization founded in 1946 to settle persons displaced by the war in Europe
- *The World Food Programme* is the world's largest international food aid organization for both emergency relief and as part of development programs.

- *The UN Population Fund* (UNFPA), which provides population assistance to developing countries
- *The UN Centre for Human Settlements* (Habitat) works to assist over 600 million people living in health-threatening housing conditions
- *The UN Conference on Trade and Development* (UNCTAD) promotes international trade, particularly by developing countries

A number of autonomous specialized agencies, some inherited from the League of Nations, have also been linked to the United Nations through specific agreements. These members of the UN family help to set standards, formulate policies, and provide technical assistance in their areas of expertise. The World Bank group is itself among these UN specialized agencies. Others that bear on health issues include:

- *The World Health Organization* (WHO),[21] which is described in more detail in a few pages
- *The International Labour Organization* (ILO), which works to improve working conditions and employment opportunities
- *The Food and Agriculture Organization* (FAO), which helps to raise levels of nutrition and standards of living, to improve agricultural productivity and food security, and to better the conditions of rural populations
- *The UN Educational, Scientific and Cultural Organization* (UNESCO), which promotes education, cultural development, protection of the world's natural and cultural heritage, and press freedom and communication
- *The International Fund for Agricultural Development* (IFAD), which mobilizes financial resources for better food production and nutrition among the poor in developing countries
- *The UN Industrial Development Organization* (UNIDO), which promotes the industrial advancement of developing countries through technical assistance, advisory services, and training

Other UN-associated agencies include the International Atomic Energy Agency (IAEA), an autonomous intergovernmental organization under the aegis of the UN that works for the safe and peaceful uses of atomic energy; the International Civil Aviation Organization (ICAO); the Universal Postal Union (UPU); the International Telecommunication Union (ITU); the World Meteorological Organization (WMO); the International Maritime Organization (IMO); the World Intellectual Property Organization (WIPO); and the World Trade Organization, which has already been mentioned (see note 16).

To promote international development the UN declared the 1960s to be the Development Decade; since then every ten years has seen a renewal. The Fourth Development Decade started in 1990. The UN has also sponsored or co-sponsored numerous international conferences that bear on health, some of which are listed on Table 3-3. These large international conferences typically generate resolutions, de-

Table 3-3. Some Major United Nations Conferences and Summits Bearing on Health[a]

Subject/Short Title[b]	Year	Site
Application of Science and Technology for the Benefit of Less Developed Areas	1963	Geneva
Human Environment	1972	Stockholm
Population (1st)	1974	Bucharest
Women (1st)	1975	Mexico City
Human Settlements (Habitat I)	1976	Vancouver, Canada
Water Supply and Sanitation	1977	Mar del Plata, Argentina;
Discrimination Against Inidgenous Peoples of the Americas	1977	Geneva
Desertification	1977	Nairobi
Primary Health Care	1978	Alma Ata, USSR[c]
Science and Technology for Development	1979	Vienna
Women (2nd)	1980	Copenhagen
Least Developed Countries	1981	Paris
Population	1983	Mexico City
Women (3rd)	1985	Nairobi
Promotion of International Cooperation in the Peaceful Uses of Nuclear Energy	1987	Geneva
Least Developed Countries (2nd)	1990	Paris
World Summit for Children	1990	New York
Nutrition	1992	Rome
Environment and Development (Rio Summit; Earth Summit)	1992	Rio de Janeiro
Human Rights (2nd)	1993	Vienna
Population and Development (5th World Conference on Population)	1994	Cairo
Sustainable Development of Small Island States	1994	Barbados
Women (4th)	1995	Beijing
World Summit for Social Development	1995	Copenhagen
Human Settlements (2nd) (Habitat II; City Summit)	1996	Istanbul
World Food Summit	1996	Rome
Earth Summit (2nd)	1997	New York
Global Warming	1997	Kyoto

[a]Many other conferences have some relation to health, such as the Conferences on Trade and Development (1964 Geneva, 1968 New Delhi, 1972 Santiago, Chile, 1990 Geneva, 1992 New York).

[b]Variously titled World Conference, Global Conference, International Conference, or UN Conference on . . . Many have long names; for example, the Nairobi Women's Conference (1985) was officially called *World Conference to Review and Appraise the Achievements of the United Nations Decade for Women: Equality, Development and Peace.*

[c]Now Alamaty, Kazakhstan.

clarations, and programs of action routinely approved by the participating countries.[22] Governments and multilateral agencies need to keep track of the accumulating commitments incurred in this way so that they can organize a coherent response.

In October 1995, the United Nations established the *Task Force on Basic Social Services for All* (TFBSSA) to help coordinate the response of the UN system to the many recommendations of recent United Nations conferences and summits.[23] The task force should focus on priority goals and objectives and strengthen the UN system's mechanisms to deliver coordinated assistance at the country and regional levels. The six key areas considered by the task force are: population (with emphasis on reproductive health and family planning services); primary health care; nutrition; basic education; drinking water and sanitation; and shelter. Within each of these topics, specific goals and targets have been established at one or another of the conferences. For example, regarding infant mortality: to reduce rates by the year 2000 by one-third of the 1990 level, and to reduce infant deaths to below 35 per 1000 live births by the year 2015.

The Task Force on Basic Social Services for All is an example of the pooling of efforts within the UN family to tackle complex problems of global importance. Another example is the Joint Programme on AIDS, which graduated from the WHO into the larger organization, combining the expertise of six separate UN agencies and programs to combat an epidemic that has struck over 30 million people worldwide. The UN System-Wide Special Initiative on Africa, a ten-year, $25 billion program, similarly unites various UN agencies to help provide basic education, health services, and food security in that continent. The Global Environment Facility, a $2 billion fund administered by UNDP, UNEP, and the World Bank, helps developing countries carry out environmental programmes. Development agencies of individual governments and even organizations in the private sector participate in some programs.

The World Health Organization

When the charter of the United Nations came into force in 1945, It contained provision[24] for the establishment of a specialized health agency with wide powers. The new General Assembly, constituted at the beginning of 1946; quickly adopted a resolution "to call an international conference to consider the scope of, and the appropriate machinery for, international action in the field of public health and proposals for the establishment of a single international health organization of the United Nations." The conference, convened in New York in June, produced the Constitution of the World Health Organization, which was ratified by member states on April 7, 1948, a date commemorated annually as World Health Day. The conference also set up a protocol for taking over the remaining duties of the old OIHP, the LNHO, and the United Nations Relief and Rehabilitation Agency[25] and established a commission to prepare for the first World Health Assembly. Although greatly expanded during the past half century, many of the basic concepts and concerns of the World Health Organization were inherited from the LNHO. The WHO is generally considered the flagship organization in the field of world health.

> Many professionals had seen the developing world during the Second World War: health care in these places was usually unjust, almost always incompetent, and rarely built on the great ethical heritage of the past . . . World health was the logical next step . . . it was expected by many that progress would be easy. This optimism was based, among other things, on exaggerated ideas of the power of the new antibiotics and the new internationalism.[26]

Structure

The work of the WHO is carried out at headquarters in Geneva, at the offices of its representatives in many countries, and at the six regional offices. These are:

Region	Headquarters City
Europe	Copenhagen
Eastern Mediterranean	Alexandria
Africa	Harare[27]
Southeast Asia	New Delhi
Western Pacific	Manila
The Americas	Washington

Policy is determined at the parliament-like World Health Assemblies (WHAs) held in Geneva in May of each year, attended by delegates of all member governments and observers from affiliated Non-Governmental Organizations (NGOs), Inter-Governmental Organizations (IGOs), and other agencies. The director-general is asked to prepare reports on subjects of current interest, the budget is discussed and approved, and many resolutions are passed. The Assembly may also make recommendations to member states. An Executive Board (EB), like a cabinet, meets at least twice a year in Geneva to prepare general work programs for the WHA, to work on budget and financial problems of the WHO, and to undertake emergency actions in the event of calamity or epidemic. The Director-General is subject to the authority of the EB, which consists of 32 technically qualified persons who serve three-year terms as representatives of their governments. Each board member is nominated by a country authorized to do so by vote of the Assembly, with care to maintain proper geographic distribution among the six regions.[28] The main functions of the EB are to give effect to the decisions and policies of the World Health Assembly, to advise it, and generally to facilitate its work. The EB is responsible for preparing the agenda for the annual meetings of the Assembly and for taking emergency actions when needed. The EB may authorize the Director-General to take steps to combat epidemics, to participate in health relief to victims of a disaster, and to undertake studies and research on urgent matters.

Doctor Gro Harlem Brundtland, former prime minister of Norway, was elected director-general by the 61st World Health Assembly in May 1998, and assumed her duties in July 1998. Between those two dates a transition team carried out a thorough study of the Organization, leading to a series of comprehensive changes to the structure and management of WHO. Fifty existing programs were reduced to 35 departments grouped into nine clusters (Figure 3-1), "each cluster sending a message of what business we are in," and each headed by an executive director. The executive directors, in turn, constitute a senior management and decision-making team called the Cabinet. Separate high profile cabinet projects were created for major new initiatives, including Roll Back Malaria in the Communicable Diseases cluster

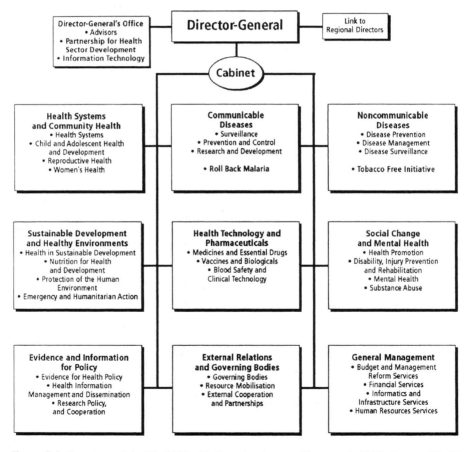

Figure 3-1 Structure of the World Health Organization as of January 1, 1999. Source: World Health Organization

and the Tobacco Free Initiative in the Noncommunicable Diseases cluster. Two new programs, the Partnership for Health Sector Development and Information Technology, were based directly in the "D-G's" office. Detailed, current information about the clusters and programs can be found on the WHO website (www.who.int/).

In 1987, 166 countries were members of the WHO, more than any other international or multilateral agency at the time, including the UN itself. Ten years later the number of members was 193 after the addition of the countries of the former Soviet Union and some smaller nations such as Andorra.[29] The budget of the WHO for the 2000–2001 biennium is projected at $1,800,854,000. The "regular budget" of about $843 million, from member country dues, is exceeded by voluntary contributions from members, with special accounts for specific programs in each of the nine clusters shown on Figure 3-1. Many projects are paid for jointly by the WHO regular budget, by the country concerned, and by funds from UNDP, UNEP, UNFPA, or UNICEF, as well as bilateral sources. These other contributions add greatly to the effectiveness of WHO programs.

The Americas represent a special case. The Pan American Sanitary Bureau (PASB), which had existed independently for 47 years, became the WHO's Regional office for the Americas in 1949, but it has also retained some independence. The Western Hemisphere is divided into six zones by PAHO, with headquarters in Mexico City, Guatemala City, Caracas, Lima, and Rio de Janeiro, as well as overall headquarters in Washington. Terminology is confusing: the Pan American Sanitary Organization changed its name to the Pan American Health Organization (PAHO) in 1958, but its secretariat, the PASB, has remained the same. Through the partial merger, a portion of PAHO's budget comes from the WHO regular budget and from UN agencies.

Functions

The mission of the WHO is spelled out very simply in article 1 of its constitution: "the attainment by all peoples of the highest possible level of health." Its specific functions are listed in article 2, as follows:

(a) To act as the directing and co-ordinating authority on international health work;

(b) To establish and maintain effective collaboration with the United Nations, specialized agencies, governmental health administrations, professional groups and such other organizations as may be deemed appropriate;

(c) To assist Governments, upon request, in strengthening health services;

(d) To furnish appropriate technical assistance and, in emergencies, necessary aid upon the request or acceptance of Governments;

(e) To provide or assist in providing, upon the request of the United Nations, health services and facilities to special groups, such as the peoples of trust territories;

(f) To establish and maintain such administrative and technical services as may be required, including epidemiological and statistical services;

(g) To stimulate and advance work to eradicate epidemic, endemic, and other diseases;

(h) To promote, in co-operation with other specialized agencies where necessary, the prevention of accidental injuries;

(i) To promote, in co-operation with other specialized agencies where necessary, the improvement of nutrition, housing, sanitation, recreation, economic or working conditions and other aspects of environmental hygiene;

(j) To promote co-operation among scientific and professional groups which contributes to the advancement of health;

(k) To propose conventions, agreements and regulations, and make recommendations with respect to international health matters and to perform such duties as may be assigned thereby to the Organization and are consistent with its objective;

(l) To promote maternal and child health and welfare and to foster the ability to live harmoniously in a changing total environment;

(m) To foster activities in the field of mental health, especially those affecting the harmony of human relations;

(n) To promote and conduct research in the field of health;

(o) To promote improved standards of teaching and training in the health, medical, and related professions;

(p) To study and report on, in co-operation with other specialized agencies where necessary, administrative and social techniques affecting public health and medical care from preventive and curative points of view, including hospital services and social security;

(q) To provide information, counsel, and assistance in the field of health;

(r) To assist in developing an informed public opinion among all peoples on matters of health;

(s) To establish and revise as necessary international nomenclatures of diseases, of causes of death and of public health practices;

(t) To standardize diagnostic procedures as necessary;

(u) To develop, establish and promote international standards with respect to food, biological, pharmaceutical and similar products;

(v) Generally to take all necessary action to attain the objective of the Organization.

The work of the WHO is divided into two major categories: central technical services and services to governments. The central services include epidemiologic intelligence; work toward international agreements concerned with health aspects of travel and commerce; international standardization of vaccines and pharmaceuticals; and the dissemination of knowledge through meetings and reports of expert committees, seminars, study groups, and publication of technical and similar literature on world health problems. Headquarters also coordinates the work of several hundred WHO collaborating centres, laboratories, and institutes throughout the world that provide expert consultation and services in many fields. An important contribution to international understanding is made by the WHO's fellowship program, under which thousands of persons have gone for brief study tours abroad in fields such as public health administration; environmental health; nursing, maternal and child health; other health services; communicable diseases; clinical medicine; and medical and allied education. These fellowships, administered through regional offices, have aided more than 3000 health workers annually in recent years.

Services to governments are provided at the request of member countries—primarily in the form of discrete projects established through the appropriate regional office. Some larger cooperative programs are set up on an interregional basis; for example: comparative studies of family planning and human reproduction, and applied research on immunization programs. Intercountry projects within a region may include a meeting of deans of faculties of medicine in the African region, in Harare; a working group on the role of nursing and midwifery in maternal and child health care in Latin America; and a cooperative plan to control pollution of the Rhone River in Europe. The heart of the WHO services lies in the thousands of individual country projects. A great proportion of these are training programs, particularly in Health Manpower Development and Strengthening of Health Services, and many are concerned with primary care or specific disease control programs.

WHO country representatives known as WRs are an important element in the functioning of the organization and coordination of its projects. Assigned to a specific country (or a few adjacent smaller ones) a WR typically has an office within the Ministry of Health and works closely with the national authorities. His or her functions include assistance to the governments in reviewing health needs and resources and in planning, cooordinating, implementing, and evaluating their national health program and policies; cooperation with the resident representatives of the United Nations Development Programme and of other agencies and donors regarding the health aspects of assistance program: representing the regional director at the country level; providing liaison to project staff; and keeping the regional director informed of all relevant actions and developments.

National Development Agencies and Official Development Assistance

The greater part of official development assistance (ODA) comes from the members of the Organization of Economic Cooperation and Development, which is made up of the wealthier industrialized countries of the world. Donor countries comprise the Development Assistance Committee (DAC) of the OECD.[30] ODA is big business, with annual flows in the range of $60 billion in recent years. In addition to programs and projects supported by the big multilateral organizations just discussed, most of the wealthier countries maintain separate official development aid organizations to fund bilateral projects—i.e., those involving one donor and one recipient government. At DAC meetings, representatives of the donors review and compare their respective national contributions to both bilateral ("foreign aid") and multilateral aid programs. The DAC also collects data and publishes annual reports on aid flows by donor, by recipient, and by sector. Detailed data are also made available on computer diskettes and tape, and on the Internet (see appendix to Chapter 5). The DAC member countries and the names of their aid agencies are:

Australia	Australian Agency for International Development (AusAID)
Austria	Austrian Development Cooperation (Österreichische Entwicklungszusammenarbeit)
Belgium	Belgian Ministry of Foreign Affairs, Foreign Trade and Development Cooperation (Ministerie van Buitenlandse Zaken, Buitenlandse Handel en Ontwikkelingssamenwerking)
Canada	Canadian International Development Agency (CIDA)
Denmark	Danish International Development Assistance, Danish Ministry of Foreign affairs (Danida)
Finland	Finnish Ministry of Foreign Affairs, Department for International Development Cooperation (FINNIDA)
France	Ministère de la Coopération, France
Germany	Deutsche Stiftung für Internationale Entwicklung (DSE) Bundesministerium für wirtschaftliche Zusammenarbeit und Entwicklung (BMZ) Kreditanstalt für Wiederaufbau (KfW) Deutsche Gessellschaft für Technische Zusammenarbeit (GTZ)
Ireland	Development Cooperation Division, Ireland
Italy	Department of Development Cooperation, Italy
Japan	Japan International Cooperation Agency (JICA)
Netherlands	Ministry of Foreign Affairs, Directorate General for International Cooperation (DGIS)
Norway	Norwegian Development Agency (NORAD)
New Zealand	Ministry of Foreign Affairs and Trade, Development Cooperation Division
Spain	Agency for International Cooperation
Sweden	Swedish International Development Authority (SIDA)
Switzerland	Département Fédéral des Affaires Étrangeres, Direction de la Coopération au Développement et de l'aide Humanitaire (DDA)
United Kingdom	Foreign and Commonwealth Office, Department for International Development (DFID) (formerly Overseas Development Administration)
United States	US Agency for International Development (USAID)

USAID

The United States, which came out of the war in the strongest relative position of any country, bypassed the nascent World Bank by independently sending massive amounts of reconstruction aid to Europe under the European Recovery Program, which came to be known as the *Marshall Plan*. The 1947 Marshall Plan is generally considered to be the beginning of the modern U.S. foreign aid program and the model for most later programs. However, the Marshall Plan did not finance "economic development" in the current sense. It provided disaster relief and humanitarian aid to Europe, which had a long tradition of commerce and technical expertise and a war-damaged infrastructure in need of reconstruction. Between 1948 and 1952 this program dispensed more than $13 billion and established a tradition of bilateral (i.e., country to country) grant assistance which has continued to the present day.

In 1949, President Harry S Truman extended the European Recovery Program to make the benefits of American scientific and industrial progress available to the lesser developed countries, and Congress passed the *Act for International Development*.[31] Thus postwar reconstruction in Europe became coupled to economic development of the so-called "Third World." Before long, the reconstruction aspect declined as Europe recovered from the war, and economic development of the many fragile new countries became the primary target over the following decades. The aid was in part truly altruistic, but it had two other tightly coupled goals tied to U.S. interests. One was political: the Cold War competition for client states. For example, initiatives of the Kennedy administration included the Peace Corps and the Alliance for Progress, which promised tens of billions of aid dollars to Latin American governments to improve their social services to the poor and undertake land reform and, not coincidentally, counter the influence of Fidel Castro and other leftist movements throughout the hemisphere.

The other interest was economic, as the emerging economies provided investment opportunities, access to raw materials, and new markets for American products. The efficiency of American agriculture led to such an abundance of surplus commodities that prices in the domestic market were severely threatened. Agricultural producers saw the developing countries as an outlet for their oversupply and a means to maintain stable price levels. Under the Agricultural Trade, Development, and Assistance Act of 1954 (Public Law or PL480) excess dairy products, wheat, and corn were sent to "assist the needy peoples of the world."[32] President Kennedy created the Food for Peace program in 1960, linking the distribution of these excess U.S. products with economic development efforts. Some food was simply donated as humanitarian aid, but much of it was given through governments for sale in commercial markets. The local currency thus generated was placed in bank accounts which were owned by the American government. This money, known as "PL480 funds" was used by the United States and local governments for a variety of cultural, educational, and development purposes. Agricultural products worth tens of billions of dollars have been sent abroad under this program, doing much good but also attracting condemnation. Critics argue that much of the donated food was simply stolen and sold by corrupt local leaders and that local farmers were injured and indigenous agriculture was ravaged by the influx of cheap American-donated commodities.

The Foreign Assistance Act of 1961, since amended several times, authorized the president to provide foreign assistance under such agency or officer of the government as he or she may direct. Accordingly, the State Department served this function until 1979, when the International Development Cooperation Agency (IDCA) was established by executive order. The director of IDCA has authority over foreign assistance, but there has been no director of IDCA since 1981, so the administrator of the USAID has also filled this role. The USAID manages many programs in about 100 countries in the developing world, central and eastern Europe, and the former USSR. Most programs are supported by Development Assistance funds or the Development Fund for Africa, which provide assistance in agriculture, health, education, family planning, science, and technology and many other fields. The Economic Support Fund (ESF) addresses economic, structural, and development problems in a small number of special countries such as Israel, Egypt, Turkey, Jordan, and Andean countries with narcotics initiatives. Other sources of funding include food aid under PL480 and special accounts for disaster assistance, private sector investments, and special initiatives including congressionally mandated programs in eastern Europe and the Newly Independent States of the former Soviet Union. Specific ODA policies and programs in the health sector are reviewed in Chapter 9.

NON-GOVERNMENTAL ORGANIZATIONS WORKING INTERNATIONALLY

Not only do individuals and commerce move across national borders, but many organizations extend their activities via the same routes. The World Bank defines NGOs as: "groups and institutions that are entirely or largely independent of government and characterized primarily by humanitarian or co-operative, rather than commercial objectives . . . that pursue activities to relieve suffering, promote the interests of the poor, protect the environment, or undertake community development."[33]

There are four major types of NGOs: (1) private voluntary organizations (PVOs), (2) philanthropic foundations, (3) professional and technical associations and societies, and (4) commercial companies.[34]

Private Voluntary Organizations (PVOs)

The thousands of PVOs are extremely diverse but share certain characteristics. Those involved in international health are non–profit making, voluntary groups dedicated to certain basic social principles, either for their own benefit (grassroots organizations) or for the benefit of others. PVOs include both religious and secular groups. In the former category are medical missions, a diverse group of institutions ranging from leprosaria to rural and urban hospitals. In addition, many other medical and humanitarian institutions such as orphanages are operated by religious denominations and are funded primarily by contributions from the wealthier countries.

The relative importance of mission hospitals has declined in many countries, where indigenous institutions and personnel are increasingly prepared to take over, but a resurgence is taking place in Sub-Saharan Africa. Many missions have been broadening their activities to include other aspects of community development, such as assistance in agriculture and animal husbandry. There are still some small, individually supported missions, but much of this work is now centralized within denominations such as the Mennonite Central Committee, Lutheran World Relief, Seventh-Day Adventist World Service, American Friends Service Committee, and Caritas International Medical Mission Board and Catholic Relief Services of the Roman Catholic Church. Some denominations are members of the Evangelical Foreign Missions Association. Others may function jointly via the Church World Service, an organization encompassing some 30 Protestant and Orthodox denominations.

Among the dozens of PVOs involved in aspects of health and development assistance there is a gradation from firmly denominational organizations to those with a generally religious orientation to the many purely secular groups offering assistance to children, refugees, or other specified beneficiaries. In the United States, many PVOs are members of the American Council of Voluntary Agencies for Foreign Service; in the 18 other member countries of OECD the International Council of Voluntary Agencies plays a similar role. The work of such groups as CARE, Oxfam, Third World First, Medicins Sans Frontièrs, and many other organizations that strive for international cooperation and understanding is commendable.

Philanthropic Foundations

Philanthropic foundations have long been active in international health work. The Rockefeller Foundation has already been discussed: Its health programs have continued to the present. One interesting initiative was the International Clinical Epidemiology Network (INCLEN), which the RF founded in 1980. The INCLEN has been an independent nonprofit organization since 1988, with headquarters in Philadelphia. The network includes clinical epidemiologists, health social scientists, biostatisticians, and clinical economists interested in the effectiveness and efficiency of health care and the factors that determine the most effective prevention and treatment strategies. The INCLEN provides training programs, global meetings, and an international communications network. It supports many young researchers and collaborative clinical studies among the centers, which are found in 22 countries.[35]

The W.K. Kellogg Foundation of Michigan is interested in developing and expanding educational programs in health and agriculture. It has funded courses that train physicians, dentists, nurses, assistants, and technicians and has provided numerous individual fellowships for study in these fields. The Kresge Foundation of Michigan makes grants for capital construction of buildings for education of professionals, for hospitals, and for health-related services. The Milbank Memorial Fund of New York is interested in the application of social and behavioral sciences to public health and preventive medicine and has supported work in demography, vital statistics, population, and general health problems. The Carnegie Corporation of New York has established programs in health technology assessment and in reduction of maternal mortality. The Ford Foundation has concentrated its work in LDCs in education, economic development and planning, food production, and population and family planning and has established programs in many countries of Asia, Africa, and Latin America. Each of these organizations has developed a specific field of interest and strives to make a meaningful contribution toward solution of a particular aspect of health-related problems.

Other private foundations in the United States have become active in supporting international health work. The David and Lucille Packard Foundation, established by one of the founders of the Hewlett-Packard Corporation (H-P), has designated $75 million to international population and reproductive health programs to help slow the rate of population growth and to expand family planning options for the poor. The William and Flora Hewlett Foundation, created by the other founder of H-P, also has a longstanding interest in issues of world population. In late 1998 the Bill and Melinda Gates Foundation, set up by the founder of the Microsoft Corporation, announced a $100 million award for a children's vaccine program to be administered by the Program for Appropriate Technology in Health (PATH) a nongovernmental organization based in Seattle, Washington. The Gates Foundation has also given several million dollars to the United Nations Population Fund (UNFPA) for its population and development programs. The greatest donation of private funds to UN organizations was made in September, 1997 by television and communications executive Ted Turner, who announced a personal gift of one billion dollars to support a variety of programs, including health. It is interesting that all of these large individual and private foundation grants for international health work arose from fortunes made in the electronics, computer, and communications industries.

Many private foundations from countries other than the United States have also been active and productive in international health work. In Britain, for instance, the Nuffield Foundation and the Wellcome Trust both support fellowships and research work in developing countries.

A noteworthy element among foundations in international health is the Aga Khan Foundation (AKF), a private, nondenominational network working to promote social development in the low-income countries of Asia and Africa. The foundation, with headquarters in Geneva, was established by H.H. the Aga Khan, 49th Imam of the Shia Imami Ismaili Muslims. Branch offices are maintained in Pakistan, India, Bangladesh, Kenya, and elsewhere. Foundation programs, spending on the order of $60 million annually, deal primarily with health, education, and rural development. More than 200 educational and 166 health institutions are supported, including the Faculty of Health Sciences at the Aga Khan University in Karachi. The foundation supports primary health care projects in several countries, including a large-scale community-based system that provides tetanus toxoid to mothers and iodinated oil to prevent goiter and cretinism in children in the rugged mountains of northern Pakistan. The foundation has sponsored large international workshops and conferences dealing with issues in primary health care, such as planning and management, application of technology, the role of hospitals, and microcomputer-based information systems.

Other Groups

Within the "aid community," the PVOs, foundations, and donor government agencies often work together. Some groups receive contributions from the general public, foundations, and government agencies. In the field of population and family planning activities, for example, the USAID has allocated hundreds of millions of dollars to PVOs such as the International Planned Parenthood Federation, the Pathfinder Fund, the Population Council, the Association for Voluntary Sterilization, and Church World Services. USAID also channels funds into many other voluntary organizations, but it is constrained by congressional restrictions that prevent support of any organization involved in promotion of abortion. Large projects may involve several major foundations in joint funding, as in Ford–Rockefeller support of the International Rice Research Institute (IRRI) in the Philippines, the International Maize and Wheat Improvement Center (CIMMYT) in Mexico, the International Center for Tropical Agriculture (CIAT) in Colombia, and the International Institute of Tropical Agriculture (IITA) in Nigeria. All of these are intended to improve health through better nutrition.

The many professional and technical associations overlapping to some extent with PVOs serve variously in the dissemination of information; in the provision of expert consultation, training, and fellowships; in the maintenance of professional standards and conditions of employment; and so forth. They may interlock with official agencies at national and international levels.

Private Industry

Private industry may provide medical care directly to employees and sometimes to their dependents, often mandated by local law. In some countries a multinational corporation may be requested to make a socially relevant contribution to the welfare of the host country, as in health care or community development. Such gestures may be considered as a good business practice by the company. In some cases where a commercial organization such as a mine or plantation provides certain services for its employees, the host country may demand that they be provided also to the surrounding community.

The role of commerce and industry in international health is complex and subject to many interpretations. Transnational and multinational enterprises provide much needed investment, employment, and access to markets. They often train local personnel in financial and personnel management and in some fields of technology. In more subtle ways they expose local people to the lifestyles and values of their expatriate staff. Much of this has been looked upon as inappropriate to local cultures and conducive to a materialistic outlook, thereby evoking familiar sorts of criticism.

Consulting

Among the entities working in international health are the many technical assistance and consulting firms that provide expertise in planning and implementing projects. Some of these are mainline NGOs and some have an NGO-like character, although most operate on a for-profit basis. Many such companies are found in Washington, D.C. and in the adjacent suburbs around the ring highway, leading to the common nickname of "beltway bandits." A large number of individual consultants in all areas of international health are employed on a subcontract basis by such companies, which may themselves receive contacts from agencies such as USAID. In many cases these professionals have the most direct contact with organizations and beneficiaries in the field. Other individual consultants make their services available, on a short- or long-term basis, to entities such as development banks. Consulting is discussed further in Chapter 15.

NOTES

1. Renamed the Pan American Sanitary Bureau in 1923.

2. Carried out to a great extent by army physicians from England, France, Italy, the United States, and other colonial powers of the time.

3. Viruses, not known with certainty at the time, were predicted to be the still mysterious "filterable agents."

4. See especially Weindling (1995) and Dubin (1995) for an extensive discussion of the LNHO and related organizations in the 1920s and 1930s.

5. Anon. (1995b).

6. Anon. (1995b).

7. Dubin (1995) referred to the United States as a "clandestine member" of the LNHO.

8. Still functioning are the Pasteur Institutes (given with year established) of: Tunis, Tunisia 1893; Algiers, Algeria 1894; Nha Trang, Vietnam 1895; Antananarivo, Madagascar 1898; Bucharest, Romania (Cantacuzene Institute) 1901; Casablanca, Morocco 1911; Athens, Greece 1919; Teheran, Iran 1920; Dakar, Senegal 1923; St. Petersburg, Russia 1923; Hanoi, Vietnam 1923; Cayenne, French Guiana 1940; Point à Pitre, Guadeloupe 1948; Papeete, Tahiti

1949; Noumea, New Caledonia 1954; Yaoundé, Cameroon 1959; Phnom Penh, Cambodia, rebuilt 1959; Bangui, Central African Republic 1961; Abidjan, Côte d'Ivoire 1972; and Rome, Italy 1976. The Bolivian Institute of High-Altitude Biology in La Paz (1963) is an associated institute.

9. Moulin (1995) described the institutes in the period between the wars.

10. Moulin (1995).

11. See Shaplen (1964), Williams (1969), and Farley (1995).

12. The Rockefeller Foundation was instrumental in founding the School of Hygiene and Public Health at Johns Hopkins University, the first professional public health school in the world.

13. World Health Organization (1994).

14. Adams (1993). This book contains a useful account of the Bretton Woods conference, its outcomes, and "North–South" relations since the 1940s.

15. A term coined by Alfred Sauvy in 1952.

16. The General Agreement on Tarriffs and Trade (GATT) served this function throughout the postwar period. Its role was always ad hoc, as it never had a proper legal foundation and was not recognized as an organization under international law. The World Trade Organization was formally (and legally) established in 1995, half a century after it was suggested at Bretton Woods. The functions of the WTO are to adminster trade agreements, serve as a forum for negotiations, handle disputes, provide technical asistance, and cooperate with other international organizations. The GATT continues to exist as one of the WTO agreements.

17. Adams (1993) describes the sometimes contentious negotiations: "the Americans, who held the purse strings, simply refused to release funds and to allow access to IMF resources in the absence of conditionality."

18. The World Bank does not give away money like an aid agency. There are, however, some small grant programs administered by the various departments.

19. In 1960 the per capita gross national product in the top 20% of countries was 30 times higher than in the bottom 20%. By 1990 the gap had increased to 60 times. See Badran (1995).

20. The founding members of CGAP are Canada, France, the Netherlands, the United States, the African Development Bank, the Asian Development Bank, the International Fund for Agricultural Development, the United Nations Development Programme, the United Nations Capital Development Fund, and the World Bank. Additional donors are Australia, Belgium, Denmark, Finland, Germany, Japan, Luxembourg, Norway, Sweden, Switzerland, the United Kingdom, the European Commission, the Inter-American Development Bank, the International Labour Office, and the United Nations Conference on Trade and Development. Each member donor has its own microfinance programs within CGAP's portfolio for sharing experience and learning on best practice. Doctor Muhammad Yunus of the Grameen Bank was elected chairman of the CGAP Policy Advisory Committee.

21. When said aloud, WHO is always pronounced as separate initials (W-H-O), *never* like the English word "who."

22. Sometimes governments express reservations about one thing or another, usually on political grounds, and these are duly recorded in the proceedings of the conference.

23. The members of the Task Force are the: UN Population Fund (UNFPA), which serves as chair; UN Secretariat; Economic Commissions for Africa (ECA), Europe (ECE), and Latin America and the Caribbean (ECLAC); Economic and Social Commissions for Asia and the Pacific (ESCAP) and Western Asia (ESCWA); Food and Agriculture Organization (FAO); International Labour Organization (ILO); International Monetary Fund (IMF); UN high commissioner for refugees (UNHCR); UN Centre for Human Settlements (Habitat); UN Chil-

dren's Fund (UNICEF); UN Development Fund for Women (UNIFEM); UN Development Programme (UNDP); UN Educational, Scientific and Cultural Organization (UNESCO); UN Environment Programme (UNEP); UN Industrial Development Organization (UNIDO); UN International Drug Control Programme (UNDCP); UN Relief and Works Agency for Palestine Refugees in the Near East (UNRWA); World Bank; World Food Programme (WFP); and World Health Organization (WHO).

24. In article 57 of the UN Charter.

25. This agency, known as UNRRA, was established in 1943 to "provide medical relief to occupied countries after their liberation, health care for displaced persons, and general support to national health administrations. It drafted emergency international sanitary conventions to take effect after the war, provided fellowships, medical literature and large quantities of drugs, and sent health missions to many countries . . . Some of these functions were later taken over by WHO" (Anon., 1995b).

26. Backett (1989).

27. Formerly in Brazzaville. The Harare office is officially considered temporary until the local situation permits a return to Brazzaville.

28. Following the 50th World Health Assembly in 1997, EB members were designated by the following countries: *Africa:* Algeria, Angola, Benin, Botswana, Burkina Faso, Burundi, Zimbabwe; *Americas:* Argentina, Barbados, Brazil, Canada, Honduras, Peru; *South-East Asia*: Bhutan, Indonesia, Sri Lanka; *Europe:* Croatia, Germany, Ireland, Netherlands, Norway, Poland, United Kingdom; *Eastern Mediterranean*: Cyprus, Egypt, Oman, United Arab Emirates; *Western Pacific*: Australia, Cook Islands, Japan, Republic of Korea. One-third of these members change each year.

29. As of 1998 essentially all independent states of the world are members. In a practical sense, the major exception is Taiwan (Republic of China), because the WHO recognizes China as a single entity represented by the government in Beijing.

30. The OECD, based in Paris, was established in 1961 to coordinate international growth, stability, and trade. It has more than 100 committees, including the DAC.

31. Title IV of the Marshall Plan amendments of 1950.

32. Distribution was handled through American private voluntary organizations (PVOs).

33. World Bank. Operational Directive on NGOs. 14.70, 1989, cited by Matthias and Green (1994).

34. Sometimes these are classified unofficially into BINGOs (Big International NGOs), CONGOS (commercial NGOs), and QUANGOs (Quasi-NGOs).

35. Argentina, Brazil, Cameroon, Canada, Chile, China, Colombia, Egypt, Ethiopia, France, India, Indonesia, Kenya, Mexico, Peru, Philippines, Spain, Thailand, Uganda, United Kingdom, United States, and Zimbabwe.

4

What We Want to Know— Data on Health

The crucial and complex subject of health-related information often suffers from neglect by those whose motivation in life is healing the sick or conducting biomedical research. The collection, dissemination, and utilization of such data may not be considered matters of great urgency, even by health services administrators. Nonetheless, accurate information is the lifeblood of decision-making, and in the present day the demand for reliable data is greater than ever. But data costs money, and as with most other things, the higher the quality, the greater the cost. In developing countries, where the need for medical services is acute and resources are perpetually inadequate, the funds allocated for collection, transmission, and analysis of data always fall short of requirements. In general, where disease occurrence is highest the numbers are the least trustworthy.

WHAT IS HEALTH?

One of the great ironies and frustrations facing persons who deal with health-related data is the absence of an acceptable definition of *health*, either at an individual or a community level. This deficiency cannot be blamed on a lack of attempts. Definitions of health in dictionaries tend to mention soundness and vigor of the body and/or the mind and freedom from disease. In this way they do not differ greatly from the ideal of Juvenal (ca. AD 60–140): *mens sana in corpore sano* (sound mind in a sound body). Most often quoted in recent years is the statement in the Preamble to the Constitution of World Health Organization: "Health is a state of complete physical, mental and social well-being and not merely the absence of disease or infirmity"—an affirmation of belief and principle rather than a quantifiable technical definition, and of limited practical use. Most people would perceive health in terms of

- Pain, fever, or other symptoms of illness
- Interference with the normal activities of life
- Deviation from a predetermined norm, and
- Ability to respond to stress and physical insult

Each of us has an adequate mental compass that points toward health and indicates deviations, but none of us can specify exactly what we mean by it, any more than we can explain the magnetism in a real compass. We may hope for a simple numerical indicator to summarize health status of individuals and populations so that we can keep track over time, compare one with another, and evaluate the effect of interventions. But beware of simple solutions: "The problem of measuring something, assuming it is health, and therefore calling it health, is not unusual with health status indicators."[1]

Even without a universal definition of *individual* health, it may be useful to have some means to depict the level of health of *populations*. Pooled figures of this kind usually involve measurable proxies such as infant mortality rate, cases of notifiable illnesses, numbers of deaths and their causes, and certain health service activities, such as immunization coverage and procedures performed. These, together with a few socioeconomic and other measures, make up the raw material for various health policy decisions. We are reminded of the little poem by Rudyard Kipling's "Just So Stories," which referred not only to international health but to everything in life:

> I keep six honest serving-men;
> They taught me all I knew.
> Their names are What and Why and When
> And How and Where and Who.

From the viewpoint of international health, the obvious questions are:

- What do we want to know?
- How can we find the data?
- What will we do with the information?

Before these are considered, however, it is important to understand why this information is being sought.

Reasons for Seeking Health Statistics

Persons responsible for health services have always required information about the kinds, quantity, and distribution of illness as guides to planning and evaluation. Six types of uses for health-related data are summarized in Table 4-1. Decision-making in many countries is becoming more sophisticated as populations, costs, medical knowledge, and information processing techniques all advance. Weighing alternative strategies for maximum effectiveness has become a task for a new kind of specialist.

The goals listed on Table 4-1 are clearly credible; but a closer look reveals many problems in the appropriate use of health indicators. Table 4-2 lists some of these considerations.

In addition to their health-related prediction and evaluation functions, statistical data about health are also needed by other branches of government at municipal, county, provincial or state, and national levels. In most countries health-related legislation originates from a perception of need that should be based on realistic and reliable information. Legal requirements for detecting, reporting, and combating locally important diseases; laws dealing with occupational and environmental hazards, regulation of hospitals, and training and licensing of professional personnel; and many similar subjects all clearly depend on relevant data. Compliance with existing laws and regulations must also be monitored.

Health statistics derived from continuous monitoring can have an early warning function. Prompt detection of outbreaks can lead to knowledge of their cause and steps to minimize the hazard. New or newly recognized conditions can be discovered early. For example, a syndrome of eye, ear, and heart damage was described in children whose mothers contracted rubella during pregnancy, and limb malformations in newborns were related to maternal use of thalidomide. In both cases, the first indications of these relationships arose not from the conventional government

Table 4-1. Some Uses for Statistical Health Measures at National Level

1. Identify emerging problems	Recognize the health issues, demographic groups, and geographic area in which they are appearing
2. Anticipate future needs	In addition to #1, follow changes in the economy, environment, and demographic composition of the population. Collect data appropriate to effective public health efforts
3. Help determine priorities	Identify the types and distribution of health problems and their impact, to design programs for priority attention
4. Estimate budgets	Determine the number of people who must be reached, their location, age, and sex, and the severity of conditions to project resource needs
5. Secure public and government	Produce trustworthy and convincing statistics for education campaigns and presentation to officials and legislators who control finances
6. Help direct progress toward goals	Have clearly defined goals. Use data to follow trends and evaluate programs. If not advancing, reconfigure toward more effective programs

Source: Adapted from Woolsey (1979).

Table 4-2. Some Questions About Health Indicators

1. At what level(s) in the health system will these be used? Village health worker, regional planning officer, provincial or central Ministry of Health, prime minister, medical college, research institute, international organization?

2. For what specific purposes? Prioritization, planning, surveillance, monitoring, evaluation, research, multiple uses?

3. If used for monitoring or evaluation, do the health programs have stated objectives, targets, or outcomes relevant to these indicators?

4. Have these or similar indicators been found useful in other programs, districts, or countries in similar circumstances?

5. Are these standard international indicators used or suggested by international or regional organizations to facilitate comparisons?

6. Is the indicator statistically valid: i.e., does it measure what it is intended to measure?

7. Is the indicator reliable and consistent? Is it sufficiently sensitive and specific?

8. Is the indicator a direct or a proxy measure?

9. What other information is needed to generate or interpret the indicator?

10. Are conditions in place to process and utilize the indicator, e.g., staff training and expertise, computer hardware and software, coding systems?

11. Are funds available to collect and manage the data and resultant information?

Source: Adapted from Graham (1986).

statistical system but from alert clinicians (in Australia and Germany, respectively). Both have resulted in worldwide awareness and control efforts. The first cases of AIDS were detected by physicians who noted an unusual number of cases of Kaposi's sarcoma and *Pneumocystis* pneumonia in a population of young homosexual males. Many similar instances could be cited.

On an international level, each country needs to know about real and potential threats to the health of its citizens, particularly from imported communicable diseases. Smallpox is now a thing of the past (Chapter 14), and the risk of widespread plague is greatly reduced, but cholera, influenza, AIDS, and other diseases still pose a hazard to many countries. Conversely, accurate figures on cases of diseases near eradication, such as polio, are crucial for monitoring progress. The health problems likely to be encountered by nationals traveling abroad also require international collation and dissemination of data.

Members of the World Health Organization are obligated under its constitution to provide certain information in the form of regular reports. They must also report annually on the action taken and progress achieved in improving the health of their people (article 61). Member states must communicate promptly to the WHO important laws, regulations, official reports, and statistics pertaining to health (article 63) and provide other statistical and epidemiological reports as determined by the World Health Assemblies (article 64). In addition, the International Health Regulations in effect since 1971 require health administrations to notify the WHO of cases or outbreaks of certain diseases and of measures taken to prevent their spread.

Many people are interested in international compilations of vital and health statistics as a yardstick to compare their country with others. Statistics concerning the ratio of population to physicians, hospital beds, etc., are often cited by advocates of one or another viewpoint, both on national and regional levels. Such data, as well as evaluations of nutritional status and similar conditions linked to socioeconomic development, are often highly sensitive and laden with political overtones. One should always be cautious in interpreting health-related data. It is difficult to define the metrics and hard to get the numbers right. There may also be certain pressures on local and regional officials and on Ministries of Health. Administrators may be tempted to overestimate the number of inoculations given or minimize reported rates of sickness or death. Concern with international trade or with the tourist industry may prompt cases of cholera to be reported as gastroenteritis, and forthcoming elections may entice a politician into uncharacteristic exaggeration. Such distortions arising from human frailty need not be overemphasized, but should be kept in mind when reading and interpreting all health-related data.

Health statistics have many uses, but they can not be used to draw causal inferences. We must distinguish between health indicators that we use on an everyday basis to describe populations and inform public health authorities about needed programs, and analytic studies designed to test hypotheses about risk factors and illnesses. Nevertheless, health statistics are woven into such investigations as essential numerator and/or denominator data.

Epidemiologic findings associating cigarette smoking with lung cancer, firearms with accidental shootings, alcohol with road accidents, and risky practices with AIDS, for example, have often been cited as arguments in favor of restrictive legislation. Proponents and opponents of tobacco, guns, alcohol, or liberated behavior have sought, identified, and interpreted data to support their particular positions. The same is true of partisans on either side of issues such as the construction of nuclear power plants or the conduct of recombinant DNA research. Health statistics are sometimes provided to officials and to the public by the advocates of one or another specific cause. The champions of a particular disease, for example, may release biased or selective information in an attempt to attract money and public interest to their cause. Diseases or conditions with determined advocates may receive disproportionate funding while others, perhaps much more destructive, languish for lack of organized proponents. The need for timely and comprehensive health statistics is unending. The global resurgence of tuberculosis occurred essentially while nobody was looking.

The overlap of medical science and public policy leads to advances in both by stimulating research designed to provide definitive data in answer to pressing questions. Certain epidemiologic information is best obtained by worldwide, multinational, or cross-cultural analyses. Detailed investigations in areas of high prevalence of specific diseases may lead to hypotheses about causation which, if confirmed elsewhere, can be translated into strategies for intervention.

It is not only official government agencies that require health-related data. Life insurance companies have a great interest in such information. Indeed, early work on mortality by demographic pioneers such as John Graunt and Edmund Halley was much more useful to underwriters than to bureaucrats. The burgeoning of commercial health insurance companies and HMOs,[2] particularly in the United States, makes the need for appropriate data on population risks of illness and accidents much more acute. In fact, any person responsible for the administration of groups of people, whether in industry, schools, the military, or elsewhere must have a certain amount of information on which to base projections of needed services, absenteeism, and other aspects of management.

Comparative information about the organization of health and medical care systems, mechanisms for their coordination and financial support, and ways in which they are utilized in other countries can provide valuable insights into the realm of human problem solving: this forms the basis of the following chapter. The training of physicians and other members of health care teams varies from one country to another, as does the utilization of auxiliary personnel such as midwives and village health workers. No nation is so omniscient that knowledge derived elsewhere can be safely ignored.

And finally there is another human characteristic that drives men and women to probe, to ask, to travel, to compare, to consider every scrap and nuance of information about the world and its contents, one that needs neither analysis nor justification, namely, curiosity.

What Kinds of Health Data Do We Need?

An infinity of variables acts to influence the health of individuals and populations. The amount of rainfall can affect nutrition by altering agricultural production and can influence subsequent rates of illness in endemic areas by controlling populations of malaria vector mosquitoes. Indeed, many people believe that global warming (if it is real) will lead to great epidemics of malaria and other vector-borne diseases. Changes in speed limits play a part in determining deaths and injuries in automobile accidents. While such variables have indirect effects on health, rainfall and speed limits do not qualify as health statistics in the conventional sense. The basic categories of generally accepted health-related statistics are:

- *Data on the population.* The number of people and their attributes, such as age, sex, ethinic origin, urbanization, geographic distribution, and similar fundamental characteristics.
- *Vital statistics.* Live births; deaths (including fetal deaths) by sex, age, and cause; marriages and divorces. (In some countries migration [internal and external], adoptions, and similar categories are also considered as vital statistics.)
- *Health statistics.* Morbidity by type, severity, and outcome of illness or accident; data on notifiable diseases, on blindness, incapacity; tumor registries, etc.

This category is not so clearly defined as the previous two and will vary from one jurisdiction to another.

- *Statistics bearing upon health services.* Numbers and types of facilities and services available; the distribution, qualifications, and functions of personnel; nature of the services and their utilization rates; hospital and health center operations; organization of government and private health care systems; costs, payment mechanisms, and related information. This large and diverse category, often subdivided into subjects of special interest, will be discussed in the following chapter.

The compilation and issuance of these data on a continuing basis entails a great deal of effort and expense for all modern governments. The situation is made far more complex, however, by the need for comparability among countries and over time. A high degree of international cooperation is required to assure that definitions, terminology, diagnostic techniques, certification practices, data-handling methods, and reporting schemes are sufficiently standardized for comparative purposes but flexible enough to take into account the variety of circumstances throughout the world.

DATA ON THE POPULATION: THE CENSUS

The basic demographic characteristics of a population literally underlie most vital and health statistics because they provide the denominators for the relevant rates and ratios (Table 4-3). Data on the population are usually obtained in two ways: by *enumeration* and by *registration*. Enumeration, when complete, is done by means of a *census of population,* which in many countries in recent times has been repeated each decade.[3] Registration, as defined by the United Nations, is the continuous, permanent, and compulsory recording of the occurrence and characteristics of vital events.

Neither enumeration nor registration is done primarily for the purpose of providing vital and health statistics. Census data have been used for millennia for purposes of taxation and conscription. The birth of Christ is said to have occurred at Bethlehem because Mary and Joseph were traveling home to Judea to be counted in a census. At about the same time (AD 2) in China a census was ordered and data were recorded on more than 12 million households, including the heads of families and the name, age, and birthplace of more than 59.5 million people.[4] In 1085 William of Normandy (William the Conqueror) ordered an official record to be made in territories that he controlled in England listing all landowners and their properties (including tenants, servants, and serfs) so that the territory could be taken from the nobility and divided among his followers. This record, known as the Domesday Book, was completed in 1086. More recently, census data have been used for determining political representation, as required for instance by the constitution of the United States (1790), as well as for many other purposes. The first census of the United

Table 4-3. Commonly Used Health Indicators

Annual crude live birth rate (= birth rate)

$$\frac{\text{Number of births occurring in a defined population during a year}}{\text{Number in that population at midyear of the same year}} \times 1000$$

Annual crude death rate (= mortality rate, death rate)

$$\frac{\text{Number of deaths occurring in a defined population during a year}}{\text{Number in that population at midyear of the same year}} \times 1000$$

Annual specific death rate (by age, sex, cause, or a combination)

$$\frac{\substack{\text{Number of deaths of a specified age (or sex, or cause)}\\ \text{occurring in a defined population during a year}}}{\text{Number of the specified age group in that population at midyear of the same year}} \times 1000$$

Annual infant mortality rate (= Infant mortality rate; IMR)

$$\frac{\text{Number of deaths under 1 year of age in a defined population during a year}}{\text{Number of live births occurring in that population during the same year}} \times 1000$$

Annual neonatal mortality rate

$$\frac{\text{Number of deaths under 28 days year of age in a defined population during a year}}{\text{Number of live births occurring in that population during the same year}} \times 1000$$

Annual postneonatal mortality rate

$$\frac{\text{Number of deaths at 28 days to 1 year of age in a defined population during a year}}{\text{Number of live births occurring in that population during the same year}} \times 1000$$

Annual fetal death rate (stillbirth rate)

$$\frac{\text{Number of deaths at 20}^{a}\text{ or more weeks gestational age in a defined population during a year}}{\text{Number of live births occurring in that population during the same year}} \times 1000$$

Annual maternal mortality rate

$$\frac{\text{Number of deaths from maternal causes}^{b}\text{ in a defined population during a year}}{\text{Number of women childbearing age in that population during the same year}} \times 100,000$$

(continued)

80

Table 4-3. Commonly Used Health Indicators (*continued*)

Proportionate mortality

$$\frac{\text{Number of deaths in a specific category in a defined population during a year}}{\text{Total number of deaths occurring in that population during the same year}} \times 100$$

Annual incidence rate for occurrence of a specified condition

$$\frac{\text{Number of new cases of the condition occurring in a defined population in a year}}{\text{Number in that population at midyear of the same year}} \times 10^{n\ \text{c}}$$

(Point) prevalence of a specified condition

$$\frac{\substack{\text{Number of cases of the specified condition existing} \\ \text{in a defined population at a particular point in time}}}{\text{Number in that population at the same point in time}} \times 10^{n}$$

Morbidity rate (crude; or specific by age, sex, occupation, etc.)

$$\frac{\substack{\text{Number of cases of a specified condition occurring in} \\ \text{specified population categories during a specified time period}}}{\text{Average population in the category during the year}} \times 10^{n}$$

[a]Varies somewhat in different jurisdictions.

[b]As listed in the latest ICD revision or defined nationally.

[c] nMultiplier varies depending on frequency of the condition.

Source: Adapted from Basch (1990), Table 3-2.

States enumerated free white males over and under 16 years of age; free white fe-males; all other free persons; and slaves, each of whom counted for three-fifths of a person.[5] The essential features of a national census of population are:

- *Sponsorship.* A legal basis must be established, with administrative machinery to ensure compliance and confidentiality.
- *Defined territory.*
- *Universality.* Every person physically present and/or residing in the territory should be included.
- *Individual enumeration.*
- *Simultaneity and specified time.* The collected date should refer insofar as possible to a single point in time.
- *Periodicity.* Censuses should be conducted at regular intervals.
- *Compilation and publication.* Raw data must be put into a useful form and published as soon as possible for maximum utlity.

The effort and expense involved in a complete census is considerable. The cost of the United States Census 2000 of Population and Housing is estimated at $34 per household (Table 4-4). The decennial expenditure just for counting each person in the United States exceeds the total per capita annual health budget of many of the world's least developed countries.

During a census, information is usually collected on a variety of topics. Specific items for inclusion recommended by the United Nations World Population Census Program censuses are indicated in Table 4-5.

The information obtained from enumeration and registration data permit a population to be characterized by a variety of classifiers, of which age and sex are most often used, as well as education and literacy status, occupation, and ethnic group. Certain categories such as age and sex will be similar everywhere; others, such as ethnicity, will vary from country to country. In the 1980 Census of Population and Housing of the United States the following self-identified categories were listed for "race": White, Black or Negro, Japanese, Chinese, Filipino, Korean, Vietnamese, Indian (American), Asian Indian, Hawaiian, Guamanian, Samoan, Eskimo, Aleut, or Other-specify. The 2000 census will have five minimum categories for data on race: American Indian or Alaska Native; Asian; Black or African American; Native Hawaiian or Other Pacific Islander; and White. There are two categories for data on ethnicity: Hispanic or Latino; and Not Hispanic or Latino.

The figures derived from the census serve as denominators for the age- and sex-specific mortality and morbidity rates defined in Table 4-6 and make possible more meaningful comparisons of the measures than can be obtained from crude (whole population) figures. As an illustration, the age and sex distributions of the populations of six countries are compared in Figure 4-1. The major functional age groups usually tracked are preschool (under 5), school age (5–14), working age (15–64),

Table 4-4. Cost, United States Census of Population and Housing, 1960 to 2000

	Cost[a]	
Year	Per household, $	Total, $ million
1960	9	523
1970	11	744
1980	20	1,795
1990	25	2,600
2000	34[b]	4,000[b]

[a]1990 dollars, except data for 2000.

[b]Estimated, current dollars.

Source: Edmonston and Schultze (1995) and Bureau of the Census.

Table 4-5. Topics Recommended by the UN World Population Census Program for Inclusion in a National Census of Population

Priority Items	Other useful items
Place of usual residence	Religion
Place at time of the census	Language
Place of birth	National/ethnic origin
Duration of residence	Live births preceding 12 months
Place of previous residence	Infants born & died last 12 months
Place of residence at [year]	Maternal orphanhood
Relationship to household head or other reference member	Educational qualifications
	Sector of employment
Sex	Time worked
Age	Income
Marital status	
Citizenship	
Children born alive	
Children living	
Duration of marriage	
Educational attainment	
Literacy	
School attendance	
Economic activity status	
Occupation	
Industry	
Status in employment/occupation	

Source: Adapted from Domschke and Goyer (1986).

and advanced age (over 65). The under-15s and over-65s are generally considered to be dependent on the population segment aged 15 to 65. The ratio of persons aged 0–14 to those aged 15–64 ($\times 100$) is called the *childhood dependency ratio*, and the *old-age dependency ratio* is calculated similarly. Table 4-5 shows how these ratios will change between 1950 and 2000 in various parts of the world. Note that whereas the proportion of children declines and that of the aged grows in most areas, the trend is exactly the reverse in (mostly sub-Saharan) Africa. The proportion of elderly almost doubles in the former USSR; it increases by 40% in North America and by 67% in Europe.[6] Such projections can be obtained only through collection of data of adequate quality.

Methodologically, it may appear that after a national census is decided on, enumerators are trained, and data processing materials are prepared, the rest is a simple matter. In actuality, appraisal of completeness and accuracy of census data calls for careful checks and sophisticated techniques. Errors and inaccuracies can infil-

Table 4-6. Childhood and Old Age Dependency Ratios, World and Major Regions, 1950, 1980, and 2000

Area	Childhood Dependency Ratio			Old Age Dependency Ratio		
	1950	1980	2000	1950	1980	2000
World	59.0	60.8	48.2	8.9	9.8	10.5
Africa	77.9	87.5	87.3	6.7	5.9	5.9
Americas						
Latin America	72.1	69.9	54.3	6.0	7.6	8.4
Northern America	41.9	34.0	32.3	12.5	16.7	17.6
Asia						
East Asia	58.0	59.6	34.3	5.9	8.5	10.9
South Asia	73.4	72.9	53.2	9.2	5.9	7.0
Europe	38.5	34.5	29.2	13.2	20.1	22.0
Oceania	47.4	47.2	40.4	11.9	12.7	14.0
USSR[a]	47.1	37.1	36.6	9.5	15.3	18.4

[a]For 2000, components of the former USSR.

Source: Adapted from United Nations (1985).

trate the raw data with great ease, particularly when questions are asked of poorly educated people unaware of the significance of the census and likely to be suspicious of its intent. The U.S. Census Bureau recognizes two types of error: *sampling error*—from selection of persons and housing units selected for certain additional questions; and *nonsampling error*—for all other errors that may occur during collection and processing of data. Coverage of large populations is never perfect, even under the best of circumstances. Each U.S. census receives thousands of official complaints from communities, all alleging undercounts which would result in lowered government subsidies and payments for education and other services based on population size. The furor over use of sampling in the 2000 census is a sign of the political sensitivity of enumeration methods.

The question of age may be taken as an example of the uncertainty inherent in census taking. Errors arise from underenumeration of certain components of the population. Children, particularly babies, are often overlooked by respondents when

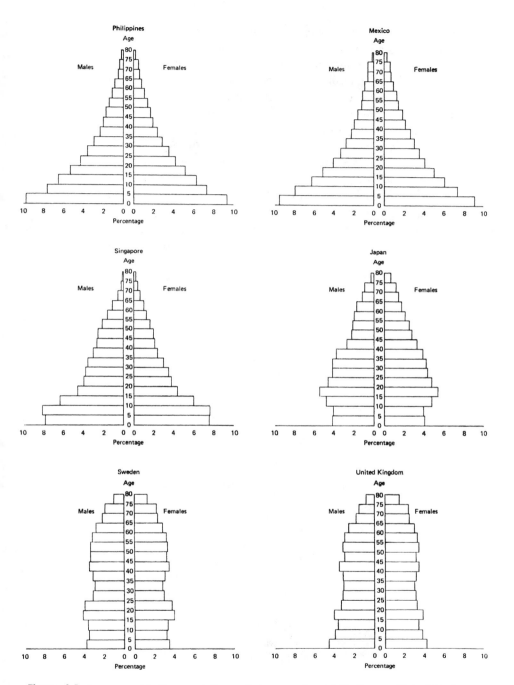

Figure 4-1 Age pyramids for populations of six countries, 1965. *Source:* United Nations, 1973.

asked about the number of people in their household. Many persons do not know their age and some may deliberately misstate the figure for one reason or another. Local customs in reckoning age also vary; some groups of Chinese, for instance, count a childs's age at birth as one rather than zero and state all ages as of the next rather than the previous birthday. In other cultures a child may not be counted at all until it has reached the age of one year. It is often considered more accurate to ask a person not for his or her current age, which changes, but for the year of birth, which is a constant more likely to be recalled correctly. Figure 4-2 illustrates graphically the strong effect of number preference in one particular case, the 1945 census of Turkey, by rounding to terminal 5 or 0. Ages ending with 1, 4, 6, and 9 were in this census commonly stated to the nearest number divisible by 5, and the even digits 2 and 8 were preferred to the odd numbers 3 and 7.

The United Nations Department of International Economic and Social Affairs, which compiles the annual *Demographic Yearbook* and other population-based sta-

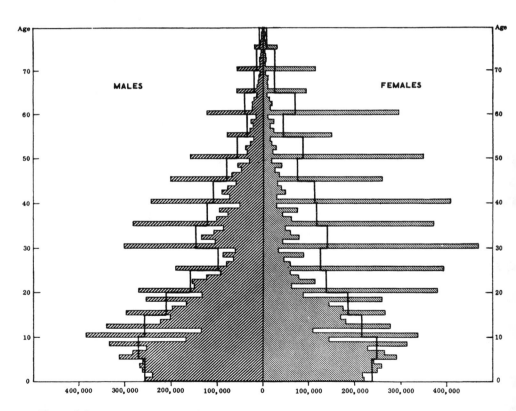

Figure 4-2 Population of Turkey, 1945, by sex, by single year of age, and 5-year age groups, according to census. *Source:* United Nations, 1955.

tistics, uses a code that takes into account four elements that affect the reliability of population estimates. These are:

- The nature of the base measurement of the population
- The time elapsed since the last measurement
- Method of time adjustment by which the base figure is updated
- Quality of adjustment

Since 1950 the proportion of the estimate of the world's population that derives from total census enumeration has risen from just over 70% to about 95%. The proportion depending on conjecture or undetermined methods has fallen proportionately.

VITAL STATISTICS

Registration of vital events is usually done at a legally designated place near the occurrence of the event. Depending on local laws and practice, this may be a police post, courthouse, municipal or district office, special civil registry office, school or other locale.

Compilation of records by administrative divisions (towns, municipalities, counties, provinces, or states) and by regions or geographic areas provides a comprehensive picture of vital events that is essential for planning and allocation of government services when a country has reached a certain level of economic development. Together with census data, vital records are essential for estimating future manpower resources and needs for schools, highways, social security, and other services including public health and medical care. Vital records have many personal and administrative uses, as shown in Table 4-7. The flow of information is very variable from one country to another, and entirely different systems may be found. Where an effective inclusive registration system exists, the availability of good quality data is often taken for granted, but it is an unfortunate fact that civil registration is still lacking or deficient in many countries.

Perhaps one-third of all births in the world are not registered, leaving people without the entitlements listed in Table 4-7. UNICEF refers to birth registration as "the first right, the right to an official identity." A survey by UNICEF found that birth registration in Latin America, central Asia, and North Africa was good, but in sub-Saharan Africa and some parts of Asia such as India and Myanmar only one-third to one-half of births were registered. Cambodia had no registration system at all, and Vietnam "did not have enough data to make even an educated guess" (see next note). "If a third of the children who are born every year are in essence non-existent in the eyes of states, then it puts them at risk. Not having a birth certificate is the functional equivalent of not having been born."[7]

Some public health functions—for example, establishing coverage of immuniza-

Table 4-7. Some Personal and Administrative Uses of Vital Records

I. *Personal uses*

  A. *Birth certificate*

    1. Establish date of birth
       Enter school, military or civil service
       Obtain work permit, marriage license, driver's license
       Qualify for voting, retirement, pension

    2. Establish place of birth
       Qualify for passport, voting. civil office
       Determine citizenship at birth

    3. Establish family relationship
       Trace descent, prove legitimacy, birth order
       Prove legal dependency
       Qualify for insurance and inheritance benefits

  B. *Marriage certificate*

    1. Qualify for housing allocation, inheritance, pension, insurance, tax deduction

    2. Prove legal responsibility of spouse, legitimacy of offspring, citizenship by marriage

  C. *Divorce certificate*

    1. Establish right to alimony or benefits

    2. Prove right to remarry

  D. *Death certificate*

    1. Establish fact of death: Claim pension, insurance, inheritance

    2. Establish cause of death: determine indemnity payment

II. *Administrative uses*

  A. *Birth records*

    1. Provide basis for child health and imunization programs, education planning, etc.

    2. Evaluate family planning programs, prenatal clinics, etc.

    3. Contribute to intercensal estimate of population size

  B. *Marriage records*

    1. Prove establishment of household for benefit programs

    2. Predict population trends

    3. Basis for construction and allocation of housing, etc.

  C. *Death records*

    1. Provide basis for cause-of-death analysis and specific prevention or control programs, particularly for infant and maternal mortality

    2. Clear files; e.g., electoral rolls, tax or military service registers, disease-case registers

    3. Contribute to intercensal estimate of population size

Source: Basch (1990) Table 2-11.

tion campaigns—are difficult to do without accurate information about the number of children in a population. Some immunization programs report more than 100% coverage because more children appeared than the official statistics had recorded.

A similar situation applies to death registration. Approximately 70% of deaths in the world are not medically certified, and registration of vital events varies greatly by region as shown in Table 4-8.

There are many reasons for this unfortunate situation. Money is in short supply everywhere, and government services are often very thinly dispersed. A population group may, for various reasons, wish its size to be either overstated or understated. In some areas there may be a lack of conviction by lower-level government officers concerning the value of collecting vital statistics. The absence of a clear administrative mandate is an impediment in some countries since responsibility for parts of this work may, for reasons of historical development, be divided among several government departments or ministries: health, finance, planning, census, social security, central statistical bureaus, or others. Trained, competent persons for this complex work are often unavailable. The Expert Committee on Health Statistics of the WHO has, over the years, issued numerous technical reports on various aspects of the problems involved.

Difficulties in obtaining data in developing countries include the isolation of rural populations or inaccessibility of registry offices, the lack of education and knowledge about the system, and the suspicion by the public that records may not be kept confidential or that they may be used by the government for taxation, enforced military service, or other purposes considered contrary to their interests. Squatters, illegal aliens, persons without identity cards, nomads having no fixed residence, persons engaged in illegal activities, and others may have strong disincentives toward

Table 4-8. Percent of Deaths Covered by Vital Registration, by Age Group, World, 1990

World Bank Region	Age at Death		
	Under 5 years	5 or More Years	Total
Established Market Economies	99.	99.	99.
Former Socialist Economies of Eastern Europe	99.	99.	99.
India	. . .[a]	. . .	. . .
China	. . .	. . .	. . .
Other Asia and Pacific Islands	2.1	13.6	10.2
Sub-Saharan Africa	0.4	1.7	1.1
Latin America and Caribbean	27.6	47.2	42.6
Middle East Crescent	12.3	27.1	21.8

[a]Sample registration only, or registration by non-medically qualified personnel.

Source: Murray and Lopez (1997a). See source for details.

registration. Fees (or bribes) may be demanded by officials for the initial registration or for copies of certificates. A legal requirement for a death certificate before authorization of burial may work a hardship in remote areas and can be easily overlooked by a bereaved family. The very same vital events to be recorded—births, marriages, and deaths—are accompanied by an infinite variety of cultural and religious traditions in human societies. These customs and rituals, developed over centuries or millennia, may be incompatible with the local government's needs for vital statistics data. Among many peoples, for instance, dissection of the dead is considered abhorrent and forbidden, thus preventing autopsy to determine cause of death.

It would seem that birth and death are both clear and unmistakable events, universally recognized and not needing a rigid definition for vital statistical purposes. But things are not so simple, especially where stillbirths and fetal deaths are concerned. It is important to distinguish whether a baby is alive at birth even if it dies moments later, not only for proper allocation and recording of the event but also for medical understanding of the events that occur during the birth process.

The recent increase in "therapeutic terminations of pregnancy" (abortions) accounts for much of the difficulty. Very early and patently nonviable fetuses may well show evidence of life, however transitory, and would qualify as live births under the strict definition. In many countries the number of abortions performed is very significant when compared with the number of live births. Inflexible application of the current definition, or variations in local interpretation and practice, can result in large discrepancies in reported rates for live births and fetal, neonatal, and infant deaths. There is no need here to discuss these technicalities in great detail, but this sort of problem must be borne in mind when comparing infant mortality data from different countries and time periods (see Chapter 7).

Recent advances in medical techniques have enabled physicians to keep alive individuals with advanced illnesses or massive injuries who under other circumstances would undoubtedly have died. The problem of defining the precise moment of death has been brought into prominence with the advent of organ transplantation and is particularly troublesome in the case of heart donors. In Japan heart transplants have almost never been done because of the prevailing belief that a person with a beating heart is not dead and therefore cannot serve as a donor. Removal of the heart would therefore constitute murder. After years of study, the Japan Medical Association decided in 1988 to accept brain death as a valid definition of death, but legislation to this effect failed in the parliament. It was not until June 1997 that a law was passed to legalize heart transplants under certain conditions. That law says that a person whose brain has stopped functioning can be defined as dead if he or she has given prior consent to donate organs for transplant. However, the patient's family has the right to veto the decision. An alternative bill to accept brain death as death was defeated. Situations of this type arising from technical advances in medical capability are likely to become more common in the future. Long-accepted definitions of death become ambiguous in the face of such unanticipated technical developments. While we presume that the removal of living hearts or other organs will never become common enough to make a significant impression on vital statistics rates, the principles involved force attention to this problem and invite review and revision of the definition of death.

United Nations definitions of birth, death, fetal death, and abortion are given in Table 4-9. These are in great need of revision.

STATISTICS ON MORTALITY

In the middle of the 17th century a London cloth merchant, John Graunt, began a study of the *Bills of Mortality,* which were parish registers of births and deaths. One may well wonder why this particular man, untrained in medicine or science, undertook such a curious hobby, but the indisputable result of Graunt's work, published in 1662, was to show that human life conforms to certain predictable statistical patterns. Graunt classified deaths by cause and found that these varied from place to place and from year to year. He described the age pattern of deaths and constructed a simple forerunner of the modern life table. It was Graunt who discovered the now universally accepted fact that the number of males born slightly but regularly exceeds the number of females. Since his time many others have undertaken similar studies, and now the volume of information available about the pattern and causes of human mortality is truly monumental.

Table 4-9. Some Vital Events, as Defined by the United Nations

Live birth is the complete expulsion or extraction from its mother of a product of conception, irrespective of the duration of pregnancy, which after such separation breathes or shows any other evidence of life such as beating of the heart, pulsation of the umbilical cord, or definite movement of voluntary muscles, whether or not the umbilical cord has been cut or the placenta is attached; each product of such a birth is considered live-born regardless of gestational age

Death is the permanent disappearance of all evidence of life at any time after live birth has taken place (postnatal cessation of vital functions without capability of resuscitation). This definition therefore excludes fetal deaths

Fetal death is death prior to the complete expulsion or extraction from its mother of a product of conception, irrespective of the duration of pregnancy; the death is indicated by that fact that after such separation the fetus does not breathe or show any other evidence of life, such as beating of the heart, pulsation of the umbilical cord, or definite movement of voluntary muscles. Late fetal deaths are those of twenty-eight or more completed weeks of gestation. These are synonymous with the events reported under the pre-1950 term stillbirth

Abortion is defined, with reference to the woman, as any interruption of pregnancy before 28 weeks of gestation with a dead fetus. There are two major categories of abortion: spontaneous and induced. Induced abortions are those initiated by deliberate action undertaken with the intention of terminating pregnancy; all other abortions are considered as spontaneous

Source: United Nations Department for Economic and Social information and Policy Analysis. Statistics Division.

Mortality statistics are in the first rank of measurements for international health studies. Because of their general unambiguity, data on mortality, where available, remain the most practical reflection of changes in the level of health of populations. The advantage of mortality statistics over other statistics relating to health, however, is mainly that they exist on a much more widespread scale throughout the countries of the world. They help to define health problems, to monitor the efficacy of health programs, and to identify the emerging problems of the public health. They provide a basis for hypotheses about different causes of death among various populations. In fact, in many regions of the world most deaths are not recorded at all, and those deaths that are recorded are not representative of mortality for the entire region. Medical certification is available for less than 30% of the 50 million or so deaths that occur in the world each year (Table 4-8). Of all child deaths 98% occur in developing countries, which also experience 83% of deaths between 15 and 59 and 59% of all deaths over 70 years of age. In wealthier countries 1.1% of girls die before their 15th birthday, while in sub-Saharan Africa it is an astounding 22%.[8]

Two Special Kinds of Mortality Rates

Because of their particular significance for international health we will now look more deeply at two categories of mortality rates listed on Table 4-3. These are infant mortality and maternal mortality. Here we will consider some methodological issues; infant and maternal mortality are discussed in greater detail in Chapter 7.

Infant mortality

The handling of deaths in the age interval between zero and one (i.e., the time period beginning at birth and ending exactly one year later) differs from all other annual age-specific death rates in several important respects. First, both numerator and denominator are derived directly from registration data, whereas the denominator for other age-specific mortality rates comes generally from census-based estimates. More importantly, the denominator of the infant mortality rate is not the number of persons in that age group at midyear but the number of live births occurring in a defined population during the year. To see why this is so, consider the temporal pattern of deaths among people during any year of adult life: say, between the 27th and the 28th birthday. Such deaths would be expected to occur randomly throughout the interval, with about one-twelfth during each month. Infant deaths, however, are not uniformly distributed over the critical year from the moment of birth until the first birthday. This leads to the second special feature of the infant mortality rate—its division into neonatal and postneonatal mortality rates, by which deaths during the first 28 days of life are compared with those during the remainder of the first year. In some jurisdictions the neonatal rate is further subdivided into first day deaths, early neonatal deaths (from birth to seven days of age), and late neonatal deaths (from the eighth through the 28th day).

A great deal of attention has been given in recent years to *perinatal* deaths. The perinatal period commences at 22 completed weeks (154 days) of gestation, when the weight is normally 500 grams, and ends at seven completed days after birth. Several conferences have dealt with this issue, whose significance is shown by the observation that the number of lives lost in the perinatal period exceeds that for the succeeding 30 years of life. The perinatal period is unique because the great majority of deaths occur through some unfavorable influence of the mother upon the fetus. Pathological processes in two separate people are involved, and they cannot be unraveled with conventional means of mortality reporting. A special certificate of perinatal death has therefore been adopted by the World Health Assembly to include information about diseases and conditions in both fetus (or infant) and mother.

Maternal mortality

A *maternal death* is defined in the ICD-10 (see below) as "the death of a woman while pregnant or within 42 days of termination of pregnancy, irrespective of the duration and the site of the pregnancy, from any cause related to or aggravated by the pregnancy or its management but not from accidental or incidental causes."

A *late maternal death* is the death of a woman from direct or indirect obstetric causes more than 42 days but less than one year after termination of pregnancy.

Maternal deaths should be subdivided into two groups:

- *Direct obstetric deaths*: those resulting from obstetric complications of the pregnant state (pregnancy, labour and puerperium), from interventions, omissions, incorrect treatment, or from a chain of events resulting from any of the above
- *Indirect obstetric deaths*: those resulting from previous existing disease that developed during pregnancy and which was not due to direct causes, but which was aggravated by physiologic effects of pregnancy

The maternal mortality rate and maternal mortalty ratio should be distinguished. The *rate* refers to the number of deaths from maternal causes per standard number of women, typically 100,000, often of a given age range; it includes both the risk of becoming pregnant and the risk of dying once pregnant. The *ratio* refers to the number of deaths from maternal causes per 1000 live births and thus measures the obstetric risk per pregnancy.

International Comparability

The need for international comparability of cause-of-death data was a prime subject of discussion at the earliest International Statistical Congresses, the first held in Brussels in 1853 and the second in Paris two years later. At the 1855 congress, William Farr of England and Marc d'Espine of Switzerland proposed tabulations that were later merged into a single list of 139 causes applicable to all countries.

That list, officially adopted by the congress, has formed the basis for subsequent classifications. The subject continued to be of great interest and four revisions appeared within the 19th century. At the 1893 meeting of the International Statistical Institute Jacques Bertillon proposed a classification which was promoted by the American Public Health Association for use in the United States, Mexico, and Canada. In 1900 the First International Conference for the Revision of the International Classification of Causes of Death was convened in Paris, and since then revisions have appeared at approximately ten-year intervals. This work, now commonly called the *International Classification of Diseases* (ICD), was greatly modified at the sixth revision (1948), with the addition of coding rubrics for morbidity (see below) as well as for causes of death. The eighth, a major revision, was adopted in 1965 and issued in 1967. Almost as soon as it appeared, work began on the ninth revision, whose worldwide use began in 1979. The United States adapted the ninth revision as the ICD-9-CM, for "clinical modification," which differed from the WHO's ICD-9 by additional coding categories and the inclusion of a third volume with an extensive list of *procedures in medicine.*

Disease classifications and procedures lists are needed for the administration of large medical care institutions such as those sponsored by health maintenance organizations, insurance companies, and government programs such as Medicare. Direct payments or cost reimbursements to health care providers depend increasingly on the efficient classification of patients into specific diagnostic categories with their related therapeutic procedures. In the United States these have come to be known as DRGs (diagnostic related groups).

The transition from one ICD revision to another always involves changes in the coding of certain categories. At each revision, some diagnoses are reassigned, resulting in sudden increases or decreases in the reported occurrences of affected categories and breaks in the comparability of statistics. For example, secondary cancer of the thoracic organs showed a drop of 61.5% between 1967 and 1968 (ICD-8/ICD-9), after average annual increases of about 15% from 1963 to 1967. Trends in cancer mortality have been studied for almost a century and are closely watched by many people searching, for instance, for clues about environmental risk factors. Changes in cause assignment or in coding rules make long-term studies much more difficult. Nevertheless, changes in the ICD are needed from time to time. New diseases such as AIDS and advances in medical knowledge and diagnostic and therapeutic technology contribute to better ways to define and distinguish among the many known diseases and possible causes of death.

In 1979, the year in which the ICD-9 came into effect, an international meeting on classification of diseases convened to start preparation of the next revision. The group felt that the unprecedented advances in knowledge of medicine and allied fields demanded a complete review of the whole approach to disease classification, which would require more than the customary decade between revisions. The ICD-10 came into effect on January 1, 1993, fourteen years after the inauguration of the

ICD-9. The new classification has more than 2036 categories and 12,159 subcategories and 12,420 codes within its 21 chapters, shown in outline on Table 4-10. Definitions of live birth, fetal death, and maternal death are retained, and new definitions are added for "pregnancy-related death" and "late maternal death."[9]

Many countries started using the ICD-10 in 1996 or 1997, but its adoption in the United States is complicated by the fact that ICD-9-CM categories and numbers are firmly embedded in hospital billing and reporting systems. The National Center for Health Statistics is developing a corresponding modification of the ICD-10 but its use for mobidity reporting is not expected before at least 2000.

Table 4-10. Major Subdivisions of the International Classification of Diseases, Tenth Revision

Chapter	Subjects	Range of Codes
I	Certain infectious and parasitic diseases	A00–A99; B00–B99
II	Neoplasms	C00–C99; D00–D49
III	Diseases of the blood and blood-forming organs and certain disorders involving immune mechanism	D50–D99
IV	Endocrine, nutritional, and metabolic diseases	E00–E99
V	Mental disorders	F00–F99
VI	Diseases of the nervous system	G00–G99
VII	Diseases of the eye and adnexa	H00–H59
VIII	Diseases of the ear and mastoid process	H60–H99
IX	Diseases of the circulatory system	I00–I99
X	Diseases of the respiratory system	J00–J99
XI	Diseases of the digestive system	K00–K99
XII	Diseases of the skin and subcutaneous tissue	L00–L99
XIII	Diseases of the musculoskeletal system and connective tissue	M00–M99
XIV	Diseases of the genitourinary system	N00–N99
XV	Pregnancy, childbirth, and the puerperium	O00–O99
XVI	Certain conditions originating in the perinatal period	P00–P99
XVII	Congenital malformations and chromosomal abnormalities	Q00–Q99
XVIII	Symptoms, signs, and abnormal clinical and laboratory findings not elsewhere classified	R00–R99
XIX	Consequences of external causes	S00–S99; T00–T99
XX	External causes of morbidity and mortality	W00–W99; X00–X99; Y00–Y99
XXI	Factors influencing health status and contact with health services	Z00–Z99

The extensive changes in the ICD-10 have required regional and national training programs throughout the world and give governments an opportunity to review
and improve the entire flow of health statistics, reformulating data processing systems and even the design of death certificates.

Certification of Death

When a death occurs, a certificate (Fig. 4-3) should be completed by the certifier.
Medical certification of cause of death is typically the responsibility of the attending physician, when there is one. In cases of sudden, violent, or suspicious death in
developed countries a coroner or other medicoloegal officer, who may or may not
be a physician, could be the certifier. In many countries the certifier may be a midwife, nurse, policeman, village chief, teacher, or layman, whose name and creden-
tial should appear on the forms actually used. Registration is not always timely or
correct. For example, police statistics in Jamaica for the years 1988, 1989, and 1990
recorded 343, 400, and 393 deaths due to motor vehicle accidents; but certified
deaths for the same years from this cause were 23, 23, and 40, respectively.[10]

INTERNATIONAL FORM OF MEDICAL CERTIFICATE OF CAUSE OF DEATH

Cause of death		Approximate interval between onset and death
I Disease or condition directly leading to death*	(a) . . . . due to (or as a consequence of)	. . . .
Antecedent causes Morbid conditions, if any, giving rise to the above cause, stating the underlying condition last	(b) . . . . due to (or as a consequence of) (c) . . . . due to (or as a consequence of) (d)	. . . .
II Other significant conditions contributing to the death, but not related to the disease or condition causing it	. . . .	. . . .

*This does not mean the mode of dying, e.g. heart failure, respiratory failure.
It means the disease, injury, or complication that caused death.

Figure 4-3 International form of medical certificate of cause of death. *Source:* World Health
Organization (1993).

The flow of information following completion of the death certificate varies among countries, but in general a centralized national statistical office eventually receives the individual records and collates the data for administrative purposes, sending summaries to Geneva for compilation by the WHO. At one point in the system the ICD coding is applied to the data by a coder or nosologist especially trained for this purpose. In the United States this is done at the state level, elsewhere usually at the national level. In some countries multiple and/or contributory causes of death are tabulated but usually only the underlying cause of death is coded, and it is this rubric under which the data finally appear in the World Health Statistics Annual and other publications. The U.S. National Center for Health Statistics has developed a computerized program[11] for automated selection of the underlying cause of death.

The underlying cause is considered to be the disease or injury that initiated the train of events leading directly to death, or the circumstances of the accident or violence which produced the fatal injury. Many problems arise with respect to accuracy of these statements, even in developed countries where most deaths are attended or certified by a physician. Questions of definition, correctness of diagnosis, proper selection of underlying cause, etc., are clearly involved. The capability of the certifying physician and presence of technical facilities (diagnostic laboratory support, pathology reports, autopsy) vary greatly and affect the reliability of certified cause of death. As people become older and accumulate more and more chronic illnesses the specific underlying cause of their death, if there is one, becomes murky or frankly undeterminable. An elderly person may die *with* heart failure (and six other serious conditions), but that does not necessarily mean that the person died *of* heart failure. Errors can also occur in application of the rules, in coding, and in transcribing.

Problems of international comparability of mortality data include all of the above, plus variations in language, terminology, and definition of disease; and local differences in medical practice and in rules for coding causes of death. In an effort to foster uniformity of diagnosis and terminology, the WHO has published a series of books with accompanying color transparencies of microscopic tissue sections as part of their project on the international histological classification of tumors. Similar publications are issued on standardized classification of atheroslerotic lesions, hypertension, and chronic ischaemic heart disease. In developing countries in general the application of such criteria is rare, for reasons already mentioned. Moreover, deaths due to these specific causes have until now been less common outside of the industrialized countries, although their number is growing rapidly (see Epidemiologic Transition, Chapter 8).

Many studies have been carried out in different parts of the world to determine the correctness of the underlying cause of death that was written on the death certificate. The obvious way to do this is to examine the body shortly after death, but it is often not feasible to perform an autopsy for this purpose. The rare confirmatory studies that have been done have found major discrepancies between stated causes of death and those determined by careful postmortem analyses. In 1987, 1060 deaths occurred in the city of Goerlitz (population 78,484) in the former East Germany, and 1023 (96.5%) of those were subjected to a thorough autopsy.[12] For each, an underlying cause of death was assigned by the pathology team, which concluded that 47% of the diagnoses on death certificates differed from those based on autopsy. In 30% of the deaths the difference crossed a major disease category—for example, the death certificate said heart failure and the pathologists found that the real cause of death was cancer, or vice versa. As expected, the extent of disagreement was higher for those who died at a great age. Physicians tended to overstate diseases of the circulatory system and hormonal and metabolic problems on the death certificates and to underrepresent cancer, infectious diseases, and respiratory, digestive, and genitourinary diseases. Many other studies have been done to determine the accuracy of death certificates, and discrepancies on the order of 30% to 50% are common.[13] Little or no training on this subject is given in most medical schools, and coronary artery disease is often the default diagnosis written on the death certificate.

National figures for deaths by cause, especially in large countries, conceal regional and ethnic differences, which may be significant. Table 4-11 shows how causes of death differ in the northeast and south of Brazil. Compared to the northeast, the south has proportionately one-fifth as many deaths from intestinal infections and less than half the homicides, but two and a half times the deaths from ischemic heart disease. Knowing nothing else about these two regions, we may make some reasonable assumptions about their relative socioeconomic status.

In many countries deaths, particularly of young children, are poorly recorded and

Table 4-11. Ten Leading Causes of Death in Regions of Brazil, 1984

Cause	National		Northeast		South	
	%	Rank	%	Rank	%	Rank
Cancer	12.2	1	9.1	3	15.1	1
Cerebrovascular disease	10.7	2	10.5	2	11.9	3
Ischemic heart disease	10.6	3	6.2	7	15.0	2
Pulmonary heart disease	6.9	4	6.5	5	7.5	4
Perinatal	6.8	5	7.4	4	4.7	6
Pneumonia, respiratory	6.4	6	6.5	6	5.5	5
Intestinal infections	4.9	7	11.0	1	2.1	13
Motor vehicle accidents	3.5	8	2.9	10	3.6	8
Other accidents	3.3	9	3.8	8	2.6	10
Homicide	3.1	10	2.6	12	1.1	19

Source: Pan American Health Organization (1988).

cause-of-death data are unreliable. In Thailand, a team of researchers carefully recorded all births and infant deaths in a rural district of 80,000 inhabitants over one year and compared their findings with official figures. The survey recorded 1258 live births (official number, 832), 28 perinatal deaths (0), 16 neonatal deaths (2), 29 infant deaths (1), and an infant mortality rate of 23.1 per 1000 live births, compared with the officially stated rate of 16.8.[14] A similar study in Jamaica showed that 94% of live births but only 13% of infant deaths were registered. The sole driving force to register an infant death is the costly certificate needed for burial, so many parents abandoned the body without registration. The surveyed infant mortality rate for 1993 was 24, but the officially reported rate was 13.[15] A household survey in Cameroon (1991–1992) found 1569 births and 106 infant deaths, while 996 births and 4 deaths were actually registered, as the families saw no benefit in doing so.[16] Such discrepancies can be found in many poorer countries. Even in the United States certificates may underreport child deaths, at least by ethnic group. A study in California found that fewer than one-third of deaths of Native American children were reported as such while the remainder were misclassified as to ethnicity.[17]

In an attempt to determine causes of death not normally recorded—for example, of children in remote areas—some investigators have resorted to the *verbal autopsy*.[18] In this technique, relatives or others who knew the child are interviewed using a structured questionnaire. Specific signs and symptoms of the deceased person elicited from the respondents are compared with carefully constructed precoded algorithms based on well-defined diagnostic criteria. The verbal autopsy shows promise of providing fairly good information on cause-specific mortality where such data are otherwise nonexistent.

Age-Adjustment

We have seen that the age structure of different populations may be very dissimilar. The "average" African population, for instance, has more than twice the proportion of under-fifteens and roughly one-fourth as many over 65 as the "average" European population (Table 4-6). It would be inappropriate and misleading to compare crude or cause-specific mortality rates between two such groups because their overall mortality experience can be expected to differ on the basis of age structure alone. In order to increase the validity of international comparisons, the crude death rate of one population is apportioned into a set of age-specific death rates, which are then applied to the proportionate age distribution of a second population. This process provides a picture of the mortality experience that population A would have had if it had the same age structure as population B; it also describes the mortality pattern if population B had the age-specific death rates of population A. In actual practice when many populations are compared, all are adjusted against a standard population which may be real or a computer model generated for the purpose of the analysis. When a number of populations are being compared, the standard population may be a composite of all. Identical procedures may of course be used for age–adjustment of morbidity rates. Various rates may be made more comparable among populations by adjusting for features other than age, such as educational attainment or economic status. The most commonly cited age-specific mortality rate, infant mortality (age zero to one year), is discussed at greater length in Chapter 7.

MEASURING HEALTH AND ILLNESS

While all societies have traditions associated with healing and persons specialized for this function, the activities of traditional or folk healers such as bomohs and curanderos, although often very important, fall outside the realm of health data as generally constituted. Very few traditional societies have corresponding roles for persons dealing with collective or community ("public") health.

Figures that track illness in populations are in many ways more germane to the needs of health analysts than are data on deaths. According to the WHO, morbidity statistics may be used for the following purposes:

- Control of communicable diseases
- Planning for development of preventive services
- Ascertainment of relationship to social factors
- Planning for provision of adequate treatment services
- Estimation of economic importance of sickness
- Research into etiology and pathogenesis
- Research on efficacy of preventive and therapeutic measures
- National and international study of distribution of diseases and impairments

The same difficulties inherent in the collection, interpretation, and comparison of vital statistics are evident, but to a far greater degree when data on health status are being considered. While at least some of the elements underlying all vital statistics are mandated by law, no such compulsion exists for most of the information related to measures of health status. One difficulty, of course, is knowing what to document or measure—that is, how to define health and ill health. Problems of definition and assessment are far more complex in health and sickness data than in mortality statistics.

In studying the distribution of particular diseases we must first define exactly what we mean—i.e., we need a strict *case definition*. For example, a case of measles may be defined as (1) generalized rash of three or more days duration and (2) fever of 101°F (38.3°C) or more and (3) cough, coryza, or conjunctivitis.[19] This clinical case definition should distinguish measles from other similar febrile illnesses. We may want a broad case definition if we are interested in any diarrhea, and a narrow one if we want to track only diarrhea caused by rotavirus, *Shigella, Salmonella*, or enteropathogenic *E. coli*. Similarly, we may be interested in any pneumonia, or in pneumonia caused by *Haemophilus* or *Streptococcus,* certain viruses, and so forth, as discussed in Chapter 7. Often it is not easy to define a "case."

When we do have a good case definition we must apply it to each suspected individual. In each instance we must see whether the individual meets the case criteria; in other words, do *case ascertainment.* Sometimes that is a relatively simple task—for example, if we are interested in collecting data on automobile injuries or falls from coconut palms. Sometimes it is very difficult. Applying the clinical case definition of measles by means of simple observation, a thermometer, and inquiring about duration of illness, we can ascertain whether a child does or does not have measles. For some other case definitions laboratory studies are needed. Costly and often impractical in the field, these may be useful in research projects, but not for routine data collection. The level of diagnostic services depends on the purpose and design of the investigation. Accurate case definition and ascertainment, tied to appropriate statistical methods, are needed to evaluate community-based interventions such as disease control programs. Alternatively, one may wish to determine whether malnutrition in under-fives exceeds, say, 5% of the population at risk, which might be the predetermined level to trigger a provincial control program. A relatively simple and inexpensive ("quick-and-dirty") clinical survey, with some laboratory backup, may be sufficient to make a yes or no decision. Such a procedure is often termed *rapid epidemiologic assessment.*

The uniform measurement and reporting of such information is complicated by the varying definition and understanding of illness and its causes among different ethnic and cultural groups (see Chapter 6). What is considered illness in one group may not be so elsewhere. For example, infection with intestinal parasites, which might horrify a middle-class American, would be considered entirely normal in many developing countries.

Many diseases exhibit a wide spectrum of clinical severity ranging from inapparent to extreme, and the overwhelming majority of infections never come to medical attention. It is in fact likely that most infections are undetected by the person harboring them or cause only generalized and nonspecific symptoms. Serological surveys to determine the prevalence of antibodies to many viruses, for instance, do not necessarily correlate with the apparent distribution of illnesses caused by them in the same population. Moreover, people have many episodes of sickness during their lifetimes, and even in the most developed countries very few persons can document their own complete health history.

Statistics on Morbidity

There are two general categories of sources for morbidity data: the records routinely compiled and accumulated by various agencies, and special surveys made to obtain information on particular issues. Morbidity statistics are numerical representations of the recognized occurrence of ill health in a population. Ideally, this information should describe ill health by diagnosis, severity and duration, distribution in place and time, and characteristics of the persons affected, such as their age, sex, occupation, and marital status. Often reliable figures are unavailable, even from international agencies. For example, published estimates of the number of people infected with leishmaniasis[20] differ by as much as 45-fold. A figure of 12 million annual cases, based on WHO sources and "amplified by unspecified reports," has been repeated in a number of publications, while several authors have used an estimate of 1.2 million (which may have originated as a decimal error). Using the best population figures and epidemiological data available, a team of investigators systematically estimated the annual incidence of visceral leishmaniasis to be 88,500 cases and for cutaneous leishmaniasis at 295,900 cases, yielding a combined total under 400,000 cases rather than the 12 million often cited.[21]

When individuals devote great time and effort, or perhaps an entire career, to research or control of a particular disease, it is understandable that they emphasize the importance of "their" subject, perhaps to the extent of subconscious exaggeration. Distortion of reality, however innocently derived, works against the scientists and administrators who must have a clear vision of the epidemiologic situation. The significance of a vaccine differs substantially if the true annual incidence is 12 million or if it is 400,000. The enthusiasm with which effort and resources are invested in research, product development, and evaluation is based on confidence in the validity of reported figures. This is a clear example of the need to be skeptical in dealing with *any* data reporting disease prevalence, especially in developing countries.

Even if prevalence estimates are grossly mistaken, certain hazards of life in poor tropical communities may be generally expected. These ubiquitous illnesses (mainly diarrheal and respiratory) are related to malnutrition, lack of sanitation and education, and similar factors associated with poverty (see Chapter 7).

The continual reporting of disease occurrence in any country is limited to certain "reportable" or "notifiable" diseases for which it is mandatory that cases be brought to the attention of health authorities. Legislation to this effect began, in modern times, with Norway in 1860, followed by the Netherlands, Sweden, Switzerland, Italy, Great Britain, France, Uruguay, Japan, and Chile, all before 1900. The 20th century has seen essentially all other countries adopt some form of compulsory notification of certain illnesses within their borders. In most cases these laws refer to highly communicable diseases that pose an immediate threat to the community, but often specific cases of other types must be reported. Botulism, which may be caused by improperly processed canned foods, is such a disease: Prompt notification may result in recall of affected production lots and thus avert additional cases. As conditions change, additional diseases may be added to the list. Epilepsy may be a notifiable disease when a driver's license is involved, and rubella became reportable after its association with birth defects was established. AIDS is reportable everywhere in the world, but the relative social isolation of many cases, the complexity of specific diagnosis, and a tangle of other reasons combine to reduce the completeness of reporting. Occupational diseases and work-related injuries are legally notifiable in many countries, in part to gather data for control purposes, and in part for validation of workmen's compensation claims. Persons legally responsible for notification may be physicians, school authorities, directors of laboratories in which positive diagnoses are made, or even heads of families. The variety of legislation governing notifiable diseases is very great. Some countries require immediate reporting of suspected cases, some only after laboratory confirmation; in some countries certain diseases must be notified only from schools, institutions, or resorts. Special regulations may require that cases or outbreaks of specified diseases in dairy farms be notified, and others may deal with nosocomial (hospital acquired) infections. In some countries otherwise-healthy carriers, particularly of typhoid organisms, must be reported and registered. The completeness of reporting often leaves much to be desired and notification is frequently neglected by busy professionals despite the legal requirement to do so.

Notification and reporting are a part of public health surveillance, defined as "the ongoing systematic collection, analysis, and interpretation of outcome-specific data for use in the planning, implementation, and evaluation of public health practice."[22] The uses of surveillance are:

- Quantitative estimation of the magnitude of a health problem
- Portrayal of the natural history of a disease
- Detection of epidemics
- Documentation of the distribution and spread of a health event
- Facilitation of epidemiologic and laboratory research
- Testing of hypotheses
- Evaluation of control and preventive measures
- Monitoring of changes in infectious agents
- Monitoring of isolation activities
- Detection of changes in health practice
- Planning

In Europe, the Maastricht treaty requires that public health surveillance be developed at the level of the European Community. A study was carried out in 1991–1992 of the surveillance systems for sexually transmitted diseases, hepatitis B, and tuberculosis in 17 European countries.[23] The survey included current national-level data collection systems with centralized analysis and dissemination of data. As expected, these varied widely. Surveillance activities were coordinated by the Ministry of Health in eight countries and by an independent national institute in nine. Seven countries had systems in which one or more public or private institutions collaborate. The main types were:

- *Mandatory notification*, in which the disease must be reported to authorities by physicians with or without patient identification

- *Voluntary notification*, where physicians and laboratories agree to notify cases
- *Sample-based systems*, in which a selected sample of physicians, clinics, laboratories, or populations is evaluated on a regular basis

The International Health Regulations define the diseases that are officially notifiable *by* health authorities (not *to* them). These diseases, termed "subject to the regulations," are cholera (including cholera caused by the El Tor vibrio), plague, and yellow fever. Smallpox, formerly a prominent member of this group, is now officially certified to be eradicated; however, if a case should be found the WHO certainly wants to hear about it! Notification is made by means of a report to the World Health Organization in Geneva within 24 hours of official awareness of the first case of a disease subject to the regulations. Before these regulations became effective in 1971, the International Sanitary Regulations had been in effect for two decades. That agreement had required international reporting of the four diseases mentioned plus louse-borne relapsing fever and louse-borne typhus. The latter two, because of diminishing importance, have now been shifted to a new group of diseases "under surveillance," which includes in addition influenza, malaria, and poliomyelitis. Reports of notifications of all these diseases, plus related information, appear in the *Weekly Epidemiological Record* of the WHO.

Another source of "continual data" on the occurrence of disease is hospital inpatient statistics which, when complete, can provide information about the following:

- The geographical sources of patients
- The age and sex distribution of different diseases and durations of hospital stay
- The distribution of diagnoses
- The associations between and among different diseases
- The period between disease onset and hospital admission
- The distribution of patients according to different social and biological factors
- The cost of hospital care
- Changing trends in the manner of diagnosis and treatment of various illnesses

Continual collection of limited types of sickness and disability records is done also by many other institutions and organizations. Among these are:

- General clinics, health centers, hospital outpatient departments
- Special clinics (e.g., sexually transmitted disease [STD], drug addiction, maternal and child health)
- School and factory dispensaries
- Voluntary health agencies
- Visiting nurses, midwives, etc.
- Physicians and dentists in private practice
- Military services and veterans hospitals

- Workmen's compensation programs
- Census bureaus
- Police and traffic organizations for road accidents
- Health insurance and life insurance companies
- Business corporations, schools, military services, etc. (physical examination on entrance)
- Registries (special registers)

The most common disease-specific registers are the *cancer registries* or *tumor registries* found in many countries, but there are also special registers of blind and disabled, handicapped children, congenital defects, and diseases of specific local importance.

The quality and completeness of these records and the length of time that they are kept vary greatly, as does their accessibility to outsiders. In many cases the information is considered confidential or privileged. This may be true especially where individual patients are identified and where the information forms the basis of legal claims for insurance, inheritance, or compensation. Annual reports with statistical summaries may be compiled on a local, district, state, or service basis and submitted to a central agency or ministry, which may be one of health, commerce and industry, social security, defense, etc., or to a central statistical office. A high degree of coordination between these agencies is seldom achieved, even in the most economically developed countries, because the information is collected differently and for different purposes, and it is compiled at different intervals. The problems of international comparability of such data are obvious, as are the frustrations that may beset a scholar who wishes to analyze them for an overview of the health situation in a particular country.

There is a growing trend in some European countries to increased privacy protection laws that some authorities feel will make much epidemiologic work impossible. Personal data of all kinds, particularly those concerned with diagnoses of mental and emotional illnesses, may be specifically sealed against such uses. The Norwegian government has decreed the destruction of past mental health registry records, sparking a conflict between patient privacy issues and epidemiologic information needs.[24]

Special surveys are undertaken to estimate the scope of illness in a particular population at a particular time, but general morbidity surveys of large populations are notably few in number. The Global Burden of Disease Project, which will be described later, has collected data about the total amount of disability throughout the world.[25] They have concluded that on average the amount of life span lived with disabilities is 8% in the wealthier countries, while in sub-Saharan Africa it is 15% of a much shorter life span.

In the United States, the National Health Survey Act of 1956 provided for the establishment and continuation of a long-term national health survey. Responsibility for development and conduct of the program is placed with the National Center for Health Statistics, a division of the Department of Health and Human Services. The studies conducted are extensive and complex, based in part on sampling methods and including interview surveys, examination surveys, and data on health facilities and institutions. Findings of these surveys are published in hundreds of reports in many different series under the general heading of *Public Health Service Publication 1000*. Some other countries, such as Finland and Canada, have also undertaken large-scale sickness surveys.

Far more common in recent years have been surveys designed to determine the prevalence of particular diseases. To date, population-based surveys depend on relatively simple, harmless, and inexpensive diagnostic tests applicable to populations. Parasitologic surveys for ascariasis or hookworm disease, for example, use the method of stool examination for the characteristic worm ova, and schistosomiasis prevalence studies are based on stool or urine examinations. Population surveys for malaria and filariasis still utilize microscopic examination of blood films, although more precise, efficient, (and costly) methods have been suggested by laboratory investigators. Some of the methods of biotechnology, such as DNA hybridization or monoclonal antibody methods, may find future application in large-scale screening for diagnostic purposes provided that costs can be greatly reduced. Trachoma, sexually transmitted diseases including AIDS, childhood diarrhea, and nutritional deficiencies are examples of other specific health problems for which large population-based survey methods are commonly employed. In many cases only defined subgroups of populations are included in specific disease surveys, as with schoolchildren or persons exposed to particular occupational hazards. The distinction is not always made clear between prevalence surveys, which demonstrate the existence of disease or infection (with or without symptoms), and screening programs, which have been undertaken in several countries for conditions such as diabetes, glaucoma, and sickle-cell trait. As surveys become more restricted in scope and size, their sponsoring organizations become more varied, health authorities have less control over content and methodology, and results become less comparable on an international basis. Medical schools, community agencies, specific disease-oriented voluntary associations, international aid organizations, missionary and other charitable groups, pharmaceutical companies planning drug trials or product marketing, government research institutes, and others may all be engaged in surveys of one kind or another within a population, often without coordination. Results may appear in official reports, journal articles, or privately circulated documents.

The Impact of Illness and the Burden of Disease

In addition to counts of disease occurrence many people have looked for ways to describe the significance of ill health for individuals, communities, and nations. Health status indicators for individuals range from simple yes/no for specific conditions (cancer, blindness) to measures that entail some assessment of "quality of life." These include the *Physical Quality of Life Index* (PQLI), Healthy Years Equivalent (HYE), Quality Adjusted Life Year (QALY), and similar measures.[26] The World Health Organization has developed a measure (WHOQOL) which produces a profile of scores from 24 facets of QOL across six broad domains.[27]

Commonly used estimates of the impact of these diseases are the years of potential life lost (YPLL) owing to each cause,[28] or, conversely, quality-adjusted years of life gained (QALY) from various interventions. Causes of death that typically strike young people, such as malaria and diarrheal or respiratory diseases will naturally be weighted far differently from the chronic diseases characteristic of the elderly. For this metric the age at death must be known, which is fairly straightforward, and also the expected age at which that person would otherwise have died, which is not so simple. Such calculations give more weight to deaths occurring at younger ages, as a person who dies in infancy or early childhood clearly loses almost all of his or her life expectancy, while an elderly person who dies loses a few years or, if old enough, none at all. Collected together the potential life lost in a population can be a powerful incentive for policy changes by governments.

The PLL technique was used in 1981 by the Ghana Health Assessment Team to demonstrate the impact of different diseases in that country (Table 4-12). The concept of healthy days of life lost was refined by Howard Barnum of the World Bank, who observed that the simple tallying of healthy days of life lost "implies comparability across age groups"; i.e., considers all years to be of equal value without considering adult productivity. Barnum took the accumulated days lost from the Ghana study and applied weightings to better indicate the actual impact of diseases. He referred to an age-productivity profile in which "the timing of health effects over the life span has implications for the economic contribution of the individual as productive days are lost from acute illness, disability and premature death."

Barnum also introduced the idea of *discounting* to the data, as it is generally agreed that a day of healthy life in the present has a greater instrinsic value to an individual than a day in the future.[29] Thus, "the time stream of healthy days of life lost to disease can be reduced to an equivalent present value through the use of a discount rate. The advantage of deriving the equivalent present value is that it allows a common comparison among diseases and thus among projects that target different diseases."[30]

By discounting at different rates (percent per year) the present value of productive life days lost to particular causes changes dramatically. For example, in the *unweighted* Ghana data malaria ranked first and cardiovascular diseases ranked 22nd in days lost. When both productivity weightings and discounting at an extreme 20% rate were applied, malaria ranked 14th and cardiovascular diseases were first in "present value of productive days of life lost income." Discounting is a complex tool of economists, little understood by most health workers, and one that stimulates great controversy.

Table 4-12. Days of Healthy Life Lost per Thousand Persons per Year for Selected Diseases, Ghana, 1970s[a]

Disease	Average Age at		Incidence[b]	Case-Fatality Ratio, %[c]	Days of Healthy Life Lost
	Onset	Death			
Malaria	1	1	40.0	2.3	32,567
Measles	2	2	9.0	3.0	23,358
Pneumonia, child	2	2	3.4	40.0	18,557
Sickle cell anemia	0	5	1.25	80.0	17,502
Accidents	15	15	7.7	10.0	14,909
Diarrhea	2	2	70.0	1.0	14,470
Tuberculosis	20	25	2.0	35.0	11,005
Cerebrovascular disease	50	50	2.3	35.0	10,477
Tetanus, neonatal	0	0	0.5	80.0	6852
Hypertension	40	50	0.75	75.0	5071
Typhoid	20	20	4.0	7.3	4755
Meningitis	10	10	1.25	20.0	4650
Pertussis	1	1	21.0	1.0	4643
Polio	3	3	0.22	5.0	1227
Cholera	15	15	0.05	7.6	65
Diphtheria	3	3	0.01	7.0	14

[a]See source for methods.

[b]Per thousand persons per year.

[c]Percent of cases who die from this disease.

Source: Adapted from Ghana Health Assessment Team (1981).

The concept of potential life lost has its critics. It is not self-evident just what the numbers mean. In the example in Table 4-13, judicious selection of expected age at death will give accidents, cancer, or heart disease the greatest "impact" in the U.S. population. Such figures can be used as arguments by specific disease advocates. Note that diabetes, the eighth leading cause of death in actual count, does not appear on any of the YPLL "top ten" lists.

In 1993 the World Bank's World Development Report (WDR93), *Investing in Health*, proposed a new composite measure called the *disability-adjusted life year* or *DALY* (rhymes with tally) as a generic indicator usable everywhere to help set health policy priorities, to facilitate comparisons between countries, and to standardize the way that decisions are made in the health sector. The DALY, defined as "the present value of the future years of disability-free life that are lost as the result of the premature deaths or cases of disability occurring in a particular year," combines four elements: levels of mortality by age, levels of morbidity by age, the value of a healthy year of life at specific ages, and a discount rate of 3%.[31]

Table 4-13. Ranking the First Ten Causes of Death by Potential Life Lost, to Selected Ages, United States, 1986[a]

Rank	Number of Deaths	Years of Potential Life Lost to Age		
		65	75	85
1	Heart	Accidents	Cancer	Heart
2	Cancer	Cancer	Heart	Cancer
3	CVD	Heart	Accidents	Accidents
4	Accidents	Sui/Hom	Sui/Hom	Sui/Hom
5	COPD	Perinatal	Perinatal	Perinatal
6	Infectious	Anomalies	Anomalies	CVD
7	Sui/Hom	SIDS	CVD	COPD
8	Diabetes	CVD	Liver	Anomalies
9	Liver	Liver	COPD	Liver
10	Perinatal	Infectious	SIDS	Infectious

[a]Anomalies = congenital anomalies; COPD = chronic obstructive pulmonary disease; CVD = cerebrovascular disease; Infectious = infectious and parasitic; Perinatal = certain causes around the time of birth; SIDS = sudden infant death syndrome; Sui/Hom = suicide, homicide, and legal intervention.

Source: Modified after Gardner and Sanborn (1990).

DALYs are applied to estimate the separate health impacts of communicable diseases, noncommunicable diseases, and injuries. The underlying assumption is that priority should go to those health problems that cause a large disease burden *and* for which generally accepted cost-effective interventions are available. Antecedents of the DALY are seen in the 1981 Ghana Health Team study and in Barnum's 1987 modification mentioned previously. The identification of priority health problems is reminiscent of the highly controversial recommendation for *selective primary health care* made 14 years earlier,[32] which is described in Chapter 7.

The accumulated DALYs are used as a sort of inverse indicator to summarize the health status of populations in each World Bank–defined region of the world and to represent the "global burden of disease," as shown in Table 4-14. Considering only data for 1990, sub-Saharan Africa was found to have the highest disease burden, 575 DALYs per 1000 population, of which 71% arise from communicable diseases; and the established market economies have the lowest, 117 DALYs per 1000 people, 78% of which arise from noncommunicable diseases. As it is intended to assist in setting health service priorities, to identify disadvantaged groups, to target health interventions, and to provide standardized measure for evaluation and planning, the DALY shows how health measures interact with economic concepts in formulating modern health policy. The principal suggestion of the WDR93 is to define a package of essential health services, which should never include a less cost-effective intervention if a more cost-effective one is not financed.

Table 4-14. Calculating DALYs and the Global Burden of Disease

1. Classify all diseases and conditions into 107 categories in 3 groups[a] and assign into 7 disability classes weighted from 0 (perfect health) to 1 (death)[b]

2. Assign all deaths to a category by age, sex, and region

3. Calculate years of life lost per death

4. Estimate all cases of disability by age, sex, region, severity (disability class), and duration (years of healthy life lost) until remission or death

5. Combine all deaths and disability losses by cause, age, sex, and region

6. Allow a discount rate of 3% so future years of healthy life are valued at progressively lower levels

7. Weight years of life lost at different ages at different relative values—less for children and aged, more for adults (the maximum value at age 25)

8. Sum all DALYs to obtain the Global Burden of Disease (GBD)

[a]Group1: communicable diseases; maternal, perinatal, and nutritional disorders. Group 2, noncommunicable diseases. Group 3, intentional and unintentional injuries.

[b]For specific severity weights and descriptions of each disabiity class see Murray and Lopez (1997b), p. 1348.

Source: Adapted from World Bank (1993).

Soon after the appearance of the WDR93, DALYs predictably came under fire from various critics on both technical and political/social grounds. The main lines of criticism[33] are:

- The DALY imposes social preferences that have not been validated. The discount rate, age weights, and disability score were selected by a small group of researchers and international professionals. They are arbitrary and do not necessarily reflect the thinking of those affected by the analysis.
- The age weights do not reflect common preferences among health specialists, economists, and the general population.The DALY values a year at age 50 at about 25% of a year at age 25; but the first year of life is valued the same as at age 25. Most scales value an adult life-year at four to seven times as much as a newborn.
- Fetal deaths are not included.
- DALYs overestimate the years of life lost in high mortality countries. Basing calculations on a life expectancy of 80 is clearly unrealistic in countries with a life expectancy of 60.
- DALYs are insensitive to the density of life-years lost. The value of 30 years lost by one individual's premature death is equated to one year lost by each of 30 individuals.
- The disability weights do not account for the different handicaps attached to some permanent disabilities in different societies. Societies differ in the degree to which they stigmatize individuals and view impairments such as psychosis, AIDS, and infertility.
- The disability due to cognitive development is not fully captured.

Despite these charges the DALY and corresponding Global Burden of Disease indicators are achieving ever more widespread application. Only repeated usage over time will determine the true utility of DALYs or any other health indicator.

As we have seen in Table 4-12, ranking the causes of death by simply counting events does not necessarily produce the same order as ranking causes of death by social value, however defined. The DALY is considered by its designers to be standardized and comparable from region to region, and it includes both years of life lost and years of life lived with disabilities. The number of DALYs by cause have been calculated for the World Bank regions and pooled to achieve global totals. The comparative rankings of major causes by numbers of deaths and number of DALYs is shown on Table 4-15.

Table 4-15 Thirty Leading Causes of Death and of DALYs, World, 1990

Rank		Cause	Number of	
Deaths	DALYs		Deaths (in thousands)	DALYs (in millions)
		All causes	50,467	
	1	Lower respiratory infections		112.9
1	5	Ischemic heart disease	6260	46.7
2	6	Cerebrovascular disease (stroke)	4381	38.5
3		Lower respiratory infections	4299	
4	2	Diarrheal diseases	2946	99.6
5	3	Perinatal disorders	2443	92.1
6	12	Chronic obstructive pulmonary disease	2211	29.1
7	7	Tuberculosis (non-HIV positive)	1960	38.4
8	8	Measles	1058	36.5
9	9	Road traffic accidents	999	34.3
10		Cancer of lung, trachea and bronchus	945	
11	11	Malaria	856	31.7
12	17	Self-inflicted injuries	786	19.0
13	25	Cirrhosis of the liver	779	13.2
14		Cancer of the stomach	752	
15	10	Congenital anomalies	589	32.9
16	29	Diabetes mellitus	571	11.1
17	19	Violence	563	17.5
18	18	Tetanus	542	17.5
19		Nephritis and nephrosis	536	
20	21	Drowning	504	15.7
21	16	War injuries	502	20.0
22		Cancer of the liver	501	

(continued)

Table 4-15 Thirty Leading Causes of Death and of DALYs, World, 1990 (*continued*)

Rank			Number of	
Deaths	DALYs	Cause	Deaths (in thousands)	DALYs (in millions)
23		Inflammatory heart disease	495	
24		Cancer of the colon and rectum	472	
25	15	Protein-energy malnutrition	372	21.0
26		Cancer of the esophagus	358	
27	23	Pertussis	347	13.4
28		Rheumatic heart disease	340	
29		Cancer of the breast	322	
30	28	HIV	312	11.2
	4	Unipolar major depression		50.8
	13	Falls		26.7
	14	Iron deficiency anemia		24.6
	20	Alcohol use (directly coded consequences)		16.7
	22	Bipolar disorder		14.3
	24	Osteoarthritis		13.3
	26	Schizophrenia		12.8
	27	Burns		11.9
	30	Asthma		10.8

Source: Adapted from Murray and Lopez (1997a), Table 3 and (1997c) Table 3.

NOTES

1. Goldsmith (1972).
2. Health Maintenance Organizations. See Chapter 12.
3. The works of Goyer and Domschke (1983) and Domschke and Goyer (1986) are indispensable references on national population censuses around the world.
4. Hookham (1972).
5. Domschke and Goyer (1986).
6. The aging of populations is discussed in Chapter 8.
7. Carol Bellamy, Executive Director of UNICEF. From an interview in the *New York Times*, July 8, 1998.
8. Murray and Lopez (1997a).
9. These categories are intended to improve the quality of maternal mortality data in order to understand women's health and reproductive health in general.
10. McCaw-Binns et al. (1996), citing official demographic statistics.
11. Automated Classification of Medical Entities, or ACME.
12. Modelmog *et al.* (1994).
13. See for example Nielsen *et al.* (1991); Lee (1994).
14. Lumbignanon *et al.* (1990).
15. McCaw-Binns *et al.* (1996).

16. Ndong *et al.* (1994).

17. Epstein *et al.* (1997).

18. Quigley *et al.* (1996) interviewed the relatives of 295 children who died in Kenya.

19. Orenstein *et al.* (1984).

20. Leishmaniasis is the name for several forms of an insect-transmitted parasitic disease that occurs many parts of the world. The cutaneous form produces skin lesions; a visceral form often called *kala azar* is a highly lethal infection that sometimes occurs in large epidemics—for example, in India and Sudan. A mucocutaneous form that affects the membranes of the mouth and nose is found mainly in South America. Leishmaniasis is one of the disease groups targeted by WHO's Special Programme for Research and Training in Tropical Diseases.

21. Ashford *et al.* (1992).

22. Teutsch and Thacker (1995).

23. Desenclos *et al.* (1993). The survey covered the 12 countries of the EC plus five COST (Cooperating in Science and Technology) countries: Austria, Finland, Norway, Sweden, and Switzerland.

24. Helgason (1992).

25. For definitions and discussion of the disability-free life expectancy (DFLE) and disability-adjusted life expectancy (DALE) see Murray and Lopez (1997b).

26. The literature on quality of life indicators is extensive. See for example Mootz (1986), Johannesson (1994), and Fitzpatrick (1996).

27. The domains are physical, psychological, level of independence, social relationships, environment, and spirituality/religion/personal beliefs. The WHOQOL has been field tested in Australia, Croatia, France, India, Israel, Japan, the Netherlands, Panama, Russia, Spain, Thailand, U.K., U.S.A., and Zimbabwe (WHOQOL Group, 1995).

28. Sometimes PLL is taken as *productive life lost* and limited to the working lifetime, usually ages 15 to 65; there are other variations to the PLL theme. See also Gardner and Sanborn (1990).

29. A Maori adage says that "Today's meal is better than tomorrow's feast."

30. Barnum (1987).

31. "DALYS from a specific condition are the sum of years of life lost because of premature mortality and years of life lived with disability, adjusted for the severity of the disability. Time lived with various short-, medium-, and long-term disabilities is weighted by a severity weight that is based on the measurement of social preferences for time lived in various states of health." Murray and Lopez (1996)—see for details about the calculations.

32. Walsh and Warren (1979).

33. From José Luis Bobadilla, personal communication. Doctor Bobadilla, of Mexico, was a principal architect of the WDR93 and of health sector studies at the World Bank and, later, at the Inter-American Development Bank (IDB). Tragically, he was killed in the crash of a commercial airliner in Peru while on duty travel for the Inter-American Development Bank.

5

From Data to Information to Decisions

The functioning of health services is often a more prominent issue in the minds of administrators, legislators, and the public than is the status of health itself. The availability and accessibility of physicians or hospital beds and the cost of medical care seem everywhere to be subjects of vigorous discussion, while the presence of disease may be tacitly considered inevitable. Here we will look at information not about births, illness, and deaths as in the previous chapter, but about the functioning of health services.[1]

the avowed goal of health systems research is the improvement of health of the target population. In this context, the health system comes all too easily to be seen as a system designed to produce health, rather than the real-life system which it is, a system of complex social institutions and relationships, within which individuals and groups have complex agendas and goals which change over time. The community wants health, and the patient wants care and cure. The patient may also need a means of validating his or her absence from work, and may need a means of claiming sickness benefit; he or she may rate this rather higher than cure at times. To some the health service is a means of providing medical care; others see it more broadly as a channel for social redistribution of resources; while others again see it as a market. The importance of the health service may lie in the service it offers the politically powerful; it may lie in the jobs it provides; it may lie in the role it plays in reducing political dissent. What becomes clear is that analysis of this system in any useful way cannot take only the "health-producing" factors out of context. It must take a broader historical and socioeconomic analysis of a system with complex roots both in the national society and culture and in the international environment.[2]

STATISTICS ON HEALTH SERVICES

The preceding chapter described some kinds of data about the health of individuals and populations. What then do we do with such data? Numbers for numbers' sake are not worth much, and their rote collection is a waste of time and resources.

the flow of information starts with data, a set of discrete observations or facts on cases, deaths, and people. When processed and analyzed by epidemiologists or statisticians, these data are converted to percentages (or proportions), incidence or mortality rates, prevalence or risk ratios, or indices, such as potential years of life lost . . . Nothing more happens, however, unless an administrator or program manager learns of the information and absorbs it as new knowledge. Action only follows if the administrator has the will and political power to act.[3]

In the past, health services generally have been characterized by insufficient planning, uncoordinated operation of their different elements, and *ad hoc* responses to novel situations. Today, most countries view information about the internal working of their own health services as an indispensable part of health statistics. With the increasing trend toward integrated, comprehensive programs, planners must have access to data about

- The characteristics of health establishments and their facilities and personnel
- Acquisition and use of commodities, supplies, and equipment
- The services provided and their utilization by the community
- The costs involved and flow of resources through the system

Nevertheless, while mortality statistics are in many places approaching a high standard and information on morbidity is improving, few countries have sufficient data to describe their health services completely. Thirty years ago a WHO working group reported that "the principal impediment to the reduction of ill-health at the present time is not the lack of medical knowledge about diseases but the problem of applying this knowledge, i.e., bringing it to bear upon the population's health needs in the most effective manner possible within the restraints imposed by economic, political, and other considerations."[4]

A generation later the application of knowledge is still a major bottleneck for health services. The WHO has taken a lead in developing health information systems by assembling a series of practical methodologies for countries to use to improve the generation, analysis, and use of health data for program and service management.

The main reasons for requiring health service statistics are:

- To support the administration, management, and coordination of local, regional, and national health services
- To create short-term and long-term plans

- To assess whether health services are accomplishing their objective (their effectiveness) and whether they are doing so in the best possible way (their efficiency)
- To provide data required by government departments and legislatures, international agencies, health service researchers, and members of the public

In view of these functions, a question arises about the degree of accuracy and completeness of information needed for effective and efficient operation of health services. Data gathering for planning and evaluation is vulnerable to criticism as an "administrative" rather than a "substantive" function of a health service, and funds for statistical purposes are likely to be kept to a minimum. This is acceptable, because *all* expenditures should be kept to a minimum, provided they are effectively and efficiently used. The amount of information needed to make policy decisions about services for health care depends on various factors, but at some point the kind and quality of data available—and the political pressures at work—will determine the practical outcome. The collecting and processing of excess information is wasteful in money and staff time. What is needed is a strategy for arriving at sound conclusions based on data that are neither too sketchy nor too costly—in other words, a way of applying techniques of decision analysis to the planning of health services. Methods for rational selection of best alternatives in the face of insufficient information have been developed by statisticians, economists, and business analysts and should be applied to a variety of public policy areas, including health. Sampling and survey methods may be used for continuous monitoring of activities (quality control); to evaluate staff effort, effectiveness, and achievement; to keep track of costs and commodities; and to determine when programs should be terminated. It is usually easier to launch a new project than to stop an old one that no longer serves the purpose for which it was designed.

Our discussion assumes that decisions are made on the basis of objective analysis rather than expediency. Acquaintance with the daily newspaper should quickly dispel the notion that health services or any other significant human enterprises are designed, operated, and utilized on entirely rational grounds. Political considerations, pride, bias, and activities of special interest groups often influence the allocation of money and effort. In practice, health services are always skewed in their economic, geographic, and programmatic distributions. Their accessibility to various groups in the population is always unequal and the problems addressed do not necessarily correspond to actual or perceived needs.

The comparison of data on health services in different countries is generally more difficult than similar studies of population, mortality, and morbidity statistics. Whereas human physiology and pathogens are essentially the same everywhere, the organizational patterns of governments and societies are very diverse. In countries where most aspects of life are regulated by a pervasive central authority, health facilities and personnel can be identified with relative clarity. Elsewhere, a variety of components forms a mosaic of official and "nonformal" health services characteristic for each area and time.

Health Establishments

Government-operated facilities range from university-based medical centers through
municipal hospitals and social security clinics to district health subcenters staffed
by auxiliary personnel on a part-time basis. Semi-official providers of health services in many developing countries include government-sanctioned missionary or
voluntary hospitals and clinics financed mainly from abroad. Industrial establishments, plantations, and estates may have their own clinics and infirmaries. Separate
nonprofit, member-financed facilities may be operated by trade unions or other
groups. The private practice of medicine may take the form of individual physicians' offices or "surgeries," joint or group practices, prepaid health programs, clinics, or large proprietary hospitals. Ancillary services such as diagnostic laboratories
may be incorporated into larger establishments or may be independent units. In many
countries individual practitioners work for the government part-time in a clinical,
teaching, or administrative capacity and also maintain their private practice for patients who pay as individuals. Pharmacists, midwives, medical assistants, dressers,
and other paramedical personnel may be the only dispensers of advice and service,
particularly in rural areas. The permutations are almost infinite, and the problem of
coding or categorizing the forms of licensed provision of health services for purposes of international comparison is truly herculean.

More difficult still is accounting for the activities of traditional healers, native
practitioners, herbalists, and the other types of nonspecific health specialists found
in all countries. The large aggregate amount of "informal" health care given in the
home by family, neighbors, and friends must also be considered. To many, perhaps
most people in the world, folk healers and family members provide the only form
of medical care experienced throughout their lives.

Health Activities

Health Services statistics deal not only with resources (facilities, personnel, financing) but also with their activities and utilization. There are few standard methods
for defining, specifying, and registering these events. The ICD-9-CM used in the
United States since 1979 included a third volume for coding of a large variety of
medical procedures. These are clearly of use to government agencies, insurance
companies, health maintenance organizations, large hospitals, and the like who need
to keep track of the numbers and costs of all categories of medical procedures, from
taking a chest X-ray to performing a quintuple coronary artery bypass operation.
Where social security or other health insurance schemes have established predetermined payment or compensation rates for certain procedures, these are categorized

and coded locally for data processing purposes. However, with the exception of some surgical operations, there has been little in the way of international standardization of preventive and curative activities. The WHO in 1978 issued for trial purposes a two-volume manual of procedures whose value has varied from one country to another. It has been decided not to issue such a coded list as part of ICD-10, primarily because revisions will be needed so frequently as medical technology advances.

International standardization of procedures is very complex. Immunizations by conventional methods using fixed doses of a standard vaccine of uniform potency may come close to the ideal of a universally comparable procedure, but what is to be said of a "physical examination"? How are users and nonusers of services to be identified and characterized, and how are outcomes of treatment to be assessed? In some way each country must face questions of these kinds if it wants to evaluate the effectiveness of its health services. When efficiency (i.e., value for investment) is considered, these questions become even more pressing.

Certain large-scale programs, international in origin and scope, have included standardization of methodologies, activities, and outcomes, and their recording. A good example is the worldwide malaria eradication program, now defunct (Chapter 14), in which field, laboratory, and clinical work as well as assessment procedures were carefully spelled out in universal protocols. Other WHO programs such as for diarrheal disease control and immunization also strive for international comparability of procedures and record keeping. Programs of this type, however, represent only a small part of the activities of health services, and in some countries, they are organized and administered separately from the other activities of the health departments or other ministries or agencies.

Reliability of Data

In most countries immunizations are given at government facilities. The procedures are discrete and clearly defined, limited in number, and should be relatively simple to track. Childhood immunization programs have been given high priority by the WHO, UNICEF, donor agencies, and governments, to whom high acceptance rates are a matter of pride. Inevitably there is some pressure to perform well, and "considerable caution is required in interpreting and making decisions on the basis of published immunization coverage estimates."[5] Table 5-1 shows such an example, which is consistent with similar comparisons from other countries.

Recalling the previous chapter, it may seem that community-based surveys are more reliable than government statistics, but that is not necessarily so. Maternal recall is often faulty, ages are confused, and, as with government officials, there may be a tendency to overstate good deeds that respondents believe interviewers would like to hear. Immunizations are not the only procedures in this category. Self-

Table 5-1. Percentage of Infants Immunized, as Reported by Ministry of Health (MOH) and by ENSMI Survey, Guatemala, 1984 to 1987[a]

Immunization	1984		1985		1986		1987	
	MOH	ENSMI	MOH	ENSMI	MOH	ENSMI	MOH	ENSMI
Measles	24.0	13.1	23.0	14.3	46.0	30.9	33.5	22.4
DPT 1	70.0	22.2	42.0	26.4	68.0	58.7	—	60.8
DPT 2	48.0	16.9	21.0	19.6	53.0	49.2	—	31.2
DPT 3	4.0	11.9	9.0	11.0	33.0	30.2	16.6	13.4
Polio 1	68.0	19.3	44.0	20.5	89.0	61.7	—	64.1
Polio 2	47.0	15.4	21.0	16.7	57.0	52.1	—	32.9
Polio 3	4.0	11.0	9.0	9.7	33.0	31.1	18.6	14.4

[a]ENSMI = Encuesta Nacional de Salud Materno Infantil (National Maternal Infant Health Survey); DPT 1, 2, 3 = first, second, and third diphtheria, pertussis, tetanus immunization; Polio 1, 2, 3 = first, second, and third polio immunization.

Source: Adapted from Goldman and Pebley (1994) Table 8. Social Science and Medicine, vol. 43. Copyright 1996. With permission from Elsevier Science.

reported adherence to "correct" behaviors, such as having Pap smears, is commonly exaggerated.[6]

HEALTH/MANAGEMENT INFORMATION SYSTEMS

Health authorities are, of course, well aware of the deficiencies of their national health information systems. As long ago as 1982 a carefully thought out national system was proposed for Zimbabwe, a country in which

> At the present time there is no specific technical body responsible for carrying out day-to-day work such as a continuous assessment of health needs, projections of expected demands, country health planning, short term and long-term programming. The Ministry of Health does not have a documentation unit (data bank). There is no centralised flow of health information nor are there standardised procedures or forms for reporting from the different facilities. In other words, a unified national health information system does not exist. Vital statistics (births and deaths) are part of the Ministry of Home Affairs; however, the information is processed by the Central Statistics Office which is part of the Ministry of Economic Planning and Development. The Ministry of Health does not control the diagnostic quality of these medical certificates nor does it influence the programming for the computer according to its needs for health information. Very little, if any, data are received from hospitals. The annual reports of the Provincial Medical Officers vary in content, are uneven in quality, but are the primary sources of information for the Ministry of Health's Annual Report. There is only incidental contact and little communication between the provincial medical officers and the district medical officers.[7]

A few years later a health records committee of the Ministry of Health of Zambia characterized the situation there:

1. There are too many forms—over 240 different ones are now in use.
2. Many forms are too complicated and result in incorrect reporting.
3. There is frequently a lapse of 4–5 years between data collection at the centre and the compilation and publication of the results.
4. Data summaries which would be useful to local health centre staff are not sent to district or local rural health centres.
5. Present recording methods on monthly report forms from rural health centres do not provide the epidemiologist with sufficient data.
6. There is a shortage of stationery and forms.
7. There is a lack of transport for the distribution of forms.
8. Completed forms are often lost or delayed in the mail.
9. There is a shortage of personnel to compile statistics at MOH headquarters, and few qualified individuals are available to train district staff in data collection and interpretation.
10. There is a lack of communication between potential data users and those collecting the data, particularly at the local level.[8]

Clearly a need existed, at least in those countries at those times, for a comprehensive information system for the health services. In the intervening years, much progress has been made on the design of such systems, but much remains to be done. In 1993 the director of the health department of the capital city of a large developing country told me that he learned of local disease outbreaks only when he read about them in the newspaper.

In an increasingly integrated health care environment the demand for health information is much broader than the reporting of clinical encounters and the movement of such data up the bureaucratic ladder. Modern health information systems (HIS) are often integrated with management information systems developed for businesses (MIS) to form H/MIS, which combine data on the status of health with information about the internal operation of the health care sector.

The WHO has identified five subsystems which can usually be found in Health and Management Information systems:[9]

- *Epidemiological Surveillance*—for detecting, reporting, and reacting to cases of notifiable infectious and communicable diseases. Sometimes these systems include non-communicable diseases and important health events and conditions (such as maternal deaths and malnourished children) and important health services such as immunization. There may be special surveys to provide figures on illness and disability by age, sex, and severity, and on mortality, by age, sex, and cause.

- *Routine Service Reporting*—all the routine service record keeping and report submission from public and nongovernment sources of care. In national service systems this would include record keeping and reporting from community health workers and posts, health centers, dispensaries, community and district hospitals, referral hospitals, and special hospitals and care services. Data may be reported by type of service, number of service units, site, and patient characteristics. In addition to routine weekly, monthly, and annual service reports there may be special reports on the use of drugs, supplies, and other resources.
- *Program Information*—All countries have special public health programs for which reports are submitted. Examples include: tuberculosis, leprosy, malaria, or other vector-borne disease control; Expanded Programme of Immunization; AIDS prevention and control; and family planning. The reporting may come through separate channels or be integrated within the routine service reporting systems, for the use of the special program managers and other officials at various levels.
- *Administrative Systems Information*—All public health services incorporate administrative systems which generate and communicate enormous amounts of data and information. The needs for operating the service include budget and financial management, inventories, accounts receivable and payable; human resources management; training; tracking and managing supplies and equipment, vehicles, and fixed facilities; research management; documentation, correspondence, and publications; management of external resources; licensing of professionals and facilities; and the administration and enforcement of various regulations. These systems each have their own record keeping, reporting, and flow of information, which may consume considerable staff time.
- *Vital or Civil Registration*—recording and reporting births, deaths, marriage, divorce, and migration may or may not be the responsibility of the health sector. However, in all countries there is usually a responsibility for health staff to support the civil registration system, such as in the registration of births and deaths. In addition, the health sector is a major user of the data produced by such systems and by the census, to provide demographic denominator information.

These information systems are, in turn, linked to databases and knowledge sources within and outside the health sector. In recent years these links have expanded to become global in scope accessible to anyone with an internet connection. Ideally, the H/MIS is a framework for the flow of information for enlightened decision-making. It is really a process, not a product, and should be exploited as much as possible.

A key resource for epidemiologic analysis is a series of microcomputer programs known as *Epi Infor,* which, together with *Epi Map* and related programs, constitutes an integrated software suite that includes word processing, data management modules suitable for health information systems. Epi Info allows the creation of a database from a questionnaire and statistical analysis and graphing capabilities. These programs were first released in 1985 under the name Epidemiology Analysis System and have been revised several times since, becoming a standard tool of field epidemiologists and public health professionals. Epi Info 2000 is a windows version designed for maximum compatibility with industry standards including databases such as Microsoft ACCESS, World Wide Web browsers, and hypertext markup language (HTML). These noncommercial programs were developed by a branch of the US Centers for Disease Control and Prevention (CDC), are all in the public domain, and may be obtained at nominal cost or downloaded from the Epi Info website, *http://www.cdc.gov/epo/epi/epiinfo.htm* without charge. A "discussion group" has been formed for exchange of information by users and several worldwide links have been established in various languages, all accessible from the website.

The Knowledge Revolution

The knowledge revolution is no less significant than the industrial revolution that preceded it. A vice-president of the World Bank has said that "Knowledge and information are destined to constitute a more important production factor than labor, raw materials, or capital."[10] The appetite for information is just as strong in the health sector as in all other aspects of human activity. The field of *health informatics* appeared in the late 1950s to integrate primary data collection with access to existing and new databases and facilitate the management of medical records. "The basic objective of Health Informatics may be described as the improvement of the quality of information available to managers (decision makers)."[11] Knowledge-based systems for health services in developing countries have been described in four categories:

- Systems that assist the medical professional in clinical decision-making
- Systems that assist health workers to use and maintain sophisticated technology and equipment
- Systems that provide intelligent services, such as checking the consistency of data, producing summaries, question answering, and discovering new connections within data
- Systems to educate health workers, including patient simulators and virtual reality applications[12]

It is argued that knowledge-based systems correlated with existing artificial intelligence techniques should be embedded within larger health information systems and the routine computing environment. Computer-based decision support systems rely on operations research techniques and will help solve logistical problems in the operation of hospitals and clinics, scheduling, staff resources, diagnosis, treatment, financial decisions, blood banking, and so on.[13] Such proposals may seem utopian and unrealistic. On a mission to a large developing country in the mid-1990s I saw recently printed paper patient-data forms that still carried the former name of the country more than two decades after independence. These outdated pages have been repeatedly reprinted since colonial days simply because nobody had taken the initiative to update them. Although such anachronisms still exist, the advance of communications technology and continuing reduction in costs make it possible, if not inevitable, that modernized health and management information systems will be generally available and widely used within a generation.

The availability of management information is intended to make the operations of the health sector more efficient—that is, to increase the output of health by using limited resources most cost-effectively and make the health sector more like a business. The essential core of business is money: Owners and investors want to maximize their intake, and customers want to minimize their expenditure consistent with the quality of the product. That is true also for the commercial aspects of the health sector such as pharmaceuticals and other products, and for privately owned medical care facilities. But the goals and incentives of the various actors in government-supported health services are more varied, as described to some extent by the quotation at the beginning of this chapter.

In information-poor countries the construction of purpose-built systems for health data analysis and planning presents an opportunity and a challenge. In general there are two categories of problems: (1) the inadequate quality, completeness, and timeliness of data produced through the routine health recording and reporting mechanisms and (2) the insufficient use of available data for planning, implementation, case and service management, monitoring, and evaluation. Health ministries must search for their own Goldilocks data system: not too little, not too much, but just right. A comparison with existing complex systems may provide a starting point.

Existing Health/Management Information Systems in Industrialized Countries

The maturing Information Technology (IT) databases and procedures in North America, Europe, Japan, and Australasia are in some ways models for nascent systems in the developing world. Not quite, because existing national information systems were cobbled together from pieces originally designed for a variety of needs, and which may not always function well together. Social security and retirement systems consume large volumes of information about illness and survival patterns. Proper payments from insurers and government agencies and billing practices of hospitals in the United States, Sweden, and some other countries required the definition and analysis of medical conditions. Data systems proliferated in hospitals and various agencies. Disease-specific registries, particularly for cancer, were es-

tablished in many regions. A partial listing of data sources useful for aging popu-
lations in the United States at the beginning of the 1990s[14] included the National
Health Interview Survey (NHIS), National Health and Nutrition Examination Sur-
vey (NHANES), NHANES I Epidemiologic Follow-up Survey, National Hospital
Discharge Survey, National Ambulatory Medical Care Survey (NAMCS), National
Nursing Home Survey (NNHS), National Mortality Statistics and National Mortality Followback Survey (NMFS), National Death Index (NDI), National Medical
Care Expenditure Surveys, National Survey of Long-Term Care/National Survey of
Caregivers, Long-Term Care Survey (LTC), Survey of Income and Program Participation (SIPP), Health and Retirement Survey (HRS), Medicare Annual Summaries, Medical Enrollment File, Medical History Sample, MEDPAR Public Use
File, and Continuous Work History Sample (CWHS). These are just some of the
relevant databases maintained by the federal government of the United States. Additional files are found in state governments, health maintenance organizations, and
the archives of health services researchers. Surely such detail is not needed everywhere for adequate decision-making.

A number of systems have been designed to provide the health sector with a tool
to help anticipate and respond to planning problems. A good example is the System for Health Area Resource Planning (SHARP) in Ontario, Canada.[15] Its seven
component models project the user population by age, sex, and characteristics; their
requirements for health care services; needed physicians, nurses, and other health
personnel; and facilities requirements into the future. The system focuses attention
on projected imbalances and on alternative policies to reduce or eliminate them.
Such a system might be transplanted with modifications into analogous programs
elsewhere in the world.

Health/Management Information Systems in Developing Countries

Based on her experience in Papua New Guinea and Nigeria, one author observed
that "the idea should be promoted that all health workers are information managers
and analysts."[16]

> In health, as elsewhere, good information facilitates sound decisionmaking. Although
> some basic health information is generated by the private sector without government
> involvement, the government has a central role in requiring, standardizing, and financ-
> ing the collection, analysis, and dissemination of health information, as well as in fi-
> nancing health systems research. Governments are already heavily involved in data col-
> lection. Unfortunately, the data are often irrelevant to policy and program design. And
> too often, the private sector is ignored when statistics are being gathered. Revamping
> health information systems is an attractive investment, both because it is relatively in-
> expensive and because poor decisions based on inadequate information can be very
> costly.[17]

An off-the-shelf H/MIS usable by health ministries in all countries seems unattainable at present. Despite the World Bank's entreaty, it is not clear just what information is needed, what kinds of management decisions are being and should be made, or what kind of training needs to be provided to decision-makers. Moreover, the structure of governments varies a great deal. Certain functions such as vital statistics may be the responsibility, e.g., of the Ministry of the Interior; medical education is in the Ministry of Education; nutrition and food inspection in the Ministry of Agriculture; vector control is in the Ministry of Environment; and the tumor registry is maintained by the private-sector National Cancer Society. Health authorities must coordinate with other agencies both within and outside the Ministry of Health, so any H/MIS should dovetail with corresponding systems in other parts of government. Furthermore, as we have seen, there is a need for coordination with donors, with other countries in the region, and with the WHO and other multilaterals at the global level.

Sometimes too much information is collected. In one Asian country in 1985

Peripheral-level health workers were expected to complete more than 30 sets of forms either on a daily or monthly basis. At the rural health center level, the local staff had to submit a set of forms with 1160 variables every month. Of these variables, 72% were requested by the Division of Disease Control, the unit responsible for epidemiological surveillance. At the next administrative level, Township Medical Officers each month had to process and review those variables, plus 786 more variables on township-level health activities, for a total of 1946 variables. The surveillance needs of the Division of Disease Control accounted for nearly 1000 of the variables sent forward by the Township Medical officer. By the time the information was received at the national level, processed and analyzed, and included in a detailed report, three years would pass. The information was then too dated to be used for decision-making. Although the surveilance report represented the time and effort of countless health workers, no one trusted the data.[18]

Three African countries in which more rational Health information systems have been introduced are Ghana, Niger, and Chad. In Ghana a variety of health information systems had been put in place which were little more than vertical reporting systems. An analysis of these systems showed that

- There was limited appreciation by staff at any level of the value of management systems.
- Goals, objectives, and targets were not clear for most programs.
- The concept of an indicator was foreign to staff.
- Staff were not adequately trained so data were not analyzed or used locally.
- Data were often of poor quality and frequently were not submitted on time.
- Raw data flowed vertically from the point of collection to the central level.
- Forms were poorly laid out and often redundant.

- Many key people were left out of the collection and reporting process.
- Feedback from higher levels was seldom forthcoming in any form.[19]

The Ministry of Health wanted to install a standardized H/MIS to monitor coverage and quality of programs, that would be easy to use, flexible to local needs, clear on goals and indicators, and that would collect and analyze only the data needed to improve decisions. A planning group assigned to meet those criteria drew up defined program components and indicators,[20] produced training materials, and tested their system.

In Niger an eight-year long program was financed by USAID. The program started with a complicated system of unrelated components in which health facilities sent separate reports for different activities directly to separate directorates within the Ministry of Health (MOH) in Niamey. Each directorate was responsible for tabulation and analysis of whatever information it received. An information audit showed that all high-level MOH staff felt a need for better management information. Accordingly, priority attention was given to tracking the allocation of personnel, vehicles, and health facilities, using customized standard databases and presentation graphics programs readily usable by MOH personnel. Only then were components for service utilization and morbidity information added to the databases.

In Chad a reported 87% of the 1989 health budget was financed by donor assistance. "Public hospitals lacked basic equipment such as beds and x-ray machines, while smaller clinics were without essentials such as soap . . . the Ministry could not muster reliable data on any aspect of its own activities and facilities . . . nor could the Ministry estimate whether its activities were meeting health needs, because the sparse epidemiological data collected were so unreliable."[21] Emerging from several decades of civil war, Chad had about as bad a health situation as could be imagined. From 1985 to 1989 the USAID provided three long-term advisors to develop a viable health information system for planning and management within the MOH. A commission was established which included the directors of all seven divisions of the Ministry of Health, other officials, and representatives of donors. Surveys of needs were conducted and a system of "compromises and trade-offs" was painstakingly hammered out. Once the system was agreed to, forms and procedures could be developed and personnel trained so that by 1990 more than 90% of all health facilities were sending regular monthly reports to the MOH. Creating a useful system was challenging:

Because most of Chad's more than 400 health centers are run by nurses with scarcely a junior high school education and with only a thermometer (if that) as a diagnostic tool, diseases had to be reported by signs and symptoms, and reporting forms had to be easy to fill out . . . as a result, Chad collects data on relatively few disease entities but has more valid and reliable information on those diseases that it follows. Nurses also report on only a limited number of their activities. So far, these limitations have posed no problems for Chadian planners, but they do irritate international organizations that have their own bureaucratic imperatives.[22]

The SHARP project in Canada is limited to the Province of Ontario, and health-related information systems in developing countries may also apply to specific regions. In China, Sichuan Province, with 107 million people, more than 7000 townships, and 14,000 health workers, is larger than many entire countries. A Provincial Health and Anti-epidemic Center with a staff of 500 is responsible for notification of 35 diseases. In 1987 a modem-based link was established with the National Health Information Center in Beijing, and by 1990 with all 21 prefectures in the province.[23] In Zimbabwe the Health Department of Harare City (population more than a million) computerized its service statistics beginning in 1986 and has expanded the system since then.[24] Many other examples could be given.

Problems of Computerization in Developing Countries

The dissemination of computers has been hailed by some as the solution to all health information system problems. Electronic data on diskette can be cleaned, duplicated, disseminated, searched, arranged, accumulated, stored, compared, transmitted, and received quickly and almost without errors. There is no doubt that computers are here to stay as the technological underpinning of information and communication systems of all kinds. Yet despite their many obvious advantages, it remains true that computerizing a bad data system leads only to a bad computerized data system.

Computer hardware and software must be subservient to the organization in which they are installed. Stand-alone machines are very useful, but hardware "islands" can never form an effective system without communication and networking capabilities. The Sichuan and Harare programs began with IBM XT and AT computers, now long outmoded. It is inadvisable to wait for the latest technology when starting a system, because a newer device or program is always around the corner. As capacity, speed, and reliability of hardware increase, costs drop substantially. Staying current with technology by updating hardware and programs is a continuing problem for all users, but the dedication of local staff will go a long way toward maintaining an effective system. In Sichuan, computer training was given only to those proficient in English. In Harare, expenditures on consultants equalled the cost of the computer hardware and software. While consultants are often needed, they must be used with caution, as many advisors seem overly enthusiastic. "Though expatriates may have good intentions, they are often eager to implement their solutions before understanding the problem."[25] Many authors remain cautious:

There is immense pressure on HMIS designers, even in developing countries, to adopt 'technological fixes' based on sophisticted computers. While it is realised that computers are a useful tool for aggregating information at higher levels, experience shows that there is nothing that can replace a solid paper and indicator-based HMIS process and basic common sense.[26]

Impediments to H/MIS

The advantages of a system for information-based planning and management are self-evident to "rational" people from wealthier countries, accustomed to high technology in their daily lives. There are economic, logistic, and technical problems to be overcome in designing, installing, and using H/MIS, but the most important obstacles are the human ones.

Western consultants and observers may express frustration that their path to progress is not always welcomed by the intended beneficiaries. Outsiders see an entrenched bureaucracy, weak planning and management, *ad hoc* decision making, and inadequate data, monitoring, and evaluation; in other words, a system in need of fixing. But while we promote new ways to improve efficiency, the recipients may see disincentives. Where we perceive intransigence, poorly trained and meagerly paid local officials may act from a sense of peril. Knowing little of the technology, insecure in their jobs, coming from a tradition of centralized authority and advancement by seniority, connections, and self-preservation, they are justifiably suspicious of sweeping changes in what they consider their domain. An information system is much more than data moving up and down the system. It is also a means to redistribute leadership, incentives, and, ultimately, power and control. Such apparent recalcitrance would become much less objectionable if we were to think how we would behave if we were in their shoes.

In one very poor country

the [Ministry of Health's] initial attitude toward the development of information systems was not universally favorable. Because approval implied that current resource allocation methods were inadequate, this plan was perceived as a threat by many of the MOH officials who were involved in making resource allocation decisions. Some officials recognized that the increased availability of information would also increase the exposure, possibly to criticism, of past and current performance. In addition, MOH personnel had little experience in planning and thus did not understand the usefulness of health and management information. As a consequence, the MOH initially blocked the design and implementation of the automated information system by creating a series of bureaucratic barriers . . . the availability of information was seen as a threat to the power base of high-level officials.[27]

In view of these difficulties the H/MIS or its local variant must be seen not only as a management tool but as a locus for discussion and consensus for all branches of the MOH at central and peripheral levels. The act of meeting to negotiate sector-wide procedures forces bureaucrats and officials to think beyond their limited piece of the system, to identify common goals and objectives, and to compromise if necessary to achieve a viable product.

To be broadly useful all systems must use common conventions such as terminology and codings. Clinical data, diagnoses, and procedures must be recorded and aggregated using universally accepted ICD codes (see previous chapter). Worldwide activities such as the Expanded Programme on Immunization, the Global Programme on AIDS, and many others depend on the collection of comparable data in uniform ways. The necessary commodities, supplies, and equipment are much the same the world over and vendors depend on standard procedures to operate their businesses. Technical specifications and protocols for communication and data exchange must be compatible everywhere. For practical purposes only English and a few other major languages are effective for international communications. Everything is being standardized and homogenized to a worldwide top-down, one-size-fits-all global network that has developed in a *ad hoc* unplanned way according to its own inevitable logic. As a consequence, cultural individuality may be lost, small and unique populations may be marginalized, and health services are likely to approach a convergence in structure and function.

COMMUNICATION

Most people in the world live and die without ever using a telephone. Hard-wired telephone systems are expensive to install. It is routine in the cities of developing countries to wait years or decades for "a line," and in many rural areas telephones are almost unknown. Is it complete folly, then, to speak of advanced electronic technology in health information systems of poor countries? Not really, because technology is advancing so rapidly that global communication has become inevitable. Every familiar product, from bread to breadboards, from pencils to penicillin, and every useful procedure and method was once a technological innovation. Viewed at first with skepticism, these products have achieved widespread diffusion and many are now considered indispensible.

The expansion of wireless networks in developing countries is hastening the spread of communication infrastructures, and satellite communication has made the globalization of ideas possible. The Internet is exploding as a *true* worldwide web. Brazil had 800 web sites in January 1995 and 77,148 in January 1997. In 1997 there were 250,000 Internet users in Malaysia. The number of households using the Internet in the United States and Canada was 15.4 million in 1996 and will reach 38.2 million in 2000.[28] South Africa had about 1 million users at the end of 1997.[29] Global Mobile Personal Communications by Satellite (GMPCS) has the potential to provide access to telecommunications to every person in the world. The information footpath of today's developing world is merging rapidly with the information superhighway already functioning in the wealthy countries.

Over the next 20 years, the cost of telecommunications may well drop to the point that it will become a virtually free commodity. In a recent study sponsored by the World Bank, the cost assumption for 2010 was on the order of 3 cents for a one hour transatlantic call. It is not implausible that by 2000, the cost of voice traffic through submarine cable links will already have dropped to one percent of its 1987 cost.[30]

The first version of this book[31] was written by hand with a pencil on a lined yellow pad. The pages were typed by a secretary and copies were made with carbon paper. Corrections were handwritten and the whole thing was retyped. It seems barely believable, even to your graying author, that this was only 20 years ago. The current edition was prepared on a computer that may seem equally archaic ten years from now. Obsolescence, the flip side of progress, affects the process as well as the hardware. By the time these words are printed and distributed the capabilities of H/MIS will have multiplied in not always predictable directions. What seems certain, however, is the primacy and expansion of communications systems. Today nurses in India are transcribing patient records dictated by physicians in New York and sending the text files back to America in a flash, all at a lower cost than could be done in the United States. Programmers from Barbados to Kyrgyzstan write lines of code for customers around the globe.

International telecommunications has been conducted via geostationary satellites since the late 1960s. Because those satellites orbit at the same speed as the earth rotates, and because they are 22,000 miles (36,000 kilometers) high, three satellites can cover the entire inhabited world. But their altitude causes a time delay and loss of signal quality and power, and a large and costly receiver dish is needed on the ground. All of that is changed with the advent of LEO (low earth orbiting) and MEO (medium earth orbiting) satellites, which orbit the earth at 700 to 10,000 kilometers. From the lower altitude it takes less power to get a signal up and back to earth, which means virtually no delay in transmission as well as much smaller and less costly antennas. Many more are needed to cover the globe but they can provide communications to people in remote areas and developing countries. Village telephones, liberated from wires, will be installed widely. The cost at first may be roughly as much as a motorcycle, then much less. Among their benefits will be routine transmissions of all kinds as well as education, disaster relief, telemedicine and environmental protection.

> Within a decade or two, most ordinary telephone conversations will cost nothing extra, whatever their duration or distance. As a result, one of the most important limits imposed by geography on human activities will eventually vanish. The demise of distance as the key to the cost of communicating may well prove the most significant economic force shaping the next half century . . . it will put more power into the homes and on to the desks of ordinary people. Voters and customers alike will find it easier to make comparisons, acquire information, by-pass gatekeepers, cross borders. The telephone is a seditious little instrument; but it will create a better-informed, more prosperous life for millions of people.[32]

Cost and technophobia are not the only obstacles to the dissemination of computer-based communication systems. Establishment of an H/MIS computer network for local and national communication immediately suggests its use for global connections. Today in many countries it is easier to send an e-mail via satellite to a distant country than to make a telephone call to the national capital. But long-distance communication is not always welcome. Totalitarian governments do not care to promote the ability of their citizens to share ideas openly within their borders, much less with outsiders. Community-minded staff in remote health centers may be under special scrutiny, so for reasons of "national security" their communications links are intentionally restricted rather than promoted.

Where communications links are open and accessible, information formerly obtainable only at great effort, or not available at all, is routinely downloaded in seconds from any of thousands of websites[33] or sent by e-mail from colleagues around the world. Through the Internet current knowledge becomes available where libraries are incomplete, inaccessible or even nonexistent. Databases such as MEDLINE and its subset ONCOLINK are available from the U.S. National Library of Medicine and at mirror sites around the world. Among the many full-text resources that can be downloaded at no charge are the *Weekly Epidemiological Record* of the WHO and the *Morbidity and Mortality Weekly Report* (MMWR) and *Emerging Infectious Diseases* from the U.S. Centers for Disease Control and Prevention. On the commercial side, for example, the journal *Health Policy and Planning,* which deals with health care issues in developing countries, is available online long before the printed version arrives in the mail. A single subscription fee covers both the electronic and paper versions.

Although costs are declining quickly it remains to be seen whether such services are affordable where resources are few. Balanced against these expenditures is the greater cost of ignorance and isolation.

Telemedicine

Telemedicine began with the first telephone call to or from a physician, and it has expanded ever since. A particularly optimistic author puts it this way:

> Telemedicine is the delivery of health care and the exchange of health care information across distances using telecommunications technology. It can include the transfer of basic patient information over computer networks (medical informatics), the transfer of images such as radiographs, CT scans . . . patient interviews and examinations, consultations with medical specialists, and health care educational activities. Recent innovations in telecommunications and computer technologies show great promise for telemedicine applications that may revolutionize health care delivery and health education on a global scale, particularly in rural and underserved areas.[34]

In the modern sense telemedicine was first applied in 1971 to provide health care services to isolated villages in Alaska using the ATS-1 satellite. Existing high-tech telemedicine links include *SatelLife/HealthNet,* a nonprofit organization working to improve communicatins and exchanges in public health, medicine, and the environment. This organization provides news, information services, collaboration, conferences, and e-mail services to health institutions in developing countries. As of late 1997, links had been established in Botswana, Burkina Faso, Cameroon, Eritrea, Ethiopia, Gambia, Ghana, Indonesia, Kenya, Malawi, Mali, Mozambique, Myanmar, Nepal, Philippines, South Africa, Sudan, Uganda, Tanzania, and Zimbabwe. Many other organizations are striving to provide such services. For example, the *Pan-Pacific Regional Telecommunications Network* Experiments and Research Satellite (PARTNERS) in Japan communicates with institutions in Cambodia, Thailand, Indonesia, Papua New Guinea, Fiji, and Hawaii.[35] In Latin America and the Caribbean a "LA&C" network has been established with cooperation of the United States, the Organization of American States, and UN agencies (WHO/PAHO, UNDP, UNESCO).[36]

Electronic communication systems can help compensate for the local absence of information and trained human resources through so-called "expert systems" that comprise a database of relevant facts and a means of applying rules of inference via algorithms to derive conclusions, provide explanations, and make recommendations.[37]

Geographic Information Systems

Just as H/MIS's may be coupled with telemedicine they can also be made to tie in with a geographic information system (GIS) which provides information about the characteristics of sites and features on maps.[38] Such systems have been used since the early 1980s in relation to research, planning, monitoring, and evaluation in agriculture, natural resources, transportation, water and sanitation, urban planning, and similar fields, but their application in the health sector has been limited. GIS techniques could be useful for analyses of disease risk factors such as vector populations, pollution (toxic plumes and runoff), and natural disasters. They can plot patterns of morbidity and mortality and the allocation of health resources. A growing number of GIS information management software packages are now commercially available. These systems generally contain two integrated databases. The first is spatial, to locate sites as digital coordinates from maps or remote sensing devices in satellites. The other gives attributes to those sites, which may be defined as residences, villages, clinics, roads, forests, rivers, census tracts or other features, and includes some information about their characteristics. The database may tell the number of beds in a clinic, children in a school, persons in a household, how many children in a village were immunized, and so forth. The programs allow for acquisition, storage, analysis, and graphical display of collected data. Many GIS programs contain digitizing systems that convert conventional paper maps into digital form usable by the computer. Some obtain geographic data by remote sensing from earth satellites such as LANDSAT and convert the data into usable maps. Weather satellites can give information about current and projected rainfall and temperature. Other kinds of data can be imported from databases or spreadsheets, or from scans of ground-based or aerial photos, from digital cameras, or even from camcorders.

Maps and information prepared by GIS systems can be used in public education and are of particular interest to persons living in the areas displayed on the computer graphics. They can also be used by health officials as an aide to monitoring and evaluation of disease distribution and control programs. Although extravagant claims are sometimes made for potential applications of GIS, these will certainly become more important components of H/MIS in the 21st century.

A cousin and component of the GIS is the *global positioning system* (GPS) which uses small handheld devices to locate any point on the earth's surface within a few meters. These have been used in village household mapping and similar activities to document the spatial distribution of disease cases down to the household level.

The application of electronic technologies, combined with improved management techniques, should lead to greater efficiency in the operation of health services worldwide, but these advances will always be limited by human attitudes and behaviors, as discussed in the following chapter.

NOTES

1. We will examine these issues in some detail in Chapters 12 and 13.
2. Barker (1995).
3. Frerichs (1991).
4. World Health Organization (1969).
5. Goldman and Pebley (1994).
6. Bowman et al. (1997).
7. Jaravaza *et al.* (1982).
8. Freund and Kalumba (1986).
9. Adapted from documents on WHO cooperation in strengthening national health information systems, especially Lwanga and Sapirie. (1995).
10. Rischard (1996). Jean-Francois Rischard is V.P. for Finance and Private Sector Development at the World Bank.
11. Salamon *et al.* (1997).
12. Tolmie and du Plessis (1997).
13. Walus *et al.* (1997).
14. Rice (1992).
15. Denton et al. (1993).
16. Hull (1994).
17. World Bank (1993).
18. Frerichs (1991).
19. Heywood and Campbell (1997).
20. Program components, each with appropriate indicators, were: medical care; communicable disease control; antenatal care; deliveries; postnatal care; family planning; child welfare and nutrition; school health; and environmental health. See Heywood and Campbell (1997) for details.
21. Foltz (1993).
22. Ibid.

23. Wang *et al.* (1993).
24. Woelk and Moyo (1995).
25. Hull (1994).
26. Heywood and Campbell (1997).
27. Mock *et al.* (1993).
28. Horwitt (1997).
29. Ibid.
30. Rischard (1996).
31. Basch (1978).
32. *Economist* (1995).
33. See a list of some useful websites in the appendix to this chapter.
34. Ferguson *et al.* (1995). See also Houtchens *et al.* (1995) for technical data.
35. Ferguson et al. (1995).
36. Mandil (1995).
37. See for example Kahen and Sayers (1997).
38. See Croner et al. (1996). A book-length discussion of GIS's in de Savigny and Wijeyaratne (1995) can be downloaded from ⟨http://www.idrc.ca/books/focus/766/⟩.

Appendix: Some World Wide Web Sites of Interest for International Health[a]

Name	URL
A	
Academy For International Health Studies Inc.	http://www.AIHS.com/
Agencies in International Aid	http://www.interaction.org/
American Medical Student Association	http://www.amsa.org/
American Public Health Association	http://www.apha.org
American Society of Tropical Medicine and Hygiene	http://www.astmh.org/
American Association of Health Plans	http://www.aahp.org
Appropriate Health Resources and Technologies Action Group	http://www.poptel.org.uk/ahrtag/index.html
Asian Development Bank	http://www.adb.org/
Australian National University Demography	http://coombs.anu.edu.au/ResFacilities/ DemographyPage.html
B	
Basic Social Services for All	http://www.undp.org/popin/wdtrends/ bss/bssatf.htm

BIREME, Latin American and Caribbean
Center on Health — http://www.bireme.br

Burden of Disease Unit — http://www.hsph.harvard.edu/
organizations/bdu/

C

Canadian Society for International Health — http://www.csih.org/

Center for International Health Information — http://www.cihi.com/

Centre for Health Economics — http://www.york.ac.uk/inst/che/welcome.htm

Christian Connections for International
Health — http://www.ccih.org/

Cochrane Collaboration — http://www.cochranelibrary.net/ccolab.htm

D

Data for Decision Making project — http://www.hsph.harvard.edu/
organizations/ddm/

Demographic and Health Surveys — http://www.macroint.com/dhs

Development Information — http://nt1.ids.ac.uk/eldis/eldis.htm

E

Emerging Infections Information Network — http://info.med.yale.edu/EIINet/

Emerging Infectious Diseases Home Page — http://www.cdc.gov/ncidod/EID/eid.htm

Epi Info — http://www.cdc.gov/epo/epi/epiinfo.htm

European Healthcare Management
Association — http://ireland.iol.ie/~ehma/index.html

F

Ford Foundation — http://www.fordfound.org/

G

G-7 Healthcare Applications — http://www.ispo.cec.be/g7/projects/
theme8.html

Global ChildNet — http://www.edie.cprost.sfu.ca/gcnet/
index.html

Global Health Council — http://www.globalhealthcouncil.org

Global Health Network — http://www.pitt.edu/HOME/GHNet/
GHNet.html

Global Population Database — http://infoserver.ciesin.org/datasets/cir/
gpopdb-home.html

Global Technology Network — http://www.usgtn.org

Guide to Family Planning, Population,
HIV/AIDS and Related Resources — http://www.jhuccp.org/netlinks.stm

GuideStar Guide to Nonprofit Organizations — http://www.guidestar.org/

H

Health and Health Statistics Websites	http://www.who.int/whosis/countrysites
Health Canada	http://www.hc-sc.gc.ca/
Health Care Information Resources	http://www.xnet.com/~hret/statind.htm
Health Economics Resources	http://www.york.ac.uk/res/herc/
Human Rights Library	http://www.umn.edu/humanrts/

I

ICD-10	http://www.who.int/nst/icd-10/index.html
Influenza Centers	http://www.who.int/cds/flu/centres.txt
Institut Pasteur	http://www.pasteur.fr/
Institute of Medicine (National Academy of Sciences) Board on International Health	http://www2.nas.edu/bih/index.html
Institute for Global Communication (PeaceNet, EcoNet, LaborNet, ConflictNet and WomensNet)	http://www.igc.org/ igc
Instituto Nacional de Salud Publica, [Mexico].	http://www.insp.mx/index.html
Inter-American Development Bank	http://www.iadb.org/
International Affairs Network list of international agencies	http://www.pitt.edu/~ian/resource/intorg.htm
International Association for Medical Assistance to Travellers	http://www.sentex.net/~iamat
International Association of Physicians in AIDS Care (IAPAC)	http://www.iapac.org
International Census Collection On-line (U. Texas Austin, Population Resrch Cntr)	http://prc.utexas.edu/
International Clearinghouse of Health System Reform I, National Institute of Public Health, Mexico	http://www.insp.mx/ichsri/
International Clinical Epidemiology Network (INCLEN)	http://www.inclen.org
International Development Research Centre (Canada)	http://www.idrc.ca
International Federation of Pharmaceutical Manufacturers Associations	http://www.ifpma.org/
International Federation of Red Cross and Red Crescent Societies	http://www.ifrc.org/
International Health Action Group American Medical Students Assn.	http://www.views.vcu.edu/amsa/namsa/ihag/
International Health Economics Assn	http://www.unh.edu/
International Health Links (University of Pennsylvania)	http://www.med.upenn.edu/~oimp/index.html

International Health Medical Education
Consortium (IHMEC) — http://www.unmc.edu/Community/ihmec/

International Health Research
Scientist database — http://www.health.ucalgary.ca/ nhr/nhrdb/ nhrdb.htm

International Healthcare Opportunities
Clearinghouse — http://library.ummed.edu/ihoc/

International Healthcare Volunteer
Opportunites — http://library.ummed.edu/ihoc/

International Medical Corps — http://www.imc-la.com/index.htm

International Monetary Fund — http://www.imf.org/

International Red Cross — http://www.icrc.ch

International Service Agencies — http://www.charity.org/type.html

International Union Against Cancer — http://www.uicc.ch/

J

Japanese International Cooperation
Administration Home Page — http://www.jica.go.jp/Index.html

K

Karolinska Institute — http://www.ki.se/

Key Fertility Rates and Statistics
(Marie Stopes International) — http://www.mariestopes.org.uk/ msi_worldwide.html

L

Library of Congress Country Studies — http://lcweb2.loc.gov/frd/cs/cshome.html

M

Medical Research Council of Canada — http://www.mrc.hwc.ca/

Medical Care Charitable Agencies — http://www.charity.org/medcare.html

Ministries of Health, Various — (at end of this list)

Multilaterals Project — http://www.tufts.edu/fletcher/multilaterals.html

N

National Council for International Health — (see Global Health Council)

NGO Link — http://www.un.org/MoreInfo/ngolink/ welcome.htm

O

Organization for Economic Cooperation
and Development (OECD) — http://www.oecd.org/

Office of Population Research (OPR),
Princeton University Data Archive — http://opr.princeton.edu/archive/

P

Packard Foundation	http://www.packard.org
Population & Family Planning Bookshelf	http://www.ssc.wisc.edu/cde/library/ books.htm
Population Index	http://popindex.princeton.edu
POPIN Worldwide Directory of Population Institutions	http://www.visitus.com/~unpopdir
Population Reference Bureau	http://www.prb.org/prb/
Popnet (Global population information)	http://www.popnet.org
PRB Glossary of Population Terms	http://www.prb.org/edu/glossary.htm
Program for Appropriate Technology in Health (PATH)	http://www.path.org
ProMed: Program for Monitoring Emerging Diseases	http://www.fas.org/promed/index.html

R

Regional donor organizations	http://nt1.ids.ac.uk/eldis/aid/rdb_lorg.htm
ReliefWeb, UN Department of Humanitarian Affairs	http://www.reliefweb.int/
ReproLine (Reproductive Health Online)	http://www.reproline.jhu.edu
Robert Wood Johnson Foundation	http://www.rwjf.org/main.html
Rockefeller Foundation	http://www.rockfound.org

S

Safe Motherhood	http://www.safemotherhood.org
SatelLife (Includes HealthNet)	http://www.healthnet.org
Social Security Programs Throughout the World	http://www.ssa.gov.statistics/ssptw97.html
Southeast Asia Ministers of Education Organization (SEAMEO) Regional Tropical Medicine and Public Health Network (TROPMED)	http://www.mahidol.ac.th/mahidol/tm/ h-tropmed.htm

T

Teaching Aids at Low Cost	http://www.ids.ac.uk/eldis/data/d021/ e02173.html

U

V

Virtual Library—Public Health	http://www.ens.gu.edu.au/eberhard/vl/ index.htm
Same: Mirror Site in Germany	http://www.uni-ulm.de/public_health/vl/ index.htm

W

Weizmann Institute	http://www.weizmann.ac.il/
World Bank	http://www.worldbank.org/
World Bank / HCO Health Issues	http://www.worldbank.org/html/hcovp/ heal/contents.html
W Bank Project Information Documents	http://www.worldbank.org/html/ pic/PIDs.html
World Factbook	http://www.odci.gov/cia/publications/ factbook/index.html
World Federation of Public Health Associations	http://www.apha.org/wfpha/basic.html
World Fertility Surveys	http://opr.princeton.edu/archive/
WWW Virtual Library—International Development	http://www.acdi-cida.gc.ca/virtual.nsf

Internet Addresses of Some Ministries of Health

[Note: Some of these web pages are in the respective national language]

Argentina: Ministry of Health and Welfare	http://www.presidencia.ar/salud.html
Australia: Department of Health	http://www.health.gov.au/
Austria: Ministry of Labor, Health and Social Affairs (in German)	http://www.bmg.gv.at/bmg
Bahrain: Ministry of Health	http://www.batelco.com.bh/mhealth/
Barbados: Ministry of Health and the Environment	http://www.uwimona.edu.jm/cesd/ barbados/barbados.htm
Bolivia: National Statistics Institute	http://www.ine.gov.bo/
Brazil: Ministry of Health	http://www.ms.gov.br/
Canada: Health Protection Branch	http://www.hwc.ca/hpb/index_e.html
Chile: Health Ministry	http://www.minsal.cl/inicio.htm
Chile: Institute of Public Health	http://www.ispch.cl/home.htm
China: Ministry of Public Health (from Hong Kong)	http://www.hkib.org.hk/china/mph.htm
Colombia: Ministry of Health	http://www.minsalud.gov.co/
Costa Rica: Ministry of Health	http://www.netsalud.sa.cr/ms/
Croatia: Ministry of Health	http://www.vlada.hr/tjela/minkab/zdrave.html
Czech Republic: Ministry of Health	http://www.mzcr.cz/
Denmark: Ministry of Health	http://www.sum.dk/uk/ukmenu.htm
Ecuador: Ministry of Public Health	http://www4.salud.org.ec/index_ms.htm
Egypt: HealthNet	http://www.idsc.gov.eg/health/
Estonia: Ministry of Social Affairs	http://www.sm.ee/welcome.html
Finland: Ministry of Social Affairs and Health	http://www.vn.fi/stm/english/index.html

France: Ministry of Health	http://www.sante.fr
Germany: Ministry of Health	http://www.bmgesundheit.de/
Guatemala: Ministry of Public Health and Welfare	http://www.concyt.gob.gt/sectpub/minist/ minsalud.htm
Guyana—Ministry of Health	http://www.guyana.org/Ministry_Health.htm
Hong Kong: Department of Health	http://www.info.gov.hk/dh/
Hungary: Ministry of the Interior	http://www.b-m.hu/english_home_page.htm
India—Minster for Health and Family Welfare	http://206.252.12.4/profiles/renuka.htm
Indonesia: Ministry of Health	http://www.depkes.go.id/english/
Ireland: Department of Health and Children	http://www.doh.ie/
Israel: Ministry of Health	http://www.israel-mfa.gov.il/health.html
Italy: Ministry of Health	http://www.sanita.interbusiness.it/
Japan: Ministry of Health and Welfare	http://www.mhw.go.jp/english/index.html
Jordan: Ministry of Health	http://www.nic.gov.jo/health/moh/moh.html
Kenya: Ministry of Health	http://www.kenyaweb.com/kenyagov/ health/health.html
Lithuania: Ministry of Health	http://www.randburg.com/li/minihealth.html
Luxembourg: Ministry of Health	http://www.santel.lu/MIN/home.html
Malaysia: Ministry of Health	http://dph.gov.my/
Malta: Ministry of Health	http://www.magnet.mt/ministries/health/
Mexico: Ministry of Health	http://www.ssa.gob.mx/
Morocco: Ministry of Public Health	http://www.mincom.gov.ma/frensh/ minister/m_san/m_san.html
Namibia: Ministry of Health and Social Service	http://www.azania.co.za/namibia/bethanie/ ministry_of_health.htm
New Zealand: Ministry of Health	http://www.health.govt.nz/moh/moh.html
Netherlands: Ministry of Health, Welfare and Sport	http://www.minvws.nl/0/home.htm
Norway: Ministry of Health	http://odin.dep.no/shd/eng/index.html
Palestine: Ministry of Health:	http://www.palnet.com/archive/health/
Philippines: Council for Health Research and Development	http://www.pchrd.dost.gov.ph/
Peru: Ministry of Health (in Spanish)	http://www.digesa.sld.pe/
Portugal: Ministry of Health	http://www.dgsaude.pt/
Russia: Public Health Institute— Ministry of Health	http://views.vcu.edu/views/fap/medsoc/ medsoc.htm
Singapore: Ministry of Health	http://www.gov.sg/moh/
Singapore: Ministry of Environment	http://www.gov.sg/env/
Slovak Republic: Ministry of Health	http://www.health.gov.sk/index_an.htm
South Africa: Ministry of Health	http://www.sacs.org.za/level4/heal.htm

Spain: Ministry of Health	http://www.insalud.es/insalud/home1.htm
St. Lucia—Ministry of Health	http://www.candw.lc/homepage/health.htm
Sweden: Social Department	http://www.sb.gov.se/info_rosenbad/departement/social/social.html
Taiwan: Ministry of Health	http://www.doh.gov.tw/english/
Thailand: Ministry of Public Health	http://www.moph.go.th/
Turkey: Ministry of Health	http://www.saglik.gov.tr/indexing.htm
United Arab Emirates: Ministry of Health	http://www.ecssr.ac.ae/03uae.ministry9.html
United Kingdom: Ministry of Health	http://www.open.gov.uk/doh/dhhome.htm
Vietnam: Ministry of Health	http://www.batin.com.vn/vninfo/ministry/h.htm

United States Government Agencies

Agency for Health Care Policy and Research (AHCPR)	http://www.ahcpr.gov/
Centers for Disease Control and Prevention	http://www.cdc.gov/
CDC Diseases Information Page	http://www.cdc.gov/diseases/diseases.html
CDC Epi Info	http://www.cdc.gov/epo/epi/epiinfo.htm
CDC International Health Bulletins	http://www.cdc.gov/epo/mmwr/international/world.html
CDC International Health Program Office	http://www.cdc.gov/ihpo/homepage.htm#
CDC Morbidity & Mortality Weekly Report	http://www.cdc.gov/epo/mmwr/mmwr.html
CDC Travel Information	http://www.cdc.gov/travel/travel.html
Census Bureau International Data Base	http://www.census.gov/ipc/www/idbnew.html
Central Intelligence Agency (CIA) CIA Publications and Factbooks	http://www.odci.gov/cia/publications/pubs.html
Food and Drug Administration (FDA) FDA International Agencies Page	http://www.fda.gov/oia/agencies.htm
Healthy People 2000 Home Page	http://odphp.osophs.dhhs.gov/pubs/hp2000/
Library of Congress Country Studies	http://lcweb2.loc.gov/frd/cs/cshome.html#toc.
MEDLINE (via Internet Grateful Med)	http://igm.nlm.nih.gov
National Center for Health Statistics	http://www.cdc.gov/nchswww/nchshome.htm
National Center for HIV, STD, and TB Prevention (NCHSTP)	http://www.cdc.gov/nchstp/od/nchstp.html
National Institute for Occupational Safety and Health (NIOSH)	http://www.cdc.gov/niosh/homepage.html
National Institutes of Health (U.S.)	http://www.nih.gov/
National Library of Medicine (U.S.) NLM Online Databases and Databanks	http://www.nlm.nih.gov/ http://www.nlm.nih.gov/publications/factsheets/online_databases.html

Statistical Abstract of the U.S.	http://www.census.gov/prod/www/abs/cc97stab.html
THOMAS—U.S. Congress on the Internet	http://thomas.loc.gov/
U.S. Agency for International Development (USAID)	http://www.info.usaid.gov/
U.S. Department of Health and Human Services	http:/dhhs.gov/
U.S. Public Health Service	http://phs.os.dhhs.gov/phs/phs.html
US State Department Travel Warnings and Consular Information Sheets	http://travel.state.gov/travel_warnings.html

United Nations Group Agencies

Pan American Health Organization (PAHO)	http://www.PAHO.org
PAHO Technical Information	http://www.paho.org/english/techinfo.htm
Population Financial Resource Flows (UNFPA/NIDI)	http://www.nidi.nl/resflows
POPIN Electronic Library	http://www.undp.org/popin/infoserv.htm
Register of Development Activities (UNESCO, UNDP, UNFPA, UNTF)	http://www.unesco.org/general/eng/infoserv/db/rda.html
United Nations	http://www.un.org/
UN Basic Social Services for All	http://www.undp.org/popin/wdtrends/bss/bss.htm
UN Development Fund for Women	http://www.unifem.undp.org
UN Development Program (UNDP)	http://www.undp.org
UNDP HIV/AIDS Publications	http://www.undp.org/hiv/hdp1d.htm
UNICEF	http://www.unicef.org/
World Health Organization (WHO)	http://www.who.int/
Global Health Situation and Estimates	http://www.who.int/whosis/globest/globest.htm
Headquarters Major Programs	http://www.who.int/home/sitemap.html
Library Catalogue	http://unicorn.who.int/uhtbin/cgisirsi/8/1/1
Regional Offices Around the World	http://www.who.int/regions/

[a]This is a sampling of some useful web sites as of early 1999. Many of these include links to other sites. New sites are added constantly. Web addresses (universal resource locators) and organization names may change. Web sites of some health ministries and agencies are in their national languages.

6

The Social Context: Sickness, Illness, and Disease

In 20,000 BC the question, "What's wrong with the child?" could be answered, "She is very warm," or, "He can't stop his bowels," or, "He is warm and has red spots all over." In 1000 BC they might have said, "She has fever," or "He has diarrhea," or "He has malaria." As recurrent patterns became recognized over time, they started to be identified by different names and to take on a sort of independent existence. *Diseases* are generalizations built up from observations on a large number of individual conditions that share certain characteristics. Diseases are often dealt with in the medical literature as if they had objective reality, similar to species of animals or plants.

An entity called *malaria* (or the equivalent) has been recognized as a disease for thousands of years. Hippocrates knew it well and described several different patterns of malaria among humans. But it was only at the end of the 1800s that the concept *malaria* was rounded out by two discoveries: that it is transmitted by mosquitoes and that a different species of pathogen is responsible for each variant. Greater knowledge led to sharper definition and *malaria* is now known to encompass at least four separate biological entities. With that knowledge the ecology of malaria may be studied very much like the ecology of a real organism, and the rules that govern its abundance and distribution can be worked out. Indeed, the predictability of disease occurrence forms the basis of the science of epidemiology and of control programs of all sorts. The specific roster of diseases recognized by our conventional western medical lore varies from place to place and time to time in part because they really differ and in part because the cultural constructs that define them reflect a certain world view which is not necessarily shared by all people. You and I probably wouldn't think of *fever* as a disease although most people probably would. We might call *diarrhea* a disease, but a medical specialist would know perhaps 13 different kinds. Everybody might agree on *measles*. Health professionals, whether feathered shamans or pediatric oncologists, each recognize a particular spectrum of diseases as part of their distinctive toolkit and job description. Diseases come and go—in reality and in concept.

One person's illness or disability will not be exactly the same as another person's, even if the two have enough in common to be *cases* of the same disease. All illnesses are individual and each is unique. Factors in the environment, including pathogens and chemicals, act in different ways on people of diverse experience and age; genetic, hormonal, and behavioral makeup; and states of health. A person may be perceived by himself, his family, or others to be feeling or acting abnormally. A healer of some kind makes a diagnosis—that is, assigns the illness to a more general, objective category of disease, by which it is related to a predictable sequence embracing causality, treatment, and prognosis. Patients and their families are concerned with the illness, which is their experience of the disease. We might say that reduction of illness is the province of the physician or healer, while control of disease belongs to public health.

What, then, is *sickness*? If disease belongs to public health and illness to medicine, sickness is the terrain of social science. An illness transforms a healthy person to a sick person. Being sick is a socially recognized state regardless of the details of the particular cause or ailment, carrying with it certain specific obligations and privileges, as we will see later in this chapter.

THE IMPORTANCE OF CULTURE

The most important aspect in this discussion of illness around the world is recognition of the central role played by culture. "Broadly speaking, culture is a group's design for living, a shared set of socially transmitted assumptions about the nature of the physical and social world, the goals of life, and the appropriate means of achieving them."[1]

It is essential at the outset to agree that not only do "they" have a culture, but we do too. For a characterization of western culture, Oswald Spengler's *Decline of the West*[2] provides a broad and useful, if somewhat metaphysical, overview. In Spengler's interpretation, each of the world's great cultures has had its unique "soul" or pattern of experience and creation, which is inherent in its art, religion, administration, commerce, thought, and behavior. Western culture is characterized as "Faustian"; its central tendency is a yearning for infinity, probing the limits of time, space, materials, and thought. This yearning is perhaps best expressed in the towering cathedrals built after about the year 900, in the mathematics that permitted their construction, in the music that was played within them, in the sermons of the everlasting life delivered there, and in the worldwide commerce that supported the entire enterprise. Science, technology, government, and social and family relations all fall within the same design for living. Although there is much room for variation within this western culture, it does provide a rough guide for comparison.

In the United States, particularly, there has developed an emphasis on continued mastery over the environment, achieved through rationalism, science, and technology. Individualism is stressed, initiative is rewarded, and achievement is the gold standard of evaluation. Efficiency and wealth are virtuous goals, achievable by constant analysis, criticism, and the willingness to adopt new methods and discard old ones. Given enough knowledge and technology, anything can be accomplished.

The *Cartesian–Newtonian paradigm*[3] is a rather heavy term for the unifying principles of western scientific thought. These include:

- *Mechanistic explanation*: Nature is a grand, complex machine functioning under relatively simple physical laws, which can be unraveled.
- *Determinism*: Natural phenomena follow causal linkages, which can be identified by methodical study of cause and effect.
- *Reductionism*: Complex phenomena are comprehensible by systematic dissection into constituent segments—that is, the whole can be understood by a study of all its parts and their relationships.
- *Materialism*: The issues susceptible to study deal only with physical entities and their interrelations, all external to the scientist.
- *Quantitative expression*: The relationships among phenomena can be expressed mathematically—that is, we can study only what we can measure.

Delete any one of these elements—for example, determinism. What kinds of investigations could we make if, in fact, there are no causal linkages, and events occur unpredictably, at random? Where would we be if we could not measure things reliably and compare them by statistical means?

Some of the same unifying principles may be advocated also by non-scientific and non-western people. For example,

- *Nature is a grand, complex machine functioning under certain laws*: Agreed, but the essence of those laws may be conceived quite differently. Trees, stones, water, and animals may have interactive souls and spirits, which must be not only respected, but perhaps appeased.
- *Natural phenomena follow causal linkages*: They certainly do: Failure to observe rituals, or the breaking of taboos, will surely result in punishment, expressed as diarrhea, mania, departure of a spouse, and so on.

The pioneering British ethnologist Sir James Frazer studied magical and religious ideas in human communities around the world. He related these concepts at the end of the 19th century in a compendium that he called *The Golden Bough*.[4] Frazer resolved the world's magical thought and practice into two patterns:

- *Imitative magic*: For example, one can try to make it rain by pouring water on the ground.
- *Associative or contagious magic*: one may try to cause injury by burning a box containing an enemy's hair or fingernail clippings or obtain advantage through contact with some powerful object. We are exposed to associative magic every time we see a product endorsement by a sports hero.

According to Frazer, imitative magic "commits the mistake of assuming that things which resemble each other are the same: contagious magic commits the mistake of assuming that things which have once been in contact with each other are always in contact."

UNDERSTANDING OTHER CULTURES

Like a fish in water, everyone is immersed in his or her local culture and, without thinking, displays appropriate attitudes and behaviors. As adaptations for functioning within a community these traits provide many positive benefits to the individual and to the group. Many culturally influenced behaviors have important health consequences. It may be our intention to try to modify the behaviors of other people in ways that we consider beneficial—that is, to immunize their children, to maintain sanitary conditions during childbirth, or to plan their families. Such efforts are unlikely to result in the desired changes if we do not understand why local conditions are as they are. A caution: We should not overinterpret culture at the expense of simple economics (i.e., poverty) in trying to understand why some people do what they do.

In many traditional societies, the overall theme of life is not to challenge nature but to harmonize with it; not to struggle for personal achievement or to thrust forward the individual but to function within prescribed roles as members of an integrated society. For example, Malay culture has been described in these terms:

> The world itself is perceived as in many ways incomprehensible, consisting of often conflicting facts. But somehow there is harmony in a live and let live sense. People too are different, and they are expected to be. Yet they must learn to live harmoniously. And by harmonious is meant gentle: one's actions must be such that they do not cause hurt or embarrassment . . . Conversation is low-keyed . . . The content of conversation too is mild. One expresses an opinion very tentatively in Malay company. No one will contradict . . . [The village chief] is not expected to display qualities of leadership. No one is. Nor is he expected to influence opinion, even less, action—no one is . . . To act aggressively is embarrassing.[5]

In traditional Shona society in rural Zimbabwe, wealth was seen as a social disorder and a deliberate effort was made to ensure that everyone was equal in material benefits and that the family lineages or segments of the clan shared their possessions equitably. The Shona frowned on change and what the modern world knows as progress, which was sacrificed for the good of the group as opposed to the interests of the individual. Peace was maintained at all costs and tensions were reduced to a minimum. If people were allowed to become acquisitive, jealousies and fighting could occur, so they were limited in the amount of wealth they could acquire.[6] Similarly, in a traditional Latin American context, the future is often viewed with fatalism and the course of events may be considered predestined. There is less faith in human ability to influence coming events. The efficiency, punctuality, and organization of Anglo-Saxon society are seen as purposeless.

Points of cultural variation with respect to health involve ideas about nosology, etiology, and therapy, or, more simply, the kinds of illnesses, how and why they occur, and what can be done about them. The official roster of western, scientifically recognized syndromes is the International Statistical Classification of Diseases, Injuries and Causes of Death, the ICD, described in Chapter 4. Its frequent revisions show that recognized types of diseases are continually changing as scientific knowledge increases and information becomes available. Moreover, changes in social and cultural factors are important, even in the developed countries: In the United States, for example, alcoholism is now generally regarded as a disease, while homosexuality is no longer considered so.

These two examples are of interest in that both represent what is often termed *deviant behavior*. The extent of socially permissible deviance varies from one culture and time to another. The sociologist Talcott Parsons, among others, has examined the concept of the definition of illness in terms of culture expectations, especially the relation of the problem of health and illness to the whole range of categories of deviant behavior. In the complex, highly differentiated western societies, obedience to institutionalized normative patterns (rules and laws) and adherence to cultural values are considered voluntary decisions for which a normal person can be held responsible. Distinctions are made between

- Deviance from commitment to accepted norms (*crime* or *illegality*)
- Deviance from accepted values (*sin* or *immorality*)
- Deviance from the capacity to perform expected tasks and roles, provided that this is involuntary (*sickness*)

Concepts of sickness, illness, and disease vary widely among peoples. The spectrum of health status is divided in different ways in different cultures, as is the visible light spectrum. Languages, which are basic tools and extensions of culture, reflect the varying types of diseases known, just as they do the numbers of discrete colors recognized. There is no one true nosology, any more than there is one true religion, one correct language, or one perfect form of music. The manifestations of an illness are generally viewed as an extension of its causation. Thus, in most cultures, the ideas of etiology and diagnosis are inseparable.

Many authors have discussed theories of illness found in cultures throughout the world. Concepts of causation are generally grouped as natural or supernatural. Natural causes arise in a way that "would appear reasonable to modern medical science": infection, stress, deterioration, accident, and human aggression. Supernatural causes are more complex and include:

- *Mystical*: an act or experience involving some impersonal causal relationship, such as *fate* (astrological influences, predestination, or bad luck), *ominous sensations* (dreams, sights, sounds thought to cause illness), *contagion* (contact with a polluting object, substance, or person), or *mystical retribution* (for violation of a taboo or moral injunction concerning food and drink, sex, behavior, ritual, property, or blasphemy).
- *Animalistic*: illness caused by the behavior of a soul, ghost, spirit, or god
- *Magical*: caused by an envious, affronted or malicious person, by sorcery or witchcraft.[7]

The apparent arbitrariness of illness and death, often striking hardest in innocent children, must be accounted for in a way that is reasonable and consistent with the system of beliefs built up by observation of nature. In traditional, pervasively religious cultures that honor few of the western values of power, progress, and material gain, but where harmony, resignation, and fatalism endure, reality resides in the world of the spirit, and it is here that the most important questions are asked and answered.

In line with the general belief that some diseases are caused by God, some by a witch, and others by a sorcerer, there is the pervasive belief that a disease caused by a sorcerer must be cured by a traditional healer. In Cameroon, for example, it is widely held that leprosy, mental illnesses, epilepsy, convulsions, and tuberculosis are in the realm of the traditional healers of the ancestors. Alternatively, diseases curable through biomedicine at the health center included diarrhea, measles, malaria, worm-caused ailments, sexually transmitted diseases, and the like.[8]

In our mechanistic experience, the usual question about causation of a person's illness is, "*How* did it happen?" In traditional societies it is usually, "*Why* did it happen? "What did the victim do wrong?" or, "Who had it in for him or her?" Some explanations for disease causality are listed in Table 6-1.

All cultures have searched for "factors" that control distribution and severity of different diseases in the population. In Europe and North America, there were repeated devastating epidemics of cholera in the 19th century. Before the era of bacteriology, the cause of this disease was the subject of much debate in the United States, where prevailing opinion held the epidemics to be "a scourge, a rod in the hand of God," and a remedy to save a once-favored nation from atheism and sin. In 1832, the disease was so strongly held to be a divine punishment that "whenever any person of substance died of cholera, it was an immediate cause of consternation, a consternation invariably allayed by reports that this ordinarily praiseworthy

Table 6-1 Some Underlying Causes to Which Human Health Problems Are Attributed

Accident

Acute poisoning or envenomation (mushroom, snake)

Allergy and immunological peculiarities

Bad habits (e.g., intemperance, masturbation, smoking)

Capricious acts of deities

Chronic poisoning (occupational exposure, pollution)

Congenital defects

Endocrine malfunction

Evil eye

Exposure to the elements

Exposure to strangers

Failure to observe ritual or breaking of taboos

Genetic or chromosomal abnormalities

Imbalance of bodily forces or humors

Jealousy

Inappropriate desires

Infections, including parasites

Intentional trauma (warfare, assault)

Mental or emotional stress

Nutritional deficiency or excess

Positions of the stars and planets

Pregnancy, labor, and childbirth

Senility

Sexual behavior

Witchcraft and spells

Any combination, including none, of the above

individual had some secret vice or else had indulged in some unwonted excess."[9] Much the same attitude can be found today with respect to AIDS.

It is not only the poor, uneducated residents of deprived countries whose health beliefs cannot stand up to modern scientific scrutiny. In every country today a certain proportion of people find it attractive to conceive of the world as controlled by external forces of good and evil, with gods and devils who must be appeased in order to keep everything, including health, on an even keel. Within the wealthy neighborhoods of European and North American cities stand many institutions founded upon the supernatural origins of illness and healing.

In the industrialized countries a great deal of money, effort, and computer time is expended in a continuing search for risk factors for cancer, cardiovascular disease, cystic fibrosis, multiple sclerosis, Alzheimer's disease, and a host of other severe illnesses. Every available scrap of information about heredity, environment, and personal behavior is examined scrupulously for some association with the occurrence of the disease in question. In the end, the primary difference between *our* "scientific" and *their* "superstitious" explanations of causality lies in the concept of statistical reasoning. Our epidemiologists crank out highly sophisticated case-control studies whose endpoint is a *P-value*, a best-guess probability that the observed difference in prevalence of disease X between populations having factor A and those lacking it is not due to the vagaries of random chance. They believe in a probabilistic universe where nothing is known with absolute certainty and are committed to abide by the results of "objective" statistical tests. In contrast, those cultures and individuals unable or unwilling to agree that the world is governed by the laws of probability are restricted to explanations involving purposeful intent. From that perspective, it is entirely logical to seek out the source of harm, whether it be enemies, gods, or spirits.

In addition to pervasive supernatural forces, many people throughout the world ascribe the cause of illnesses to disruptions in balances of vital forces. As was mentioned in Chapter 2, the European Hippocratic tradition holds that the four humors—blood, phlegm, yellow bile, and black bile—should be in proper balance. Excesses of one or another result in a person being *sanguine, phlegmatic, choleric, or melancholic* (i.e., in a bad humor)—expressions that have become part of our language, if not of our conscious thought.

The balance of hot–cold, of "heaty" and "cooling" foods, herbs, medicines, and illnesses, is considered of great importance in many parts of the world. Irrespective of their actual temperature or spiciness, some foods are thought to heat or excite the body, others to calm it. Persons with fevers should avoid heaty foods; those with weakness or needing stimulation should avoid cooling foods. Many cultures, including the Aztec, Zapotec, and Maya, developed similar concepts, apparently independently. Whereas the notion is well established in Asia, Latin America, and parts of Europe and Africa, there appears to be little agreement, even locally, about which foods belong in which category. It is generally agreed, however, that maintenance of proper health requires knowledge of inherent, impalpable attributes of foods and proper selection of a balanced diet. Many modern Americans have similar beliefs, for example, about the alleged virtues of organic food or those containing obscure nutrients with scientific-sounding names. The idea of universal opposites is pervasive in many societies and, as in the Chinese *yin* and *yang*, transcends concepts of health and body as a guiding principle for many aspects of everyday life. Contradiction is inherent in all things; right includes some wrong, and wrong includes some right.

What is considered normal in one place may be thought pathogenic elsewhere, and vice versa. More than 150 distinct conditions have been collectively termed *culture-bound syndromes*. These conditions, many of which involve the display of bizarre behavior, are sufficiently common in their own cultures to be recognizable as named diseases. In 1770 Captain James Cook observed persons with the Malayan syndrome *amok*, a "homicidal frenzy preceded by a state of brooding and ending with somnolence and amnesia."[10] Amok is tolerated, even accepted, by the community as expected behavior from someone who is placed in an unbearably embarrassing situation. This is of course the origin of the English phrase "to run amok." These entities are particularly well known to us as deriving from the more traditional areas of the world, perhaps reflecting, as much as anything, the interests and travels of western anthropologists. It must not be thought that culturally associated conditions are limited to illiterate and picturesque natives in faraway places. Americans have their fair share (Table 6-2)."

In parts of Spain and Latin America, a condition called *caída de mollera* is thought to result when the part of an infant's head directly beneath the anterior fontanelle is thought to "drop down," perhaps as a result of pulling the nipple too strongly out of the child's mouth. Vigorous maneuvers are considered necessary to restore the "fallen fontanelle" lest the infant be prevented from eating properly. In one case, a two-month-old child was held by the ankles and his head partially immersed in boiling water—a desperate attempt by his grandmother to cure a condition that she perceived as grave, but which elsewhere in the world is considered perfectly normal.

Every culture is liable to carry forward beliefs regarding health, disease, and the causes of illness that may be deemed quaint, bizarre, or grotesque by foreign observers. In recent years, several outbreaks of severe illness have occurred in the Hispanic communities of Southern California that were traced to capsules containing powdered rattlesnake meat. These capsules, called *polvo de vibora* or *vibora de cascabel*, are considered valuable for the cure of many chronic illnesses, including cancer.[11] Although the products are not known to have any medical benefit, they are often contaminated with pathogenic bacteria, particularly *Salmonella*, which is particularly dangerous to patients already debilitated by serious illness.

Sometimes rituals or practices undertaken for quite different purposes have severe adverse effects on health. One such example is the custom of foot-binding in China. From the tenth century until about 1920, millions of girls suffered the culturally sanctioned infliction of severe pain and deformation as their toes were slowly crushed by tight bandages in an attempt to produce the idealized three-inch *lotus foot*, a prized symbol of eroticism for the men, but a festering, crippling, lifelong infirmity for the women. Attempts made over the years to stop the practice were fruitless and the popularity of foot-binding among both men and women was such that even Manchurian girls imitated Chinese girls in the custom. The custom eventually succumbed to political and cultural changes at the beginning of the present century. Another example is the custom or rite or procedure of circumcision, which has been performed for thousands of years on children of both sexes.

The surgical alteration of the genitalia of females has become a prominent health issue since the late 1970s and was converted to a "cause" for feminists in western

Table 6-2. Some "Culture-Bound" Syndromes and Diseases

Name	Locality	Type[a]	Description
Amok	Malaysia	DP	Outburst of violent behavior
Anorexia nervosa	U.S. whites	A/S	Excessive preoccupation with thinness; self-starvation
Banga	Congo, Malawi		Convulsion, excitement, speech disturbance
Blackout	African Americans		Collapse, dizziness, inability to move
Boufee delirante	Haiti, W. Africa	PS	Sudden aggressive (paranoid) outbursts
Boxi	Nepal		Giddiness, headache, feeling of strangulation
Brain fag	West Africa	A/S	Fatigue from too much thinking
Brujeria	Latin America	IA	See voodoo
Bulimia	U.S. whites		Gross overeating, then vomiting or fasting
Cathard	Polynesia	DP	Similar to amok
Chronic fatigue syndrome	U.S.	A/S	Overwhelming fatigue; variable
Dhat	India	AS	Fear of loss of semen and vitality
Empacho	Hispanics		Intestinal blockage by "excess food"
Falling out	Southern U.S., Caribbean	DP	Sudden collapse; inability to see
Ghost sickness	U.S. Indians	IA	Terror, hallucinations, sense of danger or sickness from witchcraft
Grisi sicknis	Miskitos of Nicaragua, Honduras	DP	Running from attack by devils
Hex	Widespread		See voodoo
Hwa-byung	Korea	IA	Illness from suppression of anger
Hysteria	Greece		Bizarre complaints and behavior
Imu	Japan	DP	Similar to amok
Kesambel	Bali	IA	Illness or death of child from mother's fright
Koro	S. China, S.E. Asia	AS	Intense anxiety that penis is retracting into body
Latah	Malaysia, Indonesia	DP	Hypersuggestibility, trance-like behavior
Mal de pelea	Puerto Rico	DP	Similar to amok
Mal (de) ojo	Mediterranean, American Hispanic		Fitful sleep, crying, diarrhea, in children caused by evil eye of stranger
Malpuesto	Latin America	IA	See voodoo
Nangiarpok	Greenland	AS	Panic on kayaking at sea
Pibloktoq	Polar Eskimos	DP	Extreme excitement, seizures, coma

(continued)

Table 6-2. Some "Culture-Bound" Syndromes and Diseases (*continued*)

Name	Locality	Type[a]	Description
Pseudonite	Sahara	DP	Similar to amok
Qi-gong	China	PS	Acute paranoid psychotic episode
Rootwork	U.S., Caribbean	IA	See voodoo
Saka	Kenya		Anxiety, convulsion, trance-like manner
Shin-byung	Korea	DP	Anxiety, weakness, spirit possession
Suchi-bai	Bengal		Obsessive cleanliness, ritual washing
Susto	Hispanic	IA	Anxiety, trembling, phobias from sudden fright
Taijin kyofusho	Japan	AS	Anxiety that body may displease others
Type A behavior	U.S. whites		Hyperactivity, time urgency, impatience, multitasking
Voodoo	Caribbean, U.S.	IA	Various symptoms or death from witchcraft
Wagamama	Japan		Apathetic childish behavior with emotional outbursts
Waswas	Indonesia		Excessive repetition of words or gestures
Whitiko	Cree Indians	DP	Similar to amok

[a]AS = anxiety state; A/S = affective/somatoform disorder; DP = dissociative phenomenon; IA = illness of attribution; PS = psychotic state.

Source: Adapted in part from Simons and Hughes (1985) and Levine and Gaw. (1995). See originals for more synonyms.

countries in the 1980s and 1990s. The terminology alone is a sensitive issue: More moderate commentators refer to *female circumcision*, while activists prefer *female genital mutilation*, often abbreviated as FGM. Either term refers to a spectrum of procedures of varying severity,[12] performed in many traditional societies primarily in sub-Saharan and northern Africa and adjacent areas. An estimated 100 million living women have undergone ritual genital surgeries at an age varying from infancy to adulthood, depending on their specific culture. Although associated in the western mind with Islam, the practice is common in other groups; in the Moyen-Chari region of Chad, for example, it is most common (96%) among rural Catholics and least common (53%) among urban Protestants.[13] The physical and psychological consequences have been described many times[14] and appear horrifyng to many outsiders. In addition to excruciating pain there is frequent hemorrhage, infection from the use of unclean implements, and trauma to urethra, bladder, and other organs, as well as long-term pelvic inflammatory disease, fistulae, recurrent urinary tract infection, incontinence, difficult and painful intercourse, obstructed labor and/or fetal death, and a host of other dreadful sequelae. International organizations such as WHO and UNICEF have passed resolutions condemning the practice, which has been made illegal in some of the countries involved (e.g., Sudan) and in several European countries (Sweden, United Kingdom). However, powerful cultural beliefs and justifications serve to maintain female circumcision, and mothers in areas where it is practiced are overwhelmingly in favor of performing it on their daughters.[15]

> In the rural Egyptian hamlet where we have conducted fieldwork some women were not familiar with groups that did not circumcise their daughters. When they learned that the female researcher was not circumcised their response was disgust mixed with joking laughter. They wondered how she could have thus gotten married and questioned how her mother could have neglected such an important part of her preparation for womanhood. It was clearly unthinkable to them for a woman not to be circumcised.[16]

We are left impaled on the horns of a moral dilemma. On the one hand we profess respect for individual and cultural autonomy and self-determination. On the other, we feel compelled to condemn what we view as a barbaric and totally unnecessary ritual. Yet women in societies that have adhered to this practice for centuries "have found much of this Western discourse denigrating and reflective of Eurocentric preoccupations with sex, individualism, and other concerns valued in Western societies."[17] It is pointed out that the term FGM is "inflammatory and insulting," and that hundreds of thousands of American women have voluntarily undergone female mammary mutilation (breast augmentation via silicone implants) without corresponding indignation.[18]

Of course, not all traditional rituals are harmful to health. In parts of the Middle East, the practice of leishmanization has gone on for centuries, or perhaps for millennia. In this region, the disease cutaneous leishmaniasis (commonly called Oriental sore) is prevalent, characterized by a disfiguring skin lesion that may be several centimeters in diameter. Very long ago, it was observed that usually a single lesion occurred during one's lifetime. Local people concluded that some sort of immunity had been established, and so it made sense to try to simulate this process by introducing some material from a patient's lesion into the skin of an uninfected person. In this way, a discrete intentional inoculation on a young girl's buttocks could prevent a possibly disfiguring facial lesion that might make her unmarriageable (or reduce her bride-price) later in life. A similar procedure existed in the ancient practice of variolation, in which ground or powdered material from a pustule of smallpox was deliberately transferred to an uninfected person, often by inhalation. The lucky recipient became permanently immune after suffering a mild case of smallpox; the unlucky one might die. A risky business, at best.

According to an intriguing African religious belief, no blood transfusions should be given lest the sins of the donor be transmitted to the recipient. The recent history of AIDS brings a strikingly novel interpretation to that teaching.[19]

When ethnic groups are transplanted to a strange country, their traditional practices, divorced from their appropriate environment, may take on an ominous significance. Customs, universally understood at home, may be misinterpreted by the immigrants' new neighbors. In this way, many Vietnamese families have been accused of child abuse, some even put on trial, because of the time-honored practice of *cao gio* or coin rubbing. The back and chest of the patient are massaged with oil or ointment and then rubbed vigorously with a coin or similar hard object to raise small welts in the belief that circulation, respiration, and body warmth are improved. Alarmed physicians, unfamiliar with this concept, have misinterpreted the helpful intentions of the parents. The name *pseudobattering* has been given to this procedure when practiced in the United States.

BELIEF, BEHAVIOR, AND HEALTH

It is considered improper these days to "stereotype" groups of people on ethnic or cultural grounds, particularly when this is done in a pejorative sense. Individual personalities certainly vary widely in all societies: Some are more outgoing, some more taciturn, some more inquisitive whether in Madras or Tegucigalpa or Stockholm. Nevertheless, the long period of human childhood and dependency is used everywhere for learned socialization—for absorption of and indoctrination into the prevailing value structure. While modified by idiosyncrasy, the broad features of outlook and demeanor are so molded by social forces that certain generalizations or predictions can be made with some confidence.

Travelers inevitably make, and are made the objects of, comparisons of culturally determined behavior. Foreign visitors to the United States are struck by the "pace of life", the emphasis on time, efficiency, and precision; the paperwork; and the computerization of everything. Almost all non-Europeans find it hard to believe that a nine o'clock meeting is expected to start exactly at 9:00. The American attitude toward work and schooling is often different from that in the visitor's home country. A Japanese may consider the American's loyalty to his profession or occupation rather than to his employer puzzling. The elite Brazilian is amazed that wealthy North Americans will do manual work in the garden or on the car, or even help in the kitchen. Upper-class visitors from developing countries often feel that taxi drivers, salespeople, waitresses, and hotel clerks are insufficiently humble and find it extraordinary that the children of wealthy parents will take such "demeaning" jobs during the summer. The holders of these jobs in turn, do not like to be addressed as servants. In a similar vein, the Russian or Iranian student, accustomed to standing when a teacher enters the classroom, may find the informality and lack of social distance between American students and faculty a sign of unbearable disorganization.

It is in the realm of more personal relations that many cultural distinctions emerge. Public displays of affection, such as holding hands between teen-aged boys and girls, are shocking in some societies. But in Pakistan, Russia, Ethiopia, and some other countries, it is common for young men to stroll hand in hand as an innocent manifestation of friendship. Dating, courtship, and marriage are conducted under very different rules in different cultures. The rearing of children has many variants, often studied by anthropologists. While Americans try to encourage independence from an early age, an Egyptian might view a small child's sleeping in his or her own room as callous rejection by the parents. Privacy is looked on in various ways. Many people from the Middle East and Mediterranean areas, for instance, feel free to drop in and visit, or be visited, with a casualness not always appreciated elsewhere. Visitors from bustling tropical cities are struck by the emptiness of streets in American residential areas, particularly in the suburbs.

Attitudes toward women and old persons vary greatly. In many societies, women are expected to be submissive and dependent. The complex division of responsibilities between the sexes makes it at least undignified and perhaps humiliating for a man in West Africa, or much of the Caribbean or Latin America, to go marketing or profess to know anything about domestic chores. Businessmen in much of Asia may refuse to type or use a computer, which they consider the tools of a lower-class occupation. The famous Latin machismo, while an oversimplification, is real and widespread, and often matched by a complementary super-femininity. Grandparents in most countries remain with their families. In most Asian and African traditions, the seniority of age confers authority and engenders respect; persons, even of mature years, would not consider contradicting their parents or acting without their advice and support. Modern Asian countries blend traditional values with technologic pragmatism, but strongly ingrained beliefs modify health-related opinions and activities. Confucian principles of individual responsibility and family loyalty require long-term family care for the elderly, so nursing homes are very rare and serve mainly elderly persons who have no family.[20] The catalogue of cultural and behavioral diversity is endless, and these examples are only a meager sampling. The critical point is that they are all invested with meaning insofar as health and illness behavior are concerned.

Individual Behavior

Where economic conditions permit life free from the constant threat of subnutrition and contaminative diseases, health and illness are to a considerable extent determined by individual behavior. This should not imply that most people purposefully do things that are bad for them; on the contrary, good health and long life are universal goals. But, the glass raised in toast to those very goals at many weddings paradoxically may contain the seed of their negation. It is a common notion, perhaps a bit of yin and yang, that many of the things we enjoy are also a little bit harmful: "All life's pleasures are either fattening or immoral." To which one may add: or atherogenic or carcinogenic.

Although we are interested in an international perspective, the difficulty of getting suitable comparative data on "way of life" and behavioral characteristics of people in different countries is enormous. Some studies in the United States can, therefore, be cited as examples. In Alameda County, California, a questionnaire was answered by almost 7000 adults on certain of their personal habits: cigarette smoking, alcohol consumption, regularity of meals, hours of sleep, weight in relation to height, physical activity, and eating between meals. Highly significant correlations were seen between the number of "good" practices observed and the state of health.[21] In a later follow-up study[22] in the same population, the health practices were associated with mortality, showing that the average expectation of life in males reporting six to seven "good" practices was more than 11 years greater than in those reporting fewer than four; in females, the difference was seven years.

Much evidence indicates that ischemic heart disease and other atherosclerotic diseases arise primarily as a result of what is called "lifestyle." Every year, about one million persons in the United States alone experience either a myocardial infarction or sudden cardiac death, and most other industrial countries (with the notable exception of Japan and France) are reporting high levels of death due to ischemic heart disease. Of the three risk factors commonly cited, cigarette smoking is clearly a consciously chosen behavior trait; serum cholesterol level is usually related to the richness of diet, subject to genetic selection; and hypertension is associated to some degree with salt intake, weight, and perhaps stress. Additional risk factors for atherosclerosis that are commonly recognized include obesity, sedentary living (lack of exercise), and psychosocial tensions, all of which reflect cultural and behavioral characteristics.

A dramatic example of the effects of lifestyle on levels of health comes from a natural experiment involving the populations of two adjacent states in the western United States, Utah and Nevada. "Utah is inhabited primarily by Mormons, whose influence is strong throughout the state. Devout Mormons do not use tobacco or alcohol and, in general, lead stable, quiet lives. Nevada, on the other hand, is a state with high rates of cigarette and alcohol consumption and very high indexes of marital and geographic instability."[23] The adult mortality rate for all causes in Nevada is higher by about 40% to 50% than in Utah, and for the most clearly alcohol- and tobacco-related diseases, liver cirrhosis and lung cancer, the differential is as high as 600%. Many studies have shown that Mormons, Seventh-Day Adventists, Jehovah's Witnesses, and members of other groups with similar moral tenets and subdued lifestyles have far lower prevalence of many diseases than do their more indulgent neighbors. The disastrous consequences of excessive smoking and alcohol consumption in post-Soviet Russia are described in Chapter 13.

Smoking and drinking may be manifestations of reactions to life stresses, which are likely to be more common among persons attuned to achievement than among those whose life runs at a more leisurely, placid pace, one better suited to acceptance than to challenge. This is not to say that harmful health effects associated with tobacco, for example, do not occur in developing countries. By the year 2025 tobacco is expected to cause ten million adult deaths anually.

In parts of South and Southeast Asia and the Pacific, the custom of chewing betel is widespread. The *quid* is made of sliced areca nut, betel leaves, spices, lime, and sometimes tobacco in combinations that vary from place to place. In a 1973 study in Sri Lanka, betel chewing occurred in about 29% of the Sinhalese, Tamils, and Moors, but in a much smaller proportion of the more westernized Burghers. Buccal carcinoma was the most common cancer in Sri Lanka, and cancer of the esophagus was also frequent, but both were very rare among the Burgher group. Among other ethnic groups, women were found to chew more, and more heavily, than men. Contrary to the situation in western countries, esophageal carcinoma was found to be more common among women than men in Sri Lanka.[24] Betel and tobacco chewing both appear to be declining with time and improved education, but tobacco smoking is increasing. It will be interesting to observe the relative rates of oral, pharyngeal, and bronchial carcinoma in these groups over the coming years.

Other types of malignancies appear to be associated with culturally influenced human behavior. Cancer of the uterine cervix has, for over a century, been known to be extremely rare in religious sisters and other chaste women. In contrast, women in prison populations in the United States and Canada have been found to have four to six times as much cervical cancer as in the general population; and of a sample of London prostitutes in 1966, nearly 9% had uterine carcinoma in situ.[25] The association of cervical cancers with age at first intercourse and number of sexual partners has been confirmed in many parts of the world. It is now known that cervical cancer is associated with human papilloma viruses which may be sexually transmitted from male partners. The spread of sexually transmitted diseases in western populations, particularly gonorrhea, syphilis and AIDS, hardly requires documentation.

A person's behavior pattern, largely learned, can affect his or her health, even without the direct exposure to chemical or biological agents just mentioned. The effects of stress, while not yet well understood, are known to be mediated, at least in part, through changes in hormone levels. Animals, placed suddenly in dangerous situations, exhibit "fight or flight" reaction patterns characterized by release of adrenaline, localized vasoconstriction, and other rapid physiologic changes. Chronic or prolonged stress in animals may lead to longer-term adaptations such as arterial hypertension and adrenal hyperplasia. In humans, the roster of psychosomatic diseases is a long one. It has been suggested that coronary heart disease is associated with "type A" behavior, characterized by impatience; moving, walking, and eating rapidly; doing several things at once; feeling guilty when relaxing; having a sense of time urgency; and thinking of everything in numerical terms.[26] Although there is controversy about the significance of these behavior traits with respect to heart disease, it is interesting that they reflect both the impression of Americans gained by foreign visitors and Spengler's picture of the Faustian drive.

In developing countries, atherosclerotic lesions and coronary heart disease are far more rare than in many industrialized countries, even correcting for age distributions. The bimodal social structure in these countries tends to be extreme. The typically small, wealthy leadership group is usually acculturated to an internationalized lifestyle and is affected with increasing frequency by coronary artery disease. The pathologist Zilton Andrade has reported (personal communication) from Salvador, Brazil, that "clinicians who attended wealthy-class patients usually state that they frequently diagnose cases of arteriosclerotic heart disease, a condition which is virtually unknown among poor-class patients dying at similar ages and who are necropsied at the University hospital."

Developing Countries

If the low-income populations of developing countries have low rates of atherosclerosis, it should not be inferred that their lives are free from disease that is, at least in part, of their own making. Even granted the severe limitations of low income, many groups fare far worse than they should because of culturally determined practices, particularly regarding diet. "The despotism of custom," said John Stuart Mill, "is everywhere the standing hindrance to human advancement."[27] It is impossible here to chronicle the many permutations of counterproductive food taboos, which fall most heavily on those least able to tolerate them: children, pregnant women, and lactating mothers. Fish may be withheld from children for fear it may make them ill (Peru, Indonesia, Malaysia). Eggs are linked with illness (India, Lebanon, Syria); mental retardation (East Africa), late speech development (Korea), and licentiousness (various countries). In Togo and elsewhere in West Africa, eggs are kept from children on the grounds that they will come to expect luxuries and grow up to be thieves.[28] In some tropical countries, papaya and similar fruits are thought to cause worms in children. They children may develop xerophthalmia and suffer permanent blindness from the resultant avitaminosis A, an utterly needless tragedy when a papaya tree may be growing quite literally at the doorstep.

Increasing income, permitting greater expenditure for food, may actually lead to impoverishment, rather than improvement, in diet. In South Asia, food preference may go from sorghum or millet to home-polished rice to commercially polished rice. Not only thiamine and other vitamins but a good deal of protein may be lost by these refinements of natural food grains. For reasons of prestige, white corn has replaced yellow corn in parts of Latin America, with consequent loss of methionine and vitamin A; or corn (maize) tortillas may be given up entirely in favor of white bread. The "Coca-Colanization" of the world shows how rapidly cultural changes can occur. In India, more costly, but less nutritious, substitutes may replace the abundant greens, fruits, and legumes. In virtually all countries, the rapid spread of sweets, soft drinks, and other "junk" foods is well documented.

Advertising, Social Marketing, or Propaganda?

Whereas propaganda for some purposes, such as the use of automobile seat belts, may be more or less effective, constant repetition of other health messages sometimes achieves a useful behavioral change. In Jamaica, a serious veno-occlusive disease of the liver can result from drinking tea made from the plant *Crotalaria fulva*, which contains powerful alkaloids. Between 1935 and 1960, this disease was practically eliminated from the island through propaganda against drinking "bush tea."[29] (In Afghanistan, a similar disease results from eating bread contaminated with the seeds of a kind of *Heliotropium* flower.) In the United States, the proportion of adult males who smoke cigarettes has declined continuously since the late 1950s, as a result of which coronary heart disease may have peaked and begun to decline in middle-aged American men. Intensive publicity regarding the harmful effects of cigarette smoking undoubtedly played a part in this favorable trend. Not so encouraging, however, is the rise in the proportion of females who smoke cigarettes, an increase probably responsible in part for the recent tripling of female lung cancer rates in the San Francisco, California, area. Commercial advertising designed to appeal to the female market may be a powerful factor behind this increase. The portrayal of certain behaviors (such as smoking cigarettes) as glamorous, sophisticated, and attractive to the opposite sex is the stock in trade of the advertising industry everywhere. Straightening curly hair, curling straight hair, darkening light skin by tanning, and lightening dark skin by bleaching are all examples of "needs" perhaps created by culture but reinforced by advertising and the promise of satisfaction by the sponsor's product.

Commercial advertisers often have substantial resources at their disposal and can raise the prospect of rapid gratification. Public health authorities and others who try to change customary behavior in order to achieve better health usually have a more difficult road before them. Recent years have seen the introduction of "social marketing" programs in many countries based on the principles of commercial advertising. While it is clear that pest control projects in Buddhist countries are incompatible with prevailing religious belief against killing living creatures, it may not be so evident that classes for expectant mothers in Chile are inconsistent with local ideas of pride and dignity. When the classes were changed to "club meetings" and held in homes rather than in schools, they were perceived as social events and women attended readily. A series of case histories of public health projects that have encountered culturally based resistance in a variety of settings has become an anthropological classic.[30] The account of water boiling in a Peruvian village is perhaps the best known and illustrates some frustrations of cross-cultural health education.

In a village of 200 families, only 15 housewives boiled their drinking water for hygienic reasons. The local health department, noting the high incidence of water-borne disease, sent a health worker to the village to try to convince more housewives to boil their families' drinking water. After two years of effort, with the occasional support of a visiting physician, the health worker was able to influence only 11 housewives to boil drinking water. Many people resisted this change in habits, in part because boiled water was considered as suitable only for sickly people and in part because of reluctance to abandon long established traditions. In a similar vein, purification of water was resisted by Mexican villagers because water, as the creative source of life, was considered sacred; natural water, therefore, cannot be bad, and tampering with it is viewed as sacrilege.[31]

It is not only villagers in remote areas who may object to adoption of what appear to the western scientist as innocuous and obviously beneficial practices. In a modern industrial plant in Singapore, some workers refused to wear a cartridge respirator for protection from toxic fumes—not because of discomfort, but because "it looks like a pig's snout!"[32] In a poor area of northeastern Brazil, a public health poster urging cholera control (Fig. 6-1) was widely misinterpreted. The text reads, CHOLERA—DON'T CLOSE YOUR EYES TO LIFE—HELP COMBAT CHOLERA, but it aroused strong antigovernment suspicions.

> No more vivid and convincing evidence was needed, residents lamented, that the true "battle ahead" was against the "cholera poor;" they were being "identified during house-to-house searches, rounded up, tested, blindfolded, and done in." The blindfolded man depicted on the poster, we were told by informants, was "marked to die" . . . the blindfolded man and red "X" meant one thing to State Secretary of Health Cholera Control workers and something quite different to families living in poverty.[33]

Resistance to immunization is widespread, for a variety of reasons. Many educated people in western countries, including George Bernard Shaw, have campaigned against compulsory immunization. Public health authorities have launched many campaigns against measles, one of the most highly fatal diseases of young children in West Africa. In some areas, the "jet injectors" were viewed with terror, and residents made elaborate plans to avoid immunization, sometimes rehearsing for weeks to escape from the roving public health teams. The tragic aftermath of such an incident in the village of Sossobee, in the Bambara-speaking region of Mali, has been described:

> The chief who sat next to me on a straw mat said that one hundred and twenty-eight children had died in a month's time, almost half of those who had contracted measles. The epidemic began several weeks after a small girl from a neighboring village arrived in Sossobee with measles, but the chief and the elders did not draw any con-

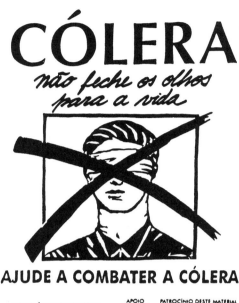

CHOLERA

Don't close your eyes
to life.

CÓLERA
*não feche os olhos
para a vida*

AJUDE A COMBATER A CÓLERA

COMISSÃO DE PREVENÇÃO E
CONTROLE DA CÓLERA

APOIO

PATROCÍNIO DESTE MATERIAL

DISQUE CÓLERA · 192187

HELP COMBAT CHOLERA

Figure 6-1 Official cholera campaign poster interpreted as war against the infected poor: marked for erradication—that is, "execution." Source: Reprinted from Nations and Monte (1996). Fig. 1. Social Science and Medicine, vol. 43. Copyright 1996, with permission from Elsevier Science.

nection between the first case and the subsequent epidemic. For them the epidemic was a manifestation of God's will, the result of an evil wind which had blown in from the swamps and plains of the delta and penetrated the skins of their children. It wasn't long before scores of children were ill with coughs, running eyes and fever and shortly thereafter rashes came out. The people of Sossobee like all the Bambara attempted to bring out the rash as quickly as possible in their children because they have over the years made the empirical observation that once the rash appears the prodromal symptoms disappear. The children were given honey by mouth and had their skins rubbed with honey, monkey feces and dirt from termite hills so that the rash would come out. Because of the tremendous concern for the rash to appear, children were not washed with water and were kept in the dark interior of their huts until the illness was over. The children were given purges of tamarind juice in order to drive the illness out of the interior of the body and into the skin. Although the sick children were dehydrated from their high fevers and from being kept in the hot unventilated huts, their parents refused to give them anything to drink for fear of impeding the development of the rash. They diminished their food intake, prohibited them from eating meat and put honey, goat's milk, tamarind juice and peanut flour solution in their eyes in the hope of preventing blinding corneal ulcers. Parents abstained from sexual relations because they believed that it worsens measles in their children. The people of Sossobee family believed that all of the practices and treatments they employed were for the benefit of their sick children and could not understand that sick children with high fevers needed protein and fluids, that serious eye infections with permanent damage resulted from the ophthalmic preparations they used, that purges were nefarious and solutions rubbed on the skin the cause of serious dermatitis. What was undertaken with the finest of intentions was in reality a major cause of the high morbidity and mortality associated with the epidemic.[34]

In a similar vein, a colleague has written to me, "In Brazil families would hide their children from health workers. What changed their tune was when they saw how beneficial vaccination was for the survival of their cattle, then they were willing to allow their children to be vaccinated."

SICKNESS

From the viewpoint of medical anthropology, culture refers to ways of perceiving and organizing ideas about health and illness as modified by the traditions of society. The concerns of the medical sociologist, by contrast, are with the relationships of individuals, the interactions between them, and their place within the context of a society's institutional structures.

To decide whether or not a person is sick is often highly situational. Infection with the parasitic worm *Schistosoma haematobium* is a common cause of blood in the urine. This sign, which would prompt most Europeans or Americans to see a physician, may be considered perfectly normal in areas in which urinary schistosomiasis is endemic. Small children with swollen bellies, characteristic of severe malnutrition, may be viewed with pride as good and fat by uneducated mothers. In contrast, a plump but healthy middle-aged housewife may decide to seek medical help for reduction of weight that she perceives as excessive only after her husband has taken an interest in a younger and slimmer woman. Standards of normality and tolerability of any particular type of perceived deviation vary from one person and community to another, and also from one time to another.

A patient (or mother) who consults a healer or physician is likely to have a tentative diagnosis in mind. The patient's and the practitioner's views often coincide, but it is possible that the two will have quite different assumptions about the nature of the episode. The medical paradigm and the patient's views may be dissonant, generally in proportion to the educational and social distance between the two parties. One might expect greater agreement when a villager consults a traditional healer, or when an educated city-dweller sees a physician, than in the opposite situations. The range of opinions of the two parties regarding the presence of any specific disease or condition can be shown as any of nine possible outcomes:

DOES A PATIENT HAVE A CONDITION?
THE PATIENT'S AND PRACTITIONER'S VIEWS

		Professional Medical Determination		
		No	Maybe	Yes
	No	NN	NM	NY
Patient's perception	*Maybe*	MN	MM	MY
	Yes	YN	YM	YY

Here, YN means that the patient believes himself (or his/her child) to have the condition, but the professional medical determination says otherwise; NY indicates just the opposite; and MM means that both parties entertain the possibility, but without great conviction.

There are four possible classes of outcome in this situation:

DOES A PATIENT HAVE A CONDITION?
THE FOUR CLASSES OF OUTCOME COMBINATIONS

Agreement	Ambiguity	Tension		Conflict
YY	MM	NM	YM	YN
NN		MN	MY	NY

The best kind of outcome is mutual agreement, in which both parties interpret the same signs and symptoms in the same way, but there may also be negotiated agreement or consensus with varying levels of persuasion, or grudging acceptance achieved through authoritarian means. Note that neither the patient's perception nor the professional determination need necessarily correspond with reality—that is, an objectively correct diagnosis. Both parties might agree, and both might be wrong.

One can readily envision a situation in which each of the nine dyads of opinion can be held. Consider the import of each combination for the diagnosis of lung cancer, pregnancy, spirit possession, malaria, sinus trouble, or your choice of condition. The therapeutic implications of the "Medical Y"—where the professional believes the condition to exist—usually can be met through the medical care system to which the professional belongs. To satisfy the needs of the "Patient Y," there may ensue some patient-initiated activity intended to reduce anxiety or uncertainty: self-treatment, seeking a second opinion, or undertaking a religious practice, for example.

The functional significance of this exercise lies in the level of patient compliance with medical advice. The outcome classes Ambiguity, Tension, and Conflict carry an increasing level of mistrust. Patients in these situations are increasingly unlikely to carry out medical instructions such as obtaining an immunization, taking a prescription correctly, or giving oral rehydration therapy to a diarrheic child. Then, if the practitioner was right and the patient wrong about the diagnosis (in an NY situation), poor patient compliance with instructions will more likely lead to an unsatisfactory outcome and the patient's mistrust will be reinforced. The reverse (YN) situation may expose the patient to unneeded or perhaps inappropriate procedures with the same unfortunate outcome. One can work out other scenarios and assess the consequences.

The interaction of doctor and patient is not an unstructured event. Each participant has a particular role to play, in the view of sociologists. Even if the two individuals have not previously met, they have learned to expect certain things and to act in certain ways provided they are similarly acculturated. Even so, the layman and the physician may have very different understandings of a particular episode of illness. The patient may find it rewarding to enter into the *sick role*, a socially institutionalized situation elaborated on in many studies by Talcott Parsons and others. In this view the patient's incapacity is held to be beyond his own power to overcome by an act of will. He can therefore not be "held responsible" for his incapacity, and being sick exempts him to some extent from normal role and task obligations. However, the sick person must recognize that she should want and try to get well and to work with others to this end; she and her family should seek competent help and cooperate with attempts to help her get well. The particular rights and obligations associated with being sick vary greatly from one culture to another and by age, sex, and status.

Since illness is recognized as an acceptable cause for withdrawing from certain role obligations, social responsibilities, and expectations, persons may be drawn to the patient role in order to obtain secondary advantages, to make claims on others for care and attention, and to provide an acceptable reason for social failure. Thus individuals may be motivated to adopt the 'sick role' . . . and others may be anxious to accord people the status of sickness in order to avoid embarrassment and social difficulties. The interpenetration between medical and other social institutions is quite complex, and often these relationships are not fully appreciated.[35]

Seeking Help

A person's decision to seek assistance from a practitioner may follow a reasoning process (largely intuitive) like the one charted in Table 6-3. It must be noted once more that many problems considered within their province by scientific physicians

Table 6-3. Stages in the Decision to Seek Treatment

1. Is there a problem?	*7. Could it be made worse by trying to alleviate it*
	a. by myself?
2. Do I know what it Is?	b. by family or friend?
	c. by a professional?
3. Is it harmful?	
	8. Will it cost a lot for treatment by
4. Is it likely to	a. myself?
a. improve by itself?	b. family or friend?
b. stay the same?	c. a professional?
c. deteriorate?	d. a God?
5. Is it remediable at all?	*9. Will the cost be in*
	a. money?
6. Can it be alleviated by	b. time?
a. myself?	c. pain?
b. family or friend?	d. embarrassment?
c. a professional?	
d. a God?	*10. Is the probable benefit worth the probable cost?*

are not perceived as such by many others. Numberless are the bowls of chicken soup prepared by persons who answer "yes" to 6a or 6b.

Data on actual rates of utilization of available medical services are hard to find for industrialized countries and pretty much nonexistent elsewhere. The few surveys that have been done have shown that a great deal of perceived minor illness is not brought to medical attention. In the United States each thousand adults 16 years and over experience about 750 episodes of some sort of illness per month, of which about 250 are brought to a physician. Two-thirds of all recognized illness in those groups are therefore treated by the individual, the family, or not at all. Conversely, many visits to physicians are not made for the cure or treatment of illness, but for insurance examinations, certification for absence from school or work, or similar reasons. Routine periodic checkups have historically taken up much physician time in the United States, but in an era of managed care their usefulness for asymptomatic adults has been seriously questioned, and they are becoming rare. Many other physician visits are for conditions that may or may not be considered as cases of any disease. Are these people sick, or ill, or both, or neither?[36] A great deal of medical effort is expended in reassuring patients about one or another worry and trying to satisfy their emotional needs. In the United States assisted reproduction via *in vitro* fertilization and other technologies is widely practiced. But is childlessness a *disease*, particularly if an older woman has deliberately resisted pregnancy during her most fertile years? Is pattern baldness in males or having smaller than desired breasts in females a disease?

The practice of esthetic surgery is not limited to wealthy southern California. In Rio de Janeiro, where physical appearance is highly prized, face-lifts and tummy tucks occupy the dreams of society matrons and the talents of 500 surgeons while thousands of children suffer from malnutrition and chronic diarrhea in the crowded *favelas* a few blocks away. Here, as in the cases of bound feet and clitoridectomy, predominant cultural values prescribe a situation viewed as normal by its participants and considered bizarre by some others.

The Clinical Encounter

A physician who is raised and educated in one culture may find it difficult or impossible to deal with patients from another culture (and vice versa) except on the most simple, mechanistic level. This is true not only with "foreign" doctors or patients but within almost all countries as well. In developing countries physicians generally come from the affluent segment of society and will probably have little in common with their poorer compatriots in their conceptualization of illness. In all countries a vague physical complaint may conceal an underlying emotional problem which is difficult for the person to express directly. The physician may interpret this as malingering. The patient, who seeks validation of his illness and legitimization of his sick role, accuses the physician of lack of sympathy. The physician may expect strict compliance with his or her instructions; for example, medication in the proper dosage to be taken at the proper intervals. The patient may expect immediate results from the drug and may see no need to continue with the prescribed course if rapid relief is obtained (or if it is not). A medically sound request for a follow-up visit may be seen by the patient as a needless waste of time and money and an instance of greed by the physician.

Some physicians and medical workers do take unfair advantage of the fears and naivete of an uneducated public. In Pakistan, for example, impoverished urban squatters and rural village residents believe that breast milk can become 'poisoned'

> by a "shadow" from the spirit world; by "evil eye" or black magic due to others' envy; by the effects of a new pregnancy; by the mother's illness or "weakness"; by her exposure to excessive cold or heat; by her dietary indiscretions . . . if a child is sickly, cries a great deal, has prolonged diarrhea, or seems reluctant to suck, mothers frequently become alarmed and suspect irreversible breastmilk "poisoning." In the latter case, a folk healer has traditionally been consulted to test the milk's quality, but in recent years pathology laboratories have increasingly taken on this function in all of the major cities of Pakistan. Not only does the mother stop breastfeeding while the milk is being tested,

but often she is unable or unwilling to resume nursing even if the milk is eventually pronounced safe to drink. This manifestation of inappropriate, child-endangring technology has gained acceptance partly because of maternal anxieties heightened by commercially-driven pressures to be "modern" and partly because of its congruence with traditional ideas surrounding breastmilk, many of which have classical antecedents.[37]

In western medical practice, particularly in the United States, the clinical encounter sometimes has overtones of confrontation, in which the physician is "challenged" to perform to the patient's expectations by implicit threat of legal action for malpractice, to which the physician responds by the excesses of defensive medicine, adding to the patient's expense and detracting from innovative (or perhaps even appropriate) treatment. This problem can perhaps be interpreted as emergence of patient and physician subcultures, with divergent goals and values.

In most traditional communities, by contrast, the patient and healer may be culturally more closely integrated, sharing the same values and outlook and often joining with family and friends to undertake the healing process. The curandero, bomoh, shaman, herbalist, or local pharmacist, while lacking in technical sophistication, generally speak the same cultural language as the patient.

SICKNESS, ILLNESS, AND SOCIETAL GOALS

Early recognition of illness or potential illness is a major goal of preventive medicine. The mobile X-ray unit, the Pap smear, mammograms, blood pressure measurements, biochemical tests for newborns, and other screening techniques are all designed to accelerate the process of becoming a patient if that is appropriate. Much attention has also been devoted in industrialized countries to reinforcing the decision to seek professional help, and quickly, as in the case of chest pain or suspicion of a warning sign of cancer. An important social role of the health care system is to minimize real illness, which is highly disruptive of individual and group functioning. In this respect, the spartan man with severe chest pains who decides to be tough and do nothing presents a greater problem in the long run than his excitable neighbor who appears for an electrocardiogram with minimal indications. The social cost of incapacitating illness and premature death is so high that a certain proportion of false alarms is readily acceptable provided the true cases are also identified. Detection of an illness in its early stages permits some medical intervention, at least in theory, to keep it from becoming (more) disruptive and expensive. This process of tracking with the intention of arresting an existing condition is known as secondary prevention. But the social system may have an equal, or greater, interest in primary prevention—that is, keeping an illness from developing at all, as by immunization, genetic counseling, water purification, ritual ceremony, observance of taboo, wearing of amulets or symbols, or other means. A comprehensive health care system must therefore be concerned with the nonpatient as well as with the patient.

NOTES

1. Paul (1955).
2. (Published 1926–1928).
3. Grenholm (1983).
4. Frazer (1950).
5. Wolff (1965).
6. Gelfand (1971).
7. Murdock (1980).
8. Azevedo et al. (1995).
9. Rosenberg (1962)
10. Levine and Gaw (1995). Many culture-bound syndromes are covered in this review.
11. One is reminded of the significance of rattlesnakes to the Aztecs and Maya, and modern-day Mexican culture. There is a rattlenake on the national flag of Mexico.
12. At a minimum part or all of the clitoris is removed, and often part or all of the labia. The stages have been categorized by Toubia (1994).
13. Leonard (1996).
14. See for example Elchal et al. (1997) .
15. Dirie and Lindmark (1991).
16. Lane and Rubinstein (1996).
17. Ibid.
18. Erwin and Hackler (1998).
19. Markos (1983).
20. Peabody *et al.* (1995).
21. Belloc and Breslow (1972).
22. Belloc (1973).
23. Fuchs (1974).
24. Senewiratne and Uragoda (1973).
25. Kessler and Aurelian (1975).
26. Friedman and Rosenman (1974) .
27. Mill (1859).
28. Berg (1973).
29. Williams and Jelliffe (1972).
30. Paul (1955).
31. Northrop (1959).
32. Phoon (1975).
33. Nations and Monte (1996).
34. Imperato (1975).
35. Mechanic (1972).
36. In later chapters we will discuss the effectiveness of health expenditures and setting priorities for publicly funded medical care.
37. Mull (1992).

7

Health on the Edge

[T]here is no doubt that the main threat to health development today is poverty. In spite of dramatic global economic growth, a quarter of the world's population today is still affected by severe poverty and the gaps between rich and poor are widening. Poverty not only increases the risk of ill-health and vulnerability of people, it also has serious implications for the delivery of effective health care such as reduced demand for services, lack of continuity or compliance in medical treatment, and increased transmission of infectious diseases. Poverty may lead to inequities in access to health care which in turn has implications both for health service capacity and costs which are reflected in, for example, higher rates of complications due to late arrival of patients. At the same time, a lack of adequate free or low cost health services for those unable to pay contributes to further impoverishment of the poor. Growing evidence suggests that health-related risk events may well be the first step towards permanent poverty.[1]

Poverty means much more than not having money. A rich person who becomes bankrupt does not become a poor person in the social/cultural sense, just as a poor person who wins the lottery does not take on the mind-set of the wealthy. Some sociologists have discerned a corresponding "culture of poverty" that "transcends regional, rural-urban and national differences and shows remarkable cross-national similarities."[2] Poverty generally includes the following elements: inadequate income; lack of education, knowledge, and skill; poor health status and lack of access to health care; poor housing; lack of access to safe water and sanitation; insufficient food and nutrition; lack of control over the reproductive process.[3] As a factor influencing health status, poverty has been given a separate ICD-10 code, Z59.5 (see Table 4-10). Some of the dimensions of poverty are shown on Table 7-1.

Poverty also has moral and ethical dimensions. It produces immense suffering

Table 7-1. Some Dimensions of Poverty

Deprivation	Lack of physical necessities, assets and income
Social subordination	Implied inferiority based, e.g., on education, language, social class, caste, religion, race or ethnic group, occupation, residence, gender, or physical, mental, or emotional status
Marginalization	Exclusion from access to social services, education and literacy, markets, employment, housing, travel, communication, contacts, information, and other forms of support that are available to others
Ill health	Disability, sickness, pain and suffering, shortened life span, reduced stamina and capacity to learn, work, and contribute to the welfare of self and others in the household and community
Exploitation	Lack of protection from, and increased susceptibility to, physical, social, and biological hazards. Economic or sexual exploitation. Low pay and few or no benefits. Charged higher prices for merchandise and services; dealt low quality goods, expired drugs. Discounts or credit unavailable
Powerlessness	Little bargaining power or ability to influence events that affect personal, household, and community welfare. Dependency on, and often victimization by, dominant individuals and groups. Inappropriate use of medicines due to inability to afford a full course of treatment
Hopelessness	Inability to advance economically and personally or to provide for family. Frustration in developing and applying talents or achieving full potential. Little optimism for future
Humiliation	Treatment by others with lack of respect, leading to reduced self-respect. Often, harrassment by police and others in authority. Family disintegration from need to find work elsewhere
Time and planning	Lack of leisure, recreational, or cultural activities because available time is needed for survival. Inability to invest or plan for the future because full attention is given to the needs of the present
Environment	Overcrowding, noise; odors; mud; pollution; exposure to elements, vectors, and pathogens; substandard housing; lack of privacy and physical security

Source: Inspired by Table 1, in Sköld (1998).

and injustice and diminishes not only those caught in its grip but the entire global society. Poverty frustrates individual potential and denies the benefits of their contributions to everyone else. Intelligence and imagination know no borders: The child that died unnecessarily in a Third World slum might have been a great scientist or engineer; another, given some schooling, could be an influential writer, teacher, or composer; and even modest means might nurture a leader in commerce or government. Poverty is a synonym for wasted human resources, thwarted ambitions, and squandered talents that are so desperately needed for everybody's benefit.

But poverty, though it do not prevent the generation, is extremely unfavourable to the rearing of children ... It is not uncommon, I have been frequently told, in the Highlands of Scotland for a mother who has borne 20 children not to have two alive ... This great mortality, however, will everywhere be found chiefly among the children of the common people, who cannot afford to tend them with the same care as those of a better station.[4]

The United Nations Development Programme has devised a *Human Poverty Index* (HPI), a composite multidimensional scale, for its annual *Human Development Report*. The HPI accounts for:

- Longevity (percent of people expected to die before 40)
- Knowledge (percent adult literacy)
- Decent standard of living
- Percent of people with access to health care and safe water
- Percent of children under five malnourished

Poverty is the single underlying cause of most ill health in the world today. It follows that relieving poverty will benefit individual, national, and global health. But economic and social policies concerning poverty are usually directed toward managing its consequences rather than toward relieving the processes that create and perpetuate it. The health sector in general has found it difficult to meet the immediate needs of the poor and has not seen the eradication of poverty as part of its mandate. Yet, after education, improved health may provide the means by which the poorest groups can help themselves to improve their situation. Therefore the ultimate means to improve human health would be an all-out attack on poverty. The UNDP 1997 report placed the cost of ridding the world of poverty at a very modest (and optimistic) $80 billion a year.

Poverty is a main cause of ill health, and the reverse can also be true. In marginal economies the illness of a breadwinner results in loss of income and earning capacity, forcing a household to borrow, often under usurious conditions, thereby becoming poorer. The derivative poverty can lead to malnutrition in children and to greater exposure and susceptibillity to infection. The illness of a child, or of its mother, can then produce further economic strain in an insoluble spiral of poverty and ill health.

Poverty is also an expensive lifestyle, in money and time. Poor people pay more for many things and they are often cheated; their property is subject to theft or destruction; they must wait for buses and medical care and most else in life. Their time horizon is short. Having nothing to spare from immediate needs they cannot invest for tomorrow, and they collect no interest or dividends as more wealthy people do. In at least in one city (Table 7-2), the cost of good water is highest to those who can least afford it, and the poor in many cities must buy low quality water from itinerant vendors. Even in areas where water is "free"—that is, in streams or ponds, there are costs in addition to the cost of contamination. Studies from several countries indicate that some poor people often spend from 100 to 300 minutes per day collecting water for domestic purposes. Therefore, considering infant mortality from diarrheal diseases, the provision of good water within easy access would have ben-

Table 7-2. Usage and Cost of Water, by Source, Lima, Peru

Relative Quality	Source	Consumption liters/Day/Person	Cost	
			Soles[a]	U.S. Dollars
Poor	Vendors	23	105	3.49
Medium	Standpipe	78	22	0.51
Good	Piped to House	152	35	0.81

[a]In 1972 $1 = 43 soles.

Source: Briscoe (1984).

efits not only in reducing infection directly but also in increasing time available for child care or other productive activities by mothers.

As mentioned, knowledge of the relationship between economic level and ill health is not new. Edwin Chadwick published careful records, made in the London of Disraeli's time, to show how the life experiences of each definable segment of society are reflected in its health, sickness, and mortality. For the highest social class of the 1840s (gentry, professional persons, and their families), the infant mortality rate was 100 per thousand live births and mean life expectancy was 44 years—both figures characteristic of the very poorest countries today. The British Registrar General has since 1911 classified occupations (not persons) in five official social classes, depending upon their general standing within the community. These are:

I   Professional, etc., occupations (e.g., law, medicine, the Church)
II   Intermediate occupations (e.g., employers, managers, farmers)
III Skilled occupations (e.g., fitters, clerks, engine drivers)
IV   Partly skilled occupations (e.g., machine minders)
V   Unskilled occupations (e.g., labourers, kitchen hands)

The designation of social class is fraught with uncertainty and conflict. In the United States the term is anathema to devotees of political correctness, and has been construed by some as a veiled proxy for ethnicity or race. In Britain, the designation of social and occupational classes is also a matter of contention and has been severely criticized.[5] Also, occupations and their classification change over time: there were no computer programmers before there were computers. Nevertheless, it is interesting to compare recent mortality rates by nominal social class in Britain (Table 7-3) with those of 1840. The Black Report, commissioned by the Labour government in England, reported in 1980 that those in the lowest social class had mortality rates twice as high as those in the highest class. "Thirty years after the National Health Service was set up in Britain, the Black Committee concluded that inequalities in health had widened, despite universal access to medical care, because the determinants of inequalities in health lay elsewhere."[6]

A comparable inverse relationship between socioeconomic status and mortality

Table 7-3. Mortality by Year and Social Class, Men Aged 15–64, England and Wales, 1930 to 1982[a]

Social Class	Year					
	1930–1932	1949–1953	1959–1963[b]	1970–1972	1979–1980[c]	1982–1983
I. Professional	90		86	75	77	66
II. Intermediate		94	92	81	81	76
IIINM. Skilled NM[d]					99	94
	97		101	100		
IIIM. Skilled manual					106	106
IV. Partly skilled		102	104	103	114	116
V. Unskilled	111	118	127	137	165	

[a]Standardized mortality ratios; all men = 100.

[b]Adjusted figures; occupations reclassified according to 1950 classification.

[c]Men aged 20–64.

[d]NM = Nonmanual.

Source: Marmot and Feeney (1997a) Table 1.

is maintained at all ages and in all countries. Note that not all specific causes of death follow this pattern. In a study of 24 types of cancer in 37 populations in 21 countries,

> More or less consistent excess risks in men in lower social strata were observed for all respiratory cancers (nose, larynx and lung) and cancers of the oral cavity and pharynx, esophagus, stomach, and, with a number of exceptions, liver, as well as for all malignancies taken together. For women, low-class excesses were consistently encountered for cancers of the esophagus, stomach, cervix uteri and, less consistently, liver. Men in higher social strata displayed excesses of colon and brain cancers and skin melanoma. In the two Latin American populations for which data were available, lung cancer was more frequent in higher social strata. Excesses in high female socioeconomic strata were seen in most populations for cancers of the colon, breast and ovary, and for skin melanoma.[7]

Throughout the history of British concern about socioeconomic differentials in death rates four suggested explanations have persisted, with continuing debates among environmentalists, hereditarians, and those emphasizing personal ignorance or irresponsibility.[8] In a thorough analysis of social inequalities in health. Marmot and Feeney[9] evaluated the following elements: medical care; health selection (i.e., poor health determines social class, not the reverse); factors operating in early life; general susceptibility to illnesses (*versus* specific factors); health-related behaviors and biological risk factors; material conditions of life; and psychosocial factors.

It is important to consider whether the observed *inequalities* are a result of *inequities*—that is, some sort of unequal, perhaps unfair, biased or neglectful treatment by society of some people in comparison with others. If that is so, such injustice may be eliminated or at least minimized by compensatory social changes of one kind or another. If that is not so, then either it is futile to expect any sort of social manipulation to even out health status and longevity among social classes, or else special attention must be given to assist the less competitive elements of the population.

Many studies in the United States have shown that low income and resultant low educational attainment are associated with low utilization of services such as childhood immunization, mammography and cervical cancer screening, and other available preventive health measures. Diets are often poor by current standards, with a surplus of carbohydrates and fats and a deficiency in fresh fruits and vegetables, smoking rates may be greater, and purposeful exercise less.

THE LIMITS OF WEALTH

If poverty induces ill health, we may ask whether greater wealth leads, in the aggregate, to continually better health. Evidence suggests that this is not so. Richard Wilkinson believes that

> Rising living standards were the basis of the historical decline of mortality in the developed world. While it is possible to argue the relative historical contributions of better nutrition, sewers, clean water supplies, improved housing, and, eventually, immunization to the long decline in mortality rates in the developed world, there can be no doubt that the enabling and sustaining power of economic growth was behind them all . . . Although it is clear that life expectancy rises steeply with increased GNPpc [gross national product per capita] among the poorer countries . . . the relationship between GNPpc and mortality peters out in the developed world. Apparently, there is some minimum level of income (around $5,000 per capita in 1990) above which the absolute standard of living ceases to have much impact on health.[10]

Furthermore, Wilkinson suggests that as countries get richer, proportional changes in income produce diminishing absolute returns in life expectancy. The countries with the highest life expectancies are not those with the greatest wealth, but those with the smallest spread of incomes and the smallest proportion of their populations in poverty. According to this theory, it is the degree of income inequality within a society, not the absolute level of income, that is correlated with levels of health and illness. The basis for such a relationship is still unexplained, although adherents have suggested that stress may play a role. Perhaps there is something detrimental about low status in a hierarchical society, including economic and social insecurity and the threat of unemployment and other causes, that have strong effects on health.

Poorly understood psychosocial mechanisms may be involved if the threat of insecurity, low social support, poor job satisfaction, and similar stressors produce ill health. Housing insecurity, debt, and other financial stress also have been linked to poorer health outcomes.

Various measures of income distribution have been proposed by economists. Perhaps the best known of these is the *Gini coefficient*, an innovation of Italian demographer Corrodo Gini, designed to indicate the degree of equality or inequality in the distribution of income within the economic deciles of a population. By this measure, if each tenth of the population received one-tenth of the income the Gini coefficient would be zero and the ideal egalitarian distribution model would be fulfilled. In contrast, the most inequitable distribution would find the upper tenth receiving all of the income and the remaining nine-tenths none, and the Gini coefficient would be 1.0. In fact, the Gini coefficient never approaches these hypothetical extremes, but an increase in the coefficient shows that income distribution is becoming less equal. Income inequality appears to be increasing almost everywhere. The U.S. Gini coefficient rose from 0.394 in 1970 to 0.456 in 1994. In Taiwan, the household Gini coefficient rose from 0.259 in 1980 0.29 in 1992.[11] Globally, 40% of the world's population receives less than 5% of the income, and 20% receives about 70% of the income. It is said that the net worth of the one thousand wealthiest people on earth is equal to the net worth of 50% of all humanity, and that even in the United States a single individual has as much wealth as the lower 40% of the population.

Everyone concedes that poor people are less healthy than rich people, but not everyone is convinced that inequitable income distribution *per se* is a determinant of ill health in a population. In a detailed study of male deaths in 11 European countries, men were classified by occupation into ten categories. The study confirmed once again the repeated finding that mortality rates were higher for manual than for nonmanual classes in all countries studied. It concluded, however, that "There is no evidence that mortality differences are smaller in countries with more egalitarian socio-economic and other policies."[12]

THE HEALTH OF CHILDREN

Since the late 1980s several international meetings have emphasized the well-being of children. The Declaration of Talloires (France), adopted in March 1988 by the Task Force for Child Survival, set a series of goals to be achieved by the year 2000.[13] The Convention on the Rights of the Child was adopted by the United Nations General Assembly in November 1989, followed in four months by the World Conference on Education for All.[14] The largest conference was the World Summit for Children, which brought 158 presidents and prime ministers to United Nations headquarters in New York in September 1990. All of these conferences have energized governments and international donors regarding the importance of early childhood development and education. One such program was launched by U.S. congressional mandate in ten sub-Saharan African countries by the U.S. Agency for International Development in cooperation with the U.S. Centers for Disease Control and Prevention. The Combatting Childhood Communicable Disease (CCCD) project, as it was called, concentrated on immunization and the treatment of diarrhea and malaria. Attention was also given to public education, health care financing, and operational research, including the training of health professionals in epidemiological methods and computerization. Numerous other large and small child health projects have been launched by various agencies. Prominent among these is UNICEF's GOBI program (standing for *G*rowth monitoring, *O*ral rehydration, *B*reastfeeding, and *I*mmunization) or its augmented form, GOBI-FFF (incorporating *F*ood supplementation, *F*emale literacy, and *F*amily planning).

Many clinics and health posts distribute printed educational materials to mothers of newborn infants. Usually these materials include a card for the mother to bring with her on each subsequent visit with her baby. These cards (Figure 7-1) often provide useful information and a place to record immunizations and other data. It also includes what is often called a "road to health" chart on which the child's weight can be plotted in relation to his or her age. Graphing is an unfamiliar concept to persons without schooling, but the charts show two lines representing upper and lower weight limits by age, the idea being that the child's data points should remain between the two lines (i.e., on the "road"). The upper line is of little consequence but declining weight that causes the child to fall below the lower line ("off the road") indicates a danger signal, as shown. These charts, printed in appropriate languages, are widely distributed throughout the developing world. Agencies such as UNICEF, UNFPA, and USAID often help to subsidize the costs of printing and distribution.

In 1955 there were 21 million deaths of children under five, and in 1997 about 10 million; 5 million are projected for the year 2025, when the world population is projected to be about 8 billion. Under-five mortality rates per thousand live births for these dates are 210, 78, and 37, respectively.[15] Improved survival does not mean that the poverty and stress that put so many children at risk of death have disappeared. Early months lived in an impoverished environment without intellectual stimulation, combined with early malnutrition, can lead to irreversible physical and emotional damage and blunted ability to learn. Too many of today's surviving children will grow up with physical, mental, social, and emotional impairents arising from adverse conditions in their earliest months and years when intelligence, personality, and social behavior are formed.

An understanding of child health requires attention to socioeconomic, behavioral, and biomedical factors, but such comprehensive studies are rarely done. One attempt at such an integrated study was the collaborative project that studied 3000 children from birth to age two in the city of Cebu in the Philippines, which gave rise to numerous reports and publications.[16]

The move toward early investments in the "whole child" is intended to benefit

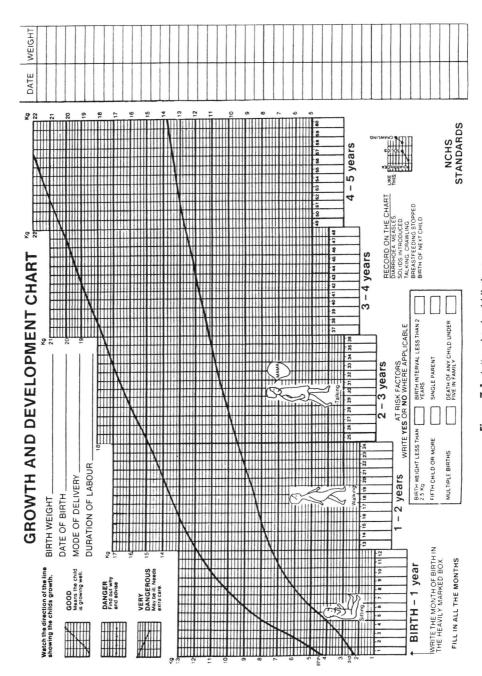

Figure 7-1 A "road to health" chart.

children, families, and the larger community, with emphasis on advancing later education. A similar integrated approach has developed within the health sector. At first called Integrated Management of the Sick Child it is now known as *Integrated Management of Childhood Illness* (IMCI). The IMCI initiative was established in the mid 1990s by the WHO Division of Child Health and Development in collaboration with many other WHO divisions and external agencies.[17] The core of the IMCI strategy is a set of guidelines for integrated case management within outpatient settings of the five most important causes of childhood deaths—acute respiratory infections, diarrhea, measles, malaria, and malnutrition—and of common associated conditions. One or more of these conditions also account for 75% of sick children seeking care at health facilities. The combination of malnutrition, diarrhea, and acute respiratory infection, which has been termed the *synergistic triad*, is said to be responsible for 69% of infant deaths and 80% of deaths of children between two and five years of age in Mexico;[18] a similar situation occurs throughout much of the developing world.

> A single diagnosis for a sick child is often inappropriate because it identifies only the most apparent problems and can lead to an associated and potentially life-threatening condition being overlooked. Treating the child may be complicated by the need to combine therapies for two or more conditions. In addition, the signs and symptoms of several of the major childhood diseases overlap substantially. Therefore, child health programmes should address the sick child as a whole and not single diseases.[19]

Table 7-4 shows the presumed causes of 12.2 million deaths among under-five-year-olds in all developing countries in 1993.

The ICMI strategy combines improved management of childhood illness with aspects of nutrition, immunization, and several other important influences on child health, including maternal health. Using a set of interventions for the integrated treatment and prevention of major childhood illnesses, the strategy aims to reduce death and the frequency and severity of illnesses and disability and to contribute to improved growth and development:

- Improvement in the case management skills of health staff through guidelines and training courses
- Improvements in the health system required for effective management of childhood illneses and drug supply
- Improvements in family health practices such as breastfeeding and community practices such as health education and mass communication—e.g., radio messages
- Improved program management tools

Far from revolutionary, the IMCI incorporates elements of existing diarrheal disease and acute respiratory infection control programs, immunization programs, and

Table 7-4. Distribution by Cause of 12.2 Million Deaths Among Under-5-Year-Olds in All Developing Countries, 1993

	Deaths	
Cause	Percent	Number (in millions)
Acute respiratory infection (ARI)	26.9	3.3
Plus measles	5.2	0.6
Plus malaria	1.6	0.2
Malaria	6.2	0.8
Measles	2.4	0.3
Diarrhea	22.8	2.8
Plus measles	1.9	0.2
ARI-associated	33.7	4.1
Diarrhea-associated	24.7	3.1
Measles-associated	9.5	1.2
Malaria-associated	7.7	0.9
Malnutrition-associated	29.0	3.6
One or more of these conditions	71.0	8.7
Other	33.1	4.0

Source: World Health Organization, 1995.

maternal and child health services. It represents another step in the trend toward presenting preplanned, integrated modular blocks to developing country health sectors and ties in to the "minimum package" strategy of the World Bank.

The clinical steps recommended in handling a sick child are: *Assess* the child for general danger signs, cough or difficult breathing, diarrhea, fever, ear problem, malnutrition, anemia. *Ask* further questions. *Look, listen, feel. Treat* the child. *Refer* when needed. *Teach the mother* to give oral drugs at home and treat local infections (eye, ear, mouth, throat). *Counsel the mother* about food and feeding problems, fluid intake during illness, when to return, and her own health. *Ask, praise, advise, check.*

Loaded with cultural, economic, and political significance, infant and maternal mortality demand close scrutiny by those interested in international health. The death of an infant or mother has profound social significance, and is often devastating for the family and immediate community. The unequivocal and universally recognized endpoint of death is likely to be remembered and in many places officially recorded.

The infant mortality rate (IMR) is often cited as the most sensitive indicator summarizing in a single number both a general level of "development" and the state of health of a population, but the maternal mortality ratio varies even more. Barring specific disasters, population IMRs span roughly a 30-fold range, from about six to about 180 deaths per thousand live births. However, in parts of sub-Saharan Africa a woman's cumulative lifetime risk of death from maternal causes is said to be about one in 20; in Asia, it is one in 54; and in Latin America, it is one in 73; in wealthy industrialized countries the corresponding risk is more like one in 10,000, leading to a 500-fold range! High rates of infant and maternal deaths reflect underlying inadequacies in socioeconomic and sanitary conditions. Appropriate education, prevention, and medical care could avert most of these deaths.

Special Features of Infant Mortality

The question of statistical artifacts—that is, whether reported rates are in fact correct always arises in considering infant deaths (see Chapter 4). Where births are seldom registered and medical attention is lacking, most infants who die are never recorded and are permanently lost to the statistical system. There is often little parental or community incentive for reporting infant deaths, particularly in areas of economic deprivation where one may expect the toll to be higher than elsewhere. Statistical coverage is often better in urban than in rural areas, distorting infant mortality and other vital rates in sometimes unpredictable ways. Infant mortality data may be reconstructed in part by questions about past pregnancy outcome on census schedules, or special retrospective surveys, but such efforts are rare and are poor substitutes for timely registration of vital events. Moreover, women who have had many pregnancies may, on questioning years later, overlook or wish to forget those who have died, particularly before becoming part of the functioning family. Culture and tradition may render the subject of deceased infants and children unsuitable for discussion, especially with strangers. It is therefore more common to obtain these data indirectly by asking primarily about the surviving children, with a question to the mother about her total number of deliveries.

Neonatal deaths (see Table 4-3 and Chapter 4) tend to be due to immaturity, certain inherent congenital conditions, or circumstances of birth that are relatively independent of postnatal care, while the later postneonatal deaths tend to result from environmental causes such as deficiencies in nutrition and from infectious disease.[20] If this is so, the ratio of neonatal to postneonatal deaths would provide a sensitive measure of adverse social, economic, and environmental conditions. A relative concentration of deaths in the neonatal period would therefore indicate more favorable conditions. In the United States and other wealthy countries the ratio of neonatal to postneonatal (NN:PNN) infant deaths is in the range of 7:3 (= 2.33), but it is typically the reverse in poor countries. The same relationship holds true within nations, and even within local areas where poorer and wealthier populations are intermixed. Table 7-5 shows data from a landmark study of infant mortality in the city of Pôrto Alegre, Brazil.[21] "Shantytown" neighborhoods were characterized by unemployment or underemployment, lack of access to medical or health services, substandard housing, inadequate nutrition, poor education, and unsanitary conditions. In 1980 more than 15% of the city's residents, and 20% of the infants, were shantytown residents. For the city, and for each of three study districts, the NN:PNN ratio was less than one among the shantytown dwellers, and exceeded one among the more affluent residents. The overall infant mortality rate of 36.5 would be high by today's standards.

Another feature of the infant mortality rate distinguishing it from other single-year age-specific death rates is that there does appear to be an irreducible lower limit that varies by place and time. This minimum mortality, consisting primarily of infants congenitally malformed or with other severe birth defects inimical to survival, is determined in part by relatively unpreventable genetic, chromosomal, developmental, or physiological mishaps during development and in part by controllable environmental factors such as maternal infection and nutrition, behavior, and prenatal care. A correlate to the concept of the irreducible minimum is the question of an acceptable minimum: At what point does society stop devoting resources such as perinatal intensive care units to ever more complex efforts at salvage of extremely ill newborns?

Sometimes attempts are made to collect data on fetal or prenatal death rates. Such

Table 7-5. Neonatal, Postneonatal, and Total Infant Mortality[a] Among "Shantytown" Residents and "Nonshantytown" Residents in the city of Pôrto Alegre, Brazil, 1980

District	Shantytown Residents				Nonshantytown Residents			
	Total	Neonatal	Postneonatal	NN:PNN	Total	Neonatal	Postneonatal	NN:PNN
North	74.0	24.2	49.8	0.49	24.3	15.4	8.9	1.73
South	80.7	35.8	44.9	0.80	25.2	17.0	8.2	2.07
Peripheral	71.6	30.9	40.7	0.76	30.0	20.0	10.0	2.00
Total	75.5	31.3	44.2	0.71	24.4	16.2	8.2	1.98

[a]Per thousand live births.
Source: Adapted from Lima Guimarães and Fischmann (1985) Figure 4.

information might be important, for example, in obtaining data on the harmful effects of certain toxic chemical or other environmental hazards. In the United States, fetal deaths are further divided into early (less than 20 weeks' gestation), intermediate (20 to 28 weeks), and late (more than 28 weeks). Methodologic problems make such data very difficult to obtain in the absence of required reporting of miscarriages or spontaneous abortions. In addition, criteria for reporting are poorly understood by the medical profession. In one study[22] of more than 1000 obstetricians in the Netherlands and Belgium, significant differences were found in their reporting, casting doubt on the international comparability of perinatal mortality figures. This is unfortunate, as such figures have often been utilized for politically based arguments about the merits of one or another system of health care. A further difficulty in deriving fetal death rates is in deciding what to use for the denominator, as it is unreasonable to maintain a registration system for pregnancies.

Correlates and Predictors of Infant Mortality

According to a useful study by Ann Millard,[23] factors leading to child mortality can be allocated to three tiers of causes. The *proximate* tier refers to the immediate biomedical causes of death such as malnutrition or certain infections (the synergistic triad). The *intermediate* tier of causes includes behavior and aspects of general living conditions that increase exposure of children to the proximate causes. Here one can find insufficient frequency of feeding, inadequate meal composition, inequitable distribution of food in the household, exposure to pathogens, and other factors tied to child care practices in the broad sense. The *ultimate* tier of causes of high rates of child mortality refers to broad economic, social, and cultural processes and structures that form the context for the other two tiers. Among these are social stratification, political and financial institutions, settlement patterns, sanitation, the division of labor in households, and opportunities for remunerative labor.

Many people have sought more specific correlates and predictors in a search for ways to reduce infant mortality. Such attempts usually have not come up empty-handed. Many factors have been cited—some more pertinent for neonatal mortality, others centering around disadvantaged personal and environmental circumstances, relating more to the postneonatal period. Among the major correlates of infant mortality are:

- *Low birth weight*: Generally defined as less than 2500 grams at live birth.[24] *Very low birth weight* is less than 1500 grams and *extremely low birth weight* is less than 1000 grams. Causes of low birth weight are many, but prematurity is among the most important. The length of gestation is clearly related to birth weight. Gestational age, often a source of confusion, is measured from the first day of the last normal menstrual period and expressed in completed days or weeks.[25] The date of the last menstrual period is often unknown, whereupon the best clinical estimate is used. It is interesting that differences in neonatal mortality between the United States and some Scandinavian countries reflect primarily differences in distribution of infant birth weights rather than in the postnatal survival of infants of a given birth weight.

- *Maternal age*: The higher mortality of infants born to very young or very old mothers is well established. Young mothers tend to have lower birth weight infants and higher infant mortality rates in general, but other factors including ethnicity are also operative. The often low level of knowledge and mothering ability and frequent lack of prenatal care among teenage mothers tends to increase postneonatal deaths. Mothers more than 35 years old at delivery also face increased risk of adverse outcome such as stillbirth and certain congenital malformations. The relationship of birth weight to maternal age is complex.

- *Birth order and plurality*: The lowest infant mortality rate occurs in second or third births, with higher risk for first births or high-order births. The relationship to maternal age and other factors needs to be clarified. Mortality is higher among children from multiple births than among singletons.

- *Sex*: The roughly 4% excess of male births over females was first pointed out in 1662 by John Graunt in his *Bills of Mortality*. During the perinatal period this numerical advantage is reduced in almost all populations by slighty higher mortality among boys, despite their greater average birth weight. As this trend continues throughout the life span, the proportion of females in the population eventually exceeds that of males. This occurs generally in the fourth decade of life in the industrialized regions but not until the seventh decade in less developed countries. The differential effect on early life survival of cultural gender preference is discussed below.

- *Interval since previous birth*: Perinatal mortality is lower when there is 18 months or more between births. One could make a case for both biological factors during pregnancy (e.g., physiological recovery of the mother) and for the amount of maternal time, attention, and resources available to the new infant.

- *Maternal education*: A powerful inverse correlate of infant mortality. More educated mothers tend to be not very young, more affluent, more interested in and willing and able to learn about and participate in health matters. More educated mothers in developing countries are more likely to be able to read posters, labels, and directions on medicines and infant formulas. Better-educated mothers will tend to be married to more-educated fathers who will probably earn a higher income and be more likely to take responsibility within the family. A study by the World Bank in Brazil determined that maternal education had more influence on reduction of childhood diarrhea than did local provision of water supply. A detailed study of 17 countries showed that the maternal education advantage in survival was less pronounced during than after the neonatal period. Poor education was associated with higher postneonatal risk, undernutrition below two years of age, and nonuse of health services, although "a large part of these associations are the result of education's strong link to household economics."[26]

- *Ethnicity and culture*: Numerous genetic and behavioral factors, sometimes difficult to distinguish from each other and from socioeconomic conditions, are lumped under this heading. Knowledge, attitudes and practice regarding nutrition, contraception, marriage, health care, and the like differ from person to person and group to group. Issues related to "family life," the roles of men and women in local society, and other attitudes are expressed variously in infant- and child-rearing practices.

  China and India have far more males in their populations than females. Both cultures throughout most of this century have practised selective neglect of female children, preference for sons, and, at times, female infanticide and mistreatment of adult women. In India, the imbalance between males and females has increased from decade to decade. In China, the disparity between males and females, which was pronounced early in the century, narrowed slightly through at least the 1960s. The male/female ratio in the population reportedly rose moderately in the 1980s, in part because of a resurgence in female infanticide after the introduction of the one-child policy and the sex-selective abortion of female fetuses since the early 1980s. The most recent censuses show that the dearth of females in India is more pronounced than in China.[27] Sex-selective abortion was facilitated by ultrasound machines that came into wide use in China in the mid-1980s and permitted visual identification of the sex of the fetus. This dreadful misapplication of technology for selective abortion of female fetuses appears to be growing also in some other countries.

- *Economic and environmental conditions, including health care*: The association of infant mortality with poverty is not new, as any reader of Charles Dickens or Friedrich Engels can testify. As long ago as 1912 a U.S. government commission reported that

  > The coincidence of a high infant mortality rate with low earnings, poor housing, the employment of the mother outside the home and large families was indicated in these studies. They all showed that there is great variation in IMR ... in different parts of the same state and in the same city, town or rural district. These differences were found to be caused by different population elements, widely varying social and economic conditions and differences in appreciation of good prenatal and infant care and the facilities available for such care.[28]

- *Maternal infection with HIV*: HIV infection and AIDS are discussed in Chapter 14 but their relationship to the infant–mother dyad must be considered here. In certain areas of sub-Saharan Africa HIV infection rates in maternity clinics can range upwards from 40%. Roughly 20% to 25% of infants born to infected mothers will themselves be infected during gestation or delivery. Approximately 1600 HIV-infected babies are born daily in the world, the majority in Africa. It is known that the drug zidovudine (AZT), given to infected mothers during the last 12 weeks of pregnancy and to their babies for 6 weeks after delivery, can reduce the rate of maternal transmission by about two-thirds. This regimen, standard in the United States, costs about $800 per patient. With the assistance of UNAIDS and the WHO the price may fall to as low as $50 per case, but this is still far too expensive for many developing countries. Ethical implications of these studies are described in Chapter 15.

Breastfeeding and HIV

In 1985 HIV was discovered in milk of infected mothers, and transmission of the virus to uninfected infants was demonstrated. It is now estimated that breastfeeding accounts for up to one-third of the 600,000 children who become HIV-positive each year, the risk increasing with greater duration of breastfeeding. Feeding with infant formula can of course avert this risk, but the infants are then exposed to other, perhaps more serious, hazards.

In the 1970s child health advocates launched a worldwide campaign against the aggressive marketing of breast-milk substitutes in developing countries. Boycotts of Nestle and other formula makers and the accompanying publicity led in 1981 to codes of conduct by formula manufacturers, who promised to cease certain promotional activities in these regions. The main concerns of activists were (1) that breastfeeding has clear nutritional and immunologic benefits to the infant, (2) that the milk powder, being expensive, was often made too dilute to be nutritious, and (3) that inadequate cleaning of bottles and nipples, mixing with contaminated water, and bottles left unprotected in hot climates resulted in diarrheal disease, dehydration, and death of thousands of infants. "Breast is Best" campaigns were launched throughout the world and breastfeeding became a pillar of international public health.

The HIV crisis has caused much anxiety. Formula manufacturers are wary of another round of vilification, while critics accuse UNICEF and similar agencies of being too wedded to breastfeeding to accept a change of policy. Formula-feeding is much more cumbersome, time-consuming, and expensive than breastfeeding: "The cost of formula for one child—when it is available in Uganda and when there is clean water to mix with it—is on average 1.5 times the sum a village family earns in a year."[29]

The HIV–breastfeeding dilemma involves a tradeoff of risks in each separate case, with no easy or universal solution.

WAR AND CIVIL DISTURBANCE

The extreme disruption caused by war and civil strife is clearly damaging to infant and child health, perhaps more so than to other age groups, but actual data are hard to find because of the turbulent situations. A rare study of this type, conducted in Somalia during a period of political and social collapse, showed that under-five mortality per 1000 children in two villages increased from 211 to 414 in just two years (1987–1989). Public health services, including immunizations, drugs, and clinics, virtually disappeared as inflation soared. Deaths were caused not by the warfare itself (e.g., injuries) but by increased threats from the usual respiratory infections, diarrhea, fever/malaria, and neonatal tetanus.[30]

The best argument that we can make to a government for instituting any program is to show that it is cost-effective—that is, that it will yield more or save more than it costs. Analyses of the economic impact of infant mortality may consider quantifiable costs to the family, such as cash outlay for prenatal care, including transportation, fees, medicines, and special foods; costs associated with delivery, including payment to clinic, doctor, or midwife; cost of ceremonies or entertainment; costs of attending to the sick infant, including fees and medicines, religious offerings, and related expenses. Non-cash costs include loss of productivity and health risks to the mother during pregnancy; reduced care to other children; time and effort devoted to the child who died by parents and other family members; and reduced productivity by parents and family during the period of mourning. The community also incurs costs such as the diversion of resources (clinic use, medical staff time, vaccines, and drugs) used for the child and loss of social contribution and future productivity of the child who died. There are of course the nonquantifiable costs of emotion, grief, loss of enthusiasm, and other psychological reactions to the infant death that may affect economic productivity and might be translated into changes in attitude or political behavior.

CAUSES OF DEATH

Protein-energy malnutrition (PEM) affects more than a third of the world's children. A review of 79 nutrition treatment centers indicated that the proportion of underweight children ranged from 8% in the best region (southern America) to 60% in the poorest (southern Asia); the proportion of stunted (small) children from 18% to 60%; and the proportion of wasted (thin) children from 2% to 17% in the same regions. Low height-for-age was estimated in 43% of under-five-year-olds in developing countries. Most tellingly, growth retardation in early childhood is associated with significant functional impairment in adult life.[31] The immense literature on nutrition, feeding, and supplementation programs to combat protein-energy malnutrition cannot be reviewed here. Although the overall rate has declined, it seems incongruous that once severe PEM has developed, the likelihood of death has changed little over the past 50 years. A review of 67 reports showed median case-fatality ratios, by decade (1950s to 1990s), to be 20%, 25.7%, 24,5%, 13.7%, and 23.5%. Questionnaires were sent to nutrition units in many countries asking about their procedures and practices in cases of severe PEM. Reponses revealed that inappropriate and faulty case-management practices are widespread and that outmoded and conflicting teaching materials are in use. The need is great for "a definitive set of user friendly, practical guidelines" with accessible and authoritative information to aid in clinical decision-making.[32]

In addition to protein-energy malnutrition, dietary deficiencies of vitamins and minerals can cause learning disabilities, mental retardation, poor health, low work capacity, blindness, and premature death. Micronutrient malnutrition is estimated to affect at least 2 billion people of all ages, but children are particularly vulnerable. All vitamins, various cofactors, and many chemical elements (e.g., zinc, manganese, cobalt) are essential in minute qualtities, but the term *micronutrient* has come to refer mainly to three substances: iodine, iron, and vitamin A. Some functional consequences of deficiency of these three major micronutrients are summarized in Table 7-6.

Iodine deficiency is the greatest single cause of preventable brain damage and mental retardation in the world. It is estimated that more than 1.5 billion people worldwide, including over 400 million in China, live in areas lacking iodine in the soils. Insufficient intake of iodine causes a variety of physical and mental disabilities collectively termed iodine deficiency disorders (IDDs). The best known of these are goiter, an enlargement of the thyroid gland, and cretinism, a severe form of mental retardation which may be associated with deaf-mutism, dwarfism, and spastic palsy of lower limbs. Iodine deficiency is the major preventable cause of intellectual handicap and can lead to spontaneous abortion and neonatal deaths. IDD is not only a public health issue but is seen as an impediment to human and economic development.

Iron deficiency is the most common nutritional disorder in the world and affects over one billion people, particularly women of reproductive age and preschool children in tropical and subtropical regions. Iron deficiency is caused by low levels of iron in the diet and can be induced by hookworm infection. Its effects include anemia, reduced work capacity, diminished learning ability, increased susceptibility to infection, and greater risk of death associated with pregnancy and childbirth. The overall anemia prevalence for women in developing countries is estimated at 42%. Severe iron deficiency may contribute to 20% of maternal deaths.

Table 7-6. Some Functional Consequences of Deficiency of Selected Micronutrients

Problem	Functional Consequences	Economic Implications
Iodine deficiency in pregnancy and early childhood	Mental retardation Growth failure Delayed maturation	Low educability and diminished productivity
Vitamin A deficiency in early childhood	Blindness Increased severity of infections Child mortality	Loss of productivity Increased health care costs
Iron deficiency anemia in children and adults	Impaired learning Low work capacity Low birthweight, increased maternal mortality	Low educability Loss of productivity Increased health care costs and loss of productivity

Source: Reprinted with permission. All rights reserved. Nutrition Reveiws, Volume 54, Number 4, Part II, page S70. ©1996 by the International Life Sciences Institute Washington, DC 20036-4810, USA.

More than 13 million people are thought to suffer night blindness or total blindness caused by vitamin A deficiency. WHO reported in 1994 that 3.1 million preschool-age children had eye damage due to a vitamin A deficiency and another 227.5 million are subclinically affected at severe or moderate level. Annually, an estimated 250,000 to 500,000 preschool children go blind from this deficiency and about two-thirds of these children die within months of becoming blind. Some investigators suggest that regular doses of vitamin A alone can reduce childhood mortality by 50% but others remain dubious and the issue remains active and controversial.[33] The level of maternal vitamin A is also important during pregnancy and lactation.

The 1990 Summit for Children endorsed three micronutrient goals for the end of the decade: the virtual elimination of iodine and vitamin A deficiencies and the reduction of iron deficiency anemia in women by one-third. The World Development Report 1993 found micronutrient programs to be among the most cost-effective of all health interventions. Most micronutrient programs cost less than $50 (U.S.) per disability-adjusted life-year (DALY) gained. Some interventions to relieve micronutrient deficiencies include:

- Education to encourage the consumption of micronutrient-rich foods, such as dark green leafy vegetables, mangoes, papayas, other carotene-rich fruits, and seafoods
- Fortification of foods such as flour and iodization of salt
- Nutritional supplementation through inexpensive pharmaceuticals
- Deworming of children to remove hookworms, roundworms, and other parasites
- Cooking in iron utensils where practicable

ACUTE RESPIRATORY INFECTIONS

Respiratory infections are caused by many different viral, bacterial, and fungal pathogens. Upper respiratory infections, mainly colds, are widespread and usually not very serious. However, acute lower respiratory infections, commonly called pneumonia, are a major cause of illness and death throughout the life span, but particularly so for the very young and the very old. There are also many agents that can cause pneumonia, but the pneumococcus, *Streptococcus pneumoniae*, may cause more fatal illness than any other single pathogen in the world. In addition to pneumonia these bacteria may cause meningitis and serious ear infections. The case-fatality ratio for invasive disease with certain serotypes may reach 40% among children under five and 50% in persons over 50. Death rates due to bacterial pneumonia have declined since the 1970s, and the case-fatality ratio has decreased, primarily because of antibiotic use. However, there is no evidence that infection rates have decreased significantly, if at all. Self-medication and indiscriminate use of antibiotics are so common in developing countries that the World Health Organization's program on acute respiratory infections has emphasized the importance of the increasing antibiotic resistance of many serotypes of *S. pneumoniae* as a major concern worldwide.

A study carried out in a low income district of Manila may be typical of the situation in urban areas of developing countries (Table 7-7). A number of children from 0 to 60 months of age were followed over a period of two years. Only 29% of the children had received all of the recommended childhood immunizations.

The children had an average of about one acute respiratory infection every two months. Infants 6 to 11 months old had almost one case of acute pneumonia each year. The duration of illness with pneumonia was 4 weeks or less in 76% of cases, 5–6 weeks in 12%, and 7–8 weeks in 6%. In a second study among children hospitalized with pneumonia,[34] clinical evidence of measles was found in 258 of 537 cases. The causative agent was identified in 235 patients: A virus was found in 121 and bacteremia was noted in 72 children. Among 55 children in whom a bacterial agent was identified, *S. pneumoniae* was the most frequent. Other bacteria found were *Haemophilus influenzae*, *Salmonella typhi*, *Staphylococcus aureus*, and *Klebsiella pneumoniae*. Many mixed viral–bacterial infections were also seen.

Control of acute respiratory infections is difficult because the viral and bacterial agents are transmitted though the air. Some, such as measles and pertussis,[35] can be reduced by immunization, but that is difficult for *S. pneumoniae* because 83 different serotypes are known, each immunologically distinct. The proportions of the different serotypes vary from place to place throughout the world. A vaccine prepared from the most important 23 serotypes (in the United States and Europe) is commercially available and recommended for individuals at special risk—for example, immunosuppressed children and adults and those over 65 years of age. Vac-

Table 7-7. Age-Specific Incidence of Acute Upper and Lower Respiratory Infections, Alabang, Metro Manila, 1985–1987[a]

Age Group (months)	No. of Child-Years at Risk	Number. of Episodes		Incidence per Child-Year		
		AURI	ALRI	AURI	ALRI	All ARI
0–5	90.4	458	56	5.1	0.6	5.7
6–11	128.8	829	122	6.4	0.9	7.3
12–23	289.3	1893	225	6.5	0.8	7.3
24–35	296.8	1660	155	5.6	0.5	6.1
36–47	310.2	1635	116	5.3	0.4	5.7
48–59	302.8	1421	73	4.7	0.2	4.9
All	1418.3	7896	747	5.6	0.5	6.1

ARI = acute respiratory infection; ALRI = acute lower respiratory infection; AURI = acute upper respiratory infection.

Source: Tupasi et al. (1990b) Table 3.

cines used in any area should contain the most prevalent serotypes in the population of that area, but it is prohibitively laborious and costly to custom-make vaccines for each region. There is a need for safe, efficacious vaccines that promote a protective immune response to invasive pneumococcal disease in young children and that could be used on a large scale. As a further complication, existing vaccines do not work well in children under two years of age, whose immune response to native pneumococcal antigens is very weak and in many cases nonexistent. However, a more complex class of vaccines, in which bacterial polysaccharides are conjugated with proteins, is protective in infants and young children. A vaccine of this more complex type, effective against *Haemophilus influenzae* type B (Hib), is now widely used.

Paradoxically, efforts to improve living standards may lead to increased childhood pneumonia. Working mothers often need to place their small children in a daycare center. However, a study in Fortaleza, Brazil, showed that attendance in a daycare center was associated with a five-fold rise in risk of pneumonia, second only to malnutrition as a risk factor. As the local government was committed to increasing the number of publicly funded daycare centers, it must also improve the design and management of such facilities to minimize the transmission of pneumonia and other illnesses.[36]

DIARRHEAL DISEASE

Perhaps the first thing to ask about diarrhea is: What is it? Simple? Not quite. Diarrhea is a sign of an illness (a *fluid-losing enteropathy*) with many different potential causes. The issue is complicated by variations in perception and definition of diarrhea from one country to another, such as:

- More than two watery or loose motions in 24 hours
- "Mother's definition"
- Five or more stools in one day preceded and followed by 1 week of normal stools
- Four loose stools or one watery or bloody stool/day
- Less than one year of age: five or more liquid or semiliquid stools/24 hours; >1 year of age: three or more liquid or semiliquid stools preceded by two weeks of normal stools
- Three or more loose stools of altered consistency or with blood or mucus in 24 hours
- Three or more liquid stools in 12 hours with or without blood, pus, or mucus
- More than four stools in 24 hours

Basic causes of diarrheas include environmental toxins, allergies, physiological states such as lactose intolerance, and nonenteric diseases such as malaria or measles.

However, by far the major agents producing diarrheas in children are enteric pathogens taken in with contaminated food, water, or formula. Some of the more important diarrhea-causing agents are listed on Table 7-8.

Despite a great deal of knowledge about these organisms, and improvements in diagnostic methods, the specific cause of a significant proportion of childhood diarrheas in developing countries remains undeterminable. It is also important to guard against "post hoc" reasoning: Finding an organism, even a known pathogen, in a stool specimen does not prove that it *caused* the episode. For this reason the term *association of an enteropathogen with diarrhea* is often employed for an organism isolated during or one day before or after a diarrheal episode. The same reasoning holds for pneumonia.

The immediate result of acute diarrhea is dehydration, which has sometimes been termed *fluid-electrolyte malnutrition*. Loss of up to about 5% of body weight is usually tolerable, although the pulse may weaken and blood pressure drop. If about

Table 7-8. Some Enteric Agents that Can Cause Acute Diarrhea

Viruses

    Rotaviruses
    Norwalk-like agents

Bacteria

    Campylobacter jejuni
    Clostridium difficile
    Escherichia coli: enterotoxigenic, enteropathogenic enterohemorrhagic, or enteroinvasive
    Salmonella species
    Shigella species
    Vibrio species, including *V. cholerae* and *V. parahaemolyticus*
    Yersinia enterocolitica

Parasites

    Protozoa

        Entamoeba histolytica
        Cryptosporidium parvum
        Cyclospora sp.
        Giardia lamblia

Worms

    Strongyloides stercoralis

10% of body weight is lost in acute diarrhea, the result may be shock, acidosis, stupor, kidney failure, and death. The effects of chronic diarrhea are multiple and include malnutrition from lowered appetite, decreased absorption of nutrients, loss of proteins in fluid stools, and increased susceptibility to infection.

In poor regions such as northeast Brazil children may have from eight to 15 diarrheal disease episodes per year in a vicious cycle of malnutrition and disease, with a profound negative impact on cognitive and motor development.

Perhaps more significant to a society than the mortality from diarrheal disease is the submerged iceberg of silent morbidity caused by numerous recurring and persistent diarrheal disease episodes among children in many developing areas in the tropics. The societal impact is greater from those who do not die, but who live through repeated bouts of dehydrating and malnourishing diarrhea in their most formative, developmental years of life.[37]

The classical clinical viewpoint would propose that treatment be directed at the cause, for which the corresponding response is to use drugs: antisecretory drugs to inhibit fluid loss, antimotility drugs to reduce intestinal movement, absorbents to soak up excess fluids, and antibiotics to stop or eliminate bacterial pathogens in the intestine. However, these drugs are often counterproductive or harmful. For example, antimotility drugs may act to keep toxins in the intestine when the body is trying to expel them via the diarrhea. Nevertheless, under some circumstances these drugs have a role, as in the case of the poor traveler with the runs who absolutely *must* get to the airport. Antibiotics such as ampicillin, tetracycline, or chloramphenicol may be appropriate and perhaps even life-saving in case of shigellosis, cholera, or typhoid, respectively. However, more harm than good may be done with such drugs. Excessive use may quickly select out resistant strains of pathogens, making the epidemiologic situation worse than before (see Chapter 14). In any event, the use of costly modern pharmaceuticals is simply not an option for millions of children in developing countries. In one review of 28 surveys of treatment patterns for childhood diarrhea it was found that private providers were less likely than public health providers to provide appropriate case management for watery diarrhea. Private providers were less likely to prescribe oral rehydration (see below) and more likely to prescribe unneeded drugs.[38]

It is likely that every group and culture has traditional remedies for acute and chronic diarrhea. Some, such as ipecacaunha bark in South America, the source of the drug emetine, are of proven pharmacologic value. Drinking green coconut water is likewise physiologically sensible. In contrast, hot pepper enemas, as used in West Africa, may be more heroic but less effective.

On a community basis the employment of medical treatment against diarrhea has not been very effective until recent years. The current treatment of choice is to counteract the dehydration that leads to the most drastic outcomes of diarrhea. This can be done by intravenous fluid therapy, which is very effective but requires sterile solutions and equipment, trained personel, fixed facilities sometimes remote from the patient, and a substantial financial investment. The introduction in recent years of *oral rehydration therapy* (ORT) using *oral rehydration solution* (ORS) has provided an effective procedure that has saved the lives of many, perhaps millions, of children in developing countries. Oral rehydration therapy replaces lost fluids by mouth rather than intravenously. It is cheap, relatively simple, requires only basic training, can be done at home by mothers or even older siblings, and involves no time delay. This method works regardless of the causative agent of the diarrhea because it counteracts the dehydration. If a cup of ORS goes in for every cup of stool lost, the body's fluid balance should remain essentially in line. According to the medical journal *Lancet*, "The discovery that sodium transport and glucose transport are coupled in the small intestine so that glucose accelerates absorption of solute and water was potentially the most important medical advance this century."[39]

The classic ORT solution contains (in grams per liter) sodium chloride 3.5, potassium chloride 1.5, sodium bicarbonate 2.5, glucose 20. Many modifications have been proposed, such as the addition of sodium citrate in place of the bicarbonate to improve keeping properties and reduce stool volumes, and glycine or other amino acids to improve fluid transport out of the intestine into the blood. Various countries have promoted the addition of local unrefined sugars, rice water, rice starch powder, or other carbohydrates and cereals. Such mixtures prepackaged in sealed foil packets are distributed widely in many countries, but may not be readily available to the majority of people in more remote areas. For this reason many public health workers have devised ways to encourage mothers to prepare their own solutions from simple materials likely to be found in the home. One such idea is the *pinch and scoop* plan, in which mothers are taught to mix two "thumb and two-finger pinches" of table salt and one "four-finger scoop" of sugar in a pint (half liter) of water.

As with any procedure, ORT is not perfect and some problems have emerged with use. For example, it is sometimes observed by untrained mothers that stool volume is increased upon feeding of ORT solutions. A natural consequence of adding fluids, this is interpreted as making the diarrhea worse. In fact, if the diarrhea should stop because the body is too dehydrated that is the worst thing that could happen. Proper education is needed to counteract this misconception. The surprising variation in the size of teaspoons, tablespoons, soupspoons, cups, and the like from one country to another make it very difficult to give specific directions to poorly educated mothers for mixing the proper formulation. One study in Nepal showed that fewer than 5% of homes possessed sugar and any type of teaspoon. For this reason several agencies have distributed double-ended plastic spoons to measure standard volumes of salt in one side and sugar in the other. Additional problems arise through

- The use of contaminated water for mixing
- Improper mixing of prepackaged powders

• Making the solution too concentrated or too dilute
• Keeping the mixed solution too long so that it serves as a culture medium for bacteria[40]

Another difficulty is the time needed to spoon-feed ORS to an ill baby, taking the mother or caretaker from other essential work. Also, ORT is not effective in persistent diarrhea, and in developing countries some 15% to 20% of acute diarrhea cases will become persistent. In shigellosis the loss of fluid may be minimal and ORT will be less effective in preventing deaths from this cause.

More ominous problems have been been described, showing just how difficult it is to apply even apparently straightforward technical advances in real field situations. In Bangladesh, the birthplace of ORT, a study was carried out for three years preceding and ten years following the introduction of an ORT program to a rural community.

> A significant increase in infant mortality due to acute watery diarrhoea was observed throughout the study period. Child mortality due to acute watery diarrhoea did not decrease during this period. The programme ensured universal knowledge of the oral rehydration solution and the availability of glucose-electrolyte sachets in every household. Yet the inadequate formulation of messages concerning the role of oral rehydration may have caused its incorrect use—oral solutions being administered to too few infants, in too small qualtities, and for too short periods.[41]

One vexing issue in the home use of ORT is the opposition of many in the medical profession. The basis of this opposition is not always evident, but may be related in part to medical conservatism. Some commentators have suspected also that physicians in developing countries are accustomed to retaining for themselves the privilege of performing all medical treatment. Doctors in training may be taught that ORT is primitive or ineffective, and other steps may be taken to discourage its use.

Because the agents of diarrhea are generally found in food and drink, it is theoretically easier to prevent diarrheas than to prevent respiratory infections. However, even when the usual cautions about water, ice, fresh vegetables, and the like are adhered to by educated travelers from wealthy countries, it is the norm for foreigners in exotic locales to experience episodes of diarrhea. The situation is far worse for children resident in such areas. Continuous exposure to fecally contaminated food, water, and environment takes its inevitable toll in the form of repeated bouts of diarrheal disease, often becoming progressively more serious in a spiral of infection and malnutrition. Bottle-feeding with powdered milk or formula mixed with bacteria-laden water may carry away infants very quickly, particularly when resistance is otherwise compromised. Preventive measures can be directed to the individual by changing biology (immunization) or behavior (training), to the community (mass education campaigns), or to the environment (water supply).

Immunization against cholera may be sought by foreign travelers, but experience has shown that such people are at low risk of contracting clinical cholera even in endemic areas.[42] Vaccines against some other diarrheal disease agents such as rotaviruses are being proposed for global use. Another strategy directed toward individuals is education, with the goal of changing behavior. In this case the target of educational programs is clearly not the infant at risk, but his or her mother. Personal or small-group training in tasks such as proper sterilization of feeding bottles and nipples where used, preparation and use of formula and ORT solutions, and general household sanitation are time- and labor-intensive. Messages through public media such as radio and television can deliver a general message but lack the one-to-one relationships and the feedback loop of trial, observation, and error correction characteristic of individual training sessions. Improved access to good water and to sanitary excreta disposal are the cornerstones of diarrheal disease control by environmental means.

Under current conditions in many developing countries water is a precious and expensive commodity. As mentioned earlier (Table 7-2), the cost of good water may be highest to those who can least afford it.

The relative value of education and water supply in reducing infant mortality was studied in urban Brazil. Increased maternal education accounted for a larger share of the mortality decline than any other single factor, including access to piped water.[43]

In addition to water supply, sanitation, and education programs, public health agencies may implement other diarrheal disease control strategies. Among these are improving childhood nutrition through encouragement of breastfeeding, proper weaning practices, promotion of ORT, and, if necessary and feasible, supplementary feeding programs. It is clear that any improvement in the health of young children will help them to resist all infectious diseases. Therefore the adoption of immunization campaigns and other health-supportive measures will increase resistance, improve maternal health consciousness, and have a salutary spillover effect on diarrheal diseases. In the long run, however, serious reductions in illness and death from diarrheal disease will occur only after substantial improvement in social and economic conditions and basic improvements in the living standards of the world's disadvantaged populations.

An example of effective reduction of diarrheal disease mortality is found in Cuba. Concerted programs to improve sanitation and nutrition, promote breastfeeding, provide medical care, and educate the public have existed on the island since 1963. Reported rates of acute diarrheal disease mortality in infants (per thousand live births) fell from 12.9 deaths in 1962 to 0.3 in 1993, while in the same period reported diarrheal mortality rates per 10,000 one-to-four-year-olds went from 6.4 to 0.1.[44]

Both respiratory and diarrheal diseases are seasonal and may compete for child deaths month by month. In the state of Rio Grande do Sul, Brazil, where a good registration system was in effect, 40,219 certified infant deaths were studied over a four-year period. Socioeconomic conditions were considered fair. The state's apparent infant mortality rate from death certificate data was 43.5/1000 live births, and estimates from other sources produced a rate of about 47, suggesting that registered deaths represented a reasonable reflection of the real situation.[45] During the study period, deaths from respiratory causes such as pneumonia, bronchitis, and influenza exceeded those from intestinal infections and diarrhea. Most of the deaths attributed to both groups of causes occurred during the first four months of life. Respiratory deaths were very high in the first month, particularly the first week. The frequency of diarrheal deaths was several times higher in the summer (January and February) than in the winter months, while respiratory deaths showed just the reverse pattern. Ambient temperature was directly associated with diarrhea mortality and inversely associated with respiratory mortality. Therefore infants born in the Southern Hemisphere spring (October to December) were at greatest risk of dying from diarrheal disease, while those born in autumn and winter were more likely to die from respiratory causes.[46] In the Gambia, 2.4 times as many children under seven die in the rainy season as compared to the dry season. Deaths from malaria, diarrheal disease, and neonatal causes were from three to 24 times higher in the rainy season; deaths from respiratory infections were roughly the same in both seasons, but deaths from meningitis were five times more common in the dry season.[47]

CHILDHOOD IMMUNIZATION

The issue of childhood immunization is extremely complicated and involves technical, financial, cultural, organizational, and other factors. It is evident that any immunization should be given before the infants are at high risk for the corresponding disease. This may vary by disease and by country; for example, measles is a threat to children less than one year old in the developing world, but usually begins much later in industrialized countries. A recommended dosage schedule for childhood immunizations is shown on Table 7-9.

A confusing complex of organized international programs is involved in childhood immunizations. The UN agencies, particularly WHO and UNICEF, have broad roles in vaccine development and utilization. WHO units in the Communicable Diseases cluster and the Health Technology and Pharmaceuticals cluster have a major interest in immunization.

The Expanded Programme on Immunization (EPI)

The EPI was launched in 1974, when there were few immunization services in most developing countries. At that time, with eradication of smallpox on the horizon, the World Health Organization turned its attention to six diseases (diphtheria, pertussis, tetanus, measles, poliomyelitis, and tuberculosis) for which proven vaccines were available. Immunization of pregnant women against tetanus is also part of the program. Only about 4% of people living in developing countries had been fully

Table 7-9. Recommended Schedule for EPI Immunizations of Normal Infants and Children, United States, and for EPI Vaccines in Developing Countries[a]

Age	United States	Developing Countries
Birth	HBV1	BCG, OPV1, HBVa1[b]
6 weeks		DPT1, OPV2, HBVa2, HBVb1[b]
1–2 months	HBV2	
2 months	DTP or DTaP1, HbCV1, OPV1	
10 weeks		DPT2, OPV3, HBVb2
14 weeks		DPT3, OPV4
4 months	DTP or DTaP2, HbCV2, OPV2	
6 months	DTP or DTaP3 (HbCV3[c])	Measles in some areas[d]
6–18 months	HBV3, polio	
9 months	Measles[e]	Measles, HBVa3/b3; YF[f]
12 months	(HbCV3[c])	
12–15 months	MMR, (HbCV4[c]), Var	
15–18 months	DTaP or DTP, OPV	
4–6 years	DTP or DTaP, OPV	
11–12 years	MMR, HBV, Var	
14–16 years	Td	
Adult women		TT (childbearing age)

[a]Consult recent issues of the MMWR for current U.S. recommendations and of the *Weekly Epidemiological Record* for WHO recommendations. Abbreviations: BCG, bacille Calmette Guerin (for tuberculosis); DPT, diphtheria toxoid, pertussis whole cell vaccine, tetanus toxoid (WHO terminology); DTP, the same (U.S. terminology); DTaP, diphtheria toxoid, tetanus toxoid, acellular pertussis vaccine; HbCV, *Haemophilus influenzae* type b conjugate vaccine; HBV, hepatitis B vaccine; OPV, oral polio vaccine; MMR, measles, mumps, and rubella; Td, tetanus toxoid, full dose, and diphtheria toxoid, reduced dose, for adults; TT, tetanus toxoid; Var., varicella (chicken pox) vaccine.

[b]Schedule a, in areas where perinatal transmission of hepatitis B is common; schedule b in places where early transmission is not a problem.

[c]Depending on manufacturer and product.

[d]In most areas.

[e]In U.S. counties at high risk of measles. Use single-antigen measles vaccine for children aged under one year and MMR for children one year or older.

[f]Yellow fever vaccine should be routinely included in countries at risk in Africa.

Source: Basch (1994) Table 2-5; Ada (1995) Table 1; CDC (1998).

immunized against all six. The program has evolved in close collaboration with UNICEF, which provides the vaccines and much of the supplies and equipment needed for their administration. Funds flow also from UN agencies, donor organizations, and governments. In addition, private groups such as the Rockefeller Foundation and the Save the Children Fund and organizations such as Rotary International contribute funds through WHO or UNICEF or provide logistic or other assistance.

The EPI is usually promoted within the context of primary health care and/or child survival programs.

Priorities are:

- Sustain what has been achieved
- Achieve disease control for polio, measles, and tetanus
- Add new vaccines such as hepatitis B
- Make the schedules of contacts for EPI and other vaccines more practical

Among other concerns, the EPI has made a major effort to improve "cold chain" technology and thermostability of vaccines for remote regions of tropical countries where continuous refrigeration is not feasible.

The eventual goal of the EPI is universal childhood immunization (UCI), which means 100% coverage,[48] but the EPI has established a target of 90% by 2000. By April 1992, using its own sources, the EPI had estimated coverage rates, by region, for each antigen (Table 7-10).

Few people believed, when the programme was created, that the 1990 goal of providing immunization for all children of the world was anything but wishful thinking. However, this initiative, like the smallpox eradication programme before it, is providing a compelling demonstration of what can be accomplished when there is unanimity of purpose . . . this has been possible because the programme is easily understood, inexpensive and easy to implement, and because it brings immediate, highly visible benefits. It is good public health and good politics.[49]

Table 7-10. Estimated Percentage of Children Immunized in the First Year of Life and Percentage of Pregnant Women Immunized Against Tetanus, by WHO Region, April 1992

Region	Percentage of Children Immunized by 12 Months of Age				Percentage of Pregnant Women Immunized
	BCG	DPT3	Polio3	Measles	Immunized
African	81	58	58	58	48
American	82	76	89	81	31
Eastern Mediterranean	86	82	81	81	62
European	74	80	82	79	2
Southeast Asian	93	88	90	80	67
Western Pacific	96	94	94	93	6
Global	88	82	84	80	39

[a]For abbreviations see Table 7-9.

Source: EPI documents.

An important element in the EPI program is the low cost of the vaccines themselves, around one dollar per immunized child (not including HBV), made possible because more than 60% of the vaccines are produced in developing countries, the remainder coming through UNICEF mainly from Canada, Japan, and Europe (but not the United States). The low cost is even more remarkable because there is about a 60% wastage rate for the EPI vaccines.[50] However, costs are increasing and some developing countries are facing a shortage of funds as some donors seek other investments to replace seemingly endless requests to fund consumable supplies. Moreover, newer vaccines such as for hepatitis B are considerably more expensive, and population growth and increasing coverage compound the problem, which some authorities consider a crisis.[51]

An analysis of approximately 30 studies on cost and cost-effectiveness of childhood immunization programs concluded that by 1994 the EPI had prevented 3.2 million child deaths from measles, neonatal tetanus, and pertussis, as well as 440,000 cases of paralytic poliomyelitis. These impressive reductions in cause-specific mortality do not tell the whole story if overall deaths are unchanged. Indeed, in the Gambia, despite immunization coverage higher than in England, infant mortality rates remained high (42 per 1000 live births) because of a shift from immunizable diseases to other causes of death, primarily malaria, acute respiratory infection (ARI), and diarrhea.[52] Such observations underscore the need for more comprehensive approaches rather than piecemeal disease-base or procedure-based programs, however worthwhile they may be.

The cost per fully immunized child (FIC) varies greatly among countries and by strategy. A study found the cost per FIC to range from $8.09 in Tanzania to $22.63 in Turkey at fixed facilities; from $15.74 to 22.63 using mobile teams; and from $11.74 to $32.69 based on national campaigns. These programs are not always affordable. Poor sub-Saharan African countries may depend on outside donors for up to 85% of immunization costs.

> Using a figure of $15 per fully immunized child, the cost of EPI at 80% coverage was estimated to be $1.4 billion per year for a sample of 50 countries. For many countries, an 80% coverage level was not affordable to governments based on allocating 0.1% of gross domestic product (GDP) to immunization services. In several African and Asian countries, a 0.4% allocation of GDP was still insufficient to cover the costs of reaching 80% coverage levels. Compared to current budgets, 80% coverage claimed between 0.31% of annual health budgets in Costa Rica to over 100% of current health budgets in Uganda. Therefore, in the short run, it appears that governments may not be able to afford some of the goals and targets of universal coverage.[53]

As the authors point out, these are costs of *providing* the services, not of *receiving* the services, which incude travel time, waiting time, possible loss of earnings, and other direct and indirect costs to families. It is essential that programs such as EPI be made as cost-effective as possible through economies of scale, reducing inefficiencies, increasing the productivity of personnel, using appropriate technologies, maintaining equipment in working order, and using it to capacity.

The Programme for Vaccine Development, initiated by the WHO in 1984, was incorporated into the Department of Vaccines and Other Biologicals of the Health Technology and Pharmaceuticals cluster in the 1998 reorganization. Additional funding comes from various governments and private foundations. Its interests are more technical, dealing more with the vaccines themselves rather than their application in the field. Its long-term goal is to minimize the number of inoculations needed, and, ultimately, to make a single children's vaccine containing many immunizing antigens all delivered in a single dose soon after birth. Its objectives are to:

- Improve existing vaccines which, because of various shortcomings such as reduced shelf life at tropical temperatures, high cost, and limited efficacy, are not totally effective in the developing world
- Develop new vaccines against major viral and bacterial diseases where no such vaccines currently exist
- Provide mechanisms for international collaboration and coordinate broad participation of the public and private sectors
- Develop general methods to improve all vaccines

Former EPI director R.H. Henderson is said to have conceived the idea of a type of "Manhattan Project" for super polio vaccines to achieve polio eradication. He promoted this concept vigorously in various agencies, including UNICEF, where the idea mutated to the concept of the "single shot" children's vaccine mentioned above. The Children's Vaccine Initiative (CVI) was founded at the World Summit for Children held at the General Assembly of the United Nations in September 1990. The founding document of the CVI is the *Declaration of New York*. It is funded primarily by UNICEF, the Rockefeller Foundation, WHO, UNDP, and the World Bank. WHO provides a small staff and office facilities in its Geneva headquarters building. The CVI promotes planning, programming, and monitoring activities for increased cooperation among potential collaborators in the public and private sectors, and in the vaccine research, development, delivery, and regulation communities.

Mass immunization campaigns have achieved some success in many countries. In 1985 attention was given to El Salvador, where the civil war was interrupted for a day in each of three successive months so that more than 300,000 children could be immunized. Despite much publicized national crash campaigns, persistent work is necessary by international, national and local staff to integrate immunization programs into ongoing primary health care in order to keep up with the 365,000 infants born in the world each day. Note that at least four separate occasions are needed to fully immunize one child. Such repeated contacts may be difficult to achieve in many parts of the world where access to health facilities is limited.

Another major goal of immunization programs is to immunize women against tetanus, both for their own protection and to protect the newborn against neonatal tetanus, a major killer in many areas of the world.

THE CHILD SURVIVAL CAMPAIGN

In 1959 the UN General Assembly designated UNICEF as the agency responsible for carrying out the principles of the newly adopted Declaration of the Rights of the Child, and this agency has become widely known as the chief architect of the *child survival and development revolution.* UNICEF priorities include growth monitoring, oral rehydration, promotion of breastfeeding, female education, child spacing, and nutrition supplementation. In 1984 a Task Force for Child Survival was established by representatives from the WHO, UNICEF, the World Bank, UNDP, and the Rockefeller Foundation. The function of this task force was to promote all effective means, including immunization, ORT, and family planning, to reduce morbidity and mortality among the world's children. As a politically unassailable subject, the campaign has gathered adherents from many countries and agencies. A goal of child survival strategists is to identify and reduce the determinants of child mortality related to maternal fertility, environmental contamination, nutrient availability, injury, and disease. One barrier to such integration is said to be the lack of communication between biomedical and social scientists, sometimes considered as great as that between different cultures. The World Summit for Children in 1990 reinforced and expanded the child survival strategy.[54]

Programs have been criticized for focusing too much on the micro or household level, which makes for a very conservative orientation, for blaming the victims, and for lack of cultural sensitivity:

> The poor are charged with ignorance and inappropriate behavior, and are asked to change their life-styles to better adjust to the circumstances in which they are embedded. For example, they are asked to adjust to the realities of contaminated water by treating diarrhea, rather than being coached in methods for demanding improved waterworks from their local governments. Despite the enormous burdens the poor already face, they are asked to sit through lectures providing answers to questions they never asked . . . *we* who provide programs tend to assume that *they* who receive programs—the targets of our campaigns—understand malnutrition, diseases, and children's mortality in much the same ways *we* do. Where differences in understanding are noted, the reflexive response is to assume that *they* are wrong, and perhaps foolish or superstitious. Very regularly, the prescribed remedy is that *they* should be administered some education, which means getting *them* to see things as *we* see them. The idea that *we* might benefit from some education regarding *their* way of understanding is rarely entertained . . . We should be fully aware of the implications of doing band-aid work where major surgery is needed.[55]

Another frequent criticism of programs aimed at disease reduction in young children is that such efforts lead to population increases in areas where resources may be insufficient for the existing population. It is contended also that saving infants only to postpone death by a few years does not benefit anyone. This is a wrenching issue that must be confronted. Common arguments in favor of infant salvage are (1) that it is a humanitarian thing to do; (2) that parents eventually will have fewer children if they can be assured of their survival (see Demographic and Epidemiologic Transitions, Chapter 8); (3) that infant mortality is emotionally, socially, and economically damaging and a waste of resources; and (4) that such efforts can be combined with family planning or other population limitation programs. Kent[56] has reviewed criticisms; for example, that growth monitoring can become ritualistic and an end in itself without leading to any actions; that oral rehydration therapy does not address the causes of diarrhea and may not affect death rates; that breast-feeding programs have not been strongly supported; that immunization programs are a centrally controlled, top-down technological fix and are contrary to community-based primary health care; and so on.

Linking family planning to child survival may be a culturally and politically sensitive matter in some countries. In the early 1980s when a major child survival program for sub-Saharan Africa was in the planning stages, there was intense discussion among the industrial-country donors concerning inclusion of family planning activities. Some potential donors, concerned that they would be accused of sponsoring genocide, resolved the impasse by providing population-related information to national development planning and health ministries to use as they saw fit.

BABIES AND THEIR MOTHERS

The Mother and Baby Package

It seems pointless to discuss infant and child health without taking account the role of the mother, as half of infant deaths are attributed to poor maternal and newborn care. A mother's death, the ultimate disaster, is said to double the death rate among her surviving sons and quadruple the death rate among her surviving daughters. The health of women in developing countries has achieved prominence in recent years and will be discussed soon, but first a formal link between infant and maternal health should be mentioned. This is the "technical tool" developed jointly between WHO and UNICEF, the *Mother and Baby Package*. The rationale for the package is that saving mothers and babies requires early detection of obstetric complications,[57] timely referrral, and effective treatment. The interventions in the package are directed at both the mother and baby during pregnancy and childbirth and after delivery and are intended to be within the capacity of local midwives. Beyond the local level, the package also contains elements for building capacity at regional and national levels, including policy formulation, funding, training, and logistic and other components. The Mother and Baby Package is tied in with existing Maternal and Child Health and Family Planning programs. Among the other close associations between child and maternal health is the observation that malnutrition and stunting in young girls can lead to obstetric risks when they grow to adulthood.

Family planning (see the following chapter) has long been a mainstay of international development efforts, but the overall role of women as providers and health agents was undervalued by the development community until the late 1970s. Some earlier family planning efforts have been expanded or converted to larger issues in women's health, and improved understanding of the important roles played by women has stimulated and followed the United Nations Decade for Women and large international conferences on women's issues in Cairo (1993) and Beijing (1995) (see Chapter 3). Despite the emphasis on empowerment, the social and economic value of women is still frequently underestimated. The low status of women may begin before birth in some developing countries, where couples rely on ultrasound or uncertain other methods for decisions about selective termination of pregnancies. Such culturally and economically based discrimination may continue in childhood, when girls receive less nutrition and health services than their brothers. Although women generally have greater life expectancy than men, they tend to have more illness and physical disability. It is estimated that ill health specifically related to reproduction accounts for 30% of the overall burden of disease and disability among women of reproductive age, compared to 12% among men. Sexually transmitted diseases alone account for 8.9% of the burden of illness in women, compared to 1.5% in men of similar ages.[58]

Gender-specific health problems associated with women's low socioeconomic status include widespread domestic violence, dowry deaths, occupational diseases and disabilities prevalent in women, and sexually transmitted diseases, including AIDS, from enforced prostitution. Their lesser education, disadvantaged social position, and lack of legal autonomy combine to maintain relative poverty and powerlessness for women in many communities. Except for a few highly retrograde regimes, the status of female education is improving in most areas of the world.

Women's poor health also affects the welfare and productivity of their households and communities. Ironically, the poorer the family, the greater its dependence on women's economic contribution. Women are the sole breadwinners in some 30 percent of the world's households, and at least 25 percent of other households depend on female earnings for more than 50 percent of total income. Women also play a critical role in their national economies, and their physical well-being determines their ability to be productive. Data on women's contribution to development, while still tentative, indicate that women are responsible for up to three-quarters of the food and cash crops produced annually in the developing world. In Africa, women produce 80 percent of the food consumed domestically and at least 50 percent of export crops. Women also constitute one-third of the world's wage labor force and one-fourth of the industrial labor force. However, women's wages for the same or similar work are substantially lower than men's. In parts of Asia and Africa, women earn 50 percent less than men. Women work longer hours than men in every country except Australia, Canada and the United States.

Therefore, female ill health has a substantial impact on productivity and economic development[59]

Safe Motherhood and Maternal Mortality

Despite the many social and economic aspects of women's health, their reproductive function continues to be the major women's issue throughout the world.

The reproductive health of women in developing countries has until recently been a relatively neglected field of study and action. It is certain that sexually transmitted diseases such as gonorrhea lead to high levels of pelvic inflammatory disease and infertility in some populations, particularly in Africa, where AIDS is taking an increasing toll of women of reproductive age. Therefore the issue of maternal mortality cannot be divorced from the more general picture of reproductive health and sexual behavior in both sexes, with repercussions in areas from family planning to the organization of health and medical services.

Improved technology and awareness and (in some areas) increased age at marriage have reduced exposure to the risks of early childbearing and extended the capability of avoiding unwanted pregnancies. The *Safe Motherhood Initiative*, launched at the Nairobi Conference (1987), focused world attention on the extent of maternal mortality in developing countries.[60] Women in developing countries spend a larger proportion of the life span in reproduction (compared to those in developed countries), with all of its associated risks of pregnancy-related complications, many of which are, or should be, preventable. Continued high levels of these conditions proves that women's health has received insufficient attention. Each year more than 50 million women in developing countries are estimated to suffer acute pregnancy-related complications, many of which remain to cause long-term disability. The impact of common infectious diseases such as malaria and hepatitis, is worsened by pregnancy.

It is increasingly realized that attention should be devoted not only to reproduction *per se* but also to efforts to improve the health, nutritional status, and general well-being of females from infancy through childhood and into the adult years. It is also important to continue efforts to improve the economic status of women— for example, through loans from microcredit organizations such as the Grameen Bank (see Chapter 3).

Great numbers of women in the developing world receive no assistance from trained health care providers through pregnancy and delivery. The majority of women of reproductive age also lack regular access to modern methods of contraception, resulting in unwanted pregnancies.

This frequently results in poorly timed or unwanted pregnancies [which] lead to between 36 and 53 million abortions around the world every year. Pregnancy termination under unsafe conditions is the cause of 115,000 to 200,000 maternal deaths each year.

In Latin America, the complications of unsafe abortion are the main cause of death among women between the ages of 15 and 39 and absorb as much as 50 percent of some hospital maternity budgets.[61]

The World Development Report 1993 listed the leading causes of DALYs lost among women aged 15–44 in developing countries: First was maternal causes (complications of pregnancy and childbirth); second was sexually transmitted diseases; third, tuberculosis; and fourth, HIV/AIDS. A broader view of reproductive deaths must take account of the interactions among these causes, such as the close relationship between tuberculosis and AIDS. Some others are not so obvious. For example, the leading cause of cancer deaths among women in developing countries is cancer of the uterine cervix. Cervical cancer is caused overwhelmingly by infection with certain strains of human papilloma virus, a sexually transmitted pathogen.

The health of infants is closely associated with that of their mothers, but until recently the issue of maternal mortality received relatively little attention. The Safe Motherhood Initiative now attracts the interest of many governmental and intergovernmental agencies as well private voluntary organizations. Activities of these groups are scattered in many directions, with interests ranging from technical aspects of fertility regulation to the politics of women's literacy, income generation, and legal empowerment. Much time and effort can be diverted by the desire to "do something," which can lead to irrelevant and unnecessary research and ineffective programs.[62]

Less than 1% of maternal deaths occur in wealthier countries, where the great majority of pregnant women receive some prenatal care. Nevertheless, the collection of data on pregnancies and their outcomes might require searching the files of all obstetricians and primary care physicians—a daunting task replete with ethical and legal caveats. Even so, many women, perhaps unaware of their pregnancy, undergo undetected early spontaneous abortions which could obviously never be recorded. Intentional abortions, particularly those with contraceptive intent, are also not widely reported, and in jurisdictions where these are not legal it is almost impossible to collect meaningful data.

The dimensions of maternal mortality have been described dramatically by Malcolm Potts, former president of Family Health International: "Every four hours, day-in, day-out, a jumbo jet crashes and all on board are killed. The 250 passengers are women, most in the prime of life, some still in their teens. They are all either pregnant or have just delivered a baby. Most of them have growing children at home, and families that depend on them."[63]

It is estimated that more than one woman dies every minute from such causes; 585,000 women every year. Country-level differences are dramatic: It is reported that one of every nine women in Ethiopia dies from pregnancy-related complications, as compared to one in 8700 in Switzerland.[64] In the Western Hemisphere the risk ranges from one in 50 in Bolivia to one in 12,990 in Canada.[65]

The true number of maternal deaths is unknown because "Most of those who die are poor, live in remote areas and their deaths are accorded little importance. In those parts of the world where maternal mortality is highest deaths are rarely recorded and even if they are, the cause of death is usually not given."[66] Of all maternally related deaths in the world more than 99% occur in the poorer countries, in which 86% of all births occur. More than half of all maternal deaths take place in Asia. Of those, three-fourths are in Bangladesh, Pakistan, and India. India alone has more maternal deaths each week than all of Europe has in a year.

- *Antenatal care*: The percentage of women who seek antenatal care at least once is 63% in Africa, 65% in Asia, and 73% in Latin America and the Caribbean. At the country level, however, use of such services can be extremely low. In Nepal, for example, only 15% of women receive antenatal care.
- *Care during childbirth*: Each year, 60 million women give birth with the help of an untrained traditional birth attendant or a family member, or with no help at all. Almost half of births in developing countries take place without the help of a skilled birth attendant (such as a doctor or midwife).
- *Care after delivery*: The majority of women in developing countries receive no postpartum care. In very poor countries and regions, as few as 5% of women receive such care.[67]

National figures do not tell the real story of maternal deaths. In South Africa during apartheid, rates of maternal death (per 100,000) were cited as 0, 38, and 52 for White, Coloured, and Black women, respectively.[68]

The many direct physiological causes of death during pregnancy, such as hemorrhage, infection, convulsions and coma (eclampsia), obstructed labor and the like, sadly catalogued in obstetric textbooks, are found with distressing frequency in the poorer countries. Fatal infections resulting from contamination during childbirth are particularly unfortunate because the means for their avoidance are available almost everywhere. In Vienna 150 years ago about 12% of women died of infection (puerperal sepsis) shortly after delivery in the General Hospital. The Hungarian physician Ignaz Semmelweis showed clearly that such deaths were caused by transmission of some infectious agent (at that time unknown) from the unwashed hands of the doctors themselves and ordered strict enforcement of basic sanitary measures, which produced a dramatic decline in deaths. Sadly, these simple rules of hygiene have not yet been adopted in some parts of the world, and the same outcome encountered by Semmelweis a century and a half ago is still all too common.

A second, and equally avoidable cause of fatal infections is unsterile, poorly performed abortions. The WHO estimated that *every minute* in the late 1990s 380 women became pregnant and 40 women had unsafe abortions. About 50 million abortions from unwanted pregnancies are performed annually, causing 13% to 20% and in some areas up to 50% of maternal deaths. Of these preventable deaths, 99%

are in developing countries, primarily in sub-Saharan Africa and Asia. These unnecessary deaths occur simply because women do not have access to the family planning services that they want and need or have no access to safe procedures or to humane treatment for the complications of abortion. Figures are particularly difficult to obtain about this cause, in large part because abortion is illegal in many countries in Latin America and elsewhere, and available data are sparse and sometimes conflicting. Complicated illegal abortion accounted for 40% of acute gynecological admissions to the Kenyatta National Hospital in Kenya, 60% of all minor surgery at the Korle Bu Hospital in Ghana, and 30%–40% of all maternal deaths in Latin America.[69]

> In Romania, abortion was made available on request in 1957; by 1965 over one million abortions per year were being performed (a lifetime rate of almost four abortions per woman). The crude birth rate fell to 14/1000 population. In 1966 dictator Nicolae Ceauşescu decreed abortion and all modern contraceptives illegal. The birth rate doubled and registered abortions fell by a factor of twenty, but by 1983, with illegal services better established, the birth rate was back to where it had been before abortion and contraception were restricted. The maternal mortality rate doubled to over 150 per 100,000 live births, ten times higher than elsewhere in Europe, with 86% of deaths due to illegal abortion. Almost one fifth of women of reproductive age became infertile, and many children were abandoned at birth and left in state orphanages. In 1989, one day after Ceauşescu was overthrown, abortion was again made available on request and contraceptives were permitted. Maternal deaths halved within a year (from 170 to 83 per 100,000 live births) and the abortion rate climbed to the highest recorded rate in the world.[70]

Other risk factors for maternal mortality include nutritional state, disease, high parity, and age below 20 or above 35. In Bangladesh, where 50% of women are married by age 15, maternal mortality among 10–14-year olds was 5 times as high as among 20–24-year olds. In the United States the risk of death, while still low, is tenfold higher at 44 than at age 24. In addition to maternal death, more than 50 million women experience maternal health problems annually. It has been estimated that more than one-quarter of all adult women living in the developing world suffer from short- or long-term illnesses and injuries related to pregnancy and childbirth.[71]

Despite the significant risks, many women in poor countries fail to seek prenatal and obstetric services because of distance from health services; cost (direct fees as well as the cost of transportation, drugs, and supplies); multiple demands on their time; and lack of decision-making power within the family. The poor quality of services, including unprofessional and unsympathetic treatment by health providers, also makes some women reluctant to use services.

A decade after the launch of the Safe Motherhood Initiative, the subject has become an international priority with the participation of governments, donors, technical agencies, nongovernmental organizations, and women's health advocates in more than 100 countries. As with any global program it has its own bureaucracy, the Safe Motherhood Inter-Agency Group (IAG), composed of the United Nations Children's Fund (UNICEF), United Nations Population Fund (UNFPA), World Bank, World Health Organization (WHO), International Planned Parenthood Federation (IPPF), and the Population Council.

A comprehensive package of services for safe motherhood should include the following:

- *During adolescence*, all young people should have information on sexuality, reproduction, contraception, decision-making skills, and gender relations in order to help them make informed decisions about sexuality and to negotiate abstinence or safer sex. Sensitive, respectful, and confidential reproductive health counselling and services for married and unmarried adolescents should emphasize the prevention of unwanted pregnancy, unsafe abortion, and sexually transmitted diseases (STDs).
- *During pregnancy*, health workers should educate women about how to stay healthy, help women and families prepare for childbirth, and raise awareness about possible pregnancy complications and how to recognize and treat them. Health workers should also identify and manage any complications early and improve women's reproductive health and well-being through preventive measures (iron supplements, tetanus immunization) and by detecting and treating existing problems (such as sexually transmitted diseases).
- *During childbirth*, every woman should be helped by a health professional who can manage a normal delivery as well as detect and manage complications such as hemorrhage, shock, and infection. Skilled attendants should have access to a functioning emergency and transport system so that they can refer women to an appropriate health facility for higher level medical care (such as caesarean delivery or blood transfusion) when necessary.
- *After delivery*, women should be seen by a health worker, preferably within three days, so that any problems (such as infection) can be detected and managed early. An additional postpartum visit within the first six weeks after delivery enables health workers to make sure that the mother and baby are doing well, to provide advice and support for breastfeeding, and to offer family planning information and services.

The Safe Motherhood guidelines specify that family planning counselling and services should be available to all couples and individuals, including adolescents and unmarried women. Family planning services should offer complete information and counselling as well as a wide choice of modern contraceptives, including emergency contraception, and should be part of a comprehensive program that addresses other sexual and reproductive health needs. In addition, high-quality services for treating and managing complications of unsafe abortion should be available through all health systems by staff who are trained and authorized to treat complications with appropriate equipment, protocols for care, and effective referral networks. This is clearly a sensitive issue in many countries where abortion is illegal. Where legal, safe services for pregnancy termination and compassionate counselling should be available. Health workers must be informed about the legal status of abortion and protocols for providing it. Appropriate technologies, including new methods such as nonsurgical abortion, should be available where feasible.

It is estimated that routine maternal care for all pregnancies, including a skilled attendant (midwife or doctor) at birth; emergency treatment of complications during pregnancy, delivery and after birth; and postpartum family planning and basic neonatal care would cost about three dollars per person per year in low-income countries.[72]

THE HEALTH OF ADULTS

Having pondered the health of children and of childbearing women, we must complete the demographics by looking at other adults. The elderly, age 60 and over, will be considered in the following chapter. Those in between form the economic backbone in all countries but have received little attention. Many health ministries, occupied with other priorities, have not emphasized work on the main causes of adult deaths; indeed, a landmark book on the subject spoke of the "adult health policy vacuum."[73] The prevalent opinion in the West is that most people in developing countries succumb to tropical infectious diseases, but

> In fact, noncommunicable diseases, rather than "tropical" or other communicable diseases, are the leading causes of adult death in developing countries. This is true even in very poor countries like Bangladesh, where the burden of communicable diseases remains high. In those countries possessing adequate data, about 72% of the mortality risk for men between 15 and 59 years (and 82% of that for women) is from noncommunicable causes, and 23% for men (and 11% for women) is from injuries. Cardiovascular diseases rank first for both men and women, and neoplasms and unintentional injuries rank in the top five for men.[74]

It is estimated that about eight million avoidable deaths between the ages of 15 and 60 occur each year. The Global Burden of Disease Study[75] reported what it termed "significant surprises," such as:

- The burdens of mental illnesses, such as depression, alcohol dependence and schizophrenia, have been seriously underestimated . . . While psychiatric conditions are responsible for little more than one per cent of deaths, they account for almost 11 per cent of disease burden worldwide.

- Adults under the age of 70 in sub-Saharan Africa today face a higher probability of death from noncommunicable disease than adults of the same age in established market economies.
- Men living in the Formerly Socialist Economies of Europe have a disturbingly poor, and deteriorating, health status, including a 28 per cent risk of death between the ages of 16 and 60.
- By 2020, tobacco is expected to kill more people than any single disease, surpassing even the HIV epidemic.[76]

In the first quarter of the 21st century the risk of death for children and adolescents is projected to decline by perhaps two-thirds in sub-Saharan Africa and South Asia. Adult women, who already outlive men almost everywhere, will see further benefits. It has become fashionable in recent years among certain circles to depict adult men as lazy, belligerent, and incompetent, but that is not always the case. Gains for adult men will be more modest worldwide, and will actually be negative in some regions because of the well known effects of tobacco and alcohol.

In addition to deaths, illnesses and injuries in the adult labor force reduce productivity and place heavy burdens on the health services because noncommunicable diseases and disabilities are usually expensive to treat. As the proportion of adults increases in populations worldwide, greater attention must be given to their health problems, particularly to education and prevention.

PRIMARY HEALTH CARE

The 30th annual World Health Assembly (1977) decided unanimously that the main social target of member governments and of the WHO itself in the succeeding decades should be "the attainment by all citizens of the world by the year 2000 of a level of health that will permit them to lead a socially and economically productive life." This clearly enunciated goal, now commonly known as *"Health for All by the Year 2000"* or simply HFA2000 quickly became a major programmatic target of the WHO. A voluminous literature, both supportive and critical, has arisen about the HFA2000 concept. Although it is generally conceded that "health for all" will not in fact be attained by the year 2000, proponents point to positive results of the HFA movement.

The HFA2000 concept was a product of the International Conference on Primary Health Care (PHC) held in September 1978 in Alma-Ata (now Almaty), the capital of Kazakhstan.[77] This conference, cosponsored by the World Health Organization (WHO) and United Nations Childrens Fund (UNICEF), was attended by representatives of 143 countries and 67 organizations, including UN agencies and nongovernmental organizations. A landmark in international health, it was at the time the largest conference ever held on any single theme. On September 12, 1978, the Declaration of Alma-Ata was adopted, stating that the key to attaining HFA2000 is *primary health care.*

The conference was no less than an international effort to expand and redirect health programs in countries throughout the world. Its goal was to make substantial, rapid, and inexpensive improvements in the delivery of preventive and curative services at the community level, primarily in rural areas. A widespread perspective at the conference identified the existing roadblocks to reaching that end as not primarily medical but essentially political, indicating that they needed to be defined and analyzed in that context.

The PHC approach was influenced by the People's Republic of China, where the Great Proletarian Cultural Revolution excoriated foreign influences and domestic professionals with the slogan "better red than expert." Chairman Mao Zedong denigrated the role of health professionals and set the stage for the era of the *barefoot doctors* (see also Chapter 12).

Tell the Ministry of Public Health it only works for 15 percent of the entire population. Furthermore, this 15% is made up mostly of the privileged. The broad ranks of the peasants cannot obtain medical treatment and also do not receive medicine. The Public Health Ministry is not a people's ministry. It should be called the Urban Public Health Ministry, or the Public Health Ministry of the Privileged, or even the Urban Public Health Ministry of the Privileged. Medical education must be reformed. It is basically useless to study so much . . . Medical education does not require senior middle school students, junior middle school students or even graduates of senior elementary school. Three years are enough. The important thing is that they study while practicing. This way doctors sent to the countryside will not overrate their own abilities, and they will be better than those doctors who have been cheating the people and better than the witch doctors. In addition the villages can afford to support them . . . At the present time the system of examination and treatment used in the medical schools is not at all suitable to the countryside. Our method of training doctors is for the cities, although China has more than 500 million peasants . . . We should keep in the cities those doctors who have been out of school for a year or two and those who are lacking in ability. The remainder should be sent to the countryside . . . In medicine and health, put the stress on the rural areas.[78]

The tone set by Chairman Mao showed that the barefoot doctor movement was established principally on political grounds as a lever to forward the cultural revolution, and secondarily as a vehicle to bring inexpensive, basic health care to the mass of people in rural areas. Although the employment of locally trained medical assistants was by then well established, e.g. in some former African colonies, barefoot doctors caught the imagination of people in many countries and were an important conceptual underpinning of the Alma-Ata conference more than a decade later.

Four lessons can be drawn from the Chinese experience. First, rely on the potential talents, enthusiasms, and creative abilities of ordinary people. Second, encourage self-reliance, which can be extended to a national scale. Third, create a new type of rural health worker, one who will retain deep roots in the village community and engage in medical work on a part-time and voluntary basis. Fourth, organize the education of rural health workers to combine theory and practice at every stage, conduct it in the countryside, and adapt it to the needs of the locality. Perhaps the most important lesson to be learned from China is that it is not impossible for a poor country to mount successful efforts against the most pervasive and damaging threats to health, that large amounts of money or of medical research are not necessarily prerequisites, and that the lack of either should not be accepted as justification for official inaction.[79]

During the 1960s many observers had become convinced, along with Chairman Mao, that conventional approaches were inadequate to provide health and medical care to a majority of the world's people. The surge of population to cities everywhere drew attention conversely to the dismal conditions of rural life in developing countries, and reevaluations of rosy postwar projections suggested that resources would never be sufficient to reach everyone. In response, the British economist E.F. Schumacher established the Intermediate Technology Development Group (ITDG) in London in 1965. Very shortly the ITDG launched a Rural Health Panel composed of a nucleus of experienced, dedicated, and influential health activists and theoreticians. Discussion of "appropriate technology" stimulated by Schumacher's book, *Small is Beautiful* (1973), became commonplace on campuses in the West, just as Rachel Carson's *Silent Spring* had earlier launched concern about the environment. The Rural Health Panel established close ties with the World Health Organization, which itself was just establishing its own program in Appropriate Technology for Health (ATH), and an Appropriate Health Resources And Technologies Action Group (AHRTAG) was developed with joint support. Numerous publications emanated from these groups, dealing with the roles of health auxiliaries, appropriate health technologies, community education, diarrheal disease control, and similar topics, all embracing simplified procedures within a community-based viewpoint.

The 1970s was a time of testing of many young countries and of often less than friendly interactions between rival East–West and North–South international blocs. The sharp rise in petroleum prices early in the decade revealed once more the emerging power of nonwestern countries. The *Group of 77*, primarily developing countries, was established in the United Nations, challenging the traditional industrialized world, and a New International Economic Order was widely discussed. The outcome of the Vietnam War in mid-decade underscored the now-permanently changed relations between industrialized and developing countries, reflected more subtly in a widely expressed emphasis on collaboration rather than aid. Newly emerged nations, most now in their second decade, were establishing their own competence through universities, government ministries and research laboratories, industry, and other institutions. Local training of professionals of all kinds, including physicians, reduced dependence upon outside experts, whose welcome was perceptibly diminished. At the same time, concerns were raised everywhere about the seemingly uncontrollable costs of medical care and its increasingly inequitable distribution.

Although the cultural revolution in China was over by the time of Alma-Ata, the barefoot doctor approach had given rise to experimentation with a variety of village or community health workers in many poorer countries. Increasing political activism was reflected in wildly differing ideas about the health significance of literacy, housing, overpopulation, and social justice. The growing popular disillusionment with high-technology approaches, particularly in the health field, found expression in other ways. Controversies over infant bottle feeding, the building of dams, use of pesticides, agricultural policies, and urbanization promoted the notion that some forms of development are bad for health and led to radical policy revisions among major international players such as the World Bank and the WHO. At the Alma-Ata conference the WHO's activist Director-General set the tone for the conference:

> It is offensive that in one country people should die young while in another they may expect to see their grandchildren grow up; that in one part of a city nutritional deficiency diseases are common, while in another, people worry about eating too much; that, despite the great advances in technology and the human sciences, there are over 500 million people in the world with incomes equivalent to $50 a year.
>
> A very important means for reducing some of these crass differences that separate human beings is the promotion of primary health care as a human right, without social or economic discrimination. This might sound like a call for the medical profession to assume a greater role. But unfortunately, it is not. In fact, the conduct of this most venerable of professions is itself one of the causes for the social ills that we are seeking to cure. This seeming paradox should unravel itself when we begin to examine the differences between "health" and "medicine": the confusion between these two words lies at the root of the crisis besetting the medical establishment in many countries.
>
> . . . We see today the fabulous medical machinery and gigantic medical establishments dedicated to treating every conceivable ill even to the point of obfuscating the distinction between life and death. The fatal attraction of summit technology has led to an obsessive concern with what I would call marginal disease, a concern that amounts to a distortion of the very concept of health as a status of physical, mental and social well-being.
>
> In these countries, for the most part Western Europe and the United States, an incredibly expensive medical industry is engaged, not in the promotion of health, but in the unlimited application of disease technology to a small number of potential beneficiaries . . . As the vast profesional establishment concentrates on the complicated problems of the few, professional education and training does likewise. The distortion of health work is therefore self-perpetuating. The whole unhealthy system finds its most grandiose expression in buildings, in disease palaces, with their ever-growing staffs and material sophistication . . . We have largely forgotten that today, more than ever before, solving our health problems depends on what people do for themselves. Helping them is the challenge facing a genuine health service as opposed to a dependence-producing medical service. Is it not strange that doctors should be accused of being the socially most alienated profession in contemporary society? [80]

He then threw down the gauntlet to attending governments in the form of challenges such as:

- Are you ready to address yourselves seriously to the existing gap between the health "haves" and the health "have nots" and to adopt concrete measures to reduce it?
- Are you ready to ensure the proper planning and implementation of primary health care in coordinated effort with other relevant sectors, in order to promote health as an indispensible contribution to the improvement of the quality of life of every individual, family and community as part of overall economic development?
- Are you ready to make preferential allocation of health resources to the social periphery as an absolute priority?
- Are you ready to introduce, if necessary, radical changes in the existing health delivery system so that it properly supports primary health care as the overriding health priority?
- Are you ready to fight the political and technical battles required to overcome any social and economic obstacles and professional resistance to the universal introduction of primary health care?
- Are you ready to make unequivocal political commitments to adopt primary health care and to mobilize international solidarity to attain the objectives of health for all by the year 2000?[81]

The consensus reached at Alma-Ata was confirmed in a resolution at the next (32nd) World Health Assembly in May 1979, and over the next few years a defined strategy was developed according to which PHC was honed as the instrument by which to achieve the goal of health for all by the year 2000. The global strategy was officially adopted by the WHO in 1981. From the beginning, PHC programs were visualized as an integral, permanent, and pervasive part of the formal health care system in any country and not as a separate add-on programs.

It should be emphasized that primary *medical* care—that is, preventive or curative personal care carried out by a primary care physician specializing in general or family practice—should not be confused with primary *health* care, as defined in conference documents: .

Essential health care based on practical, scientifically sound and socially acceptable methods and technology made universally accessible to individuals and families in the community by means acceptable to them, through their full participation and at a cost that the community and the country can afford, to maintain at every stage of their development in a spirit of self-reliance and self-determination. It forms an integral part of both the country's health system of which it is the central function and main focus of the overall social and economic development of the community. It is the first level of contact of individuals, the family and the community with the national health system, bringing health care as close as possible to where people live and work and constitutes the first element of a continuing health care process.

Despite their revolutionary appearance, neither the concept of PHC nor the means proposed to implement it were really novelties in 1978. Ideas about "basic health services," recommended many times previously, were incorporated and modified. The barefoot doctor movement in China has already been mentioned, but that was itself often predated—for example, within the Soviet Union and other countries which recommended widespread community-based health services.

The core components of PHC as defined at Alma-Ata are shown on Table 7-11. There may be differences in implementation among countries, depending upon local conditions and customs, but the underlying theory represents an integration of PHC with socioeconomic development so that each would support the other in a context of equity and social justice. The approach emphasized universal access and participation, with reallocation of resources if necessary to reduce inequalities in status and availability. Decentralization was a key, with community planning and community implementation, and all tasks performed locally insofar as possible, by local personnel appropriately trained. Methodologies for PHC were to be "scientifically sound, technically effective, socially relevant, and acceptable." The global strategy was just that: intended equally for poor and wealthy, south and north, developing and industrial.

In a widely cited paper published almost before the ink was dry on the Alma-Ata Declaration, Julia Walsh and the late Kenneth Warren[82] argued in favor of *selective PHC*. The selective approach consisted of more restrictive, specifically targeted programs for prevention and treatment of illnesses, at least as an interim measure until *comprehensive PHC* can be established. Priority for interventions would be determined on the bases of prevalence, morbidity, mortality, and feasibility of control, including efficacy and cost. Such programs, aimed at diseases with the greatest health impact, were proposed as being the most effective means of improving the health of the greatest number of people. In rebuttal, defenders of the original CPHC concept charged that the selective approach opposes the concept of commu-

Table1 7-11. The Essential Components of Primary Health Care

1. Health education
2. Environmental sanitation, especially of food and water
3. The employment of community or village health workers
4. Maternal and child health programs, including immunization and family planning
5. Prevention of local endemic diseases
6. Appropriate treatment of common diseases and injuries
7. Provision of essential drugs
8. Promotion of nutrition
9. Traditional medicine.

Source: Alma-Ata Conference Documents.

nity participation and control, selects for treatment only people with priority diseases, reinforces authoritarian attitudes, lacks a sound scientific basis, and has a questionable moral and ethical value with the imposition of foreign and elite interests over those of the people.[83] The original concept of primary health care was more akin to that of Chairman Mao: using health as a wedge to a social development strategy; SPHC had changed it to a strategy for prioritizing medical care. The key issue was control over decision-making.

Some commentators are naive and uncritical about what they consider the unlimited potential of PHC, as some people had romanticized the barefoot doctors of rural China.[84] Almost from the start, others were cynical about PHC and HFA2000, considering these programs not as *primary*, but as *primitive* health care, idealistic and unattainable, and bound to fail. Early on, even before a track record had been established, one author observed that

> There is very little real political commitment, either in the developed world or amongst the elite of the developing world, to do much for the poor. WHO now finds itself saddled with idealistic international resolutions that few countries are really keen to implement back home, whether it is in terms of coming forward with the funds required to bring health care for all, or in terms of implementing those strategies and reordering domestic health priorities. Lack of a real consituency is not the only problem. Even to prepare the intellectual framework for the change has meant antagonising such powerful actors in the existing health drama as the drug industry . . . and not least, the medical establishment.[85]

Suspicion about the motives of outsiders is common although rarely published in peer-reviewed journals. One local activist wrote about the Universal Immunization Program in India:

> One can thus discern a deeply disturbing—indeed frightening—chain of disinformation, distortion, and cheap propaganda in a bid to sell the immunization program, both globally and in India: making a case for cost-effectiveness of selective primary health care on the basis of highly questionable data; making exaggerated assessments of load of mortality and morbidity due to the six diseases; making exaggerated claims on the efficacy of the vaccines; ignoring vital epidemiological, biological, and administrtive issues in program formulation and implementation; conducting poor monitoring and surveillance; restricting or actively preventing access to the available information; and indulging in false propaganda claiming success for the program. These are many of the key elements of a totalitarian system. This account of "selling" of the immunization program in India provides an awe-inspiring instance of formation of a syndicate of medical scientists, bureaucrats, and political leaders and their mentors from abroad, who invoked the emotional cause of the plight of the children in poor countries to build a closed, monolithic, "totalitarian" program . . . Protection of children is a very desirable health action and it should indeed form an important element of primary health care activities. This is quite different from invoking the cause of children by vested market

and political interests joining some well-meaning though simplistic persons in affluent countries to impose a technocentric, high-priority, target-oriented, time-bound immunization program on a country.[86]

Well-meaning people in the West, particularly students, may be shocked and hurt by such stinging criticisms. But "we are only trying to help" is an insufficient justification in the face of deeply held suspicions by the supposed beneficiaries of primary care programs. People everywhere want to be valued and respected. While on the whole external assistance is welcome and appreciated, people resent approaches that they feel to be patronizing or belittling, especially when they feel that the supposed benefactors are responsible for putting them into poverty in the first place. Political imperialism has not been forgotten. The conceptual line between foreign investment and economic exploitation, or between expert advice and western arrogance, can be shifted by persuasive argument. It is important to know how widespread and how valid these opinions may be, and what lessons are to be learned from them. A less contentious, more genteel analysis of EPI programs has concluded that efforts to accelerate imunization coverage during the 1980s may have prevented implementation of other priority components of primary health care services, such as water and sanitation, maternal health care, health education, and family planning.[87]

The Primary Care Team

Most people believe that new approaches are needed to solve the health problems in poor areas of the world. Even within HFA no single scheme is unversally applicable, but the following elements are often suggested:

- Increased planning, coordination, and integration within the health sector for education of personnel, development of facilities, provision of services, and utilization of resources, together with national development planning in general
- Sustained attempts to make primary care services more widely available, especially in rural areas
- Greater utilization and community participation
- Broader development of health care teams, including various kinds of auxiliary medical workers.

Many job titles have been given to front-line medical auxiliaries, such as village health worker (VHW), community health worker (CHW), or traditional birth attendant (TBA) or village midwife such as the *empirica* or *parteira* (Latin America), *matrone* (French-speaking Africa), or *dai* (India). These TBAs are commonly given brief training in hygiene, nutrition, and basic first aid and provided with a kit of instruments and renewable supplies. Attempts have often been made to incorporate

practitioners of folk or traditional medicine such as *curanderos*, who understand and
have the confidence of the people they serve. It is easy for westerners to romanti-
cize community health workers, but very difficult for the CHWs to carry out their
functions, as F.M. Mburu says, with "little more than a writing pad and an empty
stomach."

> Resources at the disposal of CHW programmes are at best unreliable or minimal alto-
> gether. As a result programmes are noticeable by their prevalence, having litle or no
> impact, and, above all, by the way they rise only to fizzle out . . . Poverty, sometimes
> in abject proportions, is the real problem in most communities. It requires considerable
> resources and determination to dent it. Sending a CHW to attack poverty may have no-
> ble intent, but it is really an insignificant side-show.[88]

It is easy to make assumptions, pro or con, on ideological grounds, but evidence-
based evaluations of actual PHC programs in the field are difficult, costly, time-
consuming, and rare. A PHC program was started in the Gambia in 1981. Village
health workers and traditional birth attendants were selected and given six weeks
of training. Yet in one area a 1993 survey found significantly higher child mortality in PHC villages, where 54% of people lived, than in non-PHC villages, an outcome the authors understandably found "difficult to interpret."[89]

Despite these grim comments there are good examples of well-run projects organized by competent and charismatic leaders in which CHWs have been productive and successful. Such projects include Jamkhed in India, Gonoshasthaya Kendra
in Bangladesh, and Chimaltenango in Guatemala. Village health workers were an
important part of the national health system in Indonesia even before Alma-Ata. In
rural Java VHWs serve as liaison between households and the official health system. In a one-month study of coverage of target households and children in a village with a VHW-run nutrition program, 84% of households were reached and 71%
of children under five attended a weighing session. In two study villages about the
same number of people consulted VHWs as went to clinics. "This suggests that
VHWs can play a significant role in increasing illness care as well as in screening
and referral of cases."[90] The keys are professional interest, proper selection, well-
defined tasks, good and continued training, and adequate support and supervision

An avalanche of studies and publications on primary care has covered every aspect of this problem in many countries. Prominent in these are pictures of pyramids.
There is also the common pyramid of health services organization with the minister of health at the apex, down through the layers of bureaucracy to the many local
health installations at the base. At the local level is the *skill pyramid* within an institution, showing the physician or specialist at the top and proceeding through strata
of nurses and clerks to the most lowly and most numerous employees. Also fea-
tured in works on primary care are diagrams resembling basket starfish, with repeatedly branching arms, radiating from a central hub; these branches represent hos-

pitals, polyclinics, health centers, satellite subcenters, dispensaries, *puestos de salud*, and many other categories of medical care facilities. The greatest attention has been given to the base of the pyramid or the periphery of the radii, because that is where the frontline interactions actually occur, where the users and providers of primary health care meet face to face. What takes place during these encounters? One hopes that all, or most, of the following will occur:

- Flow of information, in both directions: to the user, education about sanitation, disease prevention, nutrition, family planning; from the user, hopes, fears, symptoms, observations, clues for an alert medical worker to use in planning better services.
- Primary prevention of disease by immunization, distribution of antimalarials, and other prophylactic measures.
- Procedures for screening real or potential health problems, especially among pregnant women and young children.
- Distribution of contraceptives to those desiring them.
- Secondary prevention by provision of medications when needed for confirmed cases of chronic illnesses such as tuberculosis. This is also a means of primary prevention for contacts of patients.
- Diagnosis, treatment, and follow-up of cases of common minor illnesses.
- First aid for trauma and other accidents.
- Arrangement for assistance with normal childbirth.
- Referral, when necessary with transportation provided, of complex, difficult, or emergency cases to better-trained workers at better-equipped facilities.
- Maintenance of records and vital statistics.

The PHC programs can often point to spectacular results. However, in evaluation of health services, as in epidemiology, it is often difficult to determine cause and effect and to know which interventions are really productive. A local infant mortality rate can be reduced quickly from 150 to 50 deaths per 1000 live births with no medical care at all by introduction of effective health-supporting measures including water supply, sanitation, better housing, improved communication, and above all by public education (see Table 7-11).

Sustainability

Often three parties are involved in PHC programs in poor countries: the government at various levels; the community; and a foreign donor, which typically is more willing to finance initial investments than to become obligated to meet endless recurrent costs. Such reluctance highlights the problem of sustainability, or the capacity of a program to continue on its own without external assistance.

All health care programs suffer from the same basic difficulty. Whereas project inputs (resources) and service outputs (number of immunizations given, number of babies delivered) can be counted, it is difficult to measure the underlying goal of improved health. The number of cases of death and specific illness can be (but rarely are) recorded before, during, and after the introduction of a PHC scheme. Questionnaires can be administered about health status, disease symptoms, social adjustment, and similar matters. Nevertheless, to quantify the total health—the mental, physical, and social well-being—of a community and to demonstrate that changes were brought about by specific PHC activities is a daunting task. Agencies, academicians, and politicians like to evaluate methods and calculate the cost-effectiveness of interventions, but when the advisers and instructors have gone home and the external support has dried up, the community will be left to depend upon its own self-reliance to maintain the program. No amount of statistical manipulation or bureaucratic argument can substitute for a community's conviction that a program is, or is not, worthwhile. If the people see the service as meaningful to their lives; if it is accessible, reliable, courteous, and productive; if it is compatible with their norms and values, if they feel a sense of ownership, and support from people they respect, then there will be an incentive and motivation to maintain it. "The feelings of those served will be the litmus test of programme effectiveness, however subjective that perception may be. After all, people rank their needs differently and assess the assistance they get in their own peculiar way."[91] Systems designed elsewhere and imposed on a community without consultation will survive only as long as their funding, and are unlikely to be missed except by those whose livelihood depended on them.

Cost

Financial aspects of health services are the concern of subsequent chapters, but we cannot ignore cost in considering primary health care. In the industrialized countries the high costs of public and private health-related activities are underwritten by general economic prosperity. In the poorer countries such a "western-style" medical care system is impossible unless the system is highly motivated and organized, as in Cuba. The classical barefoot doctor of rural China, an integral member of a rigidly hierarchical commune system, was compensated in work points donated by members of his or her production brigade. That system, peculiar to China during the cultural revolution, is no longer used. The PHC programs must therefore be operated on a monetary basis. A long-time observer of village health programs has remarked that

> There is a myth that primary health care is a cheap solution to a difficult and complex problem. Not so, and those who attempt to sell it as a cheap solution do it poor service. The two basic resources required are financial and human (trained manpower). Both commodities are in very short supply. The stratagems being proposed to overcome the

deficiencies are fallacious. Financially it is proposed that communities should be self-reliant: bluntly that they should provide their own funding. The responsibility is thus neatly transferred from central government to local government and the local community. At a stroke the national government washes its hands.[92]

That is exactly what has happened, for example, in Nigeria, where the lost decade of the 1980s took its toll, and the federal health budget for 1988 was only about a quarter of that for 1981 in real terms. Responsibility for primary care was transferred to local governments, for secondary care to the state, for tertiary care to the federal governments. On the local level per capita health spending in 1989 ranged from the equivalent of 16 to 80 U.S. cents, and about 60% of that went to salaries.[93]

Symptoms of underfinancing are evident in many countries. These include:

- Reliance on foreign donors for drugs and other supplies for primary health care
- Lack of repair and replacement of equipment and vehicles; inadequate supplies of petrol to enable the services to be properly supervised
- Gross neglect of the maintenance of buildings
- Insufficient salary levels leading to the temptation to encourage "gifts" from users with consequential effects on equity in the use of services
- Inadequate staff, particularly of nurses in urban hospitals and other staff in the more remote rural areas
- Lack of a functioning information system[94]

As one example, insufficient funding of programs in Senegal led to demoralization of personnel, chronic shortages of drugs, rapid increase in the number of private pharmacies, and a rising temptation to divert products provided for pubic sector into "parallel markets." A loss of faith in public health services has reduced attendance by the population. "Under these circumstances the primary health care strategy tends to be discredited in the eyes of the medical staff in the public sector."[95]

Community Utilization of Programs

Perhaps surprisingly, many programs are characterized by low utilization by the public. Underutilization can arise partly from logistic issues, such as location of the facilities or hours of operation; partly from cost, both monetary and in time in comparison with other pressing priorities; partly from skepticism about western medicine or the competence of health workers; partly from the expected unavailability of supplies or medicines; and partly from perceived indifference and lack of respect from the health center staff. Interviews with more than 2000 persons in an East African country revealed the average expenditures of time for medical consultations shown on Table 7-12.

Part of the problem may arise from inappropriate resource allocations by health

Table 7-12. Average Time, in Minutes, Spent in Visit to Health Facilities, Tanzania[a]

Facility	Travel Time	Time at the Facility	Total Time
Mission hospitals	63	105	231
Government hospitals	52	177	281
Government health centers	38	134	210
Government dispensaries	31	100	162

[a]Year not specified; 1992 or just prior.

Source: Adapted from Abel-Smith and Rawal (1992) Table 1.

officials. In one study it was found that whereas offical pronouncements were strongly supportive of PHC programs, 59% of the health budget was actually spent for hospitals and only 7% for rural and preventive medicine. Moreover, the local villagers themselves showed only lukewarm interest in a PHC program. In general they wanted curative medicine and were not attracted to preventive activities that show no immediate result.[96] A similar situation occurred with a rural water project in Togo:

> In about 10% of the project villages, participation in project activities has been poor. Especially in larger villages (over 2,000) conflicts between different ethnic groups, chiefs, or political factions block communal collaboration . . . Previous bad experiences with village committees (who have often served only a figurehead role) and with mismanagement of communal funds have caused the inappropriate selection of committee members and distrust or misconception of the VHC [Village Health Committee] role. Villages with a large number of politically influential citizens have often benefited from development "gifts" (schools, pharmacies) and are thus unconvinced of the need for community participation.[97]

In Latin America a decade after Alma Ata the Pan American Health Organization launched a program for local health systems (Sistemas Locales de Salud) known as SILOS specifically to carry out the PHC strategy. SILOS were intended to decentralize health services in a democratic and efficient way and coordinate local resources into a larger health web. This is not an easy task. In Bolivia many such projects have been started, but with little reported effect on the health picture. The three main components of local services were expansion of health facilities, training of health personnel, and institutional strengthening. New health centers were intended to reduce the geographical barrier to access to health care and to respond to popular demand, but existing facilities have "notoriously low" rates of utilization. Why then build new facilities that will not be used?[98] The problem of underutilization of PHC services was pondered by the editor of a leading journal in these exasperated and perhaps exaggerated terms:

It seems clear to us that the picture of rural masses hungry for medical care services is an erroneous one. From this it would appear to follow that vast expenditures on supplying services for which there is so obviously no felt need may be an extravagant waste of resources. Perhaps we have in the past too readily assumed that we knew what people ought to want, and by mental legerdemain transposed that into what we thought they really did want. Maybe we should go back to fundamentals again.

There is no doubt at all that in the developing countries there is a great need for such things as ante-natal and post-natal clinics, well-baby clinics, tuberculosis clinics. Infant and toddler mortality rates are still in too many areas unacceptably high, and only the development of appropriate care centers will reduce them. Regrettably, while we know this, the people concerned show only too clearly by their failure to use these facilities that they do not. The conventional answer is of course health education, but here arises a "chicken and egg" situation that is difficult to resolve. Do you spend money on creating facilities that people do not want and probably will not use, just so you can educate people slowly to begin to use them? Alternatively, can you educate in the absence of facilities, until you have created a consumer demand?[99]

The Inevitable Role of the PHC Worker as a Sociopolitical Agent

Programs, especially social programs in developing countries, do not occur in a vacuum. As with any human endeavor, the medium of PHC may be distorted in directions other than the ostensibly innocent one of merely providing health care to underserved populations. We have seen how barefoot doctors in China were, at least in part, a purposeful tool to break the power of the medical profession. This point need not be belabored, nor is it in any way suggested that PHC programs are primarily conspiracies, acting as a proxy for the sinister motives of one party or another. Nevertheless, some parts of the world are dangerous places in which it is better to be cautious than to be naive.

A startling perspective on the misuse of PHC described hazards faced by frontline PHC workers in several countries.[100] It is axiomatic that implementation of PHC programs requires a degree of organization in villages and communities and a critical analysis of the local root causes of ill health. However, such activities may be viewed by repressive governments as provocative or hostile acts and may be subject to reprisals, particularly if efforts are actually undertaken to combat the underlying social origins of a community's health problems. Health workers may be in danger from conflict with established elites. In some countries VHWs have been murdered for exposing corrupt practices such as the sale of free government medicines.

However, PHC programs and their health workers may be utilized to further a government's political strategy or to show "commitment" to the people and thereby to defuse community unrest. A new PHC facility may serve as a vehicle to disseminate a government's viewpoints, to "cool out" potential opposition, or to provide a base for surveillance of possible antigovernment or "liberation" movements.

A basic public health measure such as a population census or household survey may be a politically value-laden undertaking in many areas.

A government's use of health inputs as a means of social control may result in the people's suspicion of the PHC worker, particularly in sensitive areas such as family planning. Obvious foreign sponsorship may invite a degree of suspicion.

Evaluation of PHC

At their best, PHC programs can fulfill the intentions of the drafters of the Declaration of Alma Ata. Benefits can accrue not only to the health status of individuals and communities but to confidence, self-sufficiency, and awareness of the participants. In order to determine whether a particular PHC program (or any program) is effective, some mechanism for evaluation must be built in from the start.

The reality has been that PHC has been adopted spottily in the developing world, and most wealthy countries have considered that PHC and HFA do not apply to themselves, if they have considered them at all. The western biomedical establishment, including medical schools, universities, and industry, have on the whole been oblivious to the PHC issue and wary of the whole HFA approach, to which they have in general been neither invited nor encouraged to play a role. HFA2000 is ultimately about poverty, politics, and power.[101] In the broadest view, as a strategy for societal development, PHC can help to tie together the educational, environmental, and social underpinnings of health within a community, but it can do so only with the collaboration of citizens, political leaders, and professional health workers.

Experience in the field suggests that the provision of PHC is a far more complex and cumbersome process than is reflected by current strategies.[102] From the point of a view of an outside donor agency, not enough is known about the interaction between social factors and the use and effects of interventions such as oral rehydration therapy. Similarly, we need better knowledge of the interaction between the structure of health care systems and the political economy of a population—in particular, the underlying assumption that communities in developing countries require large public systems using simple technologies and paraprofesionals. As expected, many of the problems have been administrative, such as inadequate integration with existing health services; poor training and low staff morale; too much haste; insufficient attention to supervision, supplies, and logistics; and poor administrative and financial support. The biomedical and social sciences must cooperate to avoid a program that is too vague in approach on the one hand or too technology-based on the other.

Critics have declared the death, or at least grave debility, of primary health care. One public health specialist from the World Bank opined that with the retirement of Halfdan Mahler as Director General of WHO, "the spirited advocacy for PHC and HFA essentially disappeared . . . internally WHO's top management has accepted that PHC and HFA are rapidly becoming sterile concepts of the past."[103] Nevertheless WHO continues to promote HFA. Their *Third Evaluation of Progress in Implementing the Global Strategy for Health for All by the year 2000*, carried out in 1997, reports significant improvements worldwide in the following elements of primary health care since the first evaluation in 1985: immunization against the EPI target diseases; trained attendance at childbirth; local health services; and water supply and excreta-disposal facilities. In developing countries, 65% of pregnant women were said to have access to antenatal care services and 53% to skilled attendance at delivery. In rural areas, 75% of the population have access to a safe water supply, and about 34% to adequate sanitation. Immunization program that covered 5% of children in the 1970s expanded to over 80% in 1996, with a big impact on the health status of children. These improvements, however, were found to be less significant in the least developed countries. The model has been remedicalized and the ringing egalitarian oratory of Mao and Mahler and the community-based participatory decision-making of Alma Ata seem nowhere to be found. Almost two decades later the focus in the international health arena has shifted from primary health care to health sector reform (Chapter 13). Selective PHC has in essence reappeared as a "package of essential services," advocated by the World Bank in the 1993 World Development Report and later publications. Chairman Mao's dictum of "better red than expert" has been turned on its head as the "experts" have prevailed. Near the end of the century, the campaign for Health for All by the Year 2000 is promoted only halfheartedly, and the community-based social control promised by comprehensive primary health care has for the most part gone the way of the barefoot doctors.

DISASTERS

Disasters come in all sizes, durations, and levels of impact. A death is a disaster for the family involved, perhaps less so for the community, and may go unnoticed by the nation. Many deaths at once make headlines; the same number occurring slowly over time cause hardly a ripple. Some acute calamities, such as avalanches and earthquakes, are natural. Others, such as building collapses, dam failures, the Bhopal chemical tragedy, or the Chernobyl nuclear power plant explosion, are technological in origin. Though caused by humans, these are unintentional; indeed, contrary to the desires of their builders and operators. Some natural disasters, such as droughts and famines, are insidious in onset but no less devastating in effect. Similarly, technological disasters may present a continuing tragedy: By some estimates 100 million unexploded antipersonnel land mines await the unwary foot in Afghanistan, Angola, Cambodia, El Salvador, Iraq, Mozambique, Somalia, and other countries. These are all a part of international health, but they are focused problems and, though tragic to their victims, more or less straightforward as disasters go.

Recent years have seen a growing prominence of *complex humanitarian emer-*

gencies (CHEs), defined as, "Relatively acute situations affecting large civilian populations, usually involving a combination of war or civil strife, food shortages, and population displacement, resulting in significant excess mortality."[104] Manifestations of evil, these events represent the dark side of human behavior especially when they involve *genocide*, "the systematic, planned annihilation of a racial, political, or cultural group."[105]

The CHEs are the most brutal of disasters and generate the largest number of refugees, defined as "persons who flee from their own country because of war, violence, famine, or a well-founded fear of persecution for reasons of race, religion, or nationality."[106] The dismal catalogue of sites is familiar: Afghanistan, Bosnia, Cambodia, Chechnya, Eritrea, Ethiopia, Guatemala, Kurdistan, Liberia, Somalia, Sudan, and so on. In such places people have been forced against their will to flee for their lives, abandoning homes, possessions, and relatives.

> Despite the fact that to some extent these events can be seen as recurring throughout history, several developments in recent years have combined to make CHEs more frequent, more visible, and more challenging. These events include the ending of the Cold War, allowing greater access to many parts of the world but also releasing pent-up regional hostilities; advances in media outreach and technological support; and a proliferation of voluntary private aid agencies who see it as their mission to provide aid to trapped civilian populations.[107]

The international agency charged with helping the world's refugees is the *United Nations High Commissioner for Refugees* (UNHCR), created by the U.N. General Assembly in 1951. With a staff of more than 5000 in 244 offices worldwide, and an annual budget of more than one billion dollars, the UNHCR collaborates with more than 400 non-governmental organizations in implementing its relief work. The total number of "people of concern to UNHCR" increased from 17 million in 1991 to a record 27 million in 1995 and then declined to 22.3 million as of January 1, 1998 (Table 7-13). Estimates vary widely, however, and some groups state that the number, including internally displaced persons, was more than 42 million in 1995.[108] The actual number "persons of concern" is a relatively modest percentage of the global population, particularly in the Western Hemisphere, but their suffering is disproportionately large. Refugees are defined by the UNHCR as "those who have fled their countries because of a well-founded fear of persecution for reasons of their race, religion, nationality, political opinion or membership in a particular social group, and who cannot or do not want to return."

Many other agencies are concerned with refugees, including a little-known arm of WHO, the *Division of Emergency and Humanitarian Action*. Within the United States the primary responsible agency is the *Office of International and Refugee Health* of the U.S. Public Health Service. This office, with a total staff of 39 people, provides liaison with other governments and international agencies in all health

Table 7-13. Persons of Concern to the United Nations High Commission for Refugees, by Region and Category, January 1, 1998

Region	Refugees	Asylum Seekers	Returnees	Internally Displaced Persons	Total
Africa	3,481,700	37,700	2,171,700	1,694,000	7,385,100
Asia	4,730,300	15,000	824,100	1,889,100	7,458,500
Europe	2,940,700	267,400	459,400	2,389,000	6,056,500
Latin America	83,200	600	17,800	1,700	103,300
North America	668,500	626,400	—	—	1,294,900
Oceania	71,700	6,900	—	—	78,000
Total	11,975,500	954,000	3,473,000	5,973,800	22,376,300

Source: UNHCR website

matters and cooperates with the Office of Refugee Resettlement and USAID on refugee health issues and emergency response capacity.

The plight of refugees has become a routine feature of the nightly news as television crews compete to document the prevailing humanitarian emergency. Pictures of bedraggled families and acutely ill children have a profound impact on the public's perception of international health. Many citizens, including students and health professionals, are understandably motivated to help reduce the suffering by contributing money or participating personally in relief efforts.

The leading international aid organizations, funded through governments and/or public support, play a valuable role in organizing and operating refugee camps, feeding stations, and mobile clinics. But sites of civil turmoil are hazardous to refugees and helpers alike, and many aid workers have been injured or killed. Well-intentioned but inexperienced individuals and organizations in such situations are more likely to become part of the problem than to alleviate it. Many critics are scornful of undisciplined efforts to participate. For example:

In the past decade I have watched the emergency aid "business" . . . grow from a small element in the larger package of "development" into a giant, global, unregulated industry worth £2500 million a year . . . The Rwandan capital, Kigali, became the aid capital of the world with 169 agencies resident, many staffed by young people on their first mission overseas. United Nations troops issued each newcomer with a handy laminated card featuring a map of the country and useful phrases in the local language: "Hello." "Do not shoot." "My name is Bob." "Where is Kigali?" At one regional meeting I attended, 15 agency representatives, each carrying a two-way radio, turned up in white Toyota four-wheel drives. The Rwandan government official in charge of the region, whose job it was to coordinate the aid flow, had no telephone, no car, not even a bicycle . . . There is a distinction to be made between professional agencies with experience in emergency relief and those who just want to be there or do something without knowing how.[109]

Such criticisms have been a factor in stimulating a number of larger NGOs to formulate a code of conduct titled *Principles of Conduct for the International Red Cross and Red Crescent Movement and NGOs in Disaster Response Programs.*[110] The code coins the acronym NGHA for non-governmental humanitarian agency and refers specifically to those NGHAs involved in disaster relief. A disaster is defined as "a calamitous event resulting in loss of life, great human suffering and distress, and large scale material damage." The major principles of conduct (with lengthy commentaries in the original) are:

- The humanitarian imperative comes first.
- Aid is given regardless of the race, creed or nationality of the recipients and without adverse distinction of any kind. Aid priorities are calculated on the basis of need alone.
- Aid will not be used to further a particular political or religious standpoint.
- We shall endeavor not to act as instruments of government foreign policy.
- We shall respect culture and custom.
- We shall attempt to build disaster response on local capacities.
- Ways shall be found to involve program beneficiaries in the management of relief aid.
- Relief aid must strive to reduce future vulnerabilities to disaster as well as meeting basic needs.
- We hold ourselves accountable to both those we seek to assist and those from whom we accept resources.
- In our information, publicity, and advertising activities, we shall recognize disaster victims as dignified humans, not hopeless objects.

Providing relief to disaster victims and refugees is theoretically simple but logistically difficult. The needs are clear: food, protection from the elements, clothing, sanitation, medical care, consolation and reassurance to frightened people, and above all, fresh clean water. In the mistaken belief that any and all "medical supplies" are the first priority, individuals and organizations sometimes send drugs, which may be tax deductible to the donors but are often worse than useless to recipients. For example,

after the 1988 earthquake in Armenia, 5000 tons of drugs and medical supplies worth $55 million were sent, which took 50 people six months to sort out. Only 30% of the drugs were easy to identify and only 42% were relevant for an emergency situation . . . Eritrea received seven truck loads of expired aspirin tablets that took six months to burn; a container full of unsolicited cardiovascular drugs with two months to expiry; and 30,000 bottles of expired amino acid infusion . . . southern Sudan received donations of contact lens solution, appetite stimulants, drugs against hypercholesterolaemia, and expired antibiotics . . . By the end of 1995, 340 tons of expired drugs were stored in Mostar. Most of these were donated by European nations, and the Mayor has writen to the European Union requesting international help to have them destroyed.[111]

The WHO has described a standardized "emergency health kit" containing suficient drugs, disposable medical supplies, and basic equipment to care for 10,000 people for three months.[112] But arranging to get these things to the people who need them at a time of turbulence may be a nightmare. Refugees must cope with everything that accompanies sudden destitution, including humiliation, physical insecurity, and violence. Mortality rates, especially among small children, soar to many times the population baseline mainly from infections and malnutrition. Cause-specific mortality in selected refugee sites in Bangladesh, Ethiopia, Kenya, Sudan, and Tanzania in 1994 was as follows:[113]

Malaria/fevers of unknown origin	16%
Respiratory tract infections	13.7%
Nonbloody diarrhea	12.5%
Bloody diarrhea	7%
Pregnancy/neonatal causes	6%
Malnutrition	5%
Measles	2.5%
Tuberculosis	2%
All others	33.3%

The health situation can be thought of as a sudden and extreme retrogression of the epidemiologic transition (next chapter). Deficiency diseases such as scurvy, pellagra, and beriberi, which are almost unheard of under normal circumstances, have appeared in refugee camps.[114] Outbreaks of louse-borne typhus occur among people who are unable to bathe or change their clothing.

A characteristic of wartime CHEs is the flagrant infringement of human rights (see also Chapter 15). Categories of health-related human rights that are violated include inhumane treatment of medical personnel, the sick, or the wounded (torture, killing, and forced disappearance); arrest, detention, or abduction of wounded or sick people with failure to provide medical care; punishment of medical personnel or relief workers for having engaged in activities consistent with medical ethics; military attacks on medical personnel, transports, or units; and use of medical personnel for military purposes.[115] Nevertheless, considering research on tropical diseases, treatment of battlefield casualities, and other emergency medical advances, "it is one of the ironies of health care that advance is stimulated by the catastrophes of war."[116] Unfortunately, improved weapons technology assures that wars are no longer the province of armies. During World War I, 5% of casualties were estimated to have been among civilians; this figure rose to 50% for World War II, and to 80% in wars since about 1980.[117]

NOTES

1. Sköld (1998).
2. Lewis (1968).
3. Gunatilleke (1995).
4. Adam Smith in *The Wealth of Nations*, cited by Calman (1997).
5. Carr-Hill (1990).
6. Marmot and Feeney (1997b).
7. Faggiano *et al.* (1997).
8. MacIntyre (1997).
9. Marmot and Feeney (1997a).
10. Wilkinson (1994). See also Wilkinson (1992).
11. Kacapyr (1996); Hung (1996).
12. A common class scheme widely applied in Europe includes professionals, employers, administrators and managers (I and II); routine nonmanual employees (III); all self-employed men except professionals and farmers (IVa, b); farmers (IVc); foremen and skilled manual workers (V and VI); semiskilled and unskilled manual workers (VIIa); and farm laborers (VIIb). See Kunst *et al.* (1998).
13. These were the global eradication of polio; the virtual elimination of neonatal tetanus deaths; a 90% reduction in measles cases and a 95% reduction in measles deaths compared to preimmunization levels; a 70% reduction in annual deaths due to diarrhea in children under five which would occur in the year 2000 in the absence of oral rehydration therapy, and a 25% reduction in the diarrhea rate; a 25% reduction in case/fatality rates associated with acute respiratory infection in children under five; reduction of infant and under-five mortality rates in all countries by at least half (1980–2000) or to 50 and 70 respectively per 1000 live births; and a 50% reduction in maternal mortality rates.
14. Cosponsored by the World Bank, UNDP, UNESCO, and UNICEF.
15. Figures from the World Health Organization *World Health Report* (1998).
16. The project involved personnel from the University of San Carlos in Cebu, the Nutrition Center of the Philippines, and the University of North Carolina (Carolina Population Center); with funding from the U.S. National Institutes of Health, the Nestles' Coordinating Center for Nutrition Research, Wyeth International, the Ford Foundation, the U.S. National Academy of Sciences, the U.S. Agency for International Development, and the World Bank. See for example Cebu Study Team (1991).
17. These include WHO programs for control of acute respiratory infections and diarrheal diseases; units dealing with maternal and child health, nutrition, prevention of blindness, and tropical diseases; the Expanded Programme on Immunization, the Action Programme on Essential Drugs and the Global Programme on AIDS, as well as UNICEF, the World Bank, and other agencies.
18. See Millard (1994).
19. World Health Organzation (1995).
20. The greatest single cause of postneonatal deaths in the United States is sudden infant death syndrome (SIDS).
21. Lima Guimarães and Fischmann (1985).
22. Keirse (1984).
23. Millard (1994).
24. The weight should be taken within an hour of birth, as newborns often lose weight during the first few days of life.
25. By international standards, *preterm* refers to less than 37 completed weeks (259 days)

of gestation, *term* to 37 to 42 completed weeks (259 to 293 days), and *post-term* to 42 completed weeks (192 days) or more.

26. Bicego and Boerma (1993).

27. Adlakha and Banister (1995).

28. Miller (1985).

29. Specter (1998).

30. Ibrahim *et al.* (1996).

31. de Onis *et al.* (1993).

32. Schofield and Ashworth (1996).

33. See for example Rahmathullah *et al.* (1990) (pro) and Vijayaraghavan *et al.* (1990) and Fawzi *et al.* (1997) (con).

34. Tupasi *et al.* (1990b).

35. Also tuberculosis, which is a special case.

36. Fonseca *et al.* (1996). It is possible that at least some of the reported increase in pneumonia in children in daycare centers is an artifact of selection bias if those cases are more likely to be reported or hospitalized than others in the same community.

37. Guerrant (1994).

38. Muhuri *et al.* (1996).

39. *Lancet* (1978).

40. Exactly the same problems arise with use of powdered breast-milk substitutes (baby formula).

41. Fauveau *et al.* (1992).

42. And currently used cholera vaccines have low protective efficacy.

43. Merrick (1993).

44. Corteguera (1995).

45. Independent validation is a prudent step in mortality analyses in developing countries. See Chapter 4.

46. Victoria *et al.* (1985).

47. Greenwood *et al.* (1987). Rainy season = June to November; dry season = December to May.

48. A formal UCI initiative was launched in 1984.

49. Henderson (1989).

50. Ada (1995).

51. Batson *et al.* (1994).

52. Greenwood *et al.* (1987).

53. Brenzel and Claquin (1994).

54. For the early history of the child survival movement see Kent (1991), especially Chapter 4.

55. Kent (1991).

56. *Ibid.*

57. Primarily hemorrhage, eclampsia, abortion, obstructed labor, and sepsis. See Türmen (1995).

58. García-Moreno and Türmen (1995).

59. Tinker (1992).

60. The founding organizations included, among others, WHO, UNICEF, UNDP, UNFPA, the International Planned Parenthood Federation, and the Population Council.

61. Tinker (1992).

62. See Campbell *et al.* (1995) for a cogent analysis.

63. Quoted by Younger (1987).

64. World Health Organization (1996).

65. Pan American Health Organization (1993) from Table 2, p. 4.

66. Royston and Lopez (1987).

67. World Health Organization (1997a).

68. Moodley *et al.* (1996).

69. Ladipo (1989).

70. Kulczycki *et al.* (1996). The maternal mortality *ratio* was indicated.

71. UNICEF (1996).

72. World Health Organization (1997 unpublished).

73. Feachem *et al.* (1990).

74. Phillips *et al.* (1993).

75. The GBD project is based at the Harvard School of Public Health and supported financially by the World Bank, Rockefeller Foundation, Edna McConnell Clark Foundation, and WHO.

76. Murray and Lopez (1996).

77. At that time a republic of the USSR; now an independent state.

78. Edict of June 25, 1965, by Mao Zedong.

79. Horn (1969).

80. Halfdan Mahler, then Director-General (WHO, 1978).

81. Mahler (1978), speech at the opening ceremony, Alma-Ata, September 6.

82. Walsh and Warren (1979).

83. Banerji (1984), cited by Rifkin and Walt (1986).

84. A barefoot doctor training manual was translated into many languages and sold widely in western countries.

85. Agarwal (1980).

86. Banerji (1990).

87. Brenzel and Claquin (1994).

88. Mburu (1994).

89. Jaffar *et al.* (1997).

90. Berman (1984).

91. Mburu (1994).

92. Fendall (1985).

93. Adewunmi (1993).

94. Adapted from Abel-Smith and Rawal (1992).

95. Diallo *et al.* (1993).

96. van der Geest (1982) in southern Cameroon.

97. Prins (1984).

98. Darras (1997).

99. McKay (1981).

100. Stark (1985).

101. Green RH. (1991).

102. Chen (1986).

103. Pannenborg (1991).

104. Burkholder (1996).

105. Gellert (1995).

106. D'Souza (1981).

107. Leaning (1996).

108. Burkholder and Toole (1995).

109. Hilsum (1995).

110. Signatories include Caritas Internationalis, Catholic Relief Services, the International Federation of Red Cross and Red Crescent Societies, the International Save the Children Al-

liance, the Lutheran World Federation, Oxfam, the World Council of Churches, and the International Committee of the Red Cross. The text of the code can be downloaded from ⟨http://www.ifrc.org/pubs/code/⟩.

111. Hogerzeil *et al.* (1997). See page 739 for a list of Guidelines for Drug Donations.

112. World Health Organization (1990).

113. Malé (1996); see also Toole (1995) for comparable data.

114. According to Brown (1991), 18,000 cases of pellagra occurred in the previous year among refugees in Malawi.

115. See Brentlinger (1996) for a more complete discussion of "abuses of medical neutrality" in wartime.

116. Maxwell (1995).

117. Toole (1996).

8

Environment, Development, and Health

Ill health is not randomly distributed among human beings. This deceptively simple statement has enormous significance for the field of international health. It is also the underpinning of the study of the distribution and determinants of disease in human populations, or *epidemiology*. The first reason for seeking the determinants (or risk factors) of a disease is to learn how to control it. Recognition of the obvious differences in health status among individuals and groups leads to related avenues of investigation. In some cases the relationships are fairly straightforward; in others, particularly the malignant and degenerative diseases, a very large amount of work still needs to be done. A knowledge of causality can then direct efforts aimed at prevention. This logical sequence is self-evident and would not merit lengthy discussion here were it not for the crucial role that international health studies have played in all its phases. Chapter 7 presented evidence of the importance of poverty in determining population health. Here we will look at health as influenced by the environment and to economic development.

It is not only for heart disease, stroke, and cancer that wide-ranging studies are needed. Infectious disease control has also relied heavily on international comparisons. It is clearly not enough, for instance, to say that tuberculosis is caused by infection with tubercle bacilli. Such infection is a necessary, but not a sufficient, condition for production of clinical illness, and most people infected with tubercle bacilli never have symptoms or show signs of clinical tuberculosis. Other factors having to do with innate and acquired characteristics of each individual—genetics and environment, nature and nurture—determine the course of infection and severity of illness. In many situations comparative studies in different countries are indispensable because the full range of relevant conditions is unavailable in any one of them.

The association of various risk factors with atheroslerosis is a good example. Diet and serum lipids, hypertension, cigarette smoking, diabetes, psychosocial relationships, heredity, and other factors have been assessed and compared in many different localities.

The flagship international epidemiologic study is the classical work on coronary heart disease in seven countries by Ancel Keys and colleagues. Impressed by the low rates of heart disease in the Mediterranean region, they analyzed the dietary habits and heart disease experience of 13,000 middle-aged people in 16 separate cohorts in Finland, Greece, Italy, Japan, Netherlands, the United States, and Yugoslavia. Of the five characteristics measured on entry to the study, (serum cholesterol, systolic blood pressure, cigarette smoking, body mass index, and physical activity at work), only serum cholesterol was found significant in explaining the large cohort differences in age-adjusted death rates from coronary heart disease. Keys and colleagues concluded that mean serum cholesterol is the major risk factor in explaining these differences, thereby generating commentary that continues to this day.[1]

A study of global distribution may help to define determinants of fatal cancers at various sites, or at least to suggest the right questions to ask. Assuming that the figures in Table 8-1 are reasonably correct, why should Mexico have one-third the overall cancer death rate of Hungary? You may say it is because it has a younger population, until you recall that differences in population age structure are accounted for in the *age-adjustment* of rates. Why is a Chilean man seven times as likely to die of stomach cancer as a North American man, while the rates are identical for their wives? Why does China have one-fifth the female breast cancer mortality of England or Denmark and one-fourth that of the United States? Can the low rates of breast and prostate cancer, or the high rate of male stomach cancer in Japan teach us anything about causality? Why are cancer death rates always lower for women, sometimes half or less?

Among the cancers listed in Table 8-1, lung cancer stands out because its association with tobacco use has been well established since the 1960s. Lung cancer death rates have been soaring in countries where cigarette use is increasing. In the United States between 1950 and 1990, age-adjusted death rates from lung cancer almost tripled among men and rose sixfold among women. Some 3 million adult deaths each year in the world are attributed to tobacco, a number expected to rise to 10 million by 2025. It is estimated that each ton of tobacco production will eventually result in one death. Tobacco is one of the two major underlying causes of premature death that is increasing. The other is HIV.[2] While tobacco consumption in developed countries is decreasing, it is increasing in developing countries, and this has become a specific target of WHO and other international agencies. Most worrisome is the extremely high rate of tobacco consumption in eastern Europe, where because of cigarette smoking "a man living in Europe's ex-communist countries today has a greater risk of dying before the age of 60 than men in most developing

Table 8-1. Age-Adjusted Death Rates per 100,000 for Cancer at Selected Sites, Various Countries, 1992–1995[a]

Country	All Sites M	All Sites F	Breast (F)	Prostate (M)	Lung M	Lung F	Colorectal M	Colorectal F	Stomach M	Stomach F
United States	163	110	21	17	55	26	16	11	4.7	2.5
Albania	91	40	4.9	7.0	26	4.9	2.3	2.1	13	2.5
Australia	159	99	20	19	40	13	21	14	6.6	1.6
Canada	159	108	22	17	53	23	16	11	6.4	2.2
Chile	139	108	12	15	22	6.4	6.2	6.3	32	2.5
China	150	83	5	—	37	16	7.9	6.4	27	0.7
Denmark	179	139	27	20	50	25	23	17	6.8	3.3
Hungary	265	138	24	17	84	18	32	19	22	5.0
Israel	124	102	24	11	27	8.4	17	13	8.8	2.5
Japan	149	75	6.8	4.2	31	8.3	16	9.8	31	2.1
Mexico	80	77	8.7	10.5	16	5.8	3.2	3.1	9.7	2.0
Sweden	127	97	18	21	23	11	15	11	7.3	2.7
Un. Kingdom	174	121	27	17	52	21	19	13	11	2.2

F = female; M = male; — = data not available; data rounded to nearest whole digit except for values below 10. See original for details.

Source: Selected and adapted from Landis et al. (1998) Table 14. See original for additional countries and sites.

countries, including India, China and the Latin American nations. According to the WHO, smoking is responsible for "about half" the deaths of men in middle age in Eastern Europe."[3]

In addition to regional differences, the rates themselves are changing in all countries. Between 1960 and 1980 in the developed countries the age-specific death rate for cancer of the lung rose dramatically for both sexes, while that for cancer of the stomach and for cancer of the uterine cervix in females declined substantially. An American man had a greater chance of dying of stomach cancer in 1930 than a Chilean man does today. We may think that we know why these differences in space and time occur, but we cannot be certain without rigorous comparative epidemiological investigation.

"Obvious" things may not always be so obvious, and sometimes we may be fooled. Consider a native reserve in a certain country. Among a population of roughly 1000, more than 100 people had been sufficiently ill with severe bloody, mucoid diarrhea to warrant hospitalization. There had been eight deaths, including two in small children. One-third of the total population were carriers of the responsible pathogen. Conditions of nutrition and sanitation were grossly deficient. A picture such as this would not seem unusual in any of dozens of tropical countries. But this did not occur in a tropical country—it happened in northern Saskatchewan, Canada, in a closely knit population of Native Americans. And the disease was amebic dysentery.[4] It may seem strange to hear of endemic amebic dysentery in the far north, when our preconceptions hold it to be a "tropical disease." However, the causative organism, *Entamoeba histolytica*, was first described in 1875 in St. Petersburg, Russia, in a patient residing in Arkhangelsk near the Arctic Circle.

To understand the health conditions of mankind, to see them accurately and objectively, one must be willing to cast aside preconceptions. As mentioned, the notion of "tropical diseases" is largely misleading. Malaria, yellow fever, cholera, and smallpox have ravaged North America and Europe. Tens of thousands died of cholera in New York City after the Civil War. Hundreds of thousands perished in Europe at the same time. That the threat is constant may be seen in the fact that some dozens died of cholera in Italy and Portugal as recently as the 1970s. Yellow fever struck repeatedly in the United States during the 18th and 19th centuries. In one outbreak in Philadelphia 10% of the population died. The most recent epidemic in an American city struck New Orleans in 1905. Malaria was endemic in the southern states until the 1940s, and smallpox occurred in the United States until 1949.

It seems reasonable to ask how it is that these diseases have come and gone from the industrialized countries, whether they might one day return, and how others such as AIDS have appeared and spread. What is it, in fact, that determines the presence of these and other less dramatic diseases at any particular time and place? The answers are surely complex, but we can start by exploring the associations between geographic location and health and the nature of interactions between humans and their environment.

First, a caution. Although *ego*system and *eco*system are both important to health, it has become popular to speak of our external surroundings as *the* environment. But we live in many interconnected environments at once, and in that sense an economist can be just as much an environmentalist as an ecologist.

THE NATURAL ENVIRONMENT

The study of localities in relation to disease and health was well established by the time of Hippocrates, about the fifth century BC, not only in Greece but in all countries for which we have an adequate historical record from those days. The Hippocratic text titled, *Airs, Waters, Places* begins:

> Whoever wishes to pursue properly the science of medicine must proceed thus: First, he ought to consider what effects each season of the year can produce; for the seasons are not at all alike, but differ widely both in themselves and at their changes. The next point is the hot winds and the cold, especially those that are universal but also those that are peculiar to each particular region . . . For with the seasons, men's diseases, like their digestive organs, suffer change.

Geological Substrate

The soil is important to human health primarily because of its chemical makeup, affecting people directly through its contained minerals and water for drinking and cooking, and less directly by way of the vegetable food and other plants and microorganisms that may or may not grow in it.

Major minerals

The most important element for human health that is frequently absent from soils is iodine, a deficiency of which may lead to endemic goiter or endemic cretinism, as mentioned in the previous chapter. Chinese writings dating from several centuries BC attribute goiter to the quality of the water. Remarkably, seaweed (which is rich in iodine) was mentioned as an efficacious remedy for goiter in a treatise on herbs and roots attributed to Shen-Nung (third millenium BC). Many other authors of antiquity, from India to Egypt to Rome, knew of goiter. Pliny (first century AD) said that swelling of the throat of men and swine was caused mostly by the water they drink.

The most notorious goitrous centers of the world are in high mountains. The Pyrenees, Alps, Himalayas, and Andes, where the uplifted terrain has been subjected to flooding or glaciation, have been effectively leached of iodine. Cretinism, marked by mental retardation and associated deaf-mutism and stunting of growth, have been endemic. Goiter was common in pre-Columbian America, and was recorded by the Spaniards among the Incas in the high Andes. The modern significance of iodine deficiency can best be seen in the Indian subcontinent, where northern Pakistan and India, Nepal, and Bhutan constitute the "Himalayan goiter belt."

> Outright cretinism remains shockingly commonplace in the Himalayas. Nepali officials thought they had found an unparalleled incidence in the mountain hamlet of Tulibesi, where 18 percent of 750 residents are cretins. Then a survey in the nearby kingdom of Bhutan revealed two villages in which one-third of the populace are cretins ... Mentally deficient people, stunted and deaf and mute people, many moving with an awkward gait, are all about. Goiters deform every throat, sometimes reaching monstrous size.[5]

The human requirement for dietary iron makes this element extremely important in prevention of anemia, a serious problem of worldwide dimensions. Anemia owing to iron deficiency is mostly due to factors other than an iron-poor soil. Loss or destruction of red blood cells by hookworm and malaria is often accompanied by inadequate consumption of iron-rich foods (liver, green leafy vegetables). Where iron cooking pots are used, anemia is rare because sufficient iron is transferred to the foods from the pot. But a high iron intake may not always be beneficial. In what may seem a paradoxical relationship, dietary iron supplementation of anemic children in Papua New Guinea was reported to lead to increased severity of malaria.

The malaria parasites, which live on iron-containing hemoglobin, found the red cells of iron-boosted children greatly to their liking. Perhaps a similar relationship may exist in areas naturally rich in iron.[6]

Trace elements

The essential trace elements are required in small amounts for proper functioning of various enzyme systems. Associations have been suggested between soil and water chemistry and diseases such as cancer, multiple sclerosis, and sarcoidosis, but these are difficult to validate in view of the large chance for statistical artifact. Studies made in various countries have suggested an inverse correlation between mortality from cardiovascular disease and hardness of drinking water, in particular the calcium, magnesium, and sodium ions. Cadmium, lead, selenium, zinc, molybdenum, manganese, and other elements appear to be able to cause mischief in deficiency or excess.

A dramatic example is the presence of high levels of arsenic in natural aquifers in areas of Bangladesh. The cumulative effect of drinking such water over long periods begins with ulcerating sores on the hands and feet and may end fatally with several forms of cancer. Estimates of the number of persons potentially affected are as high as 18 million. Ironically, this calamity is an unintended consequence of well-intended development projects. Until the mid-1970s most villagers in affected areas obtained their domestic water from hand-dug wells or natural ponds, which were often contaminated with bacterial pathogens. Then the national government, UNICEF, and other agencies began a program of sinking tube wells and hand pumps to bring clean underground drinking water into villages, and extensive health education efforts to convince people to use that water. Unfortunately it was not realized until many years later that high levels of naturally occurring arsenic leached into this water, leading to chronic poisoning in many people who drank it.

Radioactivity

All living organisms are continually exposed to ionizing radiation from three sources: the minute inherent natural radioactivity within the body originating from inhaled air and ingested food and water; cosmic radiation; and decay of naturally radioactive minerals in the earth's crust. Health consequences of ionizing radiation may be considered under two categories: those affecting the individual and those affecting genetic material in the gametes and therefore transmissible to offspring. It is more difficult to substantiate the latter effect, which certainly occurs and which may be a major engine driving the evolution of animals and plants. The amount of natural radiation to which people are exposed varies from place to place depending largely on the isotopic composition of the substrate (and, for cosmic radiation, on altitude).

Radioactivity arising from natural decay of minerals is found also in air, particularly in mines. In the United States and several other countries a number of abandoned uranium mines have been developed commercially to accommodate cancer patients and other persons willing to pay by the hour to sit in them. The radioactive element radon (atomic number 86) is an inert, colorless gas formed when radium (atomic number 88) loses an alpha particle. In some parts of the world the soil emits radon gas, and people who live in houses built on such areas may accumulate dangerous levels in room air. The highest indoor levels of radon have been found in a region known as the Reading Prong in the states of Pennsylvania, New Jersey, and New York. Inhalation of radon in the air brings ionizing radioactivity into direct contact with lung tissue, resulting in a certain amount of cell damage which is increased by other harmful factors such as cigarette smoking. Levels of exposure over time lead to a significant increase in lung cancer rates in affected areas. By some estimates more than 10,000 deaths a year may result from exposure to radon in the United States. Soils in regions of the state of Minas Gerais, Brazil, have so much natural radioactivity that plants growing there will leave a picture of themselves when placed on photographic paper in a darkroom. In many parts of the world very little is known about radioactivity in the substrate and its effects on health.

Latitude and The Seasons

The position of the noonday sun at most places on earth makes an annual migration along a north–south path. At the solstices (June 21 and December 22) the sun is at its furthest north and south limits; at the equinoxes (March 21 and September 23) the sun is at the midpoint of its path. This annual shift is caused by the $23°27'$ tilt of the polar axis in relation to the plane of rotation. As the earth circles the sun, the direct rays appear overhead at noon at a slightly different point each day, to a limit of $23°27'$ north latitude (the Tropic of Cancer) at the northern summer solstice and the corresponding southern limit (the Tropic of Capricorn) at the northern winter solstice. The two tropics thus mark the limits of latitude at which the sun is ever directly overhead at noon. The word tropic is derived from the Greek *tropos*, meaning "turning," because the sun appears to "turn" back and forth at these imaginary lines. As one proceeds into higher latitudes north or south, the sun appears to make a smaller arc in the sky, never appearing directly overhead. This arc and the consequent duration of daylight become smaller and smaller in northern latitudes as the winter solstice approaches, and the situation is reversed south of the equator. At $66°30'$ north, daylight reaches zero on the solstsice; this is the Arctic Circle. At the corresponding latitude to the south, there are 24 hours of daylight on the same date. In general, at latitudes nearer the poles the extent of continuous darkness or light becomes slowly greater as solstice approaches.

The seasons themselves are thought to have direct effects on many people. Not only do many groups from Mongolian yurt dwellers to Michigan–Florida retirees migrate with the seasons, but differences in suicide, ischemic heart disease, and other conditions have been attributed to direct seasonal factors.

Altitude

The study of the effects of altitude on humans has been emphasized in recent years because of programs to put humans into space. Atmospheric pressure and, correspondingly, the partial pressure of oxygen in inspired air decline with increased elevation. Physiological mechanisms to deal with these changes have been investigated in the field primarily in Peru, where in some areas people live and work at extreme altitudes. Peoples native to high altitudes have high hematocrits (red blood cell volumes). They may show evidence of right ventricular enlargement and pulmonary hypertension in the presence of reduced systemic arterial pressure. The virtual absence of systemic hypertension appears to be correlated with a lack of ischemic heart disease among native high-altitude populations, although a relatively high incidence of congenital heart diseases may be present.

Barometric pressure is not the only climatic factor to vary inversely with altitude. Air temperature decreases with elevation at a rate of 1°C per 140 meters in the Alps, 165 meters in the Caucasus, and 195 meters in the equatorial Andes; in consequence the duration of cold seasons is extended. In the Alps, for instance, the period with mean temperature above freezing is six months at 2000 meters but only two months at 3100 meters. One result of this temperature decline is that habitats at increasing altitude tend to resemble those at increasing latitude so that eventually the tree line and snow line are reached in either direction. Singapore, Mombasa, Belem, Nairobi, and Quito are all within a few degrees of the equator. The climates of the first three, in Asia, Africa, and Latin America, are remarkably similar—warm and wet. Nairobi is considerably cooler, and Quito cooler still. Mombasa and Nairobi are a scant 400 kilometers (250 miles) apart horizontally but almost 2 kilometers apart vertically.

Direct Effects of Climate on Health

Effects of climate, such as relative humidity, wind, ionization, and barometric pressure, are more subtle and widespread than such obvious climatic hazards as frostbite or heatstroke. Changes in humidity and pressure can trigger arthritic attacks, affect the pain of corns on the feet due to increased pressure against shoes, and have psychological effects. High humidity retards the loss of heat by reducing the evaporative cooling effect of sweating. High temperatures increase the need for water. Under desert conditions most people can tolerate a water deficit of 5% of body weight; they become very listless with a 10% deficit, and a 15% water deficit can be fatal at 30°C (86°F). Sweat losses of more than 2 liters daily may be encountered in hot climates, and the continual dermal loss of mineral ions, especially sodium, potassium, choride, and sulfate, can be significant. The total nitrogen loss may exceed 5 grams daily, and more than 1.7 grams of amino acids may be lost in one day's perspiration. These physiologic changes bear some resemblances to the effects of acute diarrhea.

It has been shown that the prevalence of kidney stones in countries with a hot climate may reach 2% of the general population. This condition may be associated with increased sweating, evaporative loss of water from the skin and lungs, and increased concentration of calcium, oxalates, and urate in the urine.

The amount of exposure to sunshine is directly associated with production of vitamin D in the skin. Ultraviolet wavelengths of 275 to 300 nanometers are most important in this activity. In areas where both dietary vitamin D and sunlight are lacking, rickets may result. This debilitating disease, marked by defects in bone growth and extreme bowleggedness, was common in the industrial cities of England and Europe when children grew up in dark houses and narrow streets always shielded from the sunshine. The same effect is seen in some countries of the Middle East in which girls and women are always completely covered or remain indoors. On one hand, schoolchildren are exposed to artificial ultraviolet light during the long winter period of darkness in some far northern communities in Russia. On the other hand, excessive exposure to sunlight is a contributing factor to skin cancers at unprotected sites on the body, and many believe that depletion of atmospheric ozone will cause an increase in skin cancers around the world.

The totality of human endeavors has repercussions on health, and almost all aspects of life are affected by climate. Compare the uniform temperature at sea level near the equator with the dramatic seasonal changes at higher latitudes. In Singapore or Freetown the entire annual range of temperatures may be spanned within any single day. In Toronto or Moscow, however, there is no mistaking June for January. The diurnal and annual pattern of activities, the customs, the sports, and the entertainments of temperate zone populations are all correlated with the annual cycle of the seasons. From the design and construction of houses to the types of clothing worn, climatic and seasonal influences are of overriding importance, and the repercussions on the distribution and the intensity of infectious and nutritional diseases can hardly be overestimated. The pervasive effects of these basic environmental parameters extend even to the organization and administration of health services, which must be adapted to local conditions if they are to be effective.

CORRELATION OF PHYSICAL AND BIOTIC ENVIRONMENTS

The combination of soil and climate determines the particular associations of plants, animals, and microorganisms potentially present at any locality. Evolution, migration, passive dispersal, and introduction establish the actual types present at any particular location and time. Long-term environmental changes such as continental movements and glaciations are important in these processes but beyond the scope of this book. Medium-term changes such as possible ozone depletion or global warming are in the daily headlines and may have influences on nutrition, infectious diseases, and behavior of the inhabitants.

The Soil as Reservoir of Disease-Producing Agents

Spores of many potentially pathogenic fungi may be recovered from the soil. *Histoplasma capsulatum*, a fungus producing a disease resembling tuberculosis, is found in many areas of the world. Some fungi are closely associated with particular kinds of environments. The agent of San Joaquin Valley fever (coccidioidomycosis) is restricted to semiarid habitats in North, Central, and South America. These and other fungal diseases may be fatal, especially in immunodeficient persons such as AIDS patients.

Other agents associated with soil are spore-forming bacteria, such as those causing tetanus, and certain normally free-living protozoa only recently recognized as pathogens. Some amebae of the genera *Naegleria* and *Acanthamoeba* are able to enter through the nasal mucosa of people swimming in ponds or lakes and can produce a rapidly fatal infection of the brain and spinal cord. This disease, known as primary amebic meningoencephalitis, has been reported from North and South America, Europe, and Australia and seems to turn up occasionally, with disastrous effects, almost anywhere.

The enormous number of human infections with worm parasites transmitted via the soil is in contrast to the small number of known cases of amebic meningoencephalitis. The large roundworm *Ascaris*, the whipworm *Trichuris*, and the hookworms *Necator* and *Ancylostoma* are all but ubiquitous in many tropical countries, with billions of human cases, mostly in children.

Soil, Climate, and Vegetation

Germination of seeds, growth of plants, formation of flowers, setting of pollen, ripening of fruit, and nutritional value of crop are determined to a great extent by soil chemistry, temperature, moisture, and photoperiod, as well as by the genetic characteristics of the plant. It is clear that in areas of little sunlight, particularly in higher latitudes during the winter, the type and amount of plant growth are severely limited. Persons in these areas who are dependent on the environment for their daily food must make dramatic seasonal adjustments in their diet. The fisherfolk of Newfoundland and Labrador, lacking fresh vegetables over the long winter months, survived mainly on white bread and as a consequence suffered from beriberi. This severe nutritional disease results from a lack of thiamine, which is lost from overmilled flour. It was also recognized that tuberculosis was increasing and that infant mortality was unacceptably high. Legislation requiring the addition of vitamin A to margarine and of niacin, iron, thiamine, riboflavin, and calcium to white flour, together with other improvements, caused beriberi to disappear.

Seasonal malnutrition is not restricted to higher latitudes. Subsistence agriculture, using inefficient methods in an area of unreliable rainfall, has affected the inhabitants of the Nangodi region in northern Ghana. The active adult community loses, on average, 6.5% in body weight during the "hungry season" as compared to the time of the year when food is more abundant.[7] Seasonal unavailability of specific foods at any locality, such as fish, vitamin A–rich fruits like papaya, or citrus fruits, may induce recurrent deficiencies in particular nutrients. Small children after weaning are particularly susceptible to these nutritional deficiencies.

Water- and Airborne Pathogens

The pathogens transmitted by fecally contaminated water generally strike hardest at infants after weaning and at young children for whom the complex of enteric diseases, combined with malnutrition, represents the great killer in most tropical areas (see Chapter 7). Even in the industrialized countries, outbreaks of enteric disease are not infrequent. Resort areas, where limited water and sewerage systems are strained by large seasonal influxes of tourists, are particularly vulnerable to such outbreaks as typhoid fever. Giardiasis, caused by a water-borne protozoan, is the most commonly diagnosed parasitic disease in the United States. Acute outbreaks of water-borne enteric disease are not uncommon,. Tens of thousands of people contracted viral hepatitis A in Shanghai, probably from undercooked clams contaminated by raw sewage in their ocean habitat. Hundreds of thousands became ill in Milwaukee, Wisconsin, from *Cryptosporidium parvum*, a protozoan parasite transmitted through the water supply. And millions were exposed to cholera bacteria in many countries of Latin America in an ongoing epidemic that threatens to last into the 21st century.

Seasonal malnutrition arising from periodic lack of food has been mentioned, as has the combination of water- and airborne pathogens responsible for the seasonal recurrence of malnutrition in poor sub-Saharan countries. The wet weather during the rainy season encourages crowding inside houses, and the increased interpersonal contact encourages the spread of measles, lower respiratory tract infections, and diarrheas. The diarrhea and illness in marginally nourished children may lead to development of clinical malnutrition, which reaches a peak at the end of the rainy season. Seasonality of infant deaths in the Gambia and Brazil was mentioned in the previous chapter.[8] Similar situations can be documented in many other countries.

We commonly think of illnesses caused by airborne pathogens as acute febrile episodes, like colds or influenza. It may seem strange to place heart disease in this category, accustomed as we are in the West to characterizing cardiac problems as chronic illnesses of older people. But here is a different perspective:

> Any doctor who has walked the paediatric wards of hospitals in the cities of warm climate countries, e.g., Singapore, Hong Kong, Lagos, Calcutta, Mexico City, is immediately impressed with the number of school age patients with rheumatic fever or rheumatic heart disease . . . surveys among school children reveal prevalence rates of rheumatic heart disease ranging from one to 20 percent.[9]

Rheumatic fever, and the heart valve damage that sometimes ensues, are caused by group A hemolytic streptococci transmitted by inhalation or by contaminated milk or food. In Central and South America, particularly Brazil, a different form of chronic heart disease may develop from infection with the insect-transmitted protozoan *Trypanosoma cruzi*, the agent of Chagas' disease. Other widely distributed and locally common heart diseases, such as endomyocardial fibrosis, may have a viral origin.

Vector-Borne Diseases

No group of diseases is so closely correlated with environmental conditions as those requiring an insect vector for transmission. Throughout history, the biting flies have been indirectly responsible for a very large proportion of human illnesses and deaths. A good example is malaria, which is not a single entity but rather a collective term for several distinct febrile diseases, each caused by one of a group of closely related parasites. The malarias occur in many local variants, each transmitted by a specific anopheline mosquito vector. The principal climatic factors controlling malaria transmission are temperature, humidity, and rainfall; all are superimposed on the pools of infected and susceptible individuals.

For *Plasmodium vivax*, the organism causing benign tertian malaria, the time needed for the extrinsic incubation (mosquito) phase of the life cycle ranges from 55 days at 16°C (61°F) to 7 days at 28°C (83°F). The most dangerous malaria parasite, *Plasmodium falciparum*, requires a minimum of 21.6° C (70° F) for transmission. Mosquitoes are unable to regulate their internal temperature and are greatly influenced not only by heat but also by relative humidity. Therefore transmission of malaria may be just as seasonal in tropical areas with long dry spells (e.g., interior West Africa) as in temperate regions. Rainfall, besides increasing relative humidity, provides water for mosquito breeding and is thus of considerable significance in itself. Where temperatures are consistently warm and rainfall sufficient throughout the year, malaria poses a threat the year round.

Each vector-borne and zoonotic disease of humans is subject to environmental restrictions, and in many cases the reasons underlying geographic distributions are well understood. For some others much epidemiologic work remains to be done. Yellow fever is such a disease. The virus is found only in the Western Hemisphere and Africa, and there is no evidence that yellow fever has ever become established in the Asian tropics, even though many Asian mosquitoes are perfectly good vectors in the laboratory. It seems inconceivable that no introduction has ever occurred, but no convincing explanation has been offered for the absence of this disease in Asia.

Despite the vigilance of public health, customs, and agriculture officials, dangerous disease vectors sometimes are carried to new areas, where they may become established and lead to disease outbreaks. The introduction to Brazil of the notorious African malaria vector *Anopheles gambiae* was mentioned in Chapter 3. Years of costly and painstaking effort were required before this mosquito was exterminated from its new home. More recently, in the mid-1980s, specimens of the tough, aggressive Asian "tiger mosquito" *Aedes albopictus* were collected from the states of Texas, Louisiana, Mississippi, and Tennessee in the United States. As carriers of dengue fever and certain encephalitis-producing viruses, these mosquitoes are particularly worrisome.

Zoonoses and Animal Reservoirs of Disease

Zoonoses are diseases of nonhuman animals, particularly mammals and birds, that are transmissible to man. Whereas some contemporary human diseases, such as measles, syphilis, and AIDS, are not known to occur naturally in other species, a great many pathogens of mankind are shared with wild and domesticated animals. The nonhuman species harboring those infections are reservoirs of the diseases in question; a vector may or may not be involved, depending on the particular disease and circumstances. Sometimes investigators are surprised at unexpected relationships, as in the finding that armadillos in the southern United States are naturally infected with leprosy bacilli. Their role, if any, in infecting humans is unclear. More than 150 zoonoses are recognized, including some of mankind's truly great diseases. The effects on human history of zoonoses such as yellow fever, typhus, and African sleeping sickness are incalculable, as are the great plague epidemics that swept through Europe in the Middle Ages, killed millions, and left many areas virtually deserted.

No area of the world is free of zoonotic diseases. Mosquito-borne viral encephalitis may occur as epidemics in Asia from the former USSR through Korea and Japan southward to the great archipelagoes of the Philippines and Indonesia. In Japan, infection with Japanese encephalitis virus can spread rapidly in wild birds. *Culex* mosquitoes, which feed on birds, are attracted also to pigs. The pigs, kept near rural habitations, are important reservoirs and amplifiers of the virus, which can cause large-scale human outbreaks by mosquito passage.

In addition their role as reservoirs of viral and other diseases, wild birds may be important in natural spread of disease agents through their migratory habits. Millions of birds make the round trip between North and South America, Europe and

Africa, Asia and Africa, Central Asia and Sri Lanka, and other temperate and tropical areas each year. Viruses and rickettsiae may travel with them, either in their
own blood and tissues or within the mites, ticks, lice, or other ectoparasites that ride
along under the feathers. These ectoparasites and the microorganisms within them
may be transferred from one end of the flight range to the other, or left at any stopping place in between.

Of all mammals, rodents seem most intimately related to human health and disease. The role of beavers in spreading giardiasis has been well documented. The
historical association of disease outbreaks with wild and domiciliated rodents (i.e.,
living around human habitations but not intentionally kept by man) is well established. Gerbils, rats, mice, squirrels, prairie dogs, and even guinea pigs have been
incriminated as natural carriers of plague, which has been documented in about
200 species of rodents in Asia, Africa, and the Americas. Humans often become involved by intruding into the wild (or sylvatic) rodent–flea–rodent cycle. Cases of
human plague occur every year in many countries, including the United States, where
the disease is endemic in rodents in the Sierra Nevada Mountains of California and
in other southwestern states. Rodents were also responsible for the lethal outbreaks
of hanta virus disease in the southwestern United states in the early 1990s.

For most people in the world today, control over their environment is minimal.
When rains fail to come, they starve; and when the rains fail to stop, they starve
again. Biting insects and fecal contamination are inescapable aspects of daily life,
and the agents that they transmit pose a continuing menace to health and to life itself. In all countries there is a growing sensitivity to environmental deterioration.
We must consider these problems in their various aspects throughout this book and
weigh proposed courses of action. It is clear that thinking about health must be
grounded in an ecological viewpoint, for only from this direction do preventive measures arise.

THE HUMAN DIMENSION

Environmental factors, including pathogenic organisms, can affect health only
through their interactions with people. Because the genetic makeup of any species
provides the instrument on which all outside factors impinge, an understanding of
environmental forces and adaptations to them can help to reveal the inner workings
of the body in relation to health and disease. Epidemiologists attempt to correlate the
prevalence of disease with environment, behavior, and other factors. Many diseases
are known to be under direct genetic control, but the degree to which hereditary factors influence susceptibility to others poses a great challenge to investigators.

Human Genetic Adaptations

The number of combinations of genetic characters is astronomical. Each human parent donates about five billion nucleotide pairs to the offspring. In addition to the tremendous number of genetic recombinations there is a small but calculable probability of molecular copying errors (on the order of ten to 100 times) in each gamete such that every person differs from *both* parents (i.e., has mutations). An advantageous mutation, the altered form of a gene which renders its possessor more likely to survive, may spread widely in a population over several generations. Conversely, disadvantageous characters are less likely to become established in a population. Mutations leading to selectively neutral characters (if indeed there are any) may distribute themselves in populations according to the rules governing random probabilities. The survival value of any particular characteristic (other than an obviously lethal one) has meaning only in the context of a defined environment, and there is no doubt that the variety of selective forces in different regions of the world has been crucial in generating the diversity found among present-day human populations.

Genetic diseases

A "genetic" disease causes ill health only when it is expressed phenotypically as such. One universal defect in mankind is absence of the enzyme gulonolactone oxidase, resulting in inability to synthesize ascorbic acid (vitamin C). Almost all mammals other than primates possess this enzyme and are able to traverse the pathway of biochemical steps from glucose to ascorbic acid. In consequence, extended dietary deprivation does not induce scruvy in them, and they have no requirements for vitamin C in the diet. Somewhere in an early ancestral primate a mutation occurred so that functional gulonolactone oxidase was no longer produced. Given a diet rich in fruits, the loss did not confer a disadvantage; it may even have been beneficial because of the saving in metabolic energy previously expended in production of an "unnecessary" substance. Many thousands of years after the original mutations, adventurous descendants of that primate put out to sea for months, or suffered prolonged crop losses, and came down with symptoms of scurvy. The time had finally come for the mutation to show the negative aspect of its effect.

Other contemporary examples may be given of interactions between heredity and environment resulting in widespread disease states. One of the best known of the inheritable traits is governed by the gene for production of hemoglobin S, a variant of normal hemoglobin differing by a single amino acid and under simple Mendelian control. Individuals receiving this gene from both parents have a serious disease, sickle-cell anemia. When one parent donates the S gene and the other the gene for normal hemoglobin, a milder form of the disease is seen, known as sickle-cell trait. The hemoglobin S gene is distributed in a broad band across Africa south of the Sahara and north of the Zambesi and Kunene Rivers; it also occurs in the Malagasay Republic (Madagascar), parts of the Middle East, India, and the Mediterranean littoral. The gene was probably introduced into the Western Hemisphere through the slave trade. It is the most widespread and clinically important of the dozens of known hemoglobin variants. Many investigators have suggested that this "molecular disease" has become widespread because it confers partial protection from malignant tertian *(falciparum)* malaria. In an area of high malaria endemicity, the variant hemoglobin, elsewhere clearly unfavorable, appears to be selected for because persons possessing conventional hemoglobin are more likely to die of falciparum malaria. This illustration shows the intimacy of the partnership between the two environments on either side of the human skin and the evolutionary bartering, so to speak, of one disease for another.

A third example of a genetically determined disease, showing interactions of heredity, environment, and cultural traits, is favism. Fava beans *(Vicia fava)* are grown extensively for human food in parts of the Middle East and North Africa, where they may account for a substantial proportion of dietary protein. Some people, usually males, who eat the beans develop a disease characterized by fatigue, pallor, jaundice, and hemoglobin in the urine resulting from acute hemolytic anemia. Death may occur from kidney failure. The disease is found principally in young children, often in weanlings on their first exposure to the beans. Cases tend to cluster in families, and the incidence of favism varies considerably from one population to another.

Understanding the biochemical and hereditary basis of favism provides the key to explaining other conditions. For example, in some people the reaction to certain drugs such as the antimalarial primaquine includes a hemolysis similar to that found in favism, which arises from precisely the same genetic deficiency in glucose-6-phosphate dehydrogenase (G6PD) metabolism.

Untangling Heredity and Environment

Many attempts have been made to evaluate the relative contributions of heredity and environment to particular aspects of health. At one extreme lie the conditions known to be inherited according to Mendelian principles; the frequencies for relevant alleles vary from one population to another. Medical attention aside, environment plays relatively little part in the expression of many of these conditions. At the other extreme are diseases such as rabies and botulism; trauma from accident, fire, or disaster; and similar hazards against which an individual's genetic makeup offers little protection. Between the extremes lie the tendencies, conditions, and diseases that form the bulk of ill health in human populations.

Ethnicity

It is difficult and perhaps unrewarding to define ethnic groups, but insofar as these have objective reality, the attempt will inevitably be made. Incidence rates for specific diseases are often compared when different ethnic groups reside permanently in the same region. Diseases common or well known in Europeans but rare in Africans include coronary thrombosis, diabetes mellitus in children, infant leukemia, carcinoma of the breast, Cushing's syndrome, Addison's disease, and thyrotoxicosis. Africans, in contrast, have considerable excess of essential thrombocytopenia, acute polyarteritis, tropical ulcer, and myositis. The two groups have very different ways of life, particularly with respect to nutrition and exposure to infectious, insect-borne, and parasitic organisms. A comparison of these risk factors may provide working hypotheses for further investigation. In Harare, Zimbabwe, the cancer pattern of the 3% white population resembles that of Europe and North America, with high rates of breast and colorectal cancers. There is also a relatively high rate of skin cancers, common in European populations living in sunny climates at low latitudes, and somewhat high rates of bladder and liver cancers. The majority African population, by contrast, has low rates of breast and colorectal cancer and high rates of liver, prostate, esophageal, bladder, (in men) lung, and (in women) cervical cancers. The prevalence of HIV in this population has given rise to many cases of Kaposi's sarcoma, now the most common cancer of African men.[10]

Burkitt's lymphoma is a highly malignant tumor of children first described by Dennis Burkitt in 1958. The tumor is limited roughly to those parts of Africa in which the average temperature of the coolest months is at least 17.5°C (60°F) and average rainfall is greater than 508 millimeters (20 inches). In some areas, such as Uganda, this particular lymphoma accounts for fully 50% of all childhood malignancies, and it has been found also in Caucasian, Indian, and Lebanese children living in the endemic zone. Investigators have suggested the possibility that the tumor may be caused by a virus spread by an insect vector. Subsequent discovery that the same sort of tumor occurs in New Guinea and tropical South America under similar ecological conditions has greatly stimulated research efforts. A herpes-like virus, which has been isolated from Burkitt's tumor patients, may be identical to the virus that produces infectious mononucleosis in young adults in temperate areas. The growing web of associations enmeshes African children and American college students, viruses and vectors, climate and locality, and it demonstrates the complexity of relationships between man and nature.

Another example of a comparison between ethnic groups in the same area is the significant excess of hypertensive heart disease in African Americans compared with Caucasian Americans. Hypertensive heart disease is present in 20.8% of the total adult black population and 8.2% of adult whites. Although this difference has been repeatedly confirmed, causal factors are still unknown. Hypotheses include genetics, diet, environmental stress, and differences in medical care.

Complementary to studies of different ethnic groups in the same area are observations on a single ethnic group in different parts of the world. For example, persons of Japanese descent in Japan, Hawaii, and mainland United States have been subjects of repeated investigations. Traditional Japanese culture and diet have generally been retained among Hawaiian Japanese to a greater degree than among those on the mainland. In Japan, mortality rates for diseases of the heart are low when compared with white Americans, but deaths from vascular lesions of the central nervous sytem (stroke) are more common. Death rates for both heart disease and stroke are intermediate among Hawaiian Japanese. Gastric cancer is relatively common in

Japan but rare among white Americans. Among Japanese immigrants incidence of gastric cancer is lower in Hawaii than in Japan, and lower still on the U.S. mainland. The relation of this cancer to the bacterium *Helicobacter pylori* is now firmly established. In American-born ethnic Japanese the incidence of gastric cancer is about the same as in other Americans. The adaptation with respect to colon cancer is similar, although opposite in direction. It is likely that environmental conditions, perhaps food, are important in the genesis of this form of cancer and that a genetic predisposition among Japanese, if it does exist, is not expressed in the American milieu. Studies such as these are open to numerous interpretations and may raise more questions than they answer, but repeated observations in many areas over a span of years are helping to piece together the relative contributions of different factors to the genesis of many diseases.

Aspects of human biology not directly related to disease are also responding to changes in the heredity–environment complex. In girls, menarche (first menstrual period) is a well-defined event, and in a given population the distribution of ages at which it occurs follows the normal bell-shaped curve. Records from England, other European countries, and parts of America show that age at menarche has declined by three to four months per decade over the past hundred years so that puberty is now attained, on average, $2^1/_2$ to $3^1/_2$ years earlier than a century ago.[11] Although there are genetic differences among populations, the reduction in age at menarche and the increase in stature are usually attributed to improved nutrition. But exactly what environmental factors are responsible for "improved nutrition"? Is it fertilizers, tractors, food technology, marketing systems, refrigeration parental income, education, cultural change, all of these, or something else?

CHANGING ENVIRONMENTS

The surroundings in which human beings find themselves are clearly impermanent. The slow alternation of glacial and interglacial periods, imperceptible within the span of lifetimes, contrasts with the sudden earthquake or volcanic eruption, but each may have profound effects on the health of involved populations. Most environmental changes of interest to us fall within an intermediate range, taking place over periods of years or centuries. Many of these have come about as a result of human activities that were not consciously directed toward producing environmental change.

At the simplest level, virtually every human activity results in some environmental change: picking a fruit, felling a tree, building a fire, killing a bear—all leave the immediate microenvironment slightly altered. In a large area, over many years, the accumulation of small events may result in profound changes. The desertification of much of northern India, for instance, is thought to have occurred by gradual destruction of the original forest in early historic times. Parts of North Africa, now desert, were bounteous wheat fields during Roman times. It seems reasonable to

suppose that wherever and whenever a sufficient number of people have accumulated, significant changes in the environment have occurred. Technology has given
rise to an infinity of mechanical, chemical, and electrical devices that have altered
the environment of almost every human being. Automobiles, refrigerators, and computers are quite obviously inventions, and they have a impact on health. But the industrial corporations producing these items are also inventions of man, as are the
cities, governments, customs, religions, and myriad other less conspicuous gears
whose turning moves the machinery of modern society. All of these are environmental factors that interact with each other and with the minds and bodies of human population and together exert a profound influence on health.

Economic Development

The phrase *economic development* has become popular to indicate some sort of
process in the evolution of nation states. An optimistic view would say that

> Development stands for an improved quality of life through gains in health, education,
> living standards, and higher income. Development is based on economic growth or so
> it is perceived since development is found to be more advanced where greater economic
> growth has occurred. The common creed is, that those countries that have not "devel-
> oped" yet will do so in the future, or are doing so now.[12]

It is likely that most people consider economic development a good thing insofar
as it offers improved conditions of life to the majority of the population. But not
everyone agrees. Some criticize development on environmental grounds. One observer has stated that "economic development is the process by which the evil day
is brought closer when everything will be gone."[13] Considering health, development
might be described as the process by which diseases of young bowels are exchanged
for diseases of old arteries.

The unfolding of economic development involves progressive changes in many
aspects of individual, community, and national life. Because development varies
from one country to another, the degree of change in each aspect also varies, and
at any given time some countries or societies are further along certain paths than
others. Development has something to do with *socioeconomic status* (another phrase
of imprecise meaning), which refers not only to the amount of money or resources
that people have, but with their perceptions as well. Such a perception is the idea
of *modernization.* Most people will equate modernization with westernization, but
over the centuries western culture has itself had powerful accretions from elsewhere,
so what we may call *the modern consensus culture* is truly global. The core of modernization lies in the expansion of technologies and their accompanying capabilities
and attitudes. Incorporating these changes into everyday life generally leads to increased receptivity to further change.

The concept that nations follow a predetermined progression from underdeveloped through developing to developed hardly existed until after World War II. Now thousands of specialists in development are employed in departments of economics and institutes of development studies, in government and private donor agencies, at the international development banks, and in financial and commercial institutions all over the world. Early postwar definitions of development centered around industrialization, considered to be the vehicle by which people in poor countries acquire the means to emulate the consumption patterns of people in the rich countries, with the western industrialized countries as a kind of gold standard. Domestic and foreign investment in factories, agricultural projects, and infrastructure such as roads and dams was encouraged as a way in which every country could produce a surplus from which to finance both consumption and further investment.

Industrialization, urbanization, and modernization were early watchwords of countries following a western template to development, but these required educated people, opportunity for individual initiative, and social mobility, which combined into an emphasis on human development. The demonstrated value of human capital promoted investments in education, health, housing, and other aspects of social policy, and stimulated definitions of development that talked about equity as well as economics. In other countries more influenced by socialism, Marxist teachings about internal and international exploitation led to models of development that emphasized state ownership of industry, agrarian collectivism, and pervasive state planning. The important lesson for students of international health is that any area's state of development is a product of prevailing social, political, and economic systems, all of which include elements that affect people's health.

Much has been written about the inequitable division of the world's material resources. Countries have been subjected to various classifications for purposes such as recording aid flows, or for differentiation by specific standards. As mentioned in Chapter 3, multilateral agencies have compiled lists of developing countries, arranged in various categories based on their stage of development. The *most seriously affected* (MSA) *countries* are distinguished by low per capita income and sharp deterioration of current account balances.

In order to help support development programs, many poorer countries borrowed huge amounts of money from international lenders, including banks in the private sector. High interest rates, deteriorating markets for their products, reduced international aid flows, falling investment, a devalued currency, and other factors combined to render many developing countries incapable of repaying even the interest on such loans. The debt crisis of the "lost decade" of the 1980s sharply reduced the funds available for many social programs, including health services. A similar crisis developed in Russia, parts of east southeast Asia, and Latin America during the late 1990s.

Developmental Differences Among Countries

In comparing the gross national product (GNP) or gross domestic product (GDP) per capita of various countries,[14] we may assume that there is some unspecified but real relationship between the figures listed and the health status of the populations concerned. Although GNP figures provide some basis for comparing countries, the numbers are misleading for regions in which many people live outside the cash economy. Rural residents in particular, as subsistence farmers, may grow much of their own food and conduct many transactions by barter. Moreover, differences in the organization of societies and corresponding social and political relationships render the concept of GNP less useful than it might appear. For example, the per capita GNP of the People's Republic of China (PRC) or of Cuba is no greater than that of some poor countries of Africa or Asia. However, their levels of public and individual health, by all reliable indicators, are typical of countries with much higher per capita product, reflecting the activities of a highly motivated and disciplined population. Here, and perhaps in a few other countries, strong central planning, coupled with relentless public education and frequent mass campaigns (sometimes coercive), have reportedly achieved results obtained elsewhere only by the expenditure of large sums of public and private money. Such social and political realities are not revealed in the stark figures appearing in the GNP tables.

An example of a territory whose state of development confounds the traditional indicators is the state of Kerala in southwest India. With a per capita income lower than the average even for India, Kerala has attained levels of infant mortality and life expectancy equal to that of many developed countries. The key to Kerala's success has been enlightened public policy: a strong commitment to education, including girls and women, leading to universal literacy; a progressive agricultural policy; an efficient food distribution system; breakdown of the caste system; and dedicated and efficient health care workers.

The ratio of relatively poor to relatively rich persons in the world as a whole is about three or four to one, but within most developing countries the discrepancy is far greater. While it is true that simplistic divisions into "poor" and "rich" obscure many social complexities, it is also true that most developing countries are characterized by sharply dualistic structures associated with political and economic domination by elite groups. This phenomenon is certainly not new. The earliest records of Egypt and China, histories from ancient Cambodia and Indonesia, and the chronicles of the conquistadores in Mexico and Peru all attest to equivalent, or even greater, social inequalities in many times and places. In 19th-century England Benjamin Disraeli, observing a similar dichotomy, suggested that Queen Victoria actually reigned over "two nations; between whom there is no intercourse and no sympathy; who are as ignorant of each other's habits, thoughts and feelings, as if they were dwellers in different zones, or inhabitants of different planets; who are formed by a different breeding, are fed by a different food, are ordered by different manners, and are not governed by the same laws . . . the rich and the poor."[15]

There is one great difference between the pharoahs, mandarins, and Aztec rulers and the world's contemporary ruling elites. During the past few centuries, colonialism, commerce, and communication have spread a homogenizing common culture to every part of the earth. It is now the rule for strangers from different continents to attend the same international conference or business meeting, dressed alike in suit and tie or in the latest fashion, drinking the same highballs and eating the same cuisine, exchanging the same shoptalk and political gossip. They may be graduates of the same universities, employees of the same bank, intergovernmental agency or multinational corporation, or members of the same profession. The international elites share elements of a common culture that ignores national borders and ties its members together in a web of interests and affiliations.

As described in the previous chapter, poverty is a relative term and the circumstances of persons considered poor in one context (e.g., the urban United States) might be envied by many others living in crowded Third World cities. Among those urban poor, the needs for adequate housing, employment, transportation, nutrition, health care, and educational opportunities for children are essentially identical in Accra, Rio, and Bangkok. In addition, specific elements of popular culture such as films, music, and certain consumer goods may help to reinforce a certain commonality of experience and attitude among people who are unaware of each other's existence.

Intermediate in international acculturation are the middle classes: businessmen, civil servants, teachers, junior professionals, and others who share a background of moderate education, limited wealth, and strong ambition for upward mobility for themselves and for their children. This middle group is dominant in industrialized countries and is increasing in numbers in some of the developing countries, particularly in southeast Asia and Latin America.

Economic Development and Health

It seems clear that modernization and development are here to stay, are spreading, sometimes hesitatingly and imperfectly, throughout the world, and have complex interrelationships with health. In 18th-century England only half the population survived to their 15th birthday. A century later half survived to 40, and more than half the children born today can expect to see their 70th birthday.

An example of an indicator of development that may have indirect effects on health is the availability of radio and television sets in a population. The electronic media may be used by authorities to transmit overt health messages, such as those for AIDS prevention, immunization, or family planning. Perhaps more significant are advertisements (for insecticide, beer, soft drinks, automobiles, powdered milk, cosmetics, and other items of commerce) and programmatic content depicting supposedly admirable people and their lives and activities. Emulation of such models may have rapid and profound health consequences, both good and bad. Moreover, as Marshall McLuhan pointed out decades ago, the medium is often the message, and the mere presence of the radio or television receiver may lead to significant changes in personal or group behavior, independent of the nature or content of the broadcast messages.

Most commentators ascribe the great decline in childhood mortality in countries that were developing during the 18th and 19th centuries to improved nutrition, water supply, excreta disposal, and housing; legislation to control employment of women and children; and public health services in the broad sense. A case in point is the reduction in childhood mortality from measles in England and Wales from 1850 to 1970 (Fig. 8-1).[16] One conceivable explanation for this trend might be that the measles virus spontaneously became less virulent during this period. That this

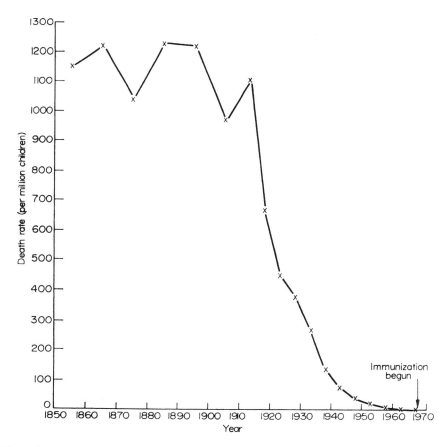

Figure 8-1 Mean annual death rate for measles of children under fifteen, England and Wales, 1850–1970. Source: McKeown and Lowe, 1974.

probably has not happened is demonstrated in West Africa, where measles today, caused by the same virus found in England, produces a very high mortality in young children. The drop in childhood mortality from measles in England is not an isolated case. Similar declines have occurred in scarlet fever, and the same sort of picture can be shown for mumps, diphtheria, whooping cough, and the other infectious "childhood" diseases. All of these declines accompanied improvements in nutrition and living conditions, and they began before there was scientific knowledge of the causative agents, mode of transmission, prevention by immunization, or means of chemotherapy. Nevertheless, immunization has had a profound effect in further reducing the burden of diseases such as measles.

However, sanitary measures and improvements in nutrition have had no beneficial effect on transmission of some diseases. It is widely believed that the prevalence of some diseases, such as paralytic poliomyelitis, has actually been fostered by improvements in standards of living. In this view, infection with poliovirus in early infancy will induce antibody formation and immunity, with relatively less likelihood of paralysis than a first infection in a susceptible older person. The virus is transmitted through the environment via the fecal-oral route, and where sanitation blocks such transmission, people are less exposed to the virus very early in life, may not develop the resulting immunity, and will be more severely affected by an encounter later on. The widespread use of poliovirus vaccines has essentially reversed this drawback of development in the wealthier countries.

Life expectancies in the tropical countries as a whole remained dismal until the time of World War II. Since then, longevity has increased dramatically with the general exception of sub-Saharan Africa.

> Within a decade in numerous instances and no more than two decades in most, many of the world's low-income nations have passed through successions of longevity stages that today's highest-income nations with the lowest mortality rates needed generations or even half-centuries to reach and leave behind. It is safe to say that nothing in world history would have prepared a pre–World War II or even a 1950 observer for the mortality trends that soon emerged—whether in terms of their size and speed; number of nations involved; diverse ecological, geographical, political, and historic context; numbers of people affected; or the mortality levels reached in relation to continued poverty and economic backwardness . . . the suggested LDR [less developed regions] gains have occurred among populations that have typically been much poorer and more economically disadvantaged than were their MDR [more developed regions] predecessors when experiencing similar gains.[17]

During the latter part of the 20th century the projected expectation of life has increased 67% in the poorest countries but less than 6% in the wealthiest countries. By 2000 the poorest countries will have life expectancies equivalent to those of some developed countries in 1950 and differentials between countries will be narrowed across the board. This narrowing of life expectancies among countries is occurring while inequalities within countries are increasing.

THE HUMAN POPULATION

The world reached "the day of 5 billion" on July 11, 1987, a day selected by Rafael Salas, then director of the UNFPA,[18] who remarked that "The birth of the five billionth baby during 1987 is a time for celebration, but it also demands the serious attention of the world community. What kind of world will it be when the five billionth child grows up—when there will be six billion people on our planet?"

The five billionth child had hardly grown up—he or she was less than 12 years old—on "the day of six billion," June 16, 1999.

The primary immediate cause for the population surge of the last 200 years has been a reduction in mortality, particularly in younger age groups. Greater survival of children will alter the age structure of a population, giving it progressively more reproductive capability, augmented further by the reduction of age at menarche and social customs permitting marriage and/or childbearing at relatively early ages. Improved health also increases fertility by reducing the effects of diseases that may cause fetal wastage and by lengthening the mother's (and the father's!) reproductive span. These effects also result from improving nutrition and living conditions as well as by preventing or treating disease. Improved health may also extend the period of a mother's lactation and thus strengthen an infant's chances of survival. Another factor enhancing the infant survival rate may be the substantial reduction in fertility that nursing mothers experience.

In 1995, the world's population increased by 9200 people per hour, more than a million more births than deaths every five days. As it continues to soar, the number of people analyzing and commenting on this growth seems to increase even faster, and readers can select from a menu of predictions ranging from extremely optimistic to utterly gloomy (see Chapter 1). While the effects of population growth on human health in the next decades are a matter for speculation, the importance of human numbers to an understanding of world health problems is not in doubt. Table 8-2 shows projections of the human population, by regions, a century into the future, based on a medium estimate. While such projections are likely to contain large errors, they probably give a fair idea of what may lie ahead.

In the late 1990s India and China together comprised 48% of the population of developing countries and 37% of the total world population. Note that the proportion of the world's population in Asia, Latin America, and Oceania is projected to remain fairly stable, but that of Europe and of North America will decline greatly.[19] The greatest gains will be in Africa, which will treble in number and almost double as a percentage of global population.

If these projections are accurate, the population of Africa in 2100 will be larger

Table 8-2. Population and Percentage Distribution, by Geographic Region, 2000, 2050, and 2100

	Population (Millions)			Percentage of World Population		
	2000	2050	2100	2000	2050	2100
World	6114	9578	10,958	100.0	100.0	100.0
Asia	3703	5638	6289	60.6	58.9	57.9
Europe	737	721	714	12.1	7.5	6.8
Africa	821	1999	2643	13.4	20.9	23.9
Latin America	512	804	883	8.4	8.4	8.2
North America	310	374	384	5.1	3.9	3.5
Oceania	31	42	45	0.5	0.5	0.4

Source: World Bank Population Projections

than the entire world population in 1950. Europe is expected to decline in actual numbers. Population decline is not an entirely new phenomenon: Ireland in 1800 had about eight million people, but after the great emigrations of the mid-19th century it has remained level at about half that number.

The reluctance of Europeans to have children is leading to extremely low birth rates and increasing proportions of older people in the population. Italy in the mid-1990s had the lowest birth rate ever recorded among humans. Countries whose total fertility rate was below replacement level of 2.1 children per woman (1995 data) are listed on Table 8-3.

Historically, the number of people on earth increased rather slowly, perhaps at 0.1% annually, from earliest times until the late 17th century, when Europe and its colonies began a rapid rise. The elements that determine population growth are complex, and the whole story is not revealed by a simple comparison of crude birth and death rates. It is unmistakably true, however, that a birth rate of 40 per thousand in a year, with 38 deaths per thousand in the same year in the same population, will result in an increase of 2 per thousand, or 0.2%. With this birth rate constant, a reduction in deaths to 20 will produce a 2% increase, and further reduction to 10 will yield 3%. Just such a general trend has occurred with rapid and significant reductions in mortality in some countries, unaccompanied by equivalent declines in natality. Any capital amount increasing at a fixed percentage x, when compounded annually, will double in about $72/x$ years. Therefore a 2% growth rate will result in a doubling in 35 years and a 3% rate in less than 24, situations that now exist in various parts of the world. The effect of mortality reduction on population growth is related to the ages and potential reproductive capacity of the deaths averted. Mortality is now very low in the so-called developed countries and expectation of life at birth for both sexes is 70 years or more. Even if death rates do fall somewhat

Tablel 8-3. Countries With Fertility Rate Below Replacement Level of 2.1 Children, 1995

Country	Fertility Rate	Country	Fertility Rate	Country	Fertility Rate
Italy	1.24	Macau	1.60	Britain	1.78
Spain	1.27	Cuba	1.60	Singapore	1.79
Germany	1.30	Belgium	1.62	Australia	1.80
Hong Kong	1.32	Ukraine	1.64	Finland	1.83
Slovenia	1.36	Latvia	1.64	Slovakia	1.85
Greece	1.38	South Korea	1.65	Norway	1.88
Austria	1.47	Croatia	1.65	Poland	1.89
Japan	1.48	Luxembourg	1.66	China	1.92
Bosnia[a]	1.50	Belarus	1.67	Yugoslavia	1.93
Romania	1.50	Czech Republic	1.68	Thailand	1.94
Portugal	1.52	Hungary	1.69	Bahamas	1.95
Switzerland	1.53	France	1.70	Sweden	2.01
Russia	1.53	Barbados	1.73	Ireland	2.01
Bulgaria	1.53	Canada	1.74	Martinique	2.05
Estonia	1.58	Denmark	1.75	United States	2.05
Netherlands	1.60	Lithuania	1.78	Malta	2.08

[a]Bosnia and Herzegovina.

Source: United Nations, 1996.

more, their effect on population growth in these countries will be negligible because the probability of survival through the normal span of fertility is already very high.

Control of Human Population Growth

It was popular in the 1960s and 1970s to make dire predictions about the world's overcrowding. Pessimists wrote books with titles like *The Population Bomb* or *Famine 1975!*[20] and predicted that the world would soon run out of everything.[21] That has not happened so far, but the dire forecasts continue. The world population is continuing to increase, but there are signs that the rate of growth is slowing. Large international data-gathering projects such as the *World Fertility Survey* and *Contraceptive Prevalence Surveys* (during the 1970s) and the *Demographic and Health Surveys*, as well as national agencies, monitor population levels. The annual rate of world population growth, estimated at 1.79% in 1950–1955, grew to 2.06% in 1965–1970, declined to 1.73% by 1980, and then remained constant for a decade. In 1995 the world population growth rate was 1.48% and total fertility had declined from 6 children per woman in 1965 to 2.96 children per woman worldwide.[22]

In Thailand, for instance, fertility plummeted 50% in 12 years; from 4.6 children per woman in 1975 to 2.3 children in 1987. In Colombia, the fertility rate fell from an average of 4.7 children per woman in 1976 to 2.8 children in 1990. In Indonesia, fertility declined 46 percent between 1971 and 1991; in Morocco, it dropped 31 percent between 1980 and 1992; in Turkey, fertility decreased 21 percent between 1978 and 1988. In eight Latin American and Caribbean countries, women today are having an average of one fewer child than women 20 years ago.[23]

But critics point out that "Many countries in sub-Saharan Africa and South Asia have not started substantial fertility reductions, deepening the gap between developing countries that are moving to lower fertility levels and those that are left behind."[24] In fact, population growth rates in sub-Saharan Africa have increased steadily during the past half century. A continuing decline in mortality combined with a sustained increase in fertility and a rejuvenated age structure led to growth rates from 2.1% around 1950 to 2.7% in 1970 to 3.2% in 1990. Both Kenya and Rwanda exceeded 4% annually during the 1980s. Fertility opposed world trends: in 1950, six countries had a total fertility rate above seven children but in 1990 ten countries did so, during a period when infant mortality rates declined from 190 to 105 per thousand live births and overall death rates from 28 to 16 per thousand inhabitants.[25]

Two things will reduce population growth: increasing mortality (an option not at present widely advocated by critics) and reducing births. One means by which it is hoped that such a fertility decline may be hastened is through *family planning*, defined as

> organized programs—mainly govermental in sponsorship, support, and administration, but often involving private efforts (family planning associations) and occasionally commercial ones—designed to provide the information, supplies, and services of (modern) means of fertility control to those interested. Such programs frequently have a persuasional component as well, advocating the small-family norm, but that element is not strong. Usually the programs more or less accept existing levels of motivation and seek to meet the existing "need" by minimizing the cost of fertility control not only monetarily but personally, by legitimizing the idea and providing services through trusted sources.[26]

Large-scale reductions in fertility have occurred in the absence of family planning programs. For example, wealthier and more educated elites in Europe had begun to control family size by the turn of the 20th century. But when the means for fertility regulation becomes readily available to those with less education and income, the process accelerates and the differential between societies disappears. In the United States the total fertility rate declined without family planning from 6 in 1842 to 3.5 in 1900, a period of 58 years. With good access to modern methods of fertility regulation (see below), the same decline occurred in Colombia in 15 years (1968–1983) and in Thailand in 8 years (1969–1977).[27]

Iran provides an interesting example of population growth and limitation. In 1979 at the time of the Islamic Revolution, Iran's population was 34 million. Pronatalist government policies and lowering the marriage age led to a population growth rate estimated as high as 3.9%. A concerned government then instituted a required course in family planning for all newly married couples, along with widespread education, distribution of free contraceptives of all kinds, with free vasectomies and tubal ligations in public clinics. A Fertility Regulation Council was established in 1990, and shortly thereafter certain benefits such as subsidized food coupons and health insurance were withdrawn after the birth of a third child. As a result of these measures population growth declined to about 1.4% by the late 1990s. In Peru a government initiative to reduce poverty by promoting birth control became a contentious issue when it was alleged that poor women were aggressively offered gifts such as clothes and food in exchange for agreeing to be sterilized. Critics said that illiterate women were coerced, or not adequately informed about the procedure, which was sometimes poorly performed. About 10,000 tubal ligations were done in Peru in 1995 and 100,000 in 1997.

The main methods of fertility control provided in family planning programs are oral contraceptives, intrauterine devices, condoms, sterilization (vasectomy and tubal ligation), and, where permitted, abortion. In addition, traditional methods such as rhythm and withdrawal are commonly practiced, especially where artificial means of contraception are restricted or prohibited. The effectiveness of such programs in the decline in world birth rates is difficult to estimate, as one must separate the effects of targeted programs from reductions that would have occurred without them, such as the tendency to increased age at marriage; general availability of contraception; changes in religious and social views, especially about the role of women; or improved communication, education, and income. Nevertheless, some studies have been carried out using true experimental designs—that is, randomizing units into different study and control groups. A meta-analysis of 16 such evaluations found positive program effects in 13, although "a much smaller effect than program proponents would like to see."[28] By 1990 the use of any contraceptive method was practiced by about 50% of eligible couples in the world, but sub-Saharan Africa still had a prevalence estimated at about 18%.

Several nations are working hard to *increase* their birth rate in certain population groups. Fearing depopulation, Sweden provides generous incentives to working parents, including cash payments, tax breaks, and flexible working hours. Despite these inducements, Sweden's fertility rate fell from 2.12 per woman in 1991 to 1.6 in 1995 and 1.42 in 1998, the same as Japan. In eastern Germany births have plunged by 50% or 60% in some areas, causing some state governments to offer cash inducements for any pregnancy. Nobody understands the reason for the decline but it seems to be related to a desire to enjoy "the good life" and unwillingness to make sacrifices for children who are viewed as an inconvenience. Also, the constant drumbeat of impending environmental disaster probably plays a role. In some countries with several competing ethnic groups each may try to assure its predominance, or survival, by trying to have more children than the other. Politics is sometimes foremost in people's minds: for example, a Palestinian woman was quoted as saying, "We must have more babies to compensate for our losses in Lebanon and to put pressure on the Jews to come to the negotiating table."[29] Among Palestinians the fertility rate has increased to 8.8 children per woman.

The literature on population and family planning is vast. Many organizations, both governmental and voluntary, are devoted to this single goal. It is not possible here to review this material, but mention may be made of the situation in the People's Republic of China, home to one-fifth of the world population. In the decades before 1980 the crude birth rate in China fell by over 50%, to about 20 per thousand, and average family size declined proportionately. In an attempt to reach a stable population of 1.2 billion with zero growth by 2000, China adopted the one-child campaign in 1979. Couples who pledge to have only one child are rewarded with economic incentives such as monthly allowances for the child, remission of certain fees and charges, and an additional pension for the parents. Conversely, the birth of additional children is accompanied by penalties.

> Rural couples in China are reluctant to stop at one child, and a large minority of them also resist stopping at two, given their perceived need for sons for farm labor, old-age support, and patrilineal family ceremonial duties. So the government modified its one-child policy in the 1980s to allow provinces to permit some couples to have two children. By 1989, 43% of China's population was still subject to the strict one-child policy, while 44% was subject to a "one-and-a-half child policy;" this means that, if a couple's first child is a boy, the couple may have no more children, but if the first child is a girl, one more birth is allowed.[30]

The one-child policy applies only to the ethnic Chinese population and is not enforced among the many minority nationalities that make up a small percentage of the population of China. The total fertility rate in Tibet, for example, has remained at about 4.5 births per woman while in all of China fertility has gone from 4.9 children per woman in 1970 to 1.8 in 1996. The population of China grew at a 1.5% annual rate during the 1980s which declined to about 1.1% in the early 1990s when fertility fell even further.

The Demographic Transition

Some experts, looking at the historical record of the present-day developed countries, have placed emphasis and high hopes on the theory of demographic transition. This term, devised by F. W. Notestein in 1945,[31] is used to describe the changes in birth and death rates that historically have accompanied the shift from a traditional to a modern society. Sharp declines in mortality have been followed, after some lag, by a reduction in fertility, as illustrated in Figure 8-2. In Notestein's classical description, a stable high stationary stage with equally high birth and death rates and little or no population growth gives way to a transitional stage of falling death rates, sustained high birth rates and rapid growth, and then a new stationary stage in which birth and death rates are low and balanced. A more recent and detailed analysis specifies five stages (LEB = life expectancy at birth; TFR = total fertility rate):

- Stage 1: mortality and fertility both high; LEB less than 45; TFR more than 6.5
- Stage 2: mortality declining, then fertility declines; LEB 45 to 55; TFR 5 to 6.5
- Stage 3: mortality and fertility decline faster; LEB 55 to 65; TFR 3.5 to 5
- Stage 4: mortality and fertility both at low levels; LEB 65 to 75; TFR 2 to 3.5
- Stage 5: mortality and fertility both very low; LEB 75 or more; TFR less than 2[32]

Besides a shrinking proportion of children, an element of the demographic transition is an increase in the median age of populations and rising life expectancy. Table 8-4 shows how life expectancy at birth has changed in the latter half of the 20th century. Note that the less developed regions have achieved greater proportionate gains than the least developed regions, and far more than the more developed regions. There has been a marked convergence in the length of human life between the rich and poor countries of the world in the second half of this century. As Mur-

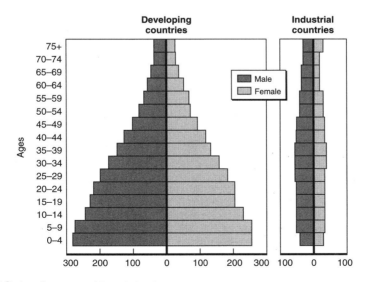

Figure 8-2 Age Structure of Population in Developing and Industrial Countries, 1995 (in millions). Source: Da Vanzo and Adamson (1998). Fig. 3.

Table 8-4. Life Expectancy at Birth, World and Major Areas, 1950–1995

Area	Life Expectancy (Years)			Percent Increase
	1950–1955	1970–1975	1990–1995	1950–1955 to 1990–1995
World	46.4	57.9	64.7	39.4
More developed regions	66.0	71.1	74.6	13.0
Less developed regions	40.7	54.5	62.4	53.3
Least developed regions	35.7	43.6	50.2	40.6
Africa	37.7	46.1	53.0	40.6
Asia	41.0	56.1	64.8	58.0
Europe	65.7	71.5	75.2	14.4
Latin America	51.4	61.1	68.0	32.1
Northern America	69.0	71.5	76.1	10.3
Australia–New Zealand	69.5	71.7	76.7	10.4

Source: United Nations (1996). Adapted from Table 38.

ray and Chen have pointed out, these declines in mortality have continued through economic upturns and downturns:

> One puzzling aspect of secular morality decline is its persistence despite major economic shocks . . . These economic insults, according to traditional theory, should have had a devastating impact on morality levels in the affected populations . . . Despite these documented cases of human suffering and perhaps pockets of mortality stagnation, the secular declines of mortality at the national level have persisted throughout the past decade.[33]

Are child survival strategies responsible for these declines? Murray and Chen find that the evidence is inconclusive; moreover, "the consistent declines in child mortality do not match temporally nor geographically the recorded coverage of immunization or oral rehydration therapy." To explain the resilience of mortality declines they propose a complex of inter-dependent factors:

- The level and distribution of national incomes
- The effectiveness of public policies
- The efficiency and effectiveness of expenditures directed toward mortality control.

During the demographic transition the age structure of the population changes dramatically, with proportionately fewer children, many more older people, and a substantial increase in median age (Fig. 8-2).

By 2150 the median age in the world is expected to be 42 years, compared with

24 years in 1990. See Figure 8-3 for a graphic illustration of how various countries of Latin America fit into the demographic transition. In Latin America and the Caribbean, for example, the population is expected to increase 4.6 times in the 80 years between 1950 and 2030, but the number of children under five will only double while those over 60 will expand more than 12 times.[34]

There is a great deal of argument over whether the currently industrialized countries are a template or road map for corresponding changes bound to come in the currently developing countries. Most observers consider this unlikely:

> Development of the poorer countries in the second half of the Twentieth Century has not been associated with the same positive change in social and health status outcomes as were observed in the late 19th and early 20th centuries in the West. Many developing countries have shown relatively small individual gains in the populations' health status. This may be due in part to rapidly increasing population levels, poor distribution of economic opportunity, and an uneven allocation of other reources including education and sanitation. A combination of these factors leads to a disproportionately large portion of the population occupying the lower socioeconomic strata associated with poor health status.[35]

Developing countries typically go through the process of demographic transition in two or three generations, or 60 to 90 years. In East Asia fertility has declined to the extent that the demographic transition has been completed in Japan, Taiwan,

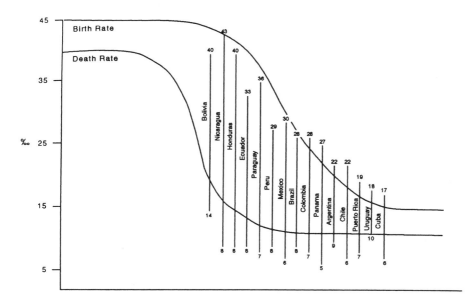

Figure 8-3 Stage of the demographic transition in Latin American countries, end of the 1980s. Source: Reprinted from Bähr and Wehrhahn (1993). Fig. 1. Social Science and Medicine, Vol. 36, Copyright 1993, with permission from Elsevier Science.

South Korea, and China. These declines have occurred in the main from the "rational choices" of couples who, with money in their pockets and assured of the survival of two or three (or fewer) children, will opt for consumer goods and better living standards instead of larger families.

> Given that numbers of surviving children were increasing and were more than sufficient to continue the family, the older generation was inclined to welcome the employment of some children in the emerging nonfarm sector, for this was likely to increase family income through remittances and provide a hedge against rural subsistence crises. As educated children stood better chances for such employment, and as the early years of primary school (at least) occurred before children had substantial labor value, the older generation was also inclined to have their children take advantage of emerging educational opportunities.[36]

Although many authors champion the idea that fertility drops spontaneously with economic development, this is still a matter of debate. A passionate advocate of an alternate viewpoint writes:

> In 1960, Korea was largely a rice farming country with a per capita income of well under US$1000 a year. The annual rate of population growth exceeded the rate of economic growth. In the early 1960s, the government and nongovernmental organizations began offering voluntary sterilization and IUD insertions by subsidizing private medical practitiners, among whom women could make their own selection. Later, the community-based distribution of subsidized pills became important. The country enjoyed de facto access to safe abortion. In 30 years the TFR plummeted from 6.0 to 1.7, and per capita income rocketed to over $5000 a year. It would be easy to suggest that such spectacular economic progress was the engine driving fertility decline, but Cuba has an economy renowned for its economic failure, where people have become poorer over the past decades; yet the mixture of contraception and safe abortion is similar to that in Korea and fertility fell in Cuba at the same rate as in Korea and to the same low level, casting doubt on the hypothesis that Korea's fertility decline was caused by its economic development.[37]

The Epidemiologic Transition

This term, proposed by Omran[38] refers to the changes in patterns of health and disease in societies, and their determinants and consequences, as they accompany the process of development. Life expectancy at birth increases and the pattern of major diseases and causes of death changes from the era of "pestilence and famine" to "receding pandemics" to "degenerative and man-made diseases." In western Europe and North America ("the classical model") the transition took approximately 100 years. In Japan and eastern Europe the transition started later but proceeded more rapidly ("the accelerated model"). Elsewhere the transition is in various phases, some nearing completion, some not ("the contemporary delayed model"). Some authors have combined the demographic and epidemiological transitions into a single *health transition*.[39]

In 1990, 7% of all DALYs[40] lost in OECD countries arose from communicable diseases, while 81% came from noncommunicable diseases. At the same time in developing countries, communicable diseases accounted for 47% of DALYs, a number expected to decline to 21% by the year 2020. Noncommunicable diseases in developing countries are expected to take the opposite direction, increasing from 38% to 58% of all DALYs by 2020. Although these figures are converging, a substantial differential will remain in the major causes of lost DALYs between OECD countries in 1990 and developing countries in 2020, suggesting that the epidemiological transition will still have a long way to go. The proportion of DALYs lost due to injuries, which is already higher in developing countries (15% versus 12%), is expected to grow to 21%, suggesting an increasingly unsafe environment.

The reduction in mortality of the early demographic transition comes mostly from prevention and management of infectious diseases at young ages with a rapid decline in infant mortality. In Chile, for example, IMR went from 82.2 per thousand live births in 1970 to 14.3 in 1992, a drop of 82%. During the same brief time period IMR in all of Latin America and the Caribbean declined by 46.3%.[41] Survival beyond the critical infectious hazards of childhood exposes people to accidents and chronic illnesses of adults.

Road fatalities are a major hazard in many developing countries because of old vehicles that carry too many people; lack of seat belts and helmets for motorcycles; poor road design and maintenance; animals, bicycles, scooters, and pedestrians on the roads; poor vehicle maintenance; inexperienced and undisciplined drivers; and alcohol. Motor accidents are a major health problem for field personnel from the Peace Corps and nongovernmental organizations working in developing countries. Between 30% and 82% of trauma admissions in developing countries come from traffic accidents, and 80% of fatalities are in males. While road traffic accidents declined by 20% in Europe between 1968 and 1983, they increased 150% in Asia and 200% in Africa. The former socialist countries of eastern Europe had, on average, the highest traffic-related mortality rates. Especially high rates of fatalities per 10,000 vehicles are found in Haiti (302), Zambia (118), Uganda (114), and Kenya (84), in comparison with Kuwait (8) Saudi Arabia (3), and Norway (1.7).[42] Growing prosperity has brought a rapid increase in automobile density to many tropical cities, resulting in traffic gridlock and widespread air pollution.

An interesting example of an epidemiological shift over a short period of time is documented for South Korea (Table 8-5), whose demographic and economic development was described previously. The infectious causes of death that were central as recently as the mid-1960s had yielded their dominance in only 15 years and by 1991 appeared to be off the "top nine" chart.

We may see an epidemiolgic transition even within the class of diseases collec-

Tablel 8-5. Rank Order of the Nine Leading Causes of Death, Republic of Korea, 1966–1991

Rank	1966	1981	1991
1	Pneumonia	Malignant neoplasms	Malignant neoplasms
2	Tuberculosis	Hypertension	Cerebrovascular
3	Cerebrovascular	Cerebrovascular	Senile disease
4	Other infectious causes	Nontraffic accidents	Pulmonary causes
5	Malignant neoplasms	Senile disease	Nontraffic accidents
6	All accidents	Chronic liver disease	Traffic accidents
7	Bronchitis	Traffic accidents	Hypertension
8	Meningitis	Tuberculosis	Chronic liver disease
9	Hypertension	Suicide	Other circulatory diseases

Source: U.S. Bureau of the Census, International Programs Center, International Data Base.

tively known as cancer. Those malignancies that are caused primarily by microorganisms, including cancers of the liver, stomach, nasopharynx, and uterine cervix, become relatively less important in developed countries, while those in which adult behaviors such as cigarette smoking, diet, delayed pregnancy, and similar risk factors predominate (lung, colon, breast) rise in incidence. Similarly, liver and pulmonary diseases, including hepatitis and pneumonias, remain well represented, although as causes of chronic adult rather than acute childhood illnesses.

As has been mentioned in previous chapters, countries are not monolithic. Different subgroups within countries represent different phases of the health transition. A leading health transition theorist, Julio Frenk of Mexico, has pointed out with respect to Omran's "eras" that

- the eras are not necessarily sequential, since two or more may overlap
- the evolutionary changes in the patterns of morbidity and mortality are reversible, giving rise to what could be called a *"counter-transition"*
- there is, in consequence, a new model of epidemiologic transition, typical of countries where the changes do not fully take place and where different types of diseases coexist in the same population; this we call a *protracted* epidemiologic transition
- the coexistence of pre- and post-transitional diseases leads, in certain countries, to an *epidemiological polarization*. The old health inequalities among social classes, which hitherto were predominantly quantitative, become qualitative with this polarization. The poorer sector of the population would not only present with higher rates of disease, but these would be of different kinds, mostly either infections or nutritional disorders.[43]

A countertransition of sorts has occurred in the former Soviet Union. In Russia and Ukraine the infant mortality rate had risen by more than 13% by 1995. Male life expectancy in Russia in 1990 was at or below the rates of the 1960s and declined further in 1993. Female life expectancy rose between 1959 and 1990 but has declined since.[44] Deteriorating economic and health conditions have encouraged a resurgence of formerly rare infectious diseases. For example, an epidemic of diphtheria swept through Russia, Ukraine, the Baltic States, and into all of the former Soviet republics, affecting many thousands with a substantial number of fatalities. Social disintegration and hopelessness have given rise to hundreds of thousands of excess deaths from accidents, homicide, suicide, and alcoholism. An epidemic of HIV infection, much of it from injection drugs, has swept through the young adult population.

Of all modern diseases, AIDS is having the greatest demographic impact, particularly in sub-Saharan Africa where 86% of all HIV-infected people reside. In addition to a drop in life expectancy, AIDS will reduce population growth rates and may actually cause certain population groups to decline in the first decades of the 21st century. In Zimbabwe, HIV infection alone will reduce the population growth rate from 3.3% per year between 1980 and 1985, to less than 1% beginning in 2000. In November, 1998 the Executive Director of the Joint United Nations Program on HIV/AIDS announced that

- In the world's nine most-affected countries (all of them located in Africa) where at least a tenth of the adult population has HIV, a child born in 2000–2005 can expect to survive only to the age of 43, instead of to age 60 as would have been expected in the absence of AIDS.
- By the first decade of next century Namibia's infant mortality rate would normally have fallen to 45 per 1000; instead, the epidemic will raise it to 72 per 1000. Already by 1996, the direct and indirect costs of AIDS represented around 8% of Namibia's gross domestic product, and the figure is set to rise much higher.
- In Côte d'Ivoire's urban households where the breadwinner has AIDS, calculations show that family income is cut by two-thirds and consumption goes down, notably for schooling, which drops by more than 50%.
- Because of AIDS, Zimbabwe expects to be burying 350 people a day in just two years' time and to have over 900 000 AIDS orphans under age 15 struggling to survive without their mothers by the year 2005. By then, AIDS patients will be occupying two-thirds of the country's public hospital beds.[45]

Further information on HIV and AIDS is given in Chapter 14.

The epidemiologic transition does not continue to change with increasing wealth. As mentioned in the previous chapter, there seems to be a break point at about

$5,000 per capita above which rising income ceases to have much impact on health. "Thus, it seems that in the later stages of industrial development countries go through a health climacteric after which the health of the vast majority of the population is no longer substantially affected by the absolute material standard of living."[46] As the pattern of disease shifts from acute/pediatric to chronic/elderly, medical care becomes far less effective in increasing life expectancy, and changes in character from what an economist would call an investment to a consumption expenditure.

Aging

The demographic and epidemiologic transitions have led to increasing numbers of older people in all parts of the world (Table 8-6). The reluctance of persons to have children is leading to extremely low birth rates and increasing proportions of older people in the population. Italy was the first nation in the world to have more people over age 60 than under age 20, and Germany, Greece, and Spain passed the same landmark in 1998. With population aging inevitable, how to pay for retirement is a major political issue everywhere. At the same time, it must not be assumed that older persons will become mere burdens on family and society. Programs for productive aging help to assure that older people, such as your industrious author, will continue to make valuable contributions to society.

Most western countries maintain an arbitrary retirement age of 65, established in 1889 by German Chancellor Otto von Bismarck, ostensibly because his advisors informed him that hardly anyone would live to that age, so the plan would rarely have

Table 8-6. Percent of Population Aged 60 and Over, 25 "Oldest" Countries, 1996

Country	Percent of Population	Country	Percent of Population
Italy	22.3	Austria	19.8
Greece	22.3	Norway	19.8
Sweden	21.9	Hungary	19.6
Belgium	21.5	Switzerland	19.5
Spain	21.2	Luxembourg	19.1
Bulgaria	21.2	Estonia	19.0
Japan	20.9	Finland	19.0
Germany	20.9	Czech Republic	18.1
United Kingdom	20.5	Belarus	17.9
France	20.3	Netherlands	17.8
Portugal	20.2	Uruguay	17.3
Denmark	19.9	Georgia	17.0
		United States	16.5

Source: U.S. Bureau of the Census, International Programs Center, International Data Base.

to pay benefits. Now it is equally rare for a person *not* to live to age 65. "In the early years of the twentieth century, when the old age pension was initiated and made available to those reaching a retirement age of 65 years in several countries of Europe, around 5% of the populations of these countries was eligible. Now roughly a quarter of the population of Europe is of pensionable age."[47]

The age at which retirement benefits are granted varies among countries. In Australia, Austria, Canada, and Greece, women receive retirement benefits at 60 and men at 65; in France it is 60 for both sexes; and in Russia and Hungary retirement comes at 55 for women and 60 for men. Denmark and Norway have mandated 67 years for both sexes, a change hotly debated in the United States. In many developing countries, such as Brazil, the mandatory retirement age remains at 55 while demographic and economic changes make this increasingly difficult to sustain financially, politically and socially.

The average life expectancy in developing countries has grown from the mid-40s in the early 1950s to the mid-60s forty years later (Table 8-4) and is projected to reach 69 by 2020. Although this figure may not seem to put much pressure on retirement funding in the poor countries, the world's over-65 population is increasing by 800,000 *per month*, 70% of whom are in the developing world. Between 1990 and 2025 the increase in the percentage of elderly (over age 65) will be phenomenal in some countries (Table 8-7). In Japan the percentage of the population over 65 (15.50%) exceeded that under 15 (15.46%) for the first time in mid-1997. Plans and budgets will need to be prepared for these changes, particularly where the increases will be several hundred percent.

While care of the elderly is traditionally a family responsibility, lower fertility means that there are fewer children (who often move away from the village) to take care of the elderly. It is unclear who will (or can) pay the costs of medical care and hospitalization for chronic illnesses of older citizens. Until now child survival campaigns have had widespread appeal and support in both developed and developing countries, but some demographers and economists predict unpleasant competition between the health needs of the young and of the old. Not only do causes of death change with age, but specific causes change over time as a proportion of deaths within age groups. Table 8-8 shows how the impact of cancer (all types) declined in the younger ages and increased in the older ages over a 20-year period as risk factors, competing causes, and medical treatment have changed.[48]

In addition to specific health needs, the general maintenance of the retired elderly is an increasing problem. Few poor countries have active old-age pension systems. In China only about 10% (all urban workers) are covered; in India, less than 8% of the population (mainly employed by the government and big corporations) falls under social security programs.[49] In midlevel countries such as Chile it is feasible to require employees to contribute 10% of salary into a privately invested pension fund, thereby converting the state pension system into individual retirement accounts. The Russian government, facing a retirement crisis in the future, has proposed a system

Table 8-7. Percent Increase in Persons Aged 65 or Older, Selected Countries, 1990–2025

Country	Percent Increase	Country	Percent Increase	Country	Percent Increase
Sweden	33	United States	101	Morocco	250
Uruguay	35	Israel	120	Philippines	254
Norway	40	Poland	121	Brazil	255
United Kingdom	45	Jamaica	126	Turkey	257
Denmark	47	Japan	129	Zimbabwe	271
Austria	50	Cuba	130	Peru	279
Belgium	54	Australia	137	Mexico	290
Bulgaria	59	Canada	141	Rep of Korea	295
Italy	63	Pakistan	146	Liberia	303
Hungary	63	Malawi	194	Malaysia	321
France	65	Bangladesh	219	Costa Rica	327
Greece	66	China	220	Thailand	337
Germany	66	Sri Lanka	238	Singapore	340
Czechoslovakia[a]	82	Egypt	238	Kenya	347
Luxembourg	96	India	242	Colombia	349
Argentina	97	Tunisia	242	Indonesia	414
New Zealand	100	Guatemala	247		

[a]Czech and Slovak Republics.

Source: Adapted from Kinsella and Taeuber (1993) Fig 2-4.

in which retiring workers will receive half their pension from the state-managed fund and half from an individual retirement account invested in a portfolio of Russian securities, but the meltdown of the Russian economy from late 1998 throws this into question. While American legislators struggle with responsibility to pay for retirement, projected pension payments over the coming decades will be less than 8% of GDP in the United States, while those Japan, Germany, France and Italy will reach 15% to 20% of GDP.

DEVELOPMENT AND ENVIRONMENT

The sanitary reformers of the 19th century dealt with polluted water, chimney smoke, animal and human waste, and other forms of pollution arising from overcrowding and lack of amenities.[50] At that time the countryside was considered more or less pristine and a refuge for those urban dwellers fortunate enough to get there. Over the past century and a half great strides have been made in cleaning up the cities of industrial countries, but people are, if anything, more distressed. Several major changes in fact and attitude have occurred. First, the organic hazards bearing hostile microorganisms have been replaced by chemical and physical threats. The in-

Table 8-8. Direction of Changes in Age-Specific Death Rates for All Cancers, by Age Group, 16 Countries, 1968–1987[a]

Age (Years)	Males		Females	
	Decrease	Increase	Decrease	Increase
0–4	15	1	15	1
5–14	16	0	14	2
15–24	16	0	15	1
25–34	15	1	14	2
35–44	13	3	15	1
45–54	9	7	13	3
55–64	6	10	10	6
65–74	6	10	7	9
75–84	0	16	4	12
85+	0	16	1	15

[a]The number of years varies from 12 to 20 within this period. See original. The countries are: Australia, Czechoslovakia, Federal Republic of Germany, Finland, France, German Democratic Republic, Greece, Hong Kong, Hungary, Israel, Italy, Japan, New Zealand, Norway, Singapore, and the United States.

Source: Bailar (1990) Table 3.

convenience of flies from the livery stable next door has been supplanted by the fear of harm from a nuclear power plant or toxic waste dump. Just as stockbrokers and investors have personalized "the market," we now have *the environment* as a distinct entity. Sanitarians have been replaced by environmentalists. At the same time that health hazards have become less local, palpable, and immediate, they have become more dispersed, intangible, and insidious. Distress about the slovenly city has given way to anxiety on a global scale, whether it be ozone depletion or the greenhouse effect. Local councils are supplanted by the Earth Summit in Rio de Janeiro (discussed below). We all share "spaceship earth," and many people feel that there is nowhere to go for relief.

We have said much about the World Bank's 1993 World Development Report (WDR), *Investing in Health*. The previous year's WDR, *Development and Environment*, also contained a great deal of health-related material. The WDR92 recommended that priority be given to environmental problems that damage health and productivity:

- The one-third of the world's population that has inadequate sanitation and the 1 billion without safe water
- The 1.3 billion people who are exposed to unsafe conditions caused by soot and smoke

- The 300 to 700 million women and children who suffer from severe indoor air pollution from cooking fires
- The hundreds of millions of farmers, forest dwellers, and indigenous people who rely on the land and whose livelihood depends on good environmental stewardship

The principal health consequences of environmental mismanagement are:

- Water pollution and water scarcity, leading to more than 2 million deaths and billions of illnesses
- Air pollution responsible for up to 700,000 premature deaths annually and for half of all childhood chronic coughing
- Solid and hazardous wastes spreading diseases through rotting garbage and blocked drains
- Soil degradation leading to reduced nutrition and greater susceptibility to drought
- Deforestation causing localized flooding
- Loss of biodiversity
- Atmospheric changes causing possible shifts in vector-borne diseases; risks from climatic natural disasters; and perhaps 3,000 additional cases of skin cancer and 1.7 million cases of cataracts attributable to ozone depletion

A full discussion of environmental health hazards related to development is beyond the scope of this text, but many useful publications are available.[51] Regularly published reports include the following:

From Official Agencies

Global Environment Outlook	UN Environment Program, Nairobi
Human Development Report	UN Development Program, New York
State of the World's Children	UNICEF, New York
State of World Rural Poverty	International Institute for Agricultural Development, Rome
UNESCO Statistical Yearbook	UNESCO, Paris
United Nations Statistical Yearbook	UN, New York
World Development Report	World Bank, Washington
World Health Report	WHO, Geneva
World Health Statistics Annual	WHO, Geneva

From Private Organizations

State of the World	Worldwatch Institute, Washington
Vital Signs	Worldwatch Institute, Washington
World Resources Report	World Resources Institute, Washington

An example of the intimate association of health, environmental conditions, and the economy is shown in Table 8-9.

As applied technology of all sorts spreads rapidly around the world, it is impossible to evaluate the eventual social benefits or detriments. But insofar as human health and welfare are concerned, we can look at some of the consequences. The world has gone through several rounds of dispersal of technology. Early Chinese development of printing, gunpowder, and the magnet, as Francis Bacon said, "changed the whole face and state of things in the world." Communication, military power, and mobility are still prime targets of technological development.

The Industrial Revolution began in Europe some two centuries ago and was itself preceded by a preparatory evolutionary development. The early groundwork included growth of the merchant, craftsman, and worker groups in European cities; establishment of market economies with wealth based on commerce and productivity (rather than land); and expansion of trade links for obtaining raw materials and distribution of manufactured products. At the same time, the flowering of scientific knowledge, from astronomy to physics and chemistry, provided a firm foundation for the rapid expansion of technologic methods and, most importantly, a built-in mechanism for sustained and continually refined diversification and for the dissemination of innovation. The closely interwoven associations between scientific, economic, political, and social forces have controlled the growth and shape not only of the western industrialized world but to a great extent that of the less developed countries as well.

Table 8-9. Infant and Child Mortality, Water Supply and Sanitation Coverage, and Gross National Product *per Capita*, Six Countries, Early 1990s

Country	Mortality Rate		Percent of Population With Access[c]		GNP/Capita[d]
	Infant[a]	Child[b]	Safe Water	Adequate Sanitation	
Sweden	5	6	100	100	24,740
Chile	15	17	96	71	3170
Philippines	39	48	84	75	850
Ghana	77	113	56	42	430
Guinea-Bissau	135	207	57	20	240
Afghanistan	159	251	10	8	<200[e]

[a]Deaths per thousand live births, 1995.

[b]Deaths per thousand children.

[c]1994 data.

[d]U.S. dollars, 1993 data.

[e]Estimated.

Source: World Health Organization (1997b) Table 1.1.

Recent decades, particularly since the end of World War II, have seen a sharp rise in industrialization in developing countries, spurred by their desire to attain as large a measure of self-sufficiency in as short a time as possible. National planners, working in concert with representatives of international development banking and lending agencies, the governments of industrialized nations, and transnational corporations, have acquired selected units of western technology for their countries. Capital investments have been made not only in extractive, manufacturing, and agricultural industries but also in military hardware, airlines, radio and television broadcasting networks, hospitals, medical schools, and other complex elements of western society.

Of all industries in LDCs, agriculture is still basic, and it is the one with the longest history of industrialization. Estate plantations were introduced on a large scale by colonial powers to provide raw materials for their expanding industry and trade: sugar, tea, coffee, rubber, palm oil, pineapples, and other agricultural products were grown, picked, processed, shipped, and used in many tropical areas. The need for workers resulted in large-scale migrations, voluntary or enforced, as with Indians from Madras to the Malay peninsula or West Africans to the Western Hemisphere—populations that not only brought pathogens with them but were often susceptible to the new diseases they encountered. Agricultural work still carries a high risk of infectious, parasitic, and zoonotic disease and often involves particular hazards such as insect-, tick-, or snakebite. Accidental injuries from falls or from cutting tools or machinery are always a danger. Long working days, poor nutrition, boredom, repetitive motions, and fatigue are closely associated with accidents. More recently, the risk of poisoning from fertilizers, herbicides, and pesticides has become significant in many areas.

Food

Although, as mentioned, predictions of imminent starvation for large segments of mankind have now been popular for some time, the true situation is difficult to assess. Food production *per capita* during the decade of the 1980s increased by 19% in India, by 33% in China, and by 12% globally, although decreases occurred in many sub-Saharan countries. Figure 8-4 shows that agricultural production has at least kept pace with population growth over the past 25 years. However, in some areas gains have not been maintained, especially in areas of civil turmoil. The countries of sub-Saharan Africa have experienced large shortfalls in food supply. As an extreme example, in Mozambique per capita daily caloric intake declined from 2075 to 1805 to 1664 in approximately 1970, 1980, and 1985, respectively.

Just because food is produced does not assure that it is distributed equitably either demographically or geographically, nor that it is of the most suitable types. Nutritionists do not agree on the optimal or minimal intake of calories, total protein, or animal protein per capita under different conditions. The situation is complicated

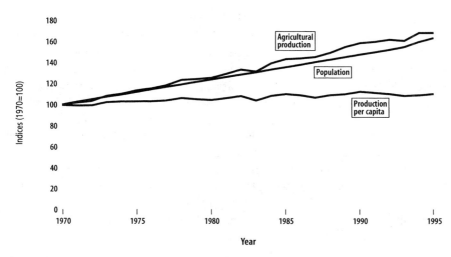

Figure 8-4 World gross agricultural production, population and production per capita
Source: World Health Organization (1997), Fig. 3-7.

by the quality of individual food items, their combination into characteristic menus, and an infinity of practices regarding food preparation and consumption. Loss of growing or stored food to rodents and insects may be very high. Seasonal factors may be important, both in respect to availability of nutrients and human activity cycles. In recent years, nevertheless, it seems that the supply of calories in relation to requirements has been less than adequate in most developing countries with the exception of Latin America, where there may be an overall excess of a few percent. Even here, however, there are many areas with severe deficiencies. The world's per capita protein supply has changed very little during the lifetime of most persons now living. The type of protein produced and consumed varies greatly from one region to another, and decisions about what to eat have far-reaching consequences. There is an almost 30-fold range in protein production per acre depending on the type of food produced there. Problems associated with production, storage, distribution, marketing, preparation, and consumption of these different foods also vary greatly from one region to another. It would be a great mistake to conclude that the world can solve its protein problems simply by growing more soybeans.

Industrialization and its consequences have health benefits, despite the problems of overcrowding, pollution, and occupational hazards. For many persons the opportunity to earn regular wages provides a route to a much higher standard of living. Better housing, environmental sanitation, wages, and medical care can result in improved nutritional status and lower prevalence of vector-borne disease in industrialized urban dwellers compared to residents of rural villages.

One type of development that has received considerable attention in recent years is the large engineering project intended to provide an infrastructural basis for further exploitation, commerce, and industrialization. Roads are certainly beneficial to health in helping to provide employment, markets, and access to facilities. In Liberia and Nigeria, however, new road networks have resulted in extension of sleeping sickness because tsetse flies concentrate wherever a road is intersected by a stream or river, extending local foci for transmission of the disease. In Brazil, the trans Amazon highway has brought workers and settlers into contact with new disease agents. Within the first two years after completion of sections of the road, a new disease syndrome called the *hemorrhagic syndrome of Altamira*, fatal in seven of the first 55 known cases, was encountered and raised fears of distribution along the new road. In some countries of sub-Saharan Africa, the AIDS virus is known to be disseminated by truck drivers who ply the few main highways and visit prostitutes in villages along the way. In a similar way, air travel has been incriminated by many epidemiologists in the transmission of the AIDS virus between nations and continents.

Dams and Health

Of all large-scale environmental engineering programs, major dams have had the most dramatic effects on health. Where the physiographic conditions permit and rainfall is abundant, impoundments provide large amounts of cheap, useful electric power. In addition, the dams serve in flood control and controlled distribution of water to irrigation networks on the downstream side. Upstream from the dam, the large impoundment of water can be used for fish production and recreation. This seems the best of all possible worlds, and there is little wonder that in the past few decades many large dams have been built in developing areas, especially in Africa.

The Akosombo Dam across the Volta River in Ghana was constructed in 1961–1964 primarily to provide electric power for an enormous aluminum smelting plant that opened in 1967. The filling of Lake Volta destroyed 739 villages, home to 14,657 households and about 80,000 persons, mostly subsistence farmers. Resettlement sites around the lake margin were inadequately planned and implemented, and the lake itself posed a severe health problem to surrounding residents. Schistosomiasis is a disease of humans caused by parasitic worms transmitted through certain aquatic snails. Prevalence in schoolchildren in some localities increased from 5% before the dam was built to 90% a few years after formation of the lake. At the same time, the prevalence of some other diseases may have been reduced. Small blackflies of the genus *Simulium* transmit the *Onchocerca* worms responsible for river blindness in vast areas of West Africa. These flies require fast-flowing water in stream rapids in order to breed, and the rising waters of Volta Lake above the dam flooded out the mainstream breeding sites. However, rapids in the stream below the dam, and in tributary rivers flowing into the lake, continue to produce blackflies. Flooding of the land adjacent to the old Volta River bed has also reduced breeding of the tsetse flies that transmit African sleeping sickness. Some other diseases, such as malaria, which has been hyperendemic in Ghana for generations, continue much as before. However, the thousands of kilometers of new lake shoreline offer numerous places suitable for breeding of the mosquitoes that transmit malaria, filariasis, and various mosquito-borne viruses.

Massive dams have been constructed on other great rivers of Africa, such as Kariba, on the Zambezi, between Zimbabwe and Zambia; Kainji, on the Niger in Nigeria; and Aswan High Dam on the Nile in Egypt, with Lake Nasser extending southward into Sudan. For each of these, tens of thousands of people have been relocated, with numerous attendant problems. Both Kariba and Aswan have resulted in massive increases of schistosomiasis incidence, and the same may occur at Kainji. Large dams have recently been built, or are under construction or being designed for the following countries: Angola, Brazil, Cambodia, China, Colombia, Congo, Ghana, India, Iran, Côte d'Ivoire, Mozambique, Nigeria, Pakistan, Senegal, Surinam, Thailand, Turkey, Uganda, and Venezuela. Health aspects of these great irrigation works must be considered no less carefully than power, irrigation, flood control, and water supply.

It is not only in developing countries that dams have been associated with disease outbreaks. Construction of the great series of hydroelectric installations on rivers in the south-central and southeastern United States were often associated with rapid buildups of local populations of malaria-carrying *Anopheles* mosquitoes and subsequent epidemics of malaria.

Environmental Pollution

Pollution is difficult to define, but the term refers to substances in the environment detrimental to the quality of human or other life. One would not usually say, for example, that high natural concentrations of fluorides, selenium, or arsenic in subsurface waters constitute pollution. Yet the same concentrations of the same elements, resulting from human activities such as mining, well drilling, or industry, would be so considered by most people. It is important to recognize that environmental pollution is not a recent development and is not restricted to industrialized societies. The great majority of harm to human health arising from pollution probably occurs in the developing countries where fecal contamination of soil and water is the most important environmental health hazard. Another major hazard is smoke. Wood, coal, straw, or animal dung fires in dwelling places, whether for warmth, cooking, or insect repellancy, have since earliest times induced pulmonary symptoms in humans. High levels of pollutants such as particulates, aldehydes, and carbon monoxide are found in poor dwellings throughout the world. Diseases of the pulmonary tree, attributable to smoke air pollution, may be the most important causes of morbidity and mortality in the New Guinea highlands. This extreme smoke pollution, together with exposure to viral and bacterial pathogens, is correlated with high rates of pneumonia in exposed infants. Although residents of industrial countries are greatly concerned with air pollution in their cities, the greatest burden of mortality from air pollution lies elsewhere (Table 8-10).

The disposal of human wastes has always been a thorny problem, particularly in cities. Travelers often remarked on the fragrance of early European towns. In the late 13th century, for example, London Bridge had 138 houses on it, providing a ready means of waste disposal for the fortunate residents. Not so lucky were the passengers of open boats plying the river, who knew well the risks of "shooting the bridge." Five hundred years later the Thames was still foul, but in recent decades a significant effort has led to cleansing of the river. Until the introduction of the automobile, the many horses in the world's cities littered the streets with great volumes of manure, attracting flies and causing severe disposal problems.

Not only in remote caves and huts but also in the cities of Europe smoke pollution has been an ever-present companion. A smoke abatement law was passed by the British Parliament in 1273, and in 1307 a commission was appointed in London to investigate the burning of coal and to punish offenders "with great fines and upon the second offence to demolish their furnaces." The pioneer demographer John Graunt in 1662 attributed the shorter life of Londoners to "smoaks, stinks, and close air." With the advent of the Industrial Revolution, forests of chimneys and stacks emitted smoke and products of inefficient combustion as well as chlorine, ammonia, and methane into the air of 19th-century Europe. It is likely that the early decades of the present century marked the high point of smoke pollution, at least in London, with gradual improvement of air quality since that time despite several acute episodes of air pollution, notably in 1952 and 1962. Chronic air quality problems

Table 8-10. Estimated Global Annual Deaths From Indoor and Outdoor Air Pollution

	Indoor Exposures		Outdoor Exposures	
	Number	Percent	Number	Percent
Developing countries				
Rural	1,876,000	67	....	....
Urban	644,000	23	186,000	93
Developed countries				
Rural	28,000	1	...	...
Urban	252,000	9	14,000	7
Total	2,800,000	100	200,000	100

Source: Adapted from World Health Organization 1997b, Fig. 4.4.

plague many areas on all continents. As the number of large cities increases in developing countries and the use of automobiles skyrockets, the situation is bound to deteriorate further.

Environment and Resources

Mankind's use for the environment has generally been for the moment, with little thought about long-term consequences. In many regions of the world soils have been eroded and depleted, forests denuded, and oceans and lakes used as sinks for wastes. Yet never before has there been a claim on the environment of such magnitude as exists today, and this will certainly accelerate in coming years. The unprecedented population growth is coupled in some areas with rising incomes and consequently increased per capita demand for all sorts of goods, a demand that agriculture, industry, and technology combine to promote as well as to meet. As a result, natural systems are everywhere strained. For the first time there seems to some a real possibility that the earth's stabilizing mechanisms may be permanently damaged by the drain, and by the wastes, of production and consumption. Needed increases in agricultural production will, for example, be accompanied by much higher total levels of environmental pollution from fertilizers and pesticides.

There is also growing concern that the supply of specific resources may become exhausted in coming decades. It is often said that the United States, with 6% of the world's population, consumes some 30% to 40% of its resources. It is therefore impossible even with today's population for the entire world to live at American standards. Energy use per capita seems to be a good proxy for development. If we examine energy use data carefully we see (1) that there is an enormous variation among countries and (2) that some countries actually fall back in energy use per capita (Table 8-11).

The energy consumption of 1 American in 1994 was approximately equivalent to that of 2 Frenchmen, 5 Mexicans, 32 Indians, 48 Nigerians, or 279 residents of Nepal. Even if the world had a stable population, far-reaching realignments would be necessary in order to meet the growing demand for greater equity in the opportunity to share in its resources.

Ecological Transition

Some observers of the demographic and epidemiological transitions have coined the imprecise term *ecological transition* to indicate the major changes wrought by human populations to their environment. Concern over the growing human population is certainly not new, as Thomas Malthus can attest, but in recent decades much interest has condensed around the health–population–environment–technology tetrad. *Appropriate technology*, a mantra of the 1970s following the publication of *Small is Beautiful*,[52] proposed that technologies must harmonize with the social system in

Table 8-11. Energy Use *Per Capita*, in Kilograms of Oil Equivalent per Year, Selected Countries, 1980 and 1994

	Energy Use per Capita	
Area	1980	1994
Low-income economies	248	369
Mozambique	93	40
Ethiopia	17	22
Nepal	12	28
Bangladesh	32	64
Nigeria	139	162
Cambodia	60	52
Mongolia	1168	1058
India	137	248
Nicaragua	270	300
Pakistan	142	254
China	421	664
Albania	1145	341
Lower-middle-income economies	1632	1449
Egypt	371	600
Bolivia	320	373
Indonesia	169	366
Guatemala	209	210
Syria	614	997
Algeria	647	906
Paraguay	175	299
Lithuania	501	2030
Belarus	5379	2392
Peru	566	367
Lebanon	259	964
Botswana	1282	387
Venezuela	426	2816
Upper-middle-income economies	1282	1544
South Africa	2074	2146
Mexico	1464	1561
Brazil	595	718
Trinidad and Tobago	3570	5436

(*continued*)

Table 8-11. Energy Use *per Capita*, in Kilograms of Oil Equivalent per Year, Selected Countries, 1980 and 1994 (*continued*)

Area	Energy Use per Capita	
	1980	1994
Malaysia	692	1699
Chile	695	1012
Saudi Arabia	3787	4566
Greece	1656	2260
High-income economies	4644	5066
Korea, Republic of	1087	2982
Spain	1837	2458
United Kingdom	3572	3772
Australia	4792	5341
Canada	7854	7854
France	3539	4042
Singapore	2651	8103
United States	7908	7819
Japan	2972	3856
World	1419	1433
Low- and middle income	686	739
Sub-Saharan Africa	249	237
East Asia and Pacific	378	593
South Asia	123	222
Europe and Central Asia	3105	2647
Middle East and North Africa	825	1220
Latin America and Caribbean	888	960

Source: Compiled from World Bank (1997), Table 8.

which they are employed. Simple tools and processes, using labor-intensive approaches based on local materials and little fossil fuel-based energy, should be promoted in most developing countries. It has become a dogma in recent decades to disturb the environment as little as possible so as to leave as much as possible for others.

A product of this environmental concern was the *World Commission on Environment and Development*, established by the United Nations and chaired by Dr. Gro Harlem Brundtland of Norway, who is now the Director-General of the World Health Organization. Widely known as the Brundtland Commission, the panel issued a report in 1987 titled *Our Common Future*, but called by everyone "The Brundtland Report." The report contained analyses and recommendations about resources, population, food, energy, the environment, and economic development. It portrayed the global interrelations of social and environmental problems related to development. The commission concluded that "a new era of economic growth" can bring a better life to all people, rich or poor, and that this can be achieved through efficient modern technologies that lower costs, reduce waste, and minimize adverse effects on the environment. The report championed the concept of *sustainable development*, which it defined as "meeting the needs of the present generation without compromising the needs of future generations." As the WDR92 stated, the idea of sustaining the earth has proved a powerful metaphor in raising public awareness and focusing on the need for better environmental stewardship.

The Brundtland Report was a prelude to the *UN Conference on Environment and Development*, or the *"Earth Summit,"* held over 12 days in June 1992 in Rio de Janeiro, Brazil. With leaders from 173 nations in attendance, it was the largest intergovernmental meeting ever held, even bigger than Alma-Ata 14 years earlier. The goal of the Earth Summit was to reach a common agreement about policy concerning climate change, biodiversity, deforestation, protection of the seas, and various other social and economic issues on the environmental agenda. The main product of the Earth Summit was *Agenda 21*, 600 pages of recommendations to governments and businesses to help ensure that economic growth does not interfere with environmental quality. *Agenda 21*, which was not legally binding, was reminiscent of the Brundtland Report issued five years previously.

In an interview after the Rio conference,[53] Dr. Brundtland gave a baseline view of sustainable development:

> Alleviating poverty should be priority number one. Very little else will matter if more than 1 billion people continue to live in absolute destitution. Only by educating people and giving them a fair chance to break out of poverty can we hope to find a sustainable relationship between population and resources. Otherwise, we will be forced, by default, to continue overusing natural resources. This is what Indira Gandhi meant when she said that "poverty is the greatest polluter."

Questions are often asked about the potential role of public health programs as a contributor to overpopulation. Many people are concerned that child survival and public health programs, however benevolently conceived, paradoxically become threats to the environment when (and because) the children grow up, use resources, and have more children. Skeptics remain unconvinced of the counterintuitive notion that preventing the death of children today will in fact prevent the birth of others tomorrow, leading to an eventual reduction in population growth rates. This subject is rarely mentioned in professional journals, perhaps because it is difficult to gather objective data to demonstrate a cause and effect relationship rather than a *post hoc* phenomenon. Also, public health professonals are understandably reluctant to view their efforts as possibly counterproductive.

Maurice King of the University of Leeds has confronted this problem head on in a series of challenging articles, beginning with one in 1990 titled "Health Is a Sustainable State."[54] King said that reducing mortality is the motivation behind many health efforts, especially in developing countries, but immense suffering will result if mortality is reduced without a corresponding reduction in the birth rate. He cited (but did not invent) the term *demographic trap*, for the situation in which a population is unable to achieve the social and economic gains needed to reduce its birth rate and becomes "trapped" as its numbers reach an unsustainable state. The entrapment would occur in three phases:

> In the *first phase* expanding human demands are well within the sustainable yield or carrying capacity of their ecosystem; in the *second phase* human demands exceed the sustainable yield, but are still expanding as the biological reserves are consumed; and in the *third phase* human consumption is forcibly reduced as the ecosystem collapses. An essential feature of a demographic transition is that it *is* a transition. The unstable second stage must be completed quickly, otherwise the population will enter the demographic trap—if the birth rate does not fall, the death rate will ultimately rise again, so the population is stuck in the trap and finds itself in an unstable state with a high birth rate and death rate, with ever increasing pressure on its resources, and with a rapidly deteriorating environment. Whether a population gets trapped depends on its rate of growth, and on the ability of the local environment to support that growth. The possible outcomes are limited: the population can: (a) die from starvation and disease; (b) flee as ecological migrants; (c) be destroyed by war or genocide; or (d) be supported by food and other resources from elsewhere, first as emergency relief and then perhaps indefinitely.[55]

From a review of the literature King concluded: "the view that if the child death rate declines sufficiently, the birth rate must decline also, and that there is a causal relation between them, is untenable . . . to the argument that the most effective way to bring down the birth rate is to lower the child death rate, the tragic reply has to be that, even if this were true, there is no certainty that a community will not destroy its ecosystem first." The lesson for the industrialized north was clear, if painful: "a sustainable lifestyle means consumption control—intensive energy conservation, fewer unnecessary journeys, more public transport . . . warmer clothes, and colder rooms . . . much more recycling and a more environmentally friendly diet." For the developing countries it means vigorous promotion of family planning programs, which is standard environmentalist doctrine; but King went a step further and suggested a reduced emphasis on child survival. Of the entire paper, one sentence stirred the juices of many readers: "If no adequately sustaining complementary measures are possible, such desustaining measures as oral rehydration should not be introduced on a public health scale, since they increase the man-years of human misery, ultimately from starvation." Although he added, "However, the individual doctor must rehydrate his patient," he had grasped the tiger firmly by the tail. The reaction was swift and mostly hostile: a typical headline in the *Guardian* newspaper read, "Doctor says let sick children die."[56]

King proposed broadening the concept of health to include its ecological foundations and cited the Brundtland Commission's concern for sustainability. Remarking that "a healthy lifestyle must now encompass a sustainable lifestyle, in that to live healthily one must also live in a sustainable relationship to one's environment. Finally he proposed a program that he called HSE2100 (Health in a Sustainable Ecosystem for the year 2100), a clear reference to HFA2000. "WHO has been exclusively concerned with the health of the *people* of the world. The recognition that their health is dependent on the health of the planet means that WHO now has a shared concern for the health of the planet as a whole."

Most authors are convinced that irreversible environmental degradation can be avoided only by limiting the human population and that the key to population limitation is unhindered access to the fullest possible range of fertility regulation methods while respecting individual choice.

THE RUSH TO THE CITIES

National statistics for persons per square kilometer range from about one in Libya or Mauritania to almost 4500 in Singapore. Almost everywhere there is a strong tendency toward greater clumping of populations, so the proportion of people living in urban areas is increasing at a rate faster than the underlying national population growth. In 1950 just over one quarter of humanity lived in urban areas. The world's population living in cities more than doubled between 1950 and 1975. Of the total global population, 42% lived in urban areas in 1985; in the late 1990s more than half of all humans live in cities of 100,000 or more. The proportion of total population living in cities is increasing in most developing countries, in large part bcause of migration from the countryside, where birth rates are still higher.

The definition of *urban* is very slippery. In Iceland it is a locality of 200 or more;

in Scotland 1000; in Ireland 1500; in the United States 2500; in Zambia 5000; in Jordan, Malaysia, Portugal, or Switzerland, 10,000; and in Japan 50,000.

Urban death rates have historically exceeded those in the countryside, at least in Europe. John Graunt demonstrated this in England in the late 17th century. The difference there became more acute with the Industrial Revolution and consequent bad living conditions in cities and towns. Prior to about 1900, urban mortality was also higher than rural in Prussia, Finland, Sweden, France, and the United States. In the present century the difference in urban–rural mortality has vanished in these countries owing to changes in society and better general standards of living, particularly improvements in sanitation and hygiene. Differences in specific causes of death tend to be small, but in general cancer rates are higher in urban areas, especially in males, and most particularly in the case of lung cancer. Whether this relative increase is a result of cigarette smoking combined with breathing city air, or better diagnosis and reporting, is not known. Tuberculosis deaths have also tended to be higher in urban areas.

Throughout the world, the proportion of persons dependent for livelihood on agriculture is declining, and those depending on industry and services is increasing. In industrialized areas there is continuing absolute decline of agricultural population; in developing countries total population growth is so great that agricultural populations are still increasing, but at a far slower pace than the growth of industrial urban areas.

Not only are more people living in cities, but cities are growing larger, particularly in the tropics. London, the world's second largest city in 1950, will not even be ranked among the 25 largest in the year 2000. Cities are growing by becoming larger rather than more intensely populated. In fact, the average population density in major cities is said to have declined by more than half since 1900.

Table 8-12 shows the ten largest cities (urban agglomerations) in 1950 and 2010. Note that the tenth largest city in 2010 will be larger than the largest city in 1950. Only one city, Tokyo, is on both lists. No city in Europe will be among the ten (or even the 20) largest. Urban growth in many countries is characterized by great concentration in one or a few large metropolitan areas. The importance of the megacities is emphasized if it is realized that as recently as 1975, 73 of 104 developing countries had *total* populations of under 10 million.

The previous chapter listed many of the characteristics of poverty, which are shared by most urban dwellers in developing countries. The growth of squatter settlements has occurred in less desirable parts of the cities, especially around the urban margins. Sometimes referred to as *septic fringes* because of their poor or nonexistent sanitary facilites, these areas are known locally as *barrios* or *barriadas* in Spanish-speaking Latin America, *favelas* in Brazil, *bidonvilles* in North Africa, *bustees* in South Asia, as *shantytowns*, and by many other names. These communities are home to hundreds of millions. Unsafe and usanitary, they are typically

Table 8-12. The 10 Largest Urban Agglomerations, 1950 and 2010

City	Population, Millions	
	1950	2010
Tokyo	6.9	28.9
São Paulo		25.0
Bombay		21.7
Shanghai	5.3	17.4
Lagos		21.1
Mexico City		18.0
Beijing		18.0
Dhaka		17.6
Jakarta		17.2
New York	12.3	17.2
London	8.7	
Paris	5.4	
Moscow	5.4	
Essen, Germany	5.3	
Buenos Aires	5.0	
Chicago	4.9	
Calcutta	4.4	

Source: United Nations (1996) Table 54.

built on undesirable land such as desert (Karachi, Lima, Dakar), polluted industrial areas (Mexico City, São Paulo), tidal swamps (Recife, Manila), or steep hillsides (Rio de Janeiro, Caracas). These regions are subject to natural disasters exemplified by the frequent torrential rainstorms that sweep away entire neighborhoods in Rio de Janeiro with great loss of life. Up to two-thirds of the nominal population in some cities in developing countries are squatters. Worldwide, squatter settlements are growing at an annual rate many times that for the world population as a whole.

In industrialized countries, particularly the United States, a "flight to the suburbs" has left city centers more or less as commercial zones, with few inhabitants at night and on weekends. The pattern is the inverse of that in developing country cities, where the wealthier people live in the city and poor in the periphery. However, the process of "urban renewal" and gentrification is bringing "upscale" residents into formerly neglected districts in many American cities.

Urbanization is a manifestation of changing societies in which the relationships of individuals, families, and communities are enmeshed. These relationships and the values of all persons, except those in the most remote regions, are touched and altered. Many observers have listed factors that induce people to leave rural areas and migrate to cities. Subsistence in the countryside may be impossible because of over-farmed land diminishing in productivity or excessive division into small plots by distribution to many heirs. Rural laborers may be displaced by technological innovation, or changes in world commodity prices may lead to economic reversals. Wars, revolution, political agitation, ethnic or religious persecution, boredom, social ferment, weakening of traditions, and natural disaster all have had roles to play in the urban trend.

The great attractions of city life are the amenities so often lacking in rural areas: a stable and adequate wage structure; public services such as health centers, water, and electricity; social interactions; shopping; museums, culture, entertainment; and perhaps above all, schools and the opportunities for education and advancement of children. Actuality rarely lives up to hope and expectation since most migrants find themselves stuck in a life of poverty and bare subsistence. Yet it is very likely that the migrants, in the great majority, arrive with a realistic view of life in the city. Many had come to live for a limited time, before returning with their families; all have heard stories from friends or relatives who have preceded them on the urban trek. They stay for a variety of reasons but mostly because conditions in the city, however poor, are still better than those from which they fled.

Health problems encountered by migrants to cities are many. Psychological and emotional stress is often extreme. In places such as southern Africa, where adult males come in large numbers as wage laborers, alcholism, violent trauma, and sexually transmitted diseases are common. The breakdown of extended family life, important in many societies, causes severe strains. Where village life had been self-sufficient, traditional, and hierarchical, city life is based on cash exchange. Everything must be bought and paid for. Women may not be able to have a garden vegetable plot or keep a cow or goat for milk for the children. The clock becomes a dominant factor where jobs are concerned.

In many ways, migration to the city is like emigration to a foreign country. New divisions of labor develop within nuclear families as both parents, and often the children, adopt what are essentially foreign ways of life. Where regional or tribal dialects are common, as in Africa, India, Indonesia, and parts of Latin America, language may be a great problem, most often accompanied by racial or ethnic discrimination. Lack of education and ignorance of town ways make life difficult and expose migrants to ridicule and victimization. Nevertheless, social conconsciousness and community organization may be strong in squatter localities, easing the problems of dislocation.

If psychological conditions in urban squatter settlements are poor, the physical environment is at least equally hazardous. The squalor has been remarked on by many. The following description of an urban slum several square kilometers in size in Jakarta, Indonesia, might have been written about any of a hundred cities of Asia, Africa, or Latin America.

The survey was conducted in a crowded slum with an average population of 12,000 per km^2 . . . The soil consists of thick clay, and the small houses, most of which are made of bamboo or wood with earthen floors and roofs of palm leaves, are usually crowded together. An average house contains one or two small sleeping rooms, a kitchen and an open veranda. There are no roads in this area; foot-paths with open earthen drains on each side form the only connexion between the houses. There is no electricity or piped water supply. Water is obtained from wells or bought from water sellers and is usually grossly polluted . . . Insanitary outdoor latrines are built here and there for common use; most consist of a hole in the ground, usually unprotected from rain and open to flies. Others are built on stilts above a canal that runs along the border of the area. Water to wash the hands after defaecation is rarely available in these latrines. Children usually defaecate in the open drains along the footpaths, and fresh faecal deposits are frequent within or on the edge of the drains. Garbage usually is left in a hole in the ground, where it is burnt from time to time, or is thrown into the canal. In the rainy monsoon the area is sometimes flooded. People of a low socioeconomic class live here, mainly new settlers who have come to Djakarta from the rural areas to earn wages. The population is therefore transient. Malnutrition and kwashiorkor are often noted among the infants[57]

It is little wonder that the 66 infants who could be followed over the full two-year period of the Jakarta study experienced 409 diarrheal episodes, an average of more than six per infant. There were 30 recorded deaths among the 156 infants who started the study despite the fact that 60 infants (some of whom may also have died) moved out of the area before the study ended.

In the more mature areas of cities in developing countries, and in temperate zone cities in general, most urban dwellers live in circumstances far better than those described. Where environmental conditions are of a high standard, most of the contaminative diseases retreat to relative insignificance. Nevertheless, considerable variations in health status, as measured, for instance, by infant mortality, can occur between cities and even within single urban areas in industrialized countries (Table 7-5). Inner city neighborhoods, often old, decrepit, and bereft of their original inhabitants, have become slums. As expected, relocation of slum families to better housing results in reduction of fecally transmitted infection by reason of better water and sanitary facilities and of less opportunity for reinfection.

Despite the many hazards of urban life, the evidence suggests that at present overall mortality is lower in the cities than in the countryside. Figures are difficult to obtain and marginally reliable, but such statistics as are available from Egypt, Senegal, Brazil, India, and elsewhere substantiate this conclusion.

NOTES

1. 1. Keys (1979).
2. Bellagio Statement on Tobaco and Sustainable Development (1995).
3. Patel (1994).

4. Eaton (1968).
5. Eckholm (1985).
6. Oppenheimer *et al.* (1986).
7. Hughes and Hunter (1970).
8. Greenwood *et al.* (1987); Victoria *et al.* (1985).
9. Cruickshank (1976).
10. Gelfand (1976); Bassett *et al.* (1995a,b) for Harare cancer data.
11. Tanner (1968).
12. Brinkmann (1994).
13. Boulding (1970).
14. See for example any World Development Report or World Bank Atlas.
15. Disraeli (1845).
16. McKeown and Lowe (1974).
17. Stolnitz (1982).
18. At that time UNFPA stood for United Nations Fund for Population Activities. UNFPA is now the United Nations Population Fund.
19. The proportion of world population in the industrialized countries of Europe, North America, and Japan was about 33% in 1950, is about 20% in the mid-1990s, and will be about 15% by 2025. Sadik (1992)
20. Ehrlich (1968, 1971), Meadows (1974), Paddock (1967).
21. This may be a good time to review the four views described in Chapter 1.
22. Total Fertility Rate (TFR) refers to the mean number of children born per woman. Technically, the number of children ever born to a woman if she were to live to the end of her childbearing years and bear children at each age in accordance with prevailing age-specific fertility rates in that population group.
23. Robey *et al.* (1993).
24. Horiuchi (1992).
25. Lesthaeghe and Jolly (1994).
26. Freedman and Berelson (1976).
27. Potts (1997).
28. Bauman (1997).
29. Friedman (1987).
30. Adlakha and Banister (1995).
31. Notestein (1945).
32. Pan American Health Organization (1994).
33. Murray and Chen (1993).
34. Mosley (1994).
35. Hertz *et al.* (1994).
36. Feeney (1994).
37. Potts (1997).
38. Omran (1971, 1982). For further details consult the large chart in Omran's 1971 paper.
39. For example, Frenk *et al.* (1989, 1991).
40. DALY = disability-adjusted life-year. See Chapter 4. Data adapted from Schieber and Maeda (1997) Figures 3 and 4, p. 4.
41. Albala and Vio (1995).
42. Söderlund and Zwi (1995) and Odero *et al.* (1997).
43. Frenk *et al.* (1989).
44. Tulchinsky and Varavikova (1996). See also UNDP (1996).

45. Dr Peter Piot, from a UNAIDS press release at ⟨www.unaids.org

46. Wilkinson (1994).

47. Dall (1994).

48. Because of the gradual aging of the population and the long-term reduction in heart disease deaths, mortality from cancer as a proportion of all deaths in the United States increased from 17.5% in 1970 to 24% in 1993. (Kranczer, 1994).

49. Social Security Programs Throughout the World on the internet—at ⟨www.ssa.gov/statistics/ssptw97.html⟩ and updates.

50. Athough their focus was on urban Europe, conditions are at least equally bad for most current inhabitants of Third World cities.

51. Two useful one-volume references sources are: World Health Organization. (1997b) and World Resources 1998–99 (1998).

52. Schumacher (1973).

53. Winner (1993).

54. King (1990); see also King (1993), King and Elliott (1993), and others by the same authors.

55. *Ibid.*

56. *Lancet* editorial (1992).

57. Lie *et al.* (1966).

9

International Programs and Projects

NORTH–SOUTH INTERACTIONS

Previous chapters have shown how relations between the North (Europe and North America) and the South (the poorer parts of the world) changed fundamentally just after World War II. Explicit colonialism was replaced by a complex of affiliations whose interpretation depends mainly on one's political viewpoint. Some perceive a mere cosmetic swap of political imperialism for economic exploitation, under the guise of paternalistically controlled "development." Others foresee the decline of the North with a shift of power to the developing economies. Still others find alarming threats from overpopulation in the Third World, domination from multilateral corporations, or environmental Armageddon. What is clear is that the interactions have become immeasurably more complex as the nations of the North, individually, through the postwar multilateral agencies, and by other routes, have cultivated new forms of relationships with the emerging countries. Chapter 3 introduced the structures and relationships of the major organizations involved in international health. In this chapter we will concentrate on their programs in the field.

Programs of the Multilateral Agencies

The World Bank
Starting with Colombia in 1949 the bank carried out a series of comprehensive studies of prospects for economic development in many countries, establishing a principle of involvement in long-term development planning. During the 1950s and 60s its loans supported mainly classical "bricks and mortar" infrastructure development projects. In the early 1970s the bank undertook a searching evaluation of its potential role in direct financing of basic health services, including field research, and of

the cost-effectiveness of different health promotion systems. Its first loan in the area of health, nutrition, and population was made in 1970 for a family planning program in Jamaica. In 1974 the bank adopted a formal health policy: While it chose not to give specific large-scale support to health services *per se*, the World Bank did decide to "strengthen its awareness of the health consequences of the projects it supports, and of opportunities for improving health that are available under present patterns of lending."

Specifically, the bank planned to:

- Minimize any adverse side effects on health resulting from its lending operations in other sectors (such as projects for irrigation, drainage, land settlement, etc.)
- Make a number of key interventions necessary for improving the health of low-income groups (for example, projects involving water supply, sewerage, nutrition, family planning, sites and services for low-cost housing, and training of health personnel)
- Conduct field experiments to test selected elements of a reformed health promotion system within rural development, population, and sites and services projects[1]

In 1980 a new policy was announced, in which the bank agreed to lend money directly for health projects:

> Health projects will aim to strengthen the recipient countries' sectoral planning and budgeting capacity, and their primary health care systems. The projects will include such elements as development of the basic health infrastructure, training of community health workers and paraprofessional staff, strengthening of logistics and supply of essential drugs, promotion of proper nutrition, provision of maternal and child health care, including family planning, prevention and control of endemic and epidemic diseases, and development of management, supervision, and evaluation teams . . . Where proposals satisfy normal Bank criteria for lending, projects to manufacture drugs, health care equipment, and other supplies will also be considered.[2]

The bank's first loan to expand basic health services followed quickly, to Tunisia in 1981. During the period 1980–1985, a total of $606 million (U.S.) was loaned for projects involving health costs and financing, hospitals, pharmaceuticals, and nutrition. Most early projects had a strong rural primary health care focus, influenced by the Alma-Ata Conference and Declaration of 1978 which launched primary health care as the dominant theme in international health for a decade. These projects included human resource and physical facilities development and about 75% had integral family planning components. Bank lending in the Health, Nutrition and Population (HNP) sector increased rapidly in the 1985–1995 decade.

Total World Bank lending in the mid-1990s is about $20 billion per year, about $16 billion of which are International Bank of Reconstruction and Development (IBRD) loans and $6 billion are International Development Association (IDA) credits (see Chapter 3). In the 1996 fiscal year Health, Nutrition and Population accounted for 11% of bank lending, with $2.4 billion in new commitments and a total of $9.2 billion committed to 154 projects in 84 countries.[3] Near the end of the century about 22 new HNP projects are proposed annually, roughly one every ten working days. The largest recipient of IBRD/IDA funding is the People's Republic of China, while India receives the largest amount for the health sector.

Although it may be unique, the World Bank is still a bank. It is populated largely by economists, who have a natural interest in the economic aspects of development, including the health sector. As the practical dilemmas of providing primary health care to thousands of millions of people became more evident, the focus of attention gradually shifted from the social sphere to the hard questions of financing and organization of health systems. Many detailed studies published by the bank in the 1980s and early 1990s paved the way for its highly influential 1993 World Development Report (WDR), *Investing in Health*.[4] The thread of health sector reform will be followed further in Chapter 13.

In late 1997 HNP issued a new *Sector Strategy* paper of 97 pages with many tables, charts, and maps. The bank established three priorities for assistance to client countries:

- Improve the health, nutrition, and population outcomes of the poor, and protect the population from the impoverishing effects of illness, malnutrition, and high fertility
- Enhance the performance of health care systems by promoting equitable access to preventive and curative health, nutrition, and population services that are affordable, effective, well-managed, of good quality, and responsive to clients
- Secure sustainable health care financing by mobilizing adequate levels of resources, establishing broad-based risk pooling mechanisms, and maintaining effective control over public and private expenditure[5]

Following the philosophy of the 1993 WDR, client governments will be encouraged to address these three HNP priorities through decentralization, greater partnerships with nongovernmental providers, and a more direct public involvement in securing sustainable financing. Governments will also be encouraged to address often neglected areas that have an impact on health, nutrition, and population outcomes such as rural and urban development, other broad-based population and social policies, education, control of tobacco and alcohol abuse, food and agricultural policies, environment, water supply, sanitation, and transportation. The bank will continue its relations with WHO and other partners, building on previous collaborations such as the UNDP/World Bank/WHO Special Programme for Research and Training in

Tropical Diseases, the Onchocerciasis (River Blindness) Control Program in West Africa, and other international health, nutrition, and population initiatives.[6]

The IMF and Structural Adjustment

Few subjects in international health have been as contentious as the effects of structural adjustment programs (SAPs[7]) in poor countries. Everyone appears to have a strong opinion on the subject, innocence of economics notwithstanding.

The type of SAPs recommended (or imposed) by the World Bank and IMF began around 1980 after a number of countries in Africa, Latin America, and Asia experienced balance-of-payment problems. The underlying causes of the crisis are generally ascribed to the rapid rise in the price of petroleum during the early 1970s followed by a boom in the prices of other commodities around 1975. Many countries then increased their consumption and investment, borrowing large amounts of money from multilateral lenders and commercial banks. When oil prices increased again in 1979 a world recession occurred and world interest rates rose sharply. Governments that had borrowed heavily found themselves short of foreign exchange to buy imported goods for direct consumption and for investment in industry and agriculture. A full-blown "debt crisis" had arrived.

Sovereign governments cannot become bankrupt, and their assets and collateral cannot be seized by foreigners to satisfy debts. But governments can default on their obligations and cause extensive economic problems both within the country and in international markets. In the early 1980s it was recognized that the economic crisis was too widespread, deep, and prolonged to be reversed by demand reduction alone. By 1982 developing country debt had passed the $500 billion mark. That year, the announcement by Mexico that it would renounce its foreign debt came as a bombshell to the international financial community. Clearly, fundamental changes were required in the structure of the economy of many countries. The Bretton Woods agencies (Chapter 3) were designed (by people who remembered the worldwide economic chaos of the 1930s) to be international arbiters, helping to work out means for debtors to repay with a minimum of disruption. In accordance with its charter, the IMF swung into action to stabilize economies. It did this by rescheduling debt and providing short-term finance to restrain immediate balance-of-payment problems. Where additional money was needed the World Bank joined the IMF in providing structural adjustment loans (SALs), defined by the bank as "non-project lending to support programmes of policy and institutional change necessary to modify the structure of the economy so that it can maintain both its growth rate and the viability of balance of payments in the medium term."[8]

The IMF/IBRD loans are designed to help countries stabilize their economies, lower inflation, restore external balance, and survive a temporary economic crisis. To help assure that this happens, the lenders impose *conditionalities*, saying in effect, "We will help you reorganize your debt and reschedule payments on your loans, but in order to get our money we insist that you do certain things." Conditionalities are time-specific targets painstakingly negotiated between the IMF/IBRD and the borrowing government. The first condition is to increase economic efficiency by imposing discipline and austerity on the government's operations. Typical strategies are to:

- Decrease imports and increase exports
- Decrease consumption and increase production
- Increase the income of the rural sector and decrease rural/urban imbalance
- Decrease government expenditures and subsidies to inefficient businesses
- Increase tax rates and tax collections and reduce corruption
- Attain a more realistic foreign exchange rate

The decontrol of foreign exchange usually leads to significant devaluation of local currency. With less domestic consumption and reduced trade barriers and tariffs, more goods can be exported to pay for essential imports, at least in theory.

A second set of conditions concerns changing government institutions and policies, including privatization, by selling off or at least demanding greater efficiency in state-owned enterprises. Following Justice Louis Brandeis' famous observation that "Sunlight is the best disinfectant," the IMF can demand greater regulation and transparency in financial markets—an end to "crony capitalism" and old secretive ways of doing business. The private sector with its open competition is to take on more of the functions previously performed by the state.

The scale of the 1980s crisis was massive, and the bankers were very busy. On average, each year during 1980–1986, there were 47 countries with IMF programs and 48 that had received adjustment lending from the World Bank, a number which had risen to 59 by 1988.[9] A decade later the whole process was reignited starting with the crisis in east and southeast Asia.

The transition to a more sustainable economic structure is painful but expected to be beneficial in the long run. "The problem is that there are sectors of society where enduring present pain for future gain is not acceptable because present suffering cannot always be offset by future improvements."[10] Immediate consequences of mandated reforms were low or negative growth, increased unemployment, and reduced government services. An early target of reduced government expenditure was the social sector, including health and welfare services. Adverse effects of such changes on welfare and health, particularly of the poor, have been profoundly and frequently criticized, often on ideological grounds, by many who consider the bank to be the *bête noire* of the development world. In an editorial, the British medical journal *Lancet* observed that "The World Bank is an easy and satisfying target for those concerned with the effects of development aid on poor-to-middle income countries. It is almost a mandate among non-govermental organisations . . . to object to the Bank's policies in strong and uncompromising terms."[11] Critics contend that

IMF policies are just a means to protect international banks and continue the exploitation of the South by the North. Others, including very sober senior officials within the financial system itself, have called for a basic rethinking of the Bretton Woods organizations, arguing that they require "tune-up" and possible complete overhaul after more than 50 years of operation.

Structural adjustment and health

In the early 1990s, critics depicted the adverse health effects of the debt crisis and resultant SAPs in the poorest countries more or less in these terms:

- Structural adjustment policies are imposed mainly to help assure that interest payments continue to flow to foreign creditors. Austerity measures commonly include currency devaluation, the cancellation of subsidies for common consumer products, and cuts in public spending for social services including education, welfare, and health. Real expenditures on health declined by as much as 50% in many poor countries during the 1980s.
- The decline in personal income and increase in unemployment leads minimum and low wage earners and their dependents to experience further deterioration in nutritional and health status.
- Decreased income and increased unemployment cause many wage earners to abandon private fee-for-service health care and to be forced to utilize free or nearly free government health services of lesser quality.
- Lowered employment leads to reduced tax collections and even less revenue for social security, health services, and other government programs.
- Inflation and devaluation lower the value of local currency and increase the cost of imports. Health budgets, already under pressure, can now afford fewer pharmaceuticals, medical supplies, vehicles, gasoline, and all other imported items needed by the health service.
- To conserve the output of service units to the public as much as possible, and because health workers are likely to be paid, even at reduced salaries, government health programs will preferentially cut or eliminate maintenance, new construction, and other forms of investment.
- The double-edged pressure of increased demand and reduced capacity results in degradation of governmental health programs, expressed as decreased output of services, deterioration in quality, or both.[12]

It is not a simple matter to define cause and effect as complex economies change over time, and *post hoc* reasoning has been widespread (Table 9-1). Analysts can only speculate about what would have happened in the absence of the adjustment program. A detailed study of the direct effects of economic reforms on health was made by John Peabody, who found that government revenues and expenditures did fall, by design, during the early stages of SAPs, and that economic reforms did af-

Table 9-1. Eight Kinds of Public Expenditure Trends, Selected Countries, 1980–1991ª

Percentage Change in Total Public Expenditures							
Increase				Decrease			
Percentage Change in Health Expenditures				Percentage Change in Health Expenditures			
Increase		Decrease		Increase		Decrease	
p/c ↗	p/c ↘	p/c ↗	p/c ↘	p/c ↗	p/c ↘	p/c ↗	p/c ↘
1	2	3	4	5	6	7	8

Countries illustrating trends 1–8

1 None

2 None

3 Brazil, Mexico, Pakistan, Papua New Guinea, Philippines, Tunisia, Turkey

4 Cameroon, Kenya, Uruguay

5 Chile, Egypt, Mauritius, Costa Rica

6 Peru, Sierra Leone

7 Indonesia

8 Bolivia, El Salvador, Morocco, Sri Lanka

p/c ↗ = per capita increase in health expenditure. p/c ↘ = per capita decrease in health expenditure.

Source: Adapted from Peabody (1996). Table 1. Social Science and Medicine, vol. 43. Copyright 1996, with permission from Elsevier Science.

fect (and decrease) the quality of care in the short run. However, effects were complex and sometimes unexpected. *Per capita* expenditures on health were not always tied to increases or decreases in the health budget as a percentage of total national expenditures. Some effects were salutary. In Indonesia the abolition of subsidies for imported drugs stimulated the growth of a domestic pharmaceutical market. In Ecuador, when *per capita* Ministry of Health spending fell by more than half, the number of private clinics grew by 75% and physicians in the private sector by 147%. Reductions in food production may or may not be reflected in increased levels of malnutrition, as currency devaluations and increased production of crops raised incomes for farmers in many countries. Consider these two divergent views of the health effects of SAPs:

> "Belt tightening" has been a euphemism for a fundamental attack on the basic elements of social well-being. African countries undergoing an SAP have been reported to have experienced rising rates of ill-health and mortality in both the urban and the rural poor. Diseases that had reportedly been eliminated, such as yaws and yellow fever in Ghana, reappeared during the SAP period.[13]

> The basic measures—such as IMR, Child and Maternal Mortality (CMR and MMR, respectively) and mortality of common infectious childhood diseases—continued to de-

cline in adjusting and nonadjusting countries. Life expectancy, despite economic setbacks and attempts at reform, has continued to improve in developing countries whether SAPs were adopted or not. Many of the alarming reversals in IMR and disease prevalence seen in the early 1980s, such as Chile, have reversed. The bottom line is that such measures and even some process measures, such as immunization rates, improved in almost all countries, regardless of whether IMF/WB participaton in economic reform occurred.[14]

The 1980s have often been called the "lost decade" for development. In Latin America, per capita income declined by 7%, consumption by 6%, and investment by 4% between 1980 and 1990. Hyperinflation occurred in much of Latin America, reaching an average of 1500% in 1990. In sub-Saharan Africa per capita GNP fell nearly 10% during the same period, when foreign investment and prices for major agricultural exports declined by 50%.[15] However, the lost decade saw life expectancy increase from 63 to 67 years and infant mortality decline by a third in Latin America; even in sub-Saharan Africa life expectancy grew by five years and infant mortality fell by 20%. Several countries, such as Indonesia, achieved good economic growth and rising investment under their SAPs, and at least five sub-Saharan countries generated steady GDP growth.[16] Nevertheless, health indices clearly declined in some countries undergoing SAPs, and real harm did occur. An influential criticism of the harshest aspects of SAPs, published under the banner of UNICEF, added the term *adjustment with a human face* to the development lexicon.[17]

> While still accepting the need for adjustment, the "human face" strategy called for a range of policies directed towards the poor. These included more expansionary macro-policies ained at sustaining levels of production and employment; meso-policies designed to ensure a fairer share of incomes and resources; sectoral policies to support small-scale production, especially among small-scale farmers, the landless, urban informal workers and women; the restructuring of social expenditure towards basic needs provision; and special support programmes such as targeted food subsidies and public works employment.[18]

Over the years lessons were learned and policies adapted. In retrospect, the bank concedes that early SAPs paid insufficient attention to protecting the poor from the damaging effects of such programs, and it has even introduced a requirement that countries increase the proportion of government revenue allocated to health as a condition for receiving HNP project loans and sector-wide support programs.

Determined to prevent a repetition of the disastrous 1930s, the international community's management of the debt crisis required intense studies of the ways that governments function. The experience of fashioning similar conditionalities for one country after another highlighted the elements common to inefficient governments. As it turned out, the experience gained in the 1980s was key to a basic change in thinking about health services. The dilemma faced by the international agencies and governments around the world was how to organize the delivery of adequate health and social services in an austerity environment of reduced expenditures. The search for a solution gave rise to the era of *health sector reform*, described in detail in Chapter 13.

The World Health Organization

Over the years and particularly in the mid-1970s, the developing countries have become more united and vocal in their demands for a greater share of world resources and world decision making. The *group of 77* countries (now much larger) was responsible for enunciating the *New International Economic Order* in the United Nations and has carried its principles into all major international organizations, including the WHO. The programs mentioned, among many others, are attempts to narrow the health gap between rich and poor nations, but much more fundamental policy changes have been imposed on the WHO by its Third World members. A resolution[19] noted "with deep concern the increasing allocation of resources of the Organization towards establishment and administrative cost" and directed the Director-General to cut down on expenditures at headquarters, streamline the professional and administrative cadres, and phase out projects "which have outlived their utility." In addition, the resolution demanded that at least 60% of the 1980 budget be devoted to technical cooperation and provision of services. This challenge required the WHO to reduce its headquarters staff by 24% by 1981 in order to devote more resources to the field. Single words can make a great difference in official resolutions, and it is no accident that the term "technical cooperation" is used in a context that some years before might have seen "technical assistance." The then Director-General interpreted technical cooperation to mean:

> activities which have a high degree of social relevance for member states, in the sense that they are directed towards defined national health goals and that they will contribute significantly to the improvement of the health status of their populations through methods that they can apply now and at a cost they can afford now. These activities should conform to the aim of "developing national self-reliance in matters of health."

The tug-of-war for resources between the periphery (in the field) and the center (WHO headquarters and regional offices) has been the focus of continuing discussion over the decades.

Several major WHO programs date from the period in the mid-1970s just before the Alma-Ata conference and have continued to the present. Some worldwide WHO initiatives, such as the Expanded Programme on Immunization (EPI), have been described in Chapter 7. Others, such as the Special Programme for Research and Training in Tropical Diseases (TDR), sponsor and coordinate vital research on diseases that elicit little interest from the world's pharmaceutical industries.[20] Space does not permit a discussion of all of the important WHO initiatives. When Dr. Gro Harlem

Brundtland's term of office as Director-General began on July 16, 1998, all WHO programs were subject to evaluation, revision, and reorganization. That process is continuing at the time of writing of this book and will certainly lead to continued changes over several years. The best way to stay abreast of these developments is to check regularly with the WHO website.[21]

The Essential Drugs program

The Essential Drugs program is an example of the complex of significant WHO programs that have been in force since the 1970s. In 1977 the World Health Organization established an action program intended to specify some 200 to 500 "essential drugs," including vaccines, salts, nutrients, and vitamins, that would satisfy the baseline pharmaceutical needs of almost any population, with variations for diseases of local importance in different areas. The first *Model List of Essential Drugs* contained 205 items. In 1981, the Action Programme on Essential Drugs (DAP) was established to support countries in developing national policies for the rational use of drugs. The DAP seeks to ensure that "people are able to obtain the drugs they need at the lowest possible price; that these drugs are safe, effective, and of high quality; and that they are prescribed and used rationally."

Until 1998 there have been nine revisions to the Model List to take account of new drugs and methods and increasing antimicrobial resistance. Many developing countries have adopted model pharmacopoeias in order to save money on imported drugs and eliminate unnecessary and irrational combinations, such as mixtures of antibiotics and vitamins popular in some regions. A large literature has evolved from these experiences, emphasizing the wasteful aspects of inappropriate purchasing, poor management, quality control and security, unnecessary prescriptions, and poor patient compliance.

Firms that distribute medicines in LDCs also frequently deal in veterinary products, fertilizers, pesticides, chemicals, cosmetics, foods, soaps, and other classes of products extending into many aspects of daily life. These companies may also be associated with the production and especially with the marketing of all types of medical supplies and hospital and scientific equipment and apparatus.

One serious problem concerning the drug industry in developing countries is the enormous proliferation of products, brands, and trade names. In countries where a few hundred different drugs are really needed, thousands or tens of thousands of different pharmaceutical products are marketed, often with little regulation. At the same time, the majority of drugs marketed by transnational corporations are those developed for the health problems and marketing patterns of the much larger markets in wealthier countries. While many billions of dollars are spent on pharmaceutical research, the actual medicinal needs of the people in the developing countries (which together account for only 14% of world consumption) may not be properly represented. The United States alone, with 5% of the world's population, is said to consume more than twice the total amount of pharmaceuticals used by

75% of the world's population. At the same time developing countries often pay a premium for their drugs, and pharmaceutical companies often sponsor meetings and conferences and provide incentives to physicians to use expensive new products. Some countries, such as Pakistan, have attempted to promote the use of cheaper generic products by abolishing trade names, but such regulations are difficult to enforce and may lead to a thriving underground of smuggled branded drugs.

Counterfeit drugs are also a problem in both developed and developing countries. In one study done by the DAP, 53.4% of samples collected in Myanmar and 26.4% in Vietnam were "unregistered" and drugs imported through unauthorized channels were found in the markets. Some drugs were similar in color, packaging, and imprints to standard products.

Reactions to WHO programs

Intended to reinforce the goals of the WHO through special emphasis on the countries and people in greatest need, such programs contribute to primary health care by engaging the issues of service delivery, coverage, access, management information systems, logistics, and disease surveillance, which strengthen local health infrastructure. Moreover, many countries had determined their own goals (such as for immunization coverage) even before the establishment of the EPI. National campaigns serve to bring people into the system, and parents are usually very supportive. Nevertheless, these programs are not without the ubiquitous critics. Much of the criticism centers around the same issues involved in the selective versus comprehensive primary health care debate—that is, community participation and control (empowerment) as opposed to imposition from above. Even though efforts are made to include developing country researchers, some critics complain that support for biomedical research goes mainly to the wealthier countries. Sustainability and fostering dependence are perennial and possibly insoluble problems.

It is not the intention here to take sides in these arguments but to emphasize that such programs must satisfy many constituencies and are more complex and controversial than may appear at first sight. As mentioned previously, it is a relatively easy matter to consider the number of service units provided (e.g., immunization or ORT coverage rates) as measures of program success, but it is not so simple to determine their effect on the health of the target populations. After the campaigns have ended a great deal of surveillance and sophisticated epidemiology is needed to evaluate the degree of disease reduction actually achieved by the programs—which is the real bottom line.

Since the early 1950s, far-sighted officers of the WHO have realized that to concentrate efforts on specialized mass campaigns would yield only temporary results in improvement of health unless they were accompanied by effective permanent health services in the poor rural and urban areas of the world. There has been a slow but definite trend toward integration of special programs with basic health services and toward the assignment of higher priorities to the strengthening of primary care.

Resolutions passed by successive World Health Assemblies have progressively stressed primary care, and the number of WHO projects in all regions directly related to this field has increased enormously. Much attention has been devoted to innovative methods for meeting the health needs of the underprivileged 80% of the populations in developing countries.

As mentioned, the WHO was completely reorganized in 1998 so there is little point in citing critiques of its earlier structure and policies. One constant, however, is serious financial constraints. Dozens of member countries pay none, or very little, of their assessment, which has put a severe stress on operations, particularly in the high-cost environment of Geneva. Gifts of private benefactors (Chapter 3) can do little to relieve this situation.

The North–South bickering that cost UNESCO the membership of the United States and several other countries has been more restrained, although not absent, in the WHO. The infant formula controversy of the late 1970s led to the adoption in 1981 of an international code of marketing of breast-milk substitutes in which breast-feeding was strongly encouraged and various restrictions were recommended on the labeling and marketing of powdered formula. That action was taken by some as the opening salvo of a war against multinational pharmaceutical companies, a perceived threat made more real by adoption by the WHO of its essential drugs program, which recommended reductions in number and kinds of drugs marketed in developing countries. Other decisions by UN agencies, such as the advocacy by UNIDO of revisions in trademark and patent laws, have added to the anxiety of some enterprise interests in industrialized countries.

Over the years ideas about international health programs have changed in concert with developing perceptions. These changes, which come about through a complex of reasons, pervade the thinking of policy planners and decision-makers in donor agencies, universities, NGOs, and the major intergovernmental organizations. Although ostensibly distinct and separate, these major players are linked into an invisible mega-agency by liaison committees, informal personal connections, international meetings and conferences, and by personnel who may transfer between them or may be assigned or seconded from one to another. The intergovernmental organizations can translate the thinking of the moment into resolutions and action programs, often signed and adopted by large numbers of member countries. For their own reasons, countries may adopt current programs and make appropriate adaptations in structure or emphasis within their ministries, but may not necessarily make fundamental changes in their thinking.

In the decade of the 1960s organized family planning programs were being promoted in a big way, but their often-limited success reduced enthusiasm in some quarters. At the same time disease control efforts were usually channeled through "vertical" programs with specific targets, such as malaria or smallpox (see Table 3-1). More clinically oriented aid programs were generally institution-based, usually in hospitals, but emphasis on basic health services by WHO, UNICEF, the

World Bank, and other major players led to a shift to more community-based programs in the early 1970s. Emphasis was put on basic health services and the integration of formerly independent vertical programs became the popular model. With Alma-Ata these gave way to the HFA and PHC programs.

In the middle 1980s it appeared that interest in PHC programs was waning in some quarters, and a renewed interest in vertical programs was exemplified by the "Child Survival" and "Safe Motherhood" initiatives which acquired widespread agency, professional, and institutional support.

Bilateral Assistance ("Foreign Aid")

In the past, colonial countries provided some health services to their colonies, but these were primarily extensions of domestic programs into their overseas empires to take care of their expatriates living abroad. The idea of official development assistance (ODA or "foreign aid") other than to colonies or former colonies is very much a latter 20th-century phenomenon which became institutionalized in the decades following World War II.

The official aid agencies of the Development Assistance Committee (DAC) of the OECD were mentioned in Chapter 3. It is important to understand that these agencies are not charities and do not necessarily give their money to those in greatest need. Although practices vary among DAC governments, all fulfill some specific policy goal through the provision of development and humanitarian aid.

The approach adopted by both donor and recipient countries beginning in the 1950s and 1960s concentrated the investment of scarce resources into agriculture and industry. Local people and local societies, the intended beneficiaries, were not involved in the process and were put into a passive position. Social problems such as disparities among classes, gender issues, or urban/rural differences were essentially ignored by developers, with negative effects on the effectiveness and sustainability of national development. During the mid-1960s to the 1970s almost all developing countries achieved some economic growth, either gradually or, in some cases, decisively. After the oil crises and falling primary commodity prices of the 1970s, developing countries became more divergent economically.

During this same period donors realized that social justice and economic growth should be targeted simultaneously in order to have long-term stability in the developing world. Multilateral agencies and bilateral donors began to speak of basic human needs (BHN) such as education, health care, sanitation, nutrition, housing, and job creation, which until then had been neglected in aid programs. The Alma-Ata conference of 1978 was a good example of the new emphasis on promoting rural development through community participation. For any hope of sustainability, the active participation of beneficiaries was needed in planning and implementation of rural development, family planning and public health, education, income boosting, and housing projects.

Over the decades, development strategy has shifted. The peak of the "foreign aid industry" was reached in 1992, when $60.9 billion was transferred as development aid. Since then, funds for development assistance have declined. "Donor fatigue" has set in, and even the stalwart Scandinavians have cut back on ODA. Meanwhile, Japan has become a prominent donor (Table 9-3). There is mounting skepticism about whether the assistance is truly helping and a growing conservative opinion that improvement of economic and social conditions "here at home" should take precedence over assistance to other countries. One of the reasons for dissatisfaction with development projects is their frequently short time schedule:

> In order to satisfy domestic political agendas, bilateral donors need to be able to show results within poitically meaningful time periods, commonly those between the election of national leaders. But real changes in infant mortality or rates of disease transmission bear no necessary relationship to presidential or parliamentary election schedules . . . Given the political presures, donors keep funding cycles short to allow for rapid response to changing political needs.[22]

Another factor in erosion of support for foreign aid is the flow of private capital as access to global markets ties all nations into a commercial meshwork. The *quid pro quo* for the money sent from north to south has changed from geopolitical advantage to financial profit. To some this is seen as merely another way to exploit poor people; others argue that investments are more efective than aid in stimulating long-term economic growth, creating jobs, and reducing poverty.

At the same time the demand has grown with new claimants for international aid, such as the newly independent states of the former Soviet Union. More and more issues, such as mounting concern for environmental protection, reproductive rights, and other causes find their way onto the aid agenda. Against this background, aid donors have come to demand that their increasingly limited resources be used more effectively and efficiently to help developing nations to develop. Increasing scrutiny has been focused on the aid-absorbing capacity of developing countries—that is, whether they are capable of using aid effectively and equitably to benefit the people most in need of aid.

In December 1989, the DAC released a *Policy Statement on Development Cooperation in the 1990s* which cited sustainable development, concern for the environment, and participatory development as the most important issues on the development aid agenda for the decade. The report states that stimulating productive energies of people, encouraging their broader participation, and a more equitable sharing of benefits must become more central in development strategies and development cooperation. Policy principles are:

- Investment in human resources in the broad sense, including education and training, meeting the needs for food and health care, and efforts to eradicate AIDS and narcotics problems

- Strengthening of political systems, government mechanisms, and legal systems in which democracy and respect of human rights are secured
- Effective use not only of central governments, but also of local organizations and self-government, nongovernmental organizations (NGOs), and the private sector
- The establishment of open and competitive market economy structures to mobilize individual initiative and dynamic private enterprise

In addition to "providing humanitarian assistance and aiding postcrisis transitions," official U.S. policy toward sustainable development assistance similarly includes four interrelated and mutually reinforcing areas:

- *Encouraging broad-based economic growth* to strengthen access to markets; expand opportunities for women, the poor, and minorities; and invest in people through improved education and health
- *Protecting the environment* by addressing the root causes of environmental harm, promoting environmentally sound patterns of growth, and supporting improved management of environmental resources including long-term threats such as climate change and loss of biological diversity
- *Building democracy* by promoting a climate of respect for human rights, peaceful competition for political power, free and fair elections, respect for the rule of law, accountable government, and an environment that encourages participation.
- *Stabilizing world population* by helping to reduce excessive population growth rates through voluntary family planning, reproductive health care, and other directly related activities.

The primary vehicle to carry out these policies is the *U.S. Agency for International Development (USAID, or simply AID)*, self-described as "an independent federal government agency that conducts foreign assistance and humanitarian aid to advance the political and economic interest of the United States."[23]

AID's health policy is based on directives contained in the Foreign Assistance Act of 1961, as amended. This legislation directs AID to emphasize cooperation with developing countries in designing and implementing basic health care delivery systems, selective disease prevention and control, adequate drinking water and sanitation systems, and related health planning and research. In their 1986 health policy paper, the stated goal of USAID's health assistance program was "to improve health status in AID-assisted countries as reflected in increased life expectancy" with an emphasis on children and mothers.

Hundreds of millions of adults suffer from chronic illness, but children are the most vulnerable group. Half of all deaths in developing countries occur in the age group of five and under. The most direct way to increase life expectancy in developing countries is by addressing the health problems of children and their mothers. Thus, within A.I.D.'s health assistance program priority will be given to support for child survival and improved maternal and child health.[24]

A decade later, USAID's goals in the population, health, and nutrition sector were similar:

to stabilize world population growth and to protect human health. In order to achieve these goals, the Agency has adopted a strategy based on four strategic objectives: reducing unintended pregnancies; reducing maternal mortality; reducing infant and child mortality; and reducing STD transmission with a focus on HIV/AIDS. These are a refinement of the historical strategic direction of the Population, Health and Nutrition sector. Looking to the future, the PHN strategy also incorporates principles from the Cairo Program of Action and reflects Agency mandates in the areas of women's empowerment. The PHN program focus, therefore, is on improving the quality, availability, and use of key family planning, reproductive health, and other health interventions in the PHN sector, with sustainability and program integration as essential crosscutting themes.

To carry out these functions, the agency provided approximately $9.7 billion in PHN assistance to developing countries from 1985 to 1996, making it the largest international donor in this sector in the world. In fiscal 1996, obligations in the sector totaled approximately $916 million, of which $356 million[25] went to population activities. The ups and downs of U.S. government support for worldwide population assistance are shown in Table 9-2.

Table 9-2. Appropriations[a] to USAID for Population Assistance, 1977–1998

Fiscal Year	Total ($000)	Fiscal Year	Total($000)
1977	144,346	1988	248,066
1978	166,540	1989	257,578
1979	191,435	1990	287,128
1980	194,975	1991	353,789
1981	208,405	1992	325,643
1982	237,750	1993	447,848
1983	243,077	1994	480,172
1984	264,236	1995	541,644
1985	317,704	1996	356,000
1986	295,548	1997	385,000
1987	286,604	1998	385,000

[a] All accounts.

Source: USAID Office of Population.

The structure of USAID, reminiscent of that of the World Bank, includes geography-based bureaus and subject-based centers. The Global Bureau and four Regional Bureaus provide technical and programmatic expertise to programs in Asia, Africa, Latin America/Caribbean, and Europe/NIS.[26] The PHN Center comprises the Office of Population and the Office of Health and Nutrition, with appropriate field and program support.

The Office of Population

- Provides a centralized system for contraceptive procurement and mangement
- Raises awareness, acceptability, and use of family planning methods and improves the managerial and technical skills of family planning and health personnel
- Expands the availability and quality of family planning and related services by strengthening government programs, local private voluntary organizations, for-profit organizations, and commercial channels
- Promotes demographic research and data collection, policy concerning population, family planning, and other reproductive health programs; strategic planning; and program evaluation
- Supports biomedical research to increase understanding of contraceptive methods and to develop new fertility regulation technologies; works to improve the delivery of family planning and reproductive health services

The Office of Health and Nutrition

- Provides technical assistance, helps develop strategies, and supports programs to reduce child morbidity and to improve infant and child nutrition, child survival, and women's health, especially maternal health
- Assists in the design, implementation, research, and evaluation of health and nutrition policy reform, management and financing issues, including health care financing, quality assurance, pharmaceuticals, private sector and data activities
- Helps to design, implement, and evaluate environmental health activities and issues, including water and sanitation, hazardous wastes, vector-borne tropical diseases, food hygiene, solid waste, air pollution, and occupational health
- Provides technical guidance and supports strategy development, program design, and implementation of HIV/AIDS control activities worldwide

Table 9-3 compares total Official Development Assistance flows from DAC member countries. Table 9-4 shows ODA commitments related to health from DAC members and from some multilateral agencies to the countries on the UN "least de-

Table 9-3. Official Development Assistance by DAC Member Countries, 1994–1995

	Total ($ Million)	Percent of GNP	Percent of All OECD ODA	Average Change 1989/90–1994/95
Australia	1194	0.36	1.9	+2.5
Austria	767	0.33	1.2	+9.3
Belgium	1034	0.38	1.5	−3.9
Canada	2067	0.38	3.7	−0.6
Denmark	1623	0.96	2.6	+3.4
Finland	388	0.32	0.6	−14.5
France	8443	0.55	14.3	+0.9
Germany	7524	0.31	0.1	−0.9
Ireland	153	0.29	0.2	+17.4
Italy	1623	0.15	3.7	−9.7
Japan	14,489	0.28	23.4	+0.2
Luxembourg	65	0.36	0.1	+14.4
Netherlands	3226	0.81	4.9	−0.8
New Zealand	123	0.23	0.2	+2.7
Norway	1244	0.87	2.0	+1.1
Portugal	271	0.27	0.5	+8.3
Spain	1348	0.24	2.2	+10.1
Sweden	1704	0.77	3.0	−1.8
Switzerland	1 084	0.34	1.7	+3.0
United Kingdom	3 157	0.28	5.4	+1.8
United States	7 367	0.10	14.6	−4.4
Total DAC	58 894	0.27	100.0	−0.9

Source: OECD website.

veloped" list and to all developing countries. The complexities of international book-keeping and the natural interrelations of such programs make these categories difficult to compare among various donor and recipient countries. However, an analysis of multilateral, bilateral, and nongovernmental external assistance to the health sector (including population) in 1990 shows that:

- Health external asistance totalled $4800 million, of which 82% originated from public sources in developed countries, and 18% from private households.
- 40% of the flow was through bilateral development agencies, 33% through UN agencies (mainly WHO, UNICEF, UNFPA), 8% through the World Bank and regional deveopment banks, 17% through NGOs, and 1.5% through foundations.
- Of total external assistance, 8.8% went to the health sector.

- External assistance accounted for 2.8% of the $170,000 million total health expenditures in the developing world.
- External assistance accounted for 10% of all health expenditures in Africa and 20% in sub-Saharan Africa (excluding South Africa).
- Africa received the largest share of donor support (38.5%), which came to $2.45 per person. China received the smallest share (6% and $0.07).
- External assistance for population was $936 million, or almost 20% of all health sector expenditures.[27]

World Bank data for 1994 for external assistance by region are shown in Table 9-5.

ODA programs have met with frequent criticism from both sides, and their effectiveness has often been less than optimal. Since the end of the Cold War, donor countries have come to demand that development aid be more effectively and efficiently implemented and have begun to seek new aid strategies to replace that based on East–West ideological conflict.

Criticism on the donor side (especially by the public) emphasizes inefficiency, corruption, excessive dependence, and ingratitude on the part of the beneficiaries. The recipient side may claim donor-country hypocrisy, excessive self-interest, export dumping and restrictive purchase agreements, exploitation, arrogance, and neo-colonialism. As experience has accumulated, the solution most commonly proposed has been to increase the channeling of aid through multilateral, regional, or global institutions rather than simple country-to-country agreements. This step, it is asserted, would reduce many of the tensions and obligations implicit in bilateral arrangements, distribute aid on the basis of need rather than political loyalty, and make assistance contingent on policy reforms backed by world opinion. While this may be so, multilateralization introduces into the ODA picture at least a third bureaucracy and consequent administrative expense and delay, and it blurs the special relationships and specific mutual interests of the parties concerned. For this reason many governmental bodies have pondered the correct posture for governments in relation to development assistance. A generation ago a U.S. presidential task force on international development suggested that "a predominantly bilateral U.S. program is no longer politically tenable in our relations with many developing countries, nor is it advisable in view of what other countries are doing in international development."[28]

The term ODA embraces work in agriculture, industry, energy, transport, education, infrastructure (roads, water supplies, etc.), health, and other sectors. Within the health field ODA is generally spent for capital construction of facilities; manpower and institutional development (including fellowships); "vertical" programs such as malaria control; maternal and child health and nutrition; or family planning.

Within the U.S. government, support for international health programs directed through multilateral channels is the primary responsibility of the Bureau of Inter-

Table 9-4. Bilateral Official Development Assistance Commitments Related to Health, by Recipient Country Groupings and Purpose[a] 1991, 1993, 1995

Aid Recipient Country Groupings (Population in Millions) and Purpose	Commitments, Millions U.S.$, by Year		
	1991	1993	1995
Least developed countries (587)			
Education	332	395	488
Health	251	275	445
Water supply and sanitation	328	377	289
Food Aid	1,186	588	796
Total	7,160	6 599	7,555
Other low-income countries (2787)			
Education	391	728	941
Health	136	324	418
Water supply and sanitation	733	885	1,023
Food aid	528	373	257
Total	19,516	12,820	15,890
Lower-middle-income countries (715)			
Education	467	745	672
Health	158	249	347
Water supply and sanitation	416	1,175	863
Food aid	800	715	358
Total	12,092	11,910	11,174
Upper-middle-income countries (412)			
Education	41	273	206
Health	37	157	146
Water supply and sanitation	66	73	210
Food aid	35	40	5
Total	1,674	1,999	1,706
High-income countries (42)			
Education	6	62	118
Health	0.5	2	1.3
Water supply and sanitation	0.1	0.1	0.1
Food aid	10.	0.4	0
Total	3,842	2,648	1,401

(continued)

314

Table 9-4. Bilateral Official Development Assistance Commitments Related to Health, by Recipient Country Groupings and Purpose[a] 1991, 1993, 1995 (*continued*)

Aid Recipient Country Groupings (Population in Millions) and Purpose	Commitments, Millions U.S.$, by Year		
	1991	1993	1995
Developing countries total (4574)			
Education	1,472	2,747	3,056
Health	652	1,095	1,884
Water supply and sanitation	1,550	2,539	2,409
Food aid	2,974	1,951	1,511
Total	45,905	39,354	42,180
Africa north of Sahara[b] (127)			
Education	56	94	59
Health	12	54	83
Water supply and sanitation	313	295	361
Food aid	361	57	76
Total	8,849	4,320	2,985
Africa south of sahara[c] (589)			
Education	444	458	486
Health	265	317	462
Water supply and sanitation	412	435	486
Food aid	1,051	532	649
Total	8,627	7,926	8,168
North and Central America[d] (156)			
Education	116	130	88
Health	66	116	171
Water supply and sanitation	45	90	206
Food aid	521	214	83
Total	2,695	1,992	2,167
South America (321)			
Education	57	184	108
Health	70	123	197
Water supply and sanitation	168	75	265
Food aid	213	137	93
Total	2,406	2,367	2,524

(*continued*)

Table 9-4. Bilateral Official Development Assistance Commitments Related to Health, by Recipient Country Groupings and Purpose[a] 1991, 1993, 1995 (*continued*)

Aid Recipient Country Groupings (Population in Millions) and Purpose	Commitments, Millions U.S.$, by Year		
	1991	1993	1995
Middle east[e] *(157)*			
Education	17	145	162
Health	16	38	39
Water supply and sanitation	17	75	126
Food Aid	60	71	24
Total	5,992	3,542	2,881
South and Central Asia[f] *(1381)*			
Education	134	148	186
Health	109	66	164
Water supply and sanitation	114	165	308
Food aid	295	547	374
Total	4,773	3,982	5,293
East Asia[g] *(1 732)*			
Education	379	937	1,208
Health	57	285	217
Water supply and sanitation	324	882	561
Food aid	94	68	61
Total	8903	10,364	12,a540
Central and Eastern European Countries and Newly Independent States of former USSR[h] *(391)*			
Education	22	56	343
Health	7	14	80
Water supply and sanitation	0	0	30
Food aid	4	1 368	212
Total	510	2,321	6,368

[a]Purpose: *Education:* educational infrastructure, services, and investment in all areas except specialized education in special sectors such as agriculture or energy reported separately. *Health:* assistance to hospitals and clinics, including specialized institutions such as those for tuberculosis, maternal and child care; other medical and dental services, including disease and epidemic control; vaccination programs; nursing; provision of drugs; health demonstration, public health administration, and medical insurance programs. *Water supply and sanitation:* all assistance given for water supply, use, and sanitation, but excluding irrigation systems for agriculture. *Food aid:* supplies of food under bilateral programs, including food aid for emergency needs. *Total:* All ODA commitments for social

(continued)

national Organization Affairs of the Department of State; those through bilateral channels, of the Agency for International Development. Certain research programs are carried out by the Fogarty International Center for Advanced Study in the Health Sciences at the National Institutes of Health, by the Comparative Studies staff of the Office of Research and Statistics of the Social Security Administration (both agencies of the Department of Health and Human Services), and by other units.

Nongovernmental and Private Voluntary Organizations

The types of nongovernmental organizations were described in Chapter 3. Some disaster and refugee relief activities and a *code of conduct* were described in Chapter 7. The roughly 3000 northern NGOs (NNGOs, based in the industrialized coun-

Table 9-5. External Assistance for Health Costs, By Region, circa 1990[a]

Region	External Assistance as Percentage of per Capita Health Expenditure
East Asia and the Pacific (excluding China)	3.7
China	0.5
Latin America and the Caribbean	3.6
Middle East and North Africa	1.5
South Asia (excluding India)	13.1
India	0.7
Sub-Saharan Africa	16.4

[a]Note: Regional data are country-weighted averages. Not enough data were available for Europe and Central Asia to prepare an estimate.

Source: Schieber and Maeda (1997) Table 3.

infrastructure and services (education, health, water shown here) and program assistance (food aid shown). Not on this table are economic infrastructure and services (energy, transport, and communications); production sectors (agriculture, industry, trade & tourism); multisector; action relating to debt; emergency assistance; and unallocated.

[b]Algeria, Egypt, Libya, Morocco, Tunisia.

[c]All other countries and territories in Africa.

[d]Mexico and all countries of Central America and the Caribbean.

[e]Bahrain, Iran, Iraq, Israel, Jordan, Kuwait, Lebanon, Oman, Palestinian Administered areas, Qatar, Saudi Arabia, Syria, United Arab Emirates, Yemen.

[f]Afghanistan, Armenia, Azerbaijan, Bangladesh, Bhutan, Georgia, India, Kazakhstan, Kyrgyz Republic, Maldives, Myanmar, Nepal, Pakistan, Sri Lanka, Tajikistan, Turkmenistan, Uzbekistan.

[g]Brunei, Cambodia, China, Chinese Taipei (= Taiwan), Hong Kong, Indonesia, Korea North, Korea South, Laos, Macao, Malaysia, Mongolia, Philippines, Singapore, Thailand, Timor, Vietnam.

[h]Belarus, Bulgaria, Czech Republic, Estonia, Hungary, Latvia, Lithuania, Moldova, Poland, Romania, Russia, Slovak Republic, Ukraine. See note f for other former Soviet republics, which are also listed individually in the source.

Source: Compiled from OECD, 1997. Geographical Distribution of Financial Flows to Aid Recipients, pages 216 to 248. See original for more details.

tries) and 30,000 to 50,000 southern NGOs (SNGOs, based in the developing countries) together with hundreds of thousands of local grassroots organizations are said to reach about 250 million people. Regardless of their overall mission, the work of most NGOs is organized into discrete projects.[29]

Without question, many NGOs have provided selfless, valuable assistance in both community development and disaster relief situations. Much of the public on both donor and recipient sides has more faith in NGOs than in official agencies, which are frequently viewed as corrupt, inefficient, or at least suspect. NGO workers are seen to have higher standards, a greater sense of mission, and to be less self-serving than goverment officials and bureaucrats. But objective studies and evaluations of NGOs are rare. The French-based organizations *Médecins sans Frontières* (Doctors Without Borders) and *Médecins du Monde* (Doctors of the World) have been closely reviewed, with general approval, from their small-scale origins until they "have grown in size, scale, range of activities, numbers of projects undertaken, theatres of operation, staff and vounter personnel, budget and financial resources, matériel and logistical capacities, means of print and electronic communication, public saliency and support, and in the complexity of their organizations."[30]

A survey of the role played by health-related NGOs in southern Africa concluded that their presumed comparative advantage must be analyzed closely. It is not clear that NGOs are more efficient or effective than the public sector on one hand and the private for-profit sector on the other.[31] Mburu[32] has made many pithy comments, pro and con, about NGOs in the health field in Africa:

- The developing world is littered with policy statements never translated into action, while failed and aborted projects are common. Sometimes one finds projects isolated from any known policies; implementors own such projects in close collaboration with public officials who enjoy personal gain for the lifetime of the project.
- With the advent of PHC virtually all agencies and professional groups consider themselves competent to proffer advocacy for change and to demonstrate how to provide selected health services . . . It is for this reason that so many NGOs are involved in health, bringing in their wake textbook notions of change.
- The best hospitals in many countries in Africa are Christian mission hospitals. They have well-trained permanent staff. They often have drugs which make medical care a reality, in contrast to government hospitals which are probably notorious for neglect, shortage of supplies and a consistently disheartened staff.
- Common health goals notwithstanding, the established, older medical professionals have felt under attack from the proliferation of NGO health projects outside the control of the Ministry of Health.

- The vast number of NGOs . . . neither have bureaucracies of their own nor work according to bureaucratic rules. They are flexible and in most situations able to respond rapidly to needs as they arise.
- Uncertain funding sources contribute to shaky NGO projects which are of short duration, locally disruptive and often unsustainable. Resources come quickly, are rapidly invested and often rapidly fizzle out.
- While NGOs have a powerful advocacy voice, a common complaint is that they are quick with the tongue, fast on foot but mean with the wallet.
- It is common for donors to employ their own nationals however ill-prepared their personnel might be . . . NGOs therefore follow conventional wisdom being seen as channels for repatriating the little foreign exchange they are supposed to leave behind.
- Anti-establishment as the NGOs are, they are in many ways the inadvertent vehicles of imperialism.

The diverse NNGOs are mostly non-profit-making and are funded from a variety of sources. Most of the smaller ones obtain their money from appeals to the public. The religion-based NGOs have their clear constituencies, and secular organizations use a variety of channels to solicit funds. Some NGOs generate income from sale of products or services. Many of the big international ones (BINGOs) receive contracts from their home government development agencies to carry out particular projects, often but not always for humanitarian relief. By the mid-1990s, NGOs were reported to have displaced governments as the primary recipients and conduits of aid for humanitarian relief and emergency assistance. Such contracting to NGOs facilitates work in the field where the funding agency lacks experience, personnel, and equipment; permits a more rapid, flexible, and informal response; circumvents inefficient and corrupt government bureaucracies; "sanitizes" the operation by displaying the NGO, rather than the sponsoring government, to recipients; and presents a more acceptable face to maintain support from the public of donor countries. At their best, committed NGOs can deliver imaginative, appropriate, and meaningful humanitarian assistance. It is estimated that about one-third of rich-country development financing now goes to NGOs, which has led to competition among SNGOs for these funds. At their worst, NGOs can become, or actually be created as, inefficient routine contract service providers with little innovation or dedication to the public welfare.

As international funding grew and state institutions contracted, large numbers of NGOs were created in response to little more than the opportunity to pursue the available resources. Older NGOs . . . felt obliged to join in the chase for funds . . . or be lost in the ocean of new NGO acronyms. The diversity of views that these organizations represented has largely been lost as they have competed with one another to become the favoured clients of international donors.[33]

The search for money is understandable in view of the precarious financial status of many NGOs, but these organizations are often seen as using their funds ineffectively. A leading critic has made a number of accusations, such as:

- An agency that contracted to deliver food to Somalia received a contract for $9 million, of which close to $1 million went to expatriate salaries and $660,000 to administrative expenses in New York.
- An NGO that advertises widely to the public collects $240 annually per child from well-meaning individuals who "sponsor" children in developing countries, but the children actually receive only $25 to $67.
- An agency that sends food to disaster areas shipped 17 tons of surplus Pop Tarts to Bosnia. The manufacturer saved the cost of warehousing and destroying the products, and also received tax benefits, good publicity and "brand-name recognition in emerging markets."[34]

A study in Bolivia "estimated that for every $100 spent on social development projects conducted by NGOs, only about $15–20 reached the designated beneficiaries. Most of the rest was used to pay administrative costs and professional salaries . . . it is apparent that commonly held assumptions about the benefits of promoting development through NGOs should not be accepted without critical scrutiny."[35]

> What these development NGOs actually do is very varied. The counterpart of expansion has been role diversification, with the sector's original specialism in relief and emergency work now counterbalanced by involvement in an increasingly wide range of development activities. These range from political advocacy and education (in both North and South) through support for people's movements, to direct and indirect participation in a bewildering variety of project work, extending from the search for sustainable development solutions, through community development and service delivery, to income generating and entrepreneurial activities, as well as the continuing provision of the crisis and emergency assistance, frequently war-related, that has been such a depressing characteristic of the 1990s.[36]

Prominent in the consciousness of all development aid workers is the search for sustainable development solutions, as was mentioned previously. Sustainability means developing local capacity to carry on without the external assistance, for which training activities are usually a large part. Training is relatively easy to do. Off-the-shelf courses can be obtained and adapted, visual aids prepared, pretests and post-tests given, and the foreign workers can derive a feeling of accomplishment. What is lacking is a demonstration that the training really makes much permanent difference. The director of an NGO development program in Uganda spoke of

> bitter disappointment for those who believed that training, as such, isolated from the actual work situation of the trainee, would provide the necessary internal managerial

capability for primary health care implementation. There is no lack of in-service training today in Uganda, and probably many other developing countries as well. In fact
most health workers spend too much time outside their districts attending workshops
organized by various agencies. What is needed . . . is a management strengthening strategy based on problem-solving, encompassing the whole local health system, and aimed
at transferring a sustainable learning process rather than ready-made products and solutions.[37]

The Sector-Wide Approach

An official of the Ministry of Health of a developing country might well comment
on its international affiliations in something like the following terms:

The Minister of Health and her delegations go to many regional and global meetings of
international organizations, where a lot of high-level horsetrading seems to go on. They vote
in favor of programs for immunization, nutrition, breastfeeding, population control, child survival, cardiovascular health, medical information systems, support for refugees, and other
things that nobody can vote against. Such well-intentioned multilateral agreements, nominally supported by our government, lead to an accumulation of often unwanted obligations.
Then we in the MOH must figure out how to accommodate all those programs within our
already debilitated budgets and staffs. We have obtained earmarked donor assistance for some
of them, and would like to carry them all out, but sometimes it is a burden when the time
comes to report on progress in each separate program and we do not have much to communicate.

There is continuing tension between determining our own national priorities and following the priorities of others. Ministry staff must meet with a stream of foreigners from bilateral and multilateral donor agencies, nongovernmental organizations, commercial companies,
universities, professional societies, and others. Each has his or her own agenda, different from
our own. There is often not enough time left to do our own work. A university dean wants
to send medical students and residents here for clinical experiences, but regrettably cannot
take our students in exchange because malpractice laws in his country would cause his insurance premiums to soar. The representative of an international electronics manufacturer
wants us to put an MRI scanner in every health center, on easy payment terms. The woman
from the Children's Protective Fund thinks that we should immunize all our children against
congenital rubella syndrome, which is found in her country but not ours. Undergraduates
from wealthy countries come to "study" our health care system, even though they know almost nothing about their own.

Developed country scholars, and some from our own universities, ask MOH staff for assistance to set up all kinds of studies in our country. We are happy to help, despite the fact
that they rarely send us reprints of their publications, much less invite us to be co-authors.
Researchers from industrialized countries want to try out their latest ideas. A professor plans
to test a new vaccine against amebiasis on our population. He is not easily dissuaded, even
though we point out that the best way to avoid amebiasis is to wash your hands and be careful what you eat. Another wants to apply the polymerase chain reaction to diagnosis of malaria.
We appreciate such scientific advances, but our rural health centers lack electric power, and
rarely have enough chloroquine. In some parts of our country we don't know within 20%

how many babies were born last year. We need research that will help us to plan, manage, and evaluate our work and make the health system more equitable, efficient, and effective.

We appreciate the interest and programs of the international donor agencies. However, we need a special staff within the ministry just for liaison with the development agencies from the various industrialized countries, to make sure that we spend their money for their own country's products, and to keep the many competing NGOs and PVOs out of each other's hair. Even different organizations within the UN system sometimes promote conflicting programs or compete for territory or influence. I see that the Minister of Public Health of Ecuador issued a policy statement for the triennium 1993–1996. Among "The Principal Obstacles to carrying out the policies of health programs" he referred specifically to (translation):

> An excess of studies, reports, projects, plans and programs, which although they develop a series of activities and require the efforts and dedication of many staff persons, both national and international, produce very few measurable results in effects and impact on the conditions of health and the life of the people.

Certain health issues have their own entrenched constituencies within our country and across national borders: AIDS, infant diarrheal disease, women's health, leprosy, generic drugs, and so on. Other problems that we think are very important are pretty much ignored by others: for example, alcoholism and family violence, accidents, and other aspects of mental health in which technology has made little impact. The health of economically active adults (ages 15 to 65) is critical for our country's productivity, but occupational health is not among the fashionable subjects. We have to account for these issues but few donors seem interested in planning, or paying, for them.

If our fictitious MOH official were to propose a solution to these headaches and inefficiencies, he or she might write a plan to relieve the fragmented nature of multiple health projects; the need for lengthy and bureaucratic planning and pre-arrangements; inadequate administration and management; their limited sustainability, and above all to evaluate their real effect on health. Underlying reasons for such lack of success are a mixture of structural features such as donor agency and host government red tape and lack of flexibility, plus ambiguities arising out of the environment in which projects are actually carried out. These include inadequate infrastructure (communications, facilities); competition among donor agencies; uncertainties about project ownership; limited local capacity to implement the scope of work, maintain equipment and records, and so on. At the same time, the overall strategies and policies of the Ministry totter for lack of support.

As the health sector becomes more complex, so do the scope and range of programs and projects. A typical developing country may have well over a dozen significant donor and technical agencies, several international NGOs, and several hundred local NGOs involved in the health sector. Although donor agencies may account for a very significant percentage of health expenditures in the poorest countries, there is growing dissatisfaction with the results of project implementation and the lack of integration of the many donor-assisted projects. The tendency of donors and their contractors to dominate project planning and execution ("After all, it's our money") stifles any feeling of ownership by the borrower or grantee. Such a distressed policy environment leads to lack of local commitment and responsibility and unsuccessful outcomes in which everyone loses. Donors and funders get poor value for their financial investment; local governments divert their scarce personnel and resources; the proposed beneficiaries derive little benefit; national impact is limited; sustainability is minimal; and there is very little evidence of a demonstration effect. What is clearly needed is better coordination—namely: "any activity or set of activities, formal or non-formal, at any level, undertaken by recipients in conjunction with donors, individually or collectively, which ensures that external inputs to the health sector enable the health system to function more effectively, and in accordance with local priorities, over time."[38]

Buse and Walt have made a detailed analysis of the coordination of external resources to the health sector. Table 9-6 lists their main points.[39]

In the mid-1950s it was realized, first by the Africa Technical Department of the World Bank, that the "project-by-project, and donor-by-donor approach has . . . proved fatal for the sustainability of many operations."[40] In a new paradigm, this approach can extend the principles of health sector reform beyond individual ministries to encompass the entire global health sector ODA network.

Governments do not feel that they are in control of projects, which are driven and designed by donors and international agencies, according to their own estimations of the

Table 9-6. Selected Trends Raising the Need for Aid Coordination in the Health Sector

Factors internal to the health sector

Increasing number and diversity of external agencies

Increasing volume and importance of health aid

Project proliferation and recipient institutional weakening

Shift from project aid to sector aid

Policy conditionality associated with sector reform and the need for leverage

Focus on efficiency, effectiveness, and equity goals

Factors exogenous to the health sector

Heightened scrutiny of developmental assistance

Increasing incidence of instability and massive relief and rehabilitation efforts

Debate over UN agency mandates

Source: Reprinted from Buse and Walt (1997) Table 1. Social Science and Medicine, vol. 45, copyright 1997, with permission from Elsevier Science.

problems in the sector. In many cases, governments are not even aware of the existence of some projects. The results can be that the projects die after the immediate implementation phase. The key issue is therefore to obtain government attachment and stakeholder ownership . . . Different donors have forced governments to pursue different often conflicting strategies, and with different implementation and accounting systems. This is confusing for the economic agents in a sector. It also needlessly spreads and overtaxes limited national implementation capacity. Because of these different donor approaches and regulations, donors and international agencies have often found it necessary to create special project units to manage their projects, staffing them with both expatriates and with government officials who are lured from their posts by significantly higher salaries, further weakening the already dispersed government implementation capacity.[41]

Dissatisfaction with these widespread problems and the meager impact of many projects has stimulated the development of a new approach to lending, variously called the Sector Wide Approach (SWAP), Sector Investment Program (SIP), or Sector Expenditure Program (SEP).[42] Of all sectors, health has been at the forefront of this approach in part because of the urgency of pressing problems, in part because of the welter of donor agencies and interest groups working in the sector, and in part because of the complexity of existing health systems and the trend toward health sector reform.

As the donor community grows in number and diversity, coordination of activities and multiple reporting requirements becomes increasingly unmanageable and disruptive to the host government. Almost in self-defense, governments are compelled to take a more systematic and sector-wide approach and to improve planning with donors if they are to achieve steady and sustainable health sector reforms. In meetings with donors, technical agencies, and NGOs, the various agencies accept responsibility for different aspects of the program within the government's overall health sector strategy. The donor agencies in effect transform themselves into a consortium of health partners that agree to use common procedures for planning, implementation, monitoring, and reporting.

The sector-wide approach is being promoted because it best enables government and the consortium of donors, technical agencies, and NGOs to deal openly with the full range of issues about public policy and the allocation of everyone's resources. The SEP approach could not have been proposed in the Era of Programs and Projects of the 1970s and 1980s, when quasi-independent units within ministries functioned in malaria control, immunization, maternal and child health, family planning, and so on, often supported by different donors. Although such constituencies are still in place, the emergence of the Era of Health Sector Reform has enabled the concept of sector-wide strategies to take root. The new approach can be described as follows:

- Policies and programs are sector-wide in scope and should include both capital expenditures and recurrent program costs.

- Policies and programs are prepared by local stakeholders, primarily from the host government, based on a clear sector policy strategy.
- All donors active in the sector should agree on common procedures and their share of the financing.[43]
- Implementation arrangements should be common for all donors.
- The use of long-term technical assistance should be minimized in favor of local personnel.

The differences between the SEP approach and conventional distinct projects are:

- Host governments assume the leadership of the SEP team.
- It is sector-wide and programmatic in scope, rather than disconnected individual projects.
- Individual donors cooperate rather than competing, and all accept common, or at least coordinated, procedures for planning, financing, execution, and evaluation.

Although an advance, in harmony with the times, the SEP aproach is not a panacea. Inherent problems include:

- Rigid, different legal and procedural systems in each of the donors and in the host government, leading to lack of flexibility.
- Political repercussions among citizens of donor countries from lack of national identification with specific projects.
- Donors contribute to implementing a comprehensive strategic plan which may be harder to conceive and accept than a carefully drafted limited project.
- The strategic plan and concept should be essentially the product of the host government, which makes most donors uncomfortable.
- The more open-ended nature of sectoral support, compared to discretely defined projects, may reduce the flow of donor government funding to bilateral agencies.
- Procurement of personnel, consultants (if used), and commodities arises from a centralized administration rather than from each donor's separate funds, limiting the repatriation of funds to each donor economy.[44]
- The role of the more technical support agencies, such as WHO and UNICEF, which provide services but are not primarily donors, needs to be clarified.

The SEP approach in the health sector has been tried, in various formats, in Pakistan, Zambia, Mozambique, Sierra Leone, Uganda, Benin, Bangladesh, and Ghana.

NOTES

1. World Bank (1975).
2. World Bank (1980).

3. Descriptions of these and other bank projects may be found on the Worldwide Web at http://www.worldbank.org/cgi-bin/##.

4. World Bank (1993), World Development Report 1993, *Investing in Health*. Prominent among the prior policy studies was the report by Akin et al. (1987). Many others could be mentioned.

5. World Bank (1997).

6. Likely candidates for such collaborations include African governments in a major effort to control the malaria epidemic; WHO and others to combat the pandemic of tuberculosis and to promote integrated management of childhood illness; and many partners to launch a Global Forum on Health Research.

7. Sometimes called Structural Adjustment Policies.

8. Greenaway and Morrissey (1993).

9. Jolly (1991).

10. Peabody (1996).

11. *Lancet* editorial (1996).

12. Adapted from Basch (1994).

13. Loewenson (1993).

14. Peabody (1996).

15. UNDP (1996).

16. *Ibid.*

17. Cornia *et al.* (1987).

18. Asthana (1994).

19. Resolution WHA 29.48 of the 29th World Health Assembly in 1976.

20. These diseases or disease groups are malaria, schistosomiasis, filariasis, typanosomiasis, leishmaniasis, and leprosy.

21. ⟨http://www.who.int⟩

22. Trostle and Simon (1992).

23. From USAID home page at ⟨http://www.info.usaid.gov/⟩.

24. USAID (1986).

25. Supplemented with $76 million transferred from the prior year.

26. NIS = Newly Independent States of the former USSR. See Chapter 13.

27. Michaud and Murray (1994).

28. Task Force on International Development (1970).

29. A useful general reference is Loos (1996).

30. Fox (1995).

31. Matthias and Green (1994).

32. Mburu (1989).

33. Arellano-Lopez and Petras (1994), cited by Charlton and May (1995).

34. Maren (1997).

35. *Ibid.*

36. Charlton and May (1995). See for an excellent review of NGO activities.

37. Stefanini (1995).

38. Buse and Walt (1996).

39. Buse and Walt (1997). See the original for an extensive discussion.

40. Harrold *et al.* (1995).

41. *Ibid.*

42. See Cassels (1996) and Cassels and Janovsky (1997).

43. Donors may include The World Bank or regional development banks, OECD member government aid agencies such as USAID or DANIDA, and non-governmental organizations.

44. This is "tied aid" which requires certain categories of purchases such as vehicles or laboratory equipment, or the hiring of expatriate personnel, to be done in the donor country.

10

Science and Technology

The technology that we use determines, to a large part, the pattern of our daily lives and the productivity of our work. Every familiar product, from bread to breadboards, from pencils to penicillin, and every useful procedure and method was once a technological innovation that has since achieved widespread diffusion.

The application of technology helps human beings to

- Locate, identify, gather, transport, and modify useful natural materials from their environment
- Protect themselves from the many hostile aspects of that same environment
- Express their creativity
- Escape from the limitations of their physical strength and their five senses
- Reduce the tyranny of risk in all human activities

Technology allows us to see farther or smaller than with the unaided eye; hear music not being made by living players; communicate and transmit information across continents and decades; travel faster; eat foods not freshly harvested or killed; and prevent and cure certain ailments. Technology does these things in a cumulative way, as each advance builds on those that preceded it. Since the earliest settlements and civilizations, the only human activities that have progressed without significant interruption are science and technology.

The first applications were probably related to assuring a stable food supply. Domestication and deliberate selective breeding of animals and plants, which required a practical understanding of biology, was certainly carried out all around the ancient world, inaugurating both agriculture and husbandry. The technology of food preservation—for example, by cooking, drying, and salting—helped to overcome times of scarcity. The control of fermentation by bacteria and fungi to make what we would now call beers and wines, yogurt, cheeses, leavened bread, and other products was certainly discovered independently at many different times and places.

If science is viewed as the organized, rational investigation of knowledge, then science has been closely associated with health since the earliest times. The writings of Hippocrates on the Greek island of Cos in the sixth century BC were based on careful observation of illness as a natural phenomenon, and many of his comments are still valid today. For example, without thermometer or microscope, Hippocrates distinguished tertian and quartan fevers so accurately that today we can recognize them as forms of malaria caused by different *Plasmodium* parasites, organisms of which he knew nothing.

During the so-called prescientific era, many other astute and pertinent observations were made by intelligent minds in all parts of the world. For example, there is evidence that some African peoples were aware of the transmission of sleeping sickness by tsetse flies, and of malaria by mosquitoes long before a Nobel Prize was awarded for the same observation. In South America native people knew that the bark of the cinchona tree cured fevers and that the bark of the ipecac tree stopped certain diarrheas without ever having heard of the true causes—the "etiologic agents" of these afflictions. As mentioned in Chapter 6, people in the eastern Mediterranean region, observing that disfiguring Oriental sores usually occurred only once in any person, rubbed material from an active lesion into the skin of their young daughters' buttocks to avert a potentially damaging sore on her face. In China, a similar train of thought led to comparable but more risky procedures with smallpox pustules.

Like the man who was surprised to learn that he had been speaking in prose all his life, the unknown originators of these procedures had no way to know that they were practicing "science and technology." It is only in more recent times, starting perhaps with Lind's demonstration of the nutritional cause of scurvy and Jenner's introduction of vaccination in the 18th century, that natural science has been pursued as a specific discipline that has become more and more closely associated with medicine and health (Chapter 3).

The 19th century in the western countries opened on a technological upbeat; ingenious mechanical devices powered by water or steam were transforming the pattern and improving the quality of life in city and farm. Industrial processes, based on advances in engineering, chemistry, and physics, were flourishing. Agriculture was becoming more efficient and less labor-intensive. Large volumes of raw materials and consumer goods crisscrossed the world. A philosophical outlook of pragmatism was becoming firmly established. Nevertheless, rational understanding of health and disease had proceeded so slowly that as late as 1851 the most learned men of Europe, debating for six months at the First International Sanitary Conference, could not agree whether cholera was or was not contagious (Chapter 2).

From such a shaky foundation, through a remarkably concerted achievement of the human intellect, a flood of discoveries poured from the world's laboratories in the latter half of the 19th century and established the cause and basic means of transmission of virtually every major bacterial and parasitic disease of mankind and of domestic animals. Within the span of one human lifetime, from about 1840 to 1910, vague theories of miasma and divine displeasure gave way to experimentally based laboratory data regarding the cause of many diseases and their effects upon the body. Knowledge of physiology, nutrition, and many other aspects of biomedical science also advanced strongly during this period, including asepsis, anesthesia, and medical applications of x-rays and radium. Repeated epidemics of cholera in Europe and continuing havoc from other communicable diseases were intense stimuli for investigators. The extreme intellectual ferment provoked by the theories of Darwin and Wallace provided a further incentive to an explosion of biological knowledge after the 1860s.

The rapid rise of microbiology depended on the chemical and technological underpinning provided by the Industrial Revolution. Refinements in microscope design produced the condensers and objective lenses of the 1880s, which are remarkably similar to those in use today. The chemistry of dye manufcture, developed for the textile industry, was incorporated into histology and bacteriology. Little by little the basis of modern biomedical science was hammered together.

The first half of the 20th century was marked by steady refinement and consolidation in all branches of science and technology, culminating perhaps in the discovery of insulin in the 1920s and of antibiotics and yellow fever vaccine in the late 1930s. Advances in electronics led to invention of television and the electron microscope in the same era. As is usually the case, war (World War II) provided a strong stimulus to scientific discovery, especially in nuclear physics. Important applications of biomedical science during this period included the widespread introduction of synthetic antimalarials, of antibiotics and associated fermentation technology, and of DDT-based insecticides.

TECHNOLOGY TRANSFER AND TECHNOLOGY ASSESSMENT

Many developing and middle-income countries have good health services with well-trained, motivated, and dedicated personnel. In others the situation is less favorable. I have been in Rural Health Centers in which the staff were unable to work for want of fuel for their motorcycles, where malaria technicians could not make blood films for lack of glass microscope slides, and where no one had been paid for months. I have visited a Basic Health Unit in a refugee camp, in which ancient posters hung on the canvas wall of the tent. It made little difference that the cardboard was bleached nearly white from age and weathering, as the writing was in English and incomprehensible to dispenser and patients alike.

The kinds of technology most useful for improving health in such places is not what people in industrialized countries think of as "biomedical technology" at all. The importation of advanced technology to the poorest areas will be unproductive until social and economic conditions attain a level at which it can be usefully employed. Under conditions of deprivation the greatest research need is for *operational research*, to establish the means by which the health sector can achieve its mission effectively. In such circumstances the health of the community would be advanced also by the promotion of schooling and literacy; by window screening, paved roads, telephones, electric lines, and clean water; by better agricultural tools, seeds, and livestock; and by similar mundane technologies.

Mention has been made earlier (Chapters 7 and 8) of *appropriate technology*. The term has come to take on many shades of meaning in political and ecologic senses but in general refers to processes and products that are feasible for use in a community and that are affordable and sustainable. Many nongovernmental organizations promote such technology, such as Teaching Aids at Low Cost and the Appropriate Health Resources and Technologies Action Group in England, and the Program for Appropriate Technology in Health (PATH) in the United States. PATH, for example, has designed, field tested, and produced numerous products ranging from dipstick tests for pregnancy and for malaria, HIV and other sexually transmitted diseases, to birthing kits for use by traditional birth attendants, baby scales with colored bands for persons who can not read numbers, cold chain monitors to determine when vaccine has become too warm, disposable vaccine injection devices, and similar items. Such products, when accompanied by relevant education, may be extremely useful in economically deprived environments. In addition to health applications, appropriate technology has been advocated in agriculture, housing, energy production, education and many other fields.

The typical government health service in a poor country, although underfunded, is not understaffed, so labor-saving but costly devices developed for the high-salary industrialized nations of the North lose their economic justification in the labor-rich countries of the South. Workers at all levels of civil service receive few rewards and have little incentive to adopt innovations that may threaten their professional stability. Lower-level technical workers are commonly trained for repetitive performance of well-defined and routine tasks. This is the case especially in vertical or monovalent services for control of specific diseases such as tuberculosis, where sputum collection, slide preparation, acid-fast staining, and microscopy can form the basis of a lifelong career. It does not make much sense to import a capital-intensive and labor-saving device economically effective in the United States into an environment of low wages, high unemployment, and scarce funds, where exactly the opposite kind of technology is needed. In that event a labor-intensive technology that creates employment would be much more appropriate. George Nelson of the Liverpool School of Hygiene and Tropical Medicine has pointed out that 60,000 people in India who make a living by reading malaria slides could be displaced by adoption of automated diagnostic methodologies. Therefore technologic innovations in unfamiliar surroundings might provoke unexpected social consequences that are quite distinct from their nominal scientific purpose. The same reasoning applies to equipment that requires great amounts of energy or imported raw materials.

Implicit in the idea of "modern technology" is innovative products or procedures that are attractive largely because of their recent development. However, novelty is itself of little value. On the one hand, although novelty is not an inherent property of the technology, every technology, however commonplace it may become to its originators, is new to someone else. On the other hand, the loss of novelty is inevitable as technologies mutate, radiate into various niches, or merge with other technologies.

For reasons well known, a child in a developing country is very much less likely to grow up to be a scientist than a child in the industrialized countries (Table 10-1). It is therefore probable that any application of modern science to such areas will be imported and will carry with it all of the features common to any item from abroad, such as a high price, foreign control, and uncertain application to local conditions.

It should not be presumed that technology transfer is one way, from North to South. Many important drugs, such as quinine and emetine, were derived from the knowledge of technologically unsophisticated people in what are now developing countries. Closer to home, methods developed in Brazil in the 1930s helped to make mass miniature radiographic screening practical. In addition, developed countries have much to learn about the organization of services to large numbers of people and the ingenuity necessary for application of "their" technologies in the pathogen-rich and resource-poor nations.

Table 10-1. Scientists and Engineers per Million Population Engaged in Research and Development, Selected Countries, Recent Years[a]

Scientists & Engineers		Scientists & Engineers	
Country	Number/Million	Country	Number/Million
Australia	2477	Greece	774
Belgium	1814	India	151
Bolivia	250	Korea, South	2636
Brazil	165	Malaysia	87
Bulgaria	4240	Mauritius	361
Canada	2322	Mexico	95
Central African Republic	55	Nepal	22
China	537	Pakistan	54
Costa Rica	539	Russian Federation	4358
Cuba	1369	Thailand	173
Ecuador	169	United Kingdom	2417
Egypt	458	United States	3732
El Salvador	19	Uzbekistan	1760
France	2537	Venezuela	208

[a]Note: Survey years 1981–1995. See source for more data.

Source: Selected from World Bank (1998) Table 5.12.

In addition to social and cultural compatibility, a compelling issue in the North–South transfer of technology is its physical adaptability to local conditions in developing countries. High-technology devices are generally not conceived with the tropical environment in mind and may not function to design specifications in conditions of unstable or intermitent electric power, high temperature and humidity, dust, insects, and similar hazards. Some machines are retrofitted with surge suppressors or other protective contrivances, but these are rarely an integral part of the basic design. The necessary chemicals, antigens, isotopes, or whatever is needed for research or for routine application may be costly to import, difficult to store properly, and impossible to dispose of without hazard to the environment.

The issue of capital versus recurrent costs is of primary importance. A visit to virtually any larger health facility in the tropical country of your choice will reveal apparatus and equipment ranging from ELISA (enzyme-linked immunosorbent assay) readers to X-ray machines disabled for want of supplies and consumables, maintenance, spare parts, or persons trained in proper use, care, and repair. Recently computers have begun to share a similar fate. It is common to see more equipment out of order than in working condition. Around the world, thousands of costly microscopes essential for diagnosis of tuberculosis, malaria, and intestinal parasites are gathering dust, rust, and fungus merely because no replacement is available for nonfunctional light bulbs.

The habitual dependence of many health ministries on foreign donors is a conduit for much imported technology but carries with it certain dangers. Funding from country J or country G or country U often entails the stipulation that the money must be expended for commodities and equipment from the donor country, a condition known as "tied aid." When the funding cycle is over, a different donor agency may continue the project with noncompatible apparatus and supplies. Ministries of Health must keep adapting as externally funded programs, layered over their own health services, come and go. The doctor or administrator who negotiated the original technology transfer may have received a fellowship for overseas study or may have been transferred to another facility or program in which he or she is busy ordering other items. The technician who took a course in implementing the procedures may for one reason or another be assigned elsewhere. In any case, when donor funds are gone there may not be sufficient foreign exchange to buy reagents or film or insecticide spray nozzles or whatever is needed to apply the technology as originally intended.

The foregoing is an argument in favor of restraint and discipline in the acceptance of complex devices and procedures, and not against the adoption of useful technology, which does indeed exist. Recently, in a village in the Fayyoum Oasis in Egypt, I watched a small ultrasound diagnostic machine, powered by a portable generator, being used to measure the extent of periportal fibrosis and renal impairment for instantaneous noninvasive evaluation of schistosomal pathology among local inhabitants. This information could have been obtained in no other way except by laparotomy, which was clearly not an option. The Egyptian investigators were absolutely correct in selecting and applying this technology, whose appropriateness is quite distinct from its complexity.

In practice, it appears that imported medical technology in most developing countries comes through several routes, generally with minimal control or oversight by any agency of the receiving government. One major channel is through internationally oriented individuals in the private sector. Wealthier physicians, either individually, in small-group practices, or in private hospitals have the resources to import materials and equipment inaccessible to the public sector and to maintain these investments in good working order. Their clients are willing and able to pay for the services received, and the entire process of the private importation and application of technology is buffered from most public-sector bureaucratic impediments.

The influence of commercial companies, particularly the pharmaceutical industry, is pervasive in most developing countries. In addition to various perks and giveaways for professionals, these firms sponsor short courses, conferences, dinners, and seminars, for which they distribute posters and programs displaying company and product names. Calendars and informational placards featuring corporate logos are often the sole adornments on the walls of health ministry offices and health facilities. I have a photo of one country's largest hospital, with its name on a large sign high on one wall. Also conspicuously present is the name of the company that paid for the sign, as the health ministry had no funds for the purpose. In such an environment, the introduction and distribution of new products and technologies is regulated mainly by corporate initiative.

Biomedical technology is also introduced through universities and research institutes, whose academic staff are in professional contact with colleagues in industrialized countries. These individuals may attend international conferences, participate as visiting scholars, send students, or otherwise become a part of the worldwide biomedical network. Additional technology may be transferred through donor agencies, mentioned previously, which are anxious to demonstrate that the capabilities and methods of their patrons can have a rapid and dramatic effect in resolving whichever problem they have chosen to tackle.

SCIENCE AND TECHNOLOGY POLICIES

> The degree of (our) development makes us fundamentally dependent on scientific and technologic research. To aspire to self-sufficiency is utopian; to seek, if you like, self-determination is fundamental . . . Let us orient our activities in science and technology toward technological self-determination, understanding this as the capacity of the country to decide, as a function of national priorities, what technologies to develop, which ones to use from abroad, and where to look for them.[1]

Above all, a new health technology should increase the productivity of the health sector—that is, it should provide more health per dollar or rupee or peso than the previous way of doing things. Relatively few developing countries are able to evaluate the multitude of technologies that have potential impact upon their health situation, and clear policies on science and technology are badly needed in the developing world. Ideally, a cost–benefit–risk–consequence equation should be applied to each innovation of potential value in each specific national context. Considering the difficulties of technology assesment in the industrialized countries, this seems a herculean task. The U.S. Office of Technology Assessment (OTA), an arm of the Congress, was permanently disbanded in September 1995, sacrificed to conspicuous but ill-considered cost-cutting by ignorant politicians. The former and much lamented OTA did not use the term *health technology* very often, but defined *medical technology* as "the set of techniques, drugs, equipment, and procedures used by health care professionals in delivering medical care to individuals and the systems within which such are delivered."

The medical care that is delivered to individuals can be considered in two parts in relation to technology. First, the *formal* (official, or licensed) personal medical services industry is replete with *procedure-related technologies* that deal directly with individuals or with materials removed from them or inserted into them. The many preventive, diagnostic, therapeutic, and rehabilitative procedures utilize reagents, vaccines and biologicals, pharmaceuticals, equipment and instruments, facilities, personnel training, electronic data processing, and so on. Authors on health technology usually focus on chronic, infectious, and metabolic diseases, surgical procedures, reproductive matters, and trauma. Less often considered as subjects for health technology are mental and behavioral health including alcoholism and other dependencies, occupational and environmental hazards, and many other common problems. Second, the *informal* personal medical services "industry" embraces familial and nonprofessional diagnosis (such as by grandmothers and curanderos) and self-treatment with natural or unlicensed products produced locally and on a small-scale, as well as vitamins, antibiotics, and other standard medicaments obtained from pharmacies without professional sanction.

A cynic might say that the main difference between formal and informal medical care is that the informal sector is characterized by inappropriate use of cheap technology, and the formal sector is characterized by inappropriate use of expensive technology.

There is another important application for health technology: public health. This is rarely discussed under the general rubric of health technology, mainly because the technologies most needed and used in public health are generally applicable ones. The diversity of public health work comprises, among other things, health promotion and education, water and sewage treatment, environmental pollution monitoring and control, epidemiologic surveillance, the collection and reporting of morbidity and mortality statistics, and so on. The growing role of information systems and communications technology in the management of health services was discussed in Chapter 5. Individually targeted, costly therapeutic health technology such as a heart transplant will completely change the life of the individual who receives it, but will have a trivial effect on the overall level of health in a country.[2] However, the benefits of broadly distributed technology-based preventive programs such as universal childhood immunization are difficult to evaluate for any individual, as it can never be known whether, in the absence of immunization, that particular person would have been ill, or died, from the disease that was avoided. Some criteria to determine relevance of health technologies in developing countries are listed in Table 10-2.

Many politicians are wary of the health sector, in part because is not possible to measure, or even to define, its product (i.e., health). Progress in other sectors is much easier to determine, as there are direct measures of output (Table 10-3). In satisfying consumer wants with technologic products and services the health sector is unlike any other. One refrigerator per household may be enough, and one or maybe two TV sets.[3] However, demand for personal medical servcies is not readily saturable. The potential consumption of health services has until recently had no reasonable endpoint except death; but even that frontier has now been breached as various spare parts are removed from transplant donors, who continue, *postmortem*, to consume the services of physicians and surgeons. On the supply side, the very ingenuity that we want to stimulate provides a limitless increase in the number of potentially useful procedures and products. Each health-related service produces a corresponding need for facilities, faculties, and financing. Politicians do not like bottomless pits.

Table 10-2. Criteria for Relevance of Health Technology in Developing Countries

- Direct application to reduction of disease prevalence or to risk of incidence
- Affordability in view of competing priorities
- Cost-effectiveness in terms of future costs averted
- Sustainability by the importing country after withdrawal of donor support
- Public demand and political benefit to the government
- Saving foreign exchange
- Contribution to national development, economic growth, and creation of employment
- Promotion of social equity
- Increase in the value of human resources
- Addition to national capacity in science and technology, training local scientists and technicians in advanced methods, and reducing emigration of scientific personnel
- Agreement with the government's established health policies and strategies and with science and technology policies (if any)
- Minimal opportunity cost. In a zero-sum budget, the totality of health gained by use of the new technology should equal or exceed the totality of health that would have been gained by different uses for the same amount of resources
- Reduced dependence on other foreign technology

Table 10-3. Measuring Progress in Various Sectors

Sector	Type[a]	Measures of Progress — Description
Agriculture	D	Volume, quality, and appropriateness of food and fiber
Industry	D	Variety, volume, and quality of products; sales
Commerce	D	Bank transactions, employment statistics, tax receipts
Education	D	Test achievement; compare output to national needs
Health	P	By resources (medical schools, hospital beds, health centers, nurses, doctors)
	P	By volume of services (immunizations, deliveries in hospitals, admissions, diagnostic procedures)
	P	By demographic indicators (infant and other mortality rates, expectation of life)
	P	By morbidity indicators (incidence and prevalence of acute and chronic diseases, lost school and work days)
	P	In personal health services: by consumer satisfaction
	P	In public health services: reduction in disease transmission, absence of outbreaks or epidemics

[a]D = direct measure; P = proxy measure.

Most people who write about the transfer of technologies to developing countries are usually either committed enthusiasts or perpetual critics, and disinterested objectivity is not easily encountered. In part this is because the real effects of technological innovation are often indirect. Consequently, relationships between technology and health are difficult to trace and subject to individual interpretation.

Just as health technologies have significant nonhealth effects, the opposite is also true, as has been pointed out several times in this text.

It is likely that most people envision transfer of health-related technologies in terms of hardware; or perhaps of "high-tech" surgical procedures and their enabling tests, materials, and methods; or of the wonders of molecular biology and biochemistry. Despite the profusion of specific applications, the critical element in transferring technology from industrialized to developing countries does not lie in shipping the box that contains a physical product but in conveying the scientific thinking that supported its development, and guides its use. Technology transfer should be more than an import–export business. Transplanted technology without science is inviable in the long term and cannot lead to an indigenous capacity to solve problems independently.

It could be said that health technology is in essence no different from other technologies. In an extended analogy, Table 10-4 shows a comparison of the role of health technology in the health sector and of fertilizer in agriculture.

Table 10-4. Health Technology Is to Health as Fertilizer Is to Agriculture

- It is merely a means to help achieve an end, not an end in itself
- There must be an appropriate mechanism to apply (spread) it
- It must have the proper composition and balance of elements in relation to the substrate and the desired product
- It should generate an economic value greater than its cost
- In appropriate amounts it may help to increase productivity, but in excess it may be injurious
- Although there is often pressure to import, it can usually be made satisfactorily at home
- There may be other, more organic, ways to achieve similar results
- Unrestrained use could result in long-term dependency
- Most of it is valuable, but some of it is just plain guano

ROLE OF THE STATE AND OTHER ACTORS IN HEALTH TECHNOLOGY POLICY

The purpose of a policy is to make informed decisions that will help to achieve objectives in an orderly and economical manner. A policy offers general guidelines to stimulate beneficial effects and retard harmful ones, from the point of view of the policy-maker. The policy should examine the range of alternatives, the expected health benefits and social and economic costs of each, and their relative desirability. Policies may deal with larger strategic issues, such as the adoption of a national position on hemodialysis or infant immunization; or they may be tactical, selecting which of two similar products to stock on the shelves of health centers. The Essential Drugs Program of WHO, interpreted for and by each country, is a good example of a health technology policy.

The Intersectoral Nature of Health Technology Policy

The entire health technology enterprise consists of a set of institutions and procedures organized to develop, produce, distribute, and use products intended to improve the health of the people and incidentally to make health services more effective and productive. These institutions, both local and foreign, include private and public sector, for-profit and academic research facilities, and the complex of mechanisms that provide them with funding, material resources, and capable workers. Each of these organizations may also have other missions: the function of universities is primarily educational; that of industrial research centres is to devise useful and profitable commodities and services. Decisions about the adoption of health technologies are made at various levels by government agencies, commercial companies, hospitals and other health facilities, medical practitioners, families, and individuals. Such conclusions may be made casually and *ad hoc,* or on the basis of a policy, whether written or informal. Some of the forces driving each of these actors are summarized in Table 10-5.

Table 10-5. Health Technology Transfer: Incentives of Actors in Developing Countries

Actor	Relation to Technology	Desired Outcomes
Government	Gatekeeper	*Promote:* social equity, use of local materials, employment and training, local investment *Restrict:* capital-intensive and dependency-producing methods, repatriation of profits abroad; negative cost-benefit; environmental damage
Local industry	Supplier	*Promote:* profit, widespread use, reduced dependency on imports *Restrict:* unfair advantage of foreign competitors; excessive regulations and control
Health professionals	User	*Promote:* selection, safety, efficacy, reliability, productivity, profit for the private sector *Restrict:* cost, complexity of use, ambiguous outcome; access by nonprofessionals
The public	Recipient	*Promote:* choice; physical and social well-being, convenience, low cost, quick and positive outcome *Restrict:* adverse individual and environmental effects; social disruption, cost and effort

Governmental Policy-Making

The existence of a policy does not guarantee success, but its absence foretells inequity and the dominance of powerful self-interest. Unenlightened policy, made unsystematically and without coordination, or for private motives, may be worse than no policy at all. Conventional descriptions of governmental policy-making usually invoke hypothetical econometric models based on need and adequacy, benefit and cost. In a less-than-ideal world, policies reflect the political realities of time and place, the interests of different parties, and fundamental attitudes of those who control the adoption process. The basic philosophy may be *laissez-faire* or authoritarian, inclusive or exclusive; that is, to permit innovations unless they are proven harmful, or to restrain them unless their benefits are clearly established.

> policies are not made for rational reasons or because of economical arguments. Policies are made because of pressures. People want something. They vote, they lobby, or they make financial contributions. Organizations also try to affect policy-making. These actions produce pressures on legislators and government officials. Policies result from very complex pressures and political processes.[4]

Even in the face of these political realities, a rational health technology policy can be designed. Such a policy should be both proactive, by identifying and supporting desirable technologies, and reactive to those who promote various technological agendas. This Janus-faced approach is not always easy: Do you first decide what you want to eat or first see what is on the menu? Other things being equal, it is probably best to know the full range of alternatives before making a choice.

In actual fact, much government policy, especially in less developed countries, sets priorities by ranking needs and pointing out problems or situations that could benefit from a technological solution. Where mortality or severe chronic disease is a factor, priorities may be establshed on the basis of YPLL (years of productive life lost) or QALY (quality-adjusted life-years)[5] gained.

Ideally, a new technology should result in an overall economic saving; however, new technologies rarely lower the price of medical care. The difficulty arises when, in a limited world, resources can be allocated to purpose A only by taking them away from purpose B. A good policy should foresee potential benefits and harm and balance the interests of various parties to further societal goals. In the event that an imported technology should produce adverse epidemiologic, economic, environmental, political, or cultural consequences, the policy should state, in broad and general terms, what should be done.

Imported technology may bring with it unanticipated benefits, such as:

- An educational significance beyond its obvious function
- Creating a consciousness in various levels of society about science and technology
- Stimulating scientific interest and investigation
- Helping to integrate science and technology into other sectors of national life
- Adding to the country's pool of skilled labor by training people to design, modify, operate, repair, and maintain equipment
- Improving managerial expertise, abilities that can be transferred to other uses in the future
- Serving as a nucleus for derivatives and spinoffs that create jobs and wealth

The Eternal Bridesmaid Syndrome

The rapid pace of technologic development may induce caution in adopting any particular technology because of the likelihood that a better one may be just around the next corner. This problem may lead to the eternal bridesmaid syndrome, in which one is unable to make a commitment while waiting for "Mr. Right" to come along. The institution that has just invested three million pesos in a new diagnostic scanner, however, may be dismayed to see the next generation of scanners advertised three months later for half the price and twice the efficiency. In contrast, the selection of a particular drug or vaccine may be easily changed once the current stock is exhausted (although an inappropriate drug can do more damage than an inappropriate scanner). The thoroughness of the prior assessment must be proportional to the degree of subsequent obligation to a particular technology.

Intellectual Property Rights

The control of intellectual property is an important lever by which the transfer of technology can be facilitated or retarded. Indeed, issues related to patents can sometimes prevent such movements altogether. Rich and poor countries often differ in their attitudes about the necessary disclosures of patentable subjects, and in many cases even in the patentability of entire categories of innovations. For example, in several countries products such as farm machinery, seeds and fertilizers, pharmaceuticals, and biologicals including hormones, vaccines, and diagnostic reagents considered to be for "the general good" of the people are simply not patentable. The foreign corporation, which has invested heavily in research and development, may be understandably reluctant to introduce its products into a country that does not uphold, or even recognize, its exclusive rights to the intellectual property.

Many other restrictions and limitations on patents are often not considered by health professionals. These laws, enacted in many developing countries, are intended to reduce the costs of importing technology and to protect local industry from foreign competition. Examples of such restrictions are prohibitions against the patenting of living organisms, limitations on the amount of patent licensing fees that can be charged, prohibition of certain patent licensing provisions, and limits on the duration of protection to as little as five years. In some countries patent protection is afforded only to processes, not products. A manufacturer in such a country could obtain a copy of the home country patent, which is a matter of public record, and make a trivial alteration in production conditions to yield the identical product that would be technically protected. Powerful trade and manufacturers' associations in industrialized countries are angered when pharmaceutical companies elsewhere legally produce drugs for their local market, even when they are patented elsewhere. More ominously, the outright piracy of processes and products within certain countries may be followed by punitive trade sanctions that can affect the entire economy.

The constraints on poor countries with a lack of resources and an abundance of health problems are easily understandable. Nevertheless, if sales prices are low and controlled, and if the expectation of profits is poor or nonexistent, it is no surprise that foreign companies are reluctant to enter the market. If that should happen the health technology policy of the potential importing country will be irrelevant because those technologies will never be made available.

Building Capacity in the Receiving Country's Research Environment

Various projects for transfer of technology have included training scientists and support staff in relevant methodologies in tasks ranging from the operation and maintenance of diagnostic hardware to the performance of complex techniques such as polymerase chain reactions, cell fusion for monoclonal antibody production, or cDNA library construction. While these abilities may be necessary in particular circumstances, the process of transferring technology must go further and help to support the development of underlying scientific capability in user countries.

In one country that I visited I was told with some derision by a local investigator that if they could, his laboratory staff would "come in at ten and leave at eleven." If true, such attitudes on the part of technicians are not easy to dispel in an atmosphere that gives little value to their work, where chances for advancement are minimal, and where financial and psychological rewards are grossly insufficient. Although local regulations often make it difficult to provide adequate incentives, motivation can be enhanced by encouraging and rewarding professionalism, reinforcing self-confidence, and building pride in the fulfillment of goals. The achievement of objectives can be aided by defining and overcoming obstacles in the scientific environment, clearing bottlenecks to progress, and strengthening local scientific capabilities. An approach to this process is not only to provide appropriate advice and materials but also to facilitate access of local investigators and students to the world scientific literature, to teach computer literacy, and to provoke discussion and intellectual curiosity about all sorts of scientific, ethical, and methodologic issues. This capacity building is costly and commonly neglected, but in the long run it is an essential part of technology transfer, and its absence can negate the potential of the most sophisticted science.

A Critical View of Technology Transfer

The former Director-General of WHO has said that "In too many instances, health technology is selected by individuals whose professional goals bear little resemblance to societies' health needs, or it is accumulated in a fortuitous and haphazard fashion . . . Technology for the sake of technology is a dangerous addiction-producing drug."[6] Others see the transfer and spread of technology as a threat rather than a benefit. Antitechnology activists work to prevent irradiation of foods, genetic engineering, nuclear power, use of pesticides, contraception, or other selected causes that they deem to be dreadful. In enlightened Switzerland, home of the WHO, a coalition of 50 environmental, animal rights, and consumer groups campaigned for two years to place broad restrictions on biomedical research involving genetically altered organisms. When put to a vote in June 1998 their proposal was defeated but it had the support of one third of the Swiss electorate.

The actual benefits to health of the application of a technology may be ambiguous and difficult to assess. Administrators often point to the resources made available (number of physicians, nurses, hospital beds, amount of money, and so forth) or the number of procedures or services provided, but these have little to do with the amount of health added to a population. Mortality and morbidity indicators may come somewhat closer to demonstrating health impact, but these lack information about the role of the technology in improving the quality of life, which after all is the main purpose of the entire enterprise.

Each technology must be considered independently for suitablility in each application, like a key and a lock. A key that works in one lock may be clearly ineffective in others. Some keys are masters, opening many different doors, while others have highly limited application. The same is true of technologies, depending on the specific goals and objectives of those who implement them. Some technologies, such as childhood immunizations, have received widespread endorsement, but even these must be reviewed periodically in each country.

In economically advanced countries, the controversy about investment and return in health care often centers on the costs and benefits of high technology hardware. Diagnostic imaging is a good example. In the 1970s it was CAT (computerized axial tomography) scanners. In the 1980s it was MRI (magnetic resonance imaging), a procedure formerly called NMR (nuclear magnetic resonance, whose name was changed through fear that the public would confuse the device with a nuclear power plant or bomb, with which it has no relation at all). These are powerful imaging techniques for scanning all or part of the body to produce cross-sectional computer-generated internal pictures useful for diagnosis. CAT and MRI are only diagnostic tools, helping to define certain problems in people who are already patients. Each machine can cost from several hundred thousand to several million dollars, plus space and personnel. Unending technical developments promise rapid obsolescence and reduction in price. There is no foreseeable limit on the devices that engineers can design or the amount of information that might possibly be of use to a physician.

Not only has expensive hardware been criticized as wasteful, but so have many sacrosanct medical procedures: the annual medical checkup, clinical laboratory tests, certain categories of surgery, intensive and coronary care units, the prescribing of drugs, and the deployment of highly trained medical personnel for routine duties. There is no foreseeable end to the types (and costs) of drugs, devices, and procedures that might benefit a patient, or that indeed may convert any imperfect citizen into a patient.

Can allegations about the irrelevance or counterproductiveness of certain medical procedures be evaluated, and can strategies be devised to correct deficiencies? One general methodology is the randomized controlled trial (RCT), a technique which allocates subjects on a statistically randomized basis to one or another group to assess the value of some procedure or intervention. Randomized controlled trials have been used to evaluate the efficacy of many modalities in prevention, diagnosis, and treatment, particularly in determination of drug regimens. It is certainly correct that the scientific method often calls for application of the RCT to pressing problems in the field of medical care, and of health services in general, but it is equally true that researchers who may wish to apply this basic decisional tool face many ethical and legal problems. How can a drug or procedure thought to be beneficial be withheld from some patients? How should a potentially useful but untried new intervention be tested in humans? These and many similar questions, often deceptively simple, are of crucial importance to the form and future of health care policies in many countries.

If excessively costly and perhaps unneeded technology constitutes one horn of a dilemma, then insufficient application of available technology represents the other. Half of the world's people have no access to modern health care at all, but, paradoxically, many available health facilities are underutilized. For various reasons, the world has many unused and underused technical capabilities for controlling disease and promoting health. In many developing countries scarce and expensive medical devices lie idle, while a significant number of physicians cannot find employment.

Parts of this chapter are adapted from Basch (1991a,b, 1993a,b).

NOTES

1. José López Portillo, former president of Mexico. Quoted by Whiting (1984).
2. Nevertheless, the economic consequences of performing many such procedures may be quite large.
3. Similarly, in the education sector, some people will get MDs and PhDs, or maybe both, but even they will finally stop.
4. Banta and Andreasen (1990).
5. See Chapter 4.
6. Mahler (1976).

11

The Cost of Sickness and the Price of Health

HEALTH AS WEALTH

One of the key issues in international health, and in national health programs for that matter, is determining how to spend available resources in the best way to achieve certain goals and objectives. Economics can help to provide a road map to get from here to there. The main issue in medical economics is not simply minimizing costs but obtaining the greatest *value* from the efficient use of resources. For a specific health problem we can try to get a better outcome for the same cost, or the same outcome at a lower cost (or, ideally, a better outcome at a lower cost).[1] Economics has become the unifying principle of international health in recent years, just as molecular science has done in biology and biomedicine.

> Health economics can be broadly defined as the application of the theories, concepts and techniques of economics to the institutions, actors and activities that affect health. It is concerned with such matters as the allocation of resources between various health-promoting activities; the quantity of resources used in health service delivery; the organisation, funding, and behaviour of health services institutions and providers; the efficiency with which resources are used for health purposes; and the effects of disease and health interventions on individuals, households, and society.[2]

The field of medical economics is vast and growing rapidly. A search of MEDLINE citations under the keyword *economics* showed 5230 entries for 1986. A decade later there were 9846 citations for the year, approximately 27 new journal articles about medical economics for every day of 1996, holidays and weekends included.

In the late 17th century there was no such deluge of information. William Petty, estimating the monetary value of a resident of England at between £69 and £90, decided that it was a good investment to take care of people's health. Later, the sanitary reformer Edwin Chadwick, in his 1842 *Report . . . on an Inquiry Into the Sanitary Condition of the Labouring Population of Great Britain*, estimated that ill health reduced national production by £14 million, at that time a great sum. As large factories developed in England and elsewhere, with workers becoming highly skilled in special tasks, managers became more and more aware of their monetary investment in the labor force. In the event of disability or death, workers and their families were faced with destitution, becoming burdens to society. Recognizing that this was not only a social problem, Chadwick wrote in 1862, "When the sentimentalist and moralist fails, he will have as a last resource to call in the aid of the economist."

At the same time, the development of life insurance in the 19th century drew further attention to the monetary value of human life. The stage was now set for the establishment, in Bismarck's Germany of 1883, of social paternalism, including compulsory health insurance for poor industrial workers and their families (see Chapter 12). Since that time, health, government, and economics have been inextricably tied together. Hector Acuña, a former Director of the Pan American Health Organization, has written:

> With the increasing role of health planning on the one hand and economic development planning on the other, the need for better understanding of how the level of health influences the economy, and for quanitification of its effects, has received ever more attention. The true integration of health plans into national development plans requires more complete knowledge than we now have of the economic gains that may be possible through improving the condition of health.[3]

Economic development is closely linked with the state of individual and public health, and health programs must be seen as part of a nation's economic development strategy. The economic costs of operating health and medical services also demands attention by government planners. However, governments and consumers are not the only players, for the commercial aspects of health are growing everywhere. The practice of medicine is moving rapidly from a profession to a business. The increasing volume of articles and books on the economics of health underscores both the significance and the attention being paid to this subject. But apparently more is needed: "While methodologists debate the elegant theoretical niceties of valuing human life, practitioners are still trying to figure out how much it costs to operate a health center, who is going to pay for it, how many people are likely to use it and how many deaths it might prevent."[4]

Because a population is made up of individuals, it may be well to look first at the microeconomic level to see the relationship between health and wealth for a person, and then try to generalize to the community and national levels.

The Monetary Value of a Life

Economists and health planners may view each human being as possessing a certain monetary value. There is first of all a cost involved in pregnancy and childbirth—loss of maternal earnings, consumption of special foods, prenatal care, and delivery. In industrialized countries this cost may be very high. In poor countries there may be little cash investment in a pregnancy, but other costs may accrue, such as the value of productive time lost by the pregnant woman, reduced attention to other children, and the time spent by family and midwives. The cost of rearing a child is recognized as an economic investment, and its death represents the loss of all these expenditures, plus parental time that was devoted to the child. In less developed countries where the economic base is already very low, and where half or more of all deaths may occur by age five, infant and child mortality represent a very great financial burden added to the severe emotional toll.

In addition to the costs of rearing and maintenance, a person's economic value can be described from one viewpoint by his or her present and future earning power (the human capital approach). When dealing with such calculations involving a long time span, economists always consider both the present and discounted monetary values. A unit of money has different values when obtained or spent at different times, and the process of discounting changes the future "stream" of earnings (or other benefits) into its present cash value. Premature death, defined as death before retirement from productive work, clearly results in the loss of all future earnings. Another approach to the value of a life is, as with any other commodity, to see how much people are prepared to pay for it; in this case, to reduce their (or another's) risk of dying.

Figure 11-1 recalls previous work on the economic value of individuals of different ages in developing countries. In the early 1970s Enke and Brown concluded that "preventing the death of a man of age 30 is ordinarily more worthwhile to his national economy than preventing the death of a young child of 5 years."[5] Although the authors acknowledge that their analysis illustrates a "dehumanized economic viewpoint," they argue for the establishment of "an explicit basis for allocating doctors' energies and clinics' resources that are financed by government. This criterion should be understandable and defensible." A quarter century later apologies are no longer offered as economic studies have come to the forefront. In the 1970s and 80s, resources to prevent premature deaths were concentrated on child survival and maternal and child health programs in developing countries. In these areas the proportion of persons under age 15 typically exceeds 40% or more of the total population, and a large proportion of all deaths are readily and cheaply preventable. Starting from a much lower baseline for their health establishments, poor countries will achieve a proportionately far higher impact for a given level of health expenditure than will wealthy countries. Cost-effectiveness is not an inherent characteristic of specific interventions but is highly sensitive to context. It is a truism that the big-

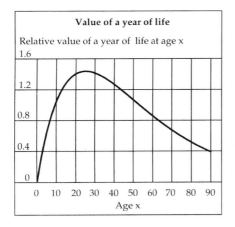
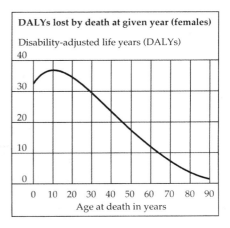

Figure 11-1 The Global Burden of Disease study (see text) recorded all deaths and estimated disabilities by age, sex, and demographic region for 1990. Death and disability losses were combined with allowance made for a discount rate of 3%, so future years of healthy life were valued at progressively lower levels; and for age weights, so that years of life lost at different ages were given different relative values. The value for each year of life lost (left hand panel) rises steeply from zero at birth to a peak at age 25 and then declines gradually with increasing age. The right-hand curve shows the number of DALYs lost by the death of a female at various ages (e.g., 32.5 DALYs at birth, 29 DALYs at age 30, and 12 DALYs at age 60). Values for males are slightly lower. See the original for details. *Source:* World Bank, World Development Report (1993). Box 1.3.

ger the existing health sector, the more money it will take to have a measurable effect. Even among high-income countries, some (e.g., Japan) apply health expenditures more efficiently than others (e.g., United States).[6]

If we accept that individuals, on average, have different economic value at different ages, then one might expect that more resources would be devoted to those at the most productive time of their lives. Considering medical expenditures alone, that is not the case. Table 11-1 shows that in the United States expenditures are moderate, and increasing least rapidly, for middle-aged people. Not unexpectedly, the elderly consume a very high proportion of all health expenditures. Here, social and cultural considerations clearly precede the strictly economic in establishing priorities, as one would expect that large medical expenditures near the end of life would not be a very profitable investment.

Due to substantial reduction in child mortality, nearly 90 percent of children in developing countries survive to be adults, even in some of the poorest countries of sub-Saharan Africa. Too many of these adults still die relatively young . . . and too many suffer from chronic impairments and frequent illnesses and injuries. Their ill-health imposes a major burden on health services as well as large, negative consequences on families, communities, and societies. Demographic trends and changes in exposure to risk

Table 11-1. Average Annual Health Spending and Increase in Health Spending, by Age, United States, 1963 and 1987

Age Group	Spending, $ per capita[a] 1963	1987	Average Annual Increase in Health Spending, % 1963 to 1987
Under 1	236	2503	9.8
1–4	164	655	5.8
5–14	175	466	4.1
15–24	353	881	3.8
25–34	435	1058	3.7
35–44	456	1095	3.6
45–54	566	1742	4.7
55–64	571	2410	6.0
65–74	622	3874	7.6
75–84	689	4694	8.0
85+	447	5650	10.6

[a]Average spending is in real (1987) dollars using the GDP deflator.

Source: Cutler and Meara (1997) Appendix Table A-1.

factors have had the effect of increasing the absolute and relative importance of adults and their health problems. Nevertheless, policy development in the area of adult health is weak, and the research necessary to support sound policy decisions has been neglected.[7]

Such remarks should not suggest a tug-of-war for resources between the humanitarian child advocates of UNICEF and the "cold-hearted accountants" of the World Bank. What they indicate is a steady shift in interpreting the significance and solution of international health issues.

It is clear that policy decisions about the distribution of resources to health services for specific segments of the population must be linked to decisions about family planning, education, economic growth, employment, the environment, and all of the other interlocking elements that comprise national planning in any country. All of these are aspects of investment in the future, and all require a future-oriented pattern of thinking, which is not equally developed in all countries.

Health as an Investment: The Individual

Illness in sufficient degree results in loss of working time (disability) and in reduced effectiveness or productivity (debility), both leading to economic loss. In addition, money may be spent on medical care, drugs, special foods, or devices necessary to cope with an illness. Hence the cost of ill health has at least two aspects: direct expenses to alleviate the condition and indirect losses from unrealized production, lost schoolwork, and the like. Where the individual is not covered by any sort of insurance or social welfare scheme, these costs must be borne privately, usually within the household.

It is in the interest of society to minimize the costs of ill health, disability, and premature death, and that is a major justification for preventive, curative, and rehabilitative health care. Insofar as expenditures for health lead to increased productivity and earnings, or reduce the need for later medical care, they are an investment. Insofar as such expenditures serve only to eliminate trivial symptoms or to enchance social status (e.g., by cosmetic surgery) they can be considered as consumption, equal to the purchase of any other commodity. The relationships between the investment and the consumption aspects of health expenditures have occupied many economists: How are improvements in the quality of life and the quality of people to be considered?

Compare the investment in health with that in education. Both forms of investment increase an individual's productivity, effectiveness, and future labor product, and they also enhance his function as a consumer. Better health improves the investment in education not only by reducing absences from school, and perhaps improving learning ability, but also by increasing the life span, thus providing a greater long-term return from schooling. It has been shown many times that education, especially for girls, leads to better family health. The inverse relationship between infant mortality and maternal education has been well established.[8] Investments in both health and education have external benefits to the community at large. In both cases, active participation of the family and individual is important. The preservation and restoration of health come not only from "being doctored" any more than learning comes only from "being taught."

Public Goods, Private Goods, and Externalities

Economists separate *public goods* from *private goods*. The idea behind public goods is that use by one person does not leave less available for others to consume. For example, if an area is sprayed against malaria-carrying mosquitoes the benefit to any person is the same regardless of the benefit to any other person in the same area. Clean air, road safety, fluoridation, education, and the knowledge from research are other examples of public goods. Private markets in general do not work in this way, because individuals buy and consume items from a limited pool. Private markets by themselves provide too little of the public goods necessary for health, and therefore government involvement is needed to increase the supply of these goods. Private goods benefit only the persons who consume them. If they are consumed by one person they cannot be consumed by another. Most medical services and commodities such as drugs are private goods.

Some health-related goods have an effect on other people who may not consume them directly. These effects are called *externalities*. For example, in infectious disease epidemiology there is a phenomenon called *herd immunity*. As the amount of, say, circulating measles virus diminishes in a population, the likelihood is reduced that an unimmunized person will get measles. As more people become immune and removed as a potential source of virus, others will be relatively more protected. When my child is immunized against measles, that protects your child to some extent: that is a *positive health externality*. Immunization programs carry large positive externalities; pollution of air and water or sale of alcohol to drivers creates *negative health externalities*. Behaviors that carry positive externalities should be encouraged, and those with negative externalities should be discouraged by financial, legal, or other disincentives.

ECONOMIC ANALYSIS IN THE HEALTH SECTOR

Economic studies reflect a recognition that resources of all kinds (human, financial, material, informational) have limits and that they can be squandered or used productively. Improvements in knowledge and technology are presenting more alternative ways to do things, forcing choices to be made. Economic analysis offers one basis upon which to make such choices.

Cost–Benefit Analysis

People responsible for planning and financing any project want to know the return that they may expect on their investment. Implicit in their decision-making is the idea that costs and benefits can be measured, or at least estimated and projected. The business investor can usually tell just how much profit (or loss) has accrued from a transaction. as costs and benefits are stated in money terms. Investments in health cannot furnish such exact figures because the monetary benefit often comes in the form of averted future costs. We spend something today in the hope of avoiding losses from illness, disability, and death and the medical expenses that these would have incurred. The main problem is that while immediate costs can be stated easily, the future savings are difficult to demonstrate with accuracy. There are of course noncash benefits in better health, increased well-being, and longevity that are even harder to quantitate.

Preventive measures that avert future costs altogether seem clearly the best ways to spend health money. It is paradoxical that such programs are most valuable, but least visible, precisely when nothing happens. Parents do not notice it when their child does get hepatitis or diphtheria or is not paralyzed by polio, nor do they recognize the "extra" money that was not spent on them. That stability and tranquility is the goal and purpose of pubic health, but when there is no epidemic it is difficult to convince those who pay that they are getting their money's worth. If an immunization program has reduced the incidence of measles by 95%, the absence of big outbreaks may suggest to government officials that there no longer is any problem, and they may decide to spend their money on some other pressing problem. But it is precisely then that continued control is needed. If control work is stopped for reasons of politics or false economy, measles could return in an epidemic wave and the previous investment in measles control would have been wasted.

In the absence of any apparent urgency for a particular health expenditure, the choice is frequently to do nothing, especially where there are many competing calls for resources. However, doing nothing may incur an eventual cost greater than that of the preventive measure. Many people find it too burdensome to brush and floss their teeth because they seem all right today, but in the long run inadequate dental hygiene can lead to the need for costly dentures and other painful consequences. In choosing among alternative programs, none at all is an important option, and perhaps the most expensive in the long run.

Other forms of prevention, particularly immunization, have been favorite subjects of health economists because fairly specific data are often available. But before vaccines can be used they must be developed. A study of research expenditures on poliomyelitis vaccines estimated that the most likely rate of return is about 11% to 12% per year, without counting benefits outside the United States.[9]

The prime example of a successful vaccination program is the worldwide campaign against smallpox (see Chapter 14). D.A. Henderson, formerly director of the World Health Organization Smallpox Campaign, has estimated that eradication of smallpox saves the world's governments more than one billion dollars annually, forever. Moreover, the elimination of vaccination and smallpox quarantine measures saved the United States alone, in less than 30 months, every penny contributed to the World Health Organization since its founding 28 years before. To this monetary saving must be added the averted loss of lives and the blindness, disfigurement, and other effects of smallpox.

Detailed estimates of the cost–benefit ratio were made during a five-year (1979–1984) immunization campaign in Indonesia.[10] Pregnant women were immunized against tetanus, and infants against tuberculosis with BCG; and against diphtheria, pertussis, and tetanus with DPT vaccine. Costs included the total program expenditures minus the remainder at termination. Benefits were allocated as follows:

- Avoided treatment costs, traditional and western
- Value of mothers' time spent in home care
- Avoided loss of agricultural wages, depending upon season
- Income gains from prevented mortality

It was concluded that benefits would continue to accrue for years after the formal termination of the campaign. Between the start of the program in 1979, and continuing to 1993, a total of about 3.5 million cases and 250,000 deaths would be averted. Total program costs of around 13 billion rupiahs would yield an extended benefit to 1993 of about 59 billion rupiahs, with a net present value (at 15%) of more than 12 billion rupiahs of positive benefit. These estimates represent a conservative analysis of benefits and do not include societal benefit from reduced transmission of the diseases, completion of schoolwork by immunized children, or reduction of maternal mortality by protection against tetanus.

We cannot enter into a discussion of the enormous literature on costs and benefits of procedures in clinical medicine, including drug therapy and surgery, except to point out that this is an area of active investigation and clashing opinions.

Cost–benefit analyses are useful only when both costs and benefits can be defined in roughly equivalent terms and estimated by some rational method. Moreover, the presence of a disease in an area does not inevitably result in measurable economic loss, nor does the availability of a vaccine necessarily bring cost savings. In many instances a good case cannot be made for implementation of a control campaign: there is a good deal of controversy, for example, about the advisability of large-scale use of chickenpox vaccine

Cost–benefit analyses suffer from several drawbacks that limit their usefulness as a guide to decisions on health policy. Many published studies are retrospective, perhaps justifying past programs in the defense of health planners. More significantly, it is not really so easy to quantify costs and benefits. Creative bookkeeping can skew figures one way or the other. Many procedures depend on the prior existence of facilities, trained personnel, and the total related infrastructure. How can this be accounted for in the calculations? The significance of the time element is often neglected—that is, assets are valued at purchase, not replacement cost, and depreciation and discounting are not done or are done incorrectly. The cost of purchasing additional units of the service (marginal cost) should normally be used rather than just totaling all costs and dividing by the number of units produced (average cost); similarly, all costs should be figured, not just monetary outlays.[11]

Cost–benefit analyses are done not only on personal health services but also on engineering projects such as water supplies and dams, where benefits come not only in improved health status but as electric power and irrigation, both of which have powerful indirect feedback benefits on health. As mentioned earlier, dams in tropical Africa may also have a down side, as the lakes formed upstream can provide breeding sites for malaria-carrying mosquitoes and snail hosts of schistosomiasis; and the rapids downstream can foster blackflies that transmit river blindness. In fact any intervention, however useful, may have unintended drawbacks and side effects. This introduces into the equation a third factor, risk. Dams may spread disease, and vaccines have unavoidable adverse effects. Vaccination against smallpox carries a small but calculable risk (about 12.3 per million) of vaccinial encephalitis with possible permanent brain damage, and death may occur once per million vaccinations. At some point in an effective control effort the risks may come to outweigh the benefits. When the U.S. Public Health Service observed that no known case of smallpox had been brought into the U.S. in the previous two decades, the risk from vaccination was judged greater than the risk of introduction of smallpox in the absence of vaccination, and the program for routine childhood smallpox vaccination was terminated.[12] Cost–benefit–risk analysis is thus seen as a tool with which to discontinue as well as to introduce health programs.

A strident anti-immunization campaign has long been waged in some European countries based on reported cases of permanent brain damage or death from whole-cell pertussis vaccine. The Swedish government decided in 1979 to terminate the routine use of whole-cell pertussis (whooping cough) vaccine in infants because of its reputed adverse effects. As a result, many cases of pertussis occurred in the unprotected children. In 1981, safer acellular pertussis vaccines with reduced incidence of adverse effects were licensed for routine use in Japan. Accordingly, a field trial of two Japanese acellular vaccines was set up in Sweden and the benefits of the new vaccines were verified. These improved vaccines have now been licensed in many countries, including the United States, with a monitoring and surveillance system set up to detect and report possible adverse events among the large pool of routine recipients. This is an example of how advances in technology can affect the cost–benefit–risk equation. Some ethical aspects of these trials are discussed in Chapter 15.

Cost-Effectiveness Analysis

Cost–benefit analysis, at home in the corporate boardroom, is a strategy for identifying maximum return on investment. Cost-beneficial programs should of course be promoted by health planners, but their investment decisions must also be based on a determination of social needs. The aim of health planning is the achievement of certain policy goals for improvement of the health of the population. Once these are determined, planners must find the best means to reach them. For this purpose the tool of cost-effectiveness analysis is often used. This type of analysis leads to a decision as to the best way to expend resources in order to achieve a particular predefined goal.

A good illustration of the use of cost-effectiveness analysis involved 15 years of studies and 150 publications about schistosomiasis control on the Caribbean island of St. Lucia.[13] One intention of the study, funded by the Rockefeller Foundation, was to determine the most cost-effective way to reduce transmission of the parasite *Schistosoma mansoni* among residents of the island.[14]

Three intensive experimental programs were undertaken, each in different valleys on the island, to evaluate three basic strategies for control. These were: (1) snail control by mollusciciding (= poisoning), to reduce populations of the intermediate host; (2) provision of domestic water supplies, plus in some areas communal laundry and shower units and swimming pools, to reduce exposure to infection in rivers and streams; and (3) chemotherapy, to reduce contamination of the environment with parasite eggs shed by infected people. Summarized results are shown in Table 11-2. Note that capital and operational costs per resident vary greatly from one control method to another and bear little relationship to the efficacy of control. Each method has its own external benefits and drawbacks, and the total picture must be considered before programmatic decisions can be made. In this lengthy study external funds were expended, quite successfully, for purposes of research. That is a quite a different matter from the expenditure of local government funds for an operational program, but without the prior research, funds for a control program might well be misspent.

Screening programs have also been analyzed from the cost-effectiveness viewpoint. Here the purpose is not primary prevention of disease but the identification of undetected early or inapparent cases so that further pathology can be reduced and a costly clinical illness avoided.[15] Tests for early tuberculosis and trachoma are in this category, as are Pap smears and mammograms to reduce risk of invasive cervical and breast cancer, respectively. In some tropical areas, community-wide screening for filariasis can lead to early treatment of those found infected and prevent the development of elephantiasis. This condition is not only painful and disfiguring but leads to loss of economic productivity. For HIV infections or other conditions for which no cure is currently available, early detection is still economically beneficial if the infected person can be treated and avoid transmission to others,

Table 11-2. Comparative Costs and Effectiveness of Alternative Schistosomiasis Control Strategies, St. Lucia, 1970–1980

	Strategy		
	Water Supply	Snail Control	Chemotherapy
Number of subjects	2000	5000	3000
		Costs, $	
Capital	72,266	2,727	0
Per person per year	1.81	0.12	0
Operational (recurrent)	23,943	74,338	11,904
Per person per year	2.99	3.24	1.00
Total per person per year	4.80	3.36	1.00
Reduction in transmission	32%	46%	88%

Source: Adapted from Jordan (1985).

who would incur further illness, loss of productivity, and medical expenses. An additional benefit of screening programs is that the epidemiological information they generate is useful in planning public health control measures.

It must be emphasized that a program or procedure may be highly cost-beneficial and cost-effective and still not be *affordable*.

The Idea of Insurance

Preventive practices such as immunization and screening are intended to reduce health risks and their costs. We will never know if the immunized child would have gotten measles, or polio, in the absence of the vaccine, but we are willing to pay for the procedure and endure the small risk of adverse effects to increase the probability that the illness will be avoided. In the same way you will never know whether a lifetime of spartan denial, exercise, and rabbit food really staved off that dreaded coronary that didn't happen or whether your earnest sacrifices actually made no difference.

If we knew exactly what would happen to our health we could make specific arrangements, but any of us can be hit by a car or a virus when we least expect it. While the degree of uncertainty that exists for individuals is great, it is less so for populations, in which risks can be projected with a fair degree of confidence. Conversely, at the individual level events are definable and definitive. You get lung cancer or you do not; you die of congestive heart failure or you do not. In contrast to clear-cut outcomes for individuals, probabilities obtain at the group level. Many people have difficulty in understanding the difference between group probabilities imposed on everyone to generate a pooled risk, and the actual experience of each person within that group.

The idea of risk evokes thoughts of insurance and the experience of professional risk managers. Health insurance in one form or another has been around for centuries, but the recent expansion of health maintenance organizations (HMOs) in the United States and elsewhere assures that insurors and health professionals will have a lot more to say to each other. The key element to insurors is their expectation of certain events based on the illness, disability, or mortality patterns of large pools of individuals. Based on their experience the insuror averages all the individual risks over the entire pool of policyholders to come up with the expected number of payouts in any time period. They do not know, or really care, what happens to any one person. Their risk is financial and based on the proportion of policyholders to undergo a covered event and incur an expense.

Individuals, in contrast, are not interested in the group's experience but in their own health and survival, including their financial survival. Private insurors who find that an applicant has an increased risk of illness or death will charge a higher premium, or delay or reduce benefits, or may deny coverage altogether. That is called risk selection and is the norm in unregulated markets and for voluntary personal coverage. The differences in risk between one individual and another are surprisingly large. In the United States just 1% of persons under age 65 use 27% of all the resources spent for health in that age group, and 10% of people under 65 use 70% of the resources.[16] The costliest 10% of infants, prematures with acute conditions, account for 89% of excess expenditures.[17] Publicly funded insurance programs will not select individuals on the basis of risk as a matter of policy and to promote equity. Their regulations may require private insurors to accept everyone and charge level premums, particularly if the insurance coverage is compulsory.[18] Conversely, if a person knows himself to be at high risk of serious illness, he will want to get the coverage for precisely the same reason that the insuror does not want to give it.

Insurors understand that a person who is completely covered against all risk may behave less prudently than if he or she lacked the coverage. The term *moral hazard* is used to describe the tendency of policyholders to take less care to reduce hazards against which they are insured.[19] The cost of such behavior is transferred to all other policyholders in the form of increased premiums or reduced benefits, regardless of whether the insurance is provided by governments through taxation, through the private sector, or a combination of the two. Insured people also tend to use their benefits liberally: "After all, it's free!" To discourage excessive use through hypochondria or malingering, and to save money for all taxpayers, policyholders or health plan members, the insuror may require some form of cost sharing such as a copayment or fee at each visit. The insuror may also place limits on certain types of claims, or insure for limited periods of time with frequent renewability of coverage. It seems improbable that people will intentionally neglect their health or take on risky behaviors just because they have health insurance, but that certainly does happen.

Public health services are paradoxical. Prevention has often been demonstrated to be relatively cost-effective. Unfortunately, paying for a public health service is sometimes considered like paying for insurance. Some people feel that their annual insurance premium was wasted if they did not have an accident during that year. Therefore they may decide, *ex post facto*, that they probably can get by the next year without the expense of the insurance premium. Perhaps they will, but having a major accident without insurance is a hard way to learn. The same is true of expenditures for sustained basic public health work.

HOW MUCH IS ENOUGH?

We have seen that some programs, such as routine childhood smallpox vaccination in the United States, reached a negative cost–benefit balance and were then terminated. It is often a more difficult matter to know when the societal goals of a program have been achieved so that money and effort can be devoted to other ends. Such decisions can not be made by a computer or abstract formula because they must reflect the prevailing spirit and culture. Nevertheless there are certain general principles of risk management that can apply to public policy. Say that you are a government official who must decide on the maximum acceptable number of workers to be injured in industrial accidents in your country. If your answer is zero, then the next question is: How much are you willing to pay to achieve zero injuries, and how could you do it? Reducing accidents to some very small number may be achievable at a reasonable cost to society. But there is a number below which the incremental cost of preventing the next accident will be more than the cost to society of letting the next accident occur. The same is true of infant deaths. Can the infant mortality rate ever become too low?

Before giving a categorical negative answer to this question, we must look at the causes, consequences, and control of infant mortality. Neonatal deaths are often caused by congenital anomalies, prematurity, and trauma at delivery. We have seen in Chapter 7 that socioeconomic development is often accompanied by a rapid decline in infant mortality, most of which is in the postneonatal period. In the process, expenditures attributable to health services in the broad sense are largely in the areas of promotion and prevention: water supply, sanitation, immunization, maternal care and education, and so on, which are low on a *per capita* basis. In terms of added years of life, these expenditures in developing countries are highly cost-beneficial and cost-effective.

In developed countries where infant mortality rates are already very low, a different picture is found, and early infant deaths predominate. Some further reductions in infant deaths may be achieved by improving prenatal care; better nutrition; education to reduce use of tobacco, alcohol, and other drugs; and careful maternal monitoring. Further reductions may result from better delivery room techniques, but there is a residue of cases arising from genetic defects or developmental anomalies whose rescue may require heroic medical effort. As clinical expertise and technology improve, an increasing proportion of such births becomes salvageable. Life support systems can maintain many infants, who formerly would have died, until they can manage on their own. Some may survive with handicaps, either correctable by surgery or requiring lengthy (or permanent) medical care. Some may pull through and develop normally, but these individuals may carry genes that will necessitate similar medical efforts a generation later, fostering dependence on medical technology. The struggle for ever-greater minimization of infant mortality also involves genetic counseling, fetal monitoring, amniocentesis, and therapeutic abortion, and such indirect steps as maternal immunization against rubella and tetanus. The remaining stubborn core of deaths becomes a subject of ever more complex research.

Clearly, the cost per life saved now increases very rapidly, and it is likely that the average quality of saved lives also declines. Is there a point at which society is willing to accept a certain level of infant deaths in order to devote the resultant savings to other purposes? Many groups have struggled with this question. In the United States the 1982 court case of "Baby Doe," a severely ill infant with spina bifida, mandated that all possible efforts must be made to keep the child alive regardless of cost. A decade later in Singapore a Ministerial Committee on Health Policies concluded that physicians must judge whose need is greater and who can benefit most, "taking into account the medical condition of individual patients and working within the overall resource constraints." They decided not to pay for several procedures[20] and left the following decisions to professional judgment:

- Aggressive treatment of incurable diseases where there is no chance of survival
- Long term life-support for severely brain-damaged patients with no chance of recovery
- Intensive care for very premature newborns who are unlikely to survive and whose long term prospects, even if they survive, are uncertain

Risk can never be eliminated from life. Achieving a zero risk will incur an infinite cost. If zero cases is not a reasonably achieveable option, what number is? Is it possible that being too risk free is not worth the cost? The decisions of society to spend its resources to reduce health risks may not be the most cost-effective ones, and it is likely that collectively we pay more than we should for gains that are less than we could achieve because we misinterpret risks.

Economists use the concept of the *margin*—the amount of benefit that will accrue from a given additional expenditure—as a fundamental tool. This concept has been discussed for health expenditures by Fuchs, who points out the difference between the economist's and the health professional's view of the "optimum" level of health:

> For the health professional, the "optimum" level is the highest level technically attainable, regardless of the cost of reaching it. The economist is preoccupied with the social optimum, however, which he defines as the point at which the value of an additional increment of health exactly equals the cost of the resources required to obtain that increment. For instance, the first few days of hospital stay after major surgery might be extremely valuable for preventing complications and assisting recovery, but at some point the value of each additional day decreases. As soon as the value of an additional day falls below the cost of that day's care, according to the concept of social optimum, the patient should be discharged.[21]

On a global scale the reduction in infant mortality discussed above is paralleled by reductions in mortality at other ages also. Figure 11-2 shows a series of survivorship curves that span the entire range of patterns of human mortality. The mortality experienced by India early in the present century lies near the maximum sustainable by a human population. Per thousand live births, about the same number

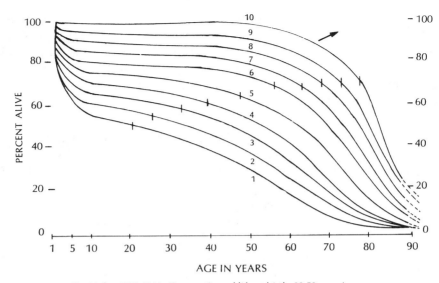

Figure 11-2 Survivorship curves, by age and sex, selected countries, 1861–1974. The small vertical bars on each line represent the expectation of life at birth.
Source: Basch (1990). Fig. 8-2.

would survive to age one for Indian males in 1901–1911 as to age 70 for Swedish females in 1974. It seems possible for any population eventually to approach or perhaps surpass line 10, moving the curve in the direction of the arrow. The policy question is: Where shall we set our goals, and how much are we willing to pay (i.e., what else are we willing to give up) to achieve them? The economic questions are: How much will it cost? How can sufficient money be obtained? And how should the expenditures be allocated?

Both the policy and the economic questions are clouded by uncertainty, in part because we do not know how much of the increases in life expectancy (or reductions in mortality) are due to general socioeconomic development, to behavior patterns and ways of life, to the effects of health services, or to other factors. Even within the health services sector, we do not know the relative benefits of public health, prevention, or medical care. Despite the analyses detailed on the preceding pages, the alliance between economics and health may be more of a shotgun wedding than an undying romance. In 1972 it was observed that:

> In this brave new world where emphasis is on quantitative planning, the health sector is often regarded as a backward, underdeveloped area. Indeed, there is a tendency for the economic planner to treat the health planner as a dunce, ignorant as he often is of econometrics and innocent of regression analysis . . . It is because the doctor often suspects the economist of being incapable of thinking beyond economic criteria that the dialogue between [them] is so often unfruitful.[22]

Twenty-five years later an economist confirmed the point: "Perhaps because the subject has been dominated by health professionals, much if not most of the world's thinking about health system organization is uncontaminated by economic insight."[23]

Even though it is difficult to determine the best basis for making decisions in the health sector, we can ask whether most health services are doing a good job at their assigned tasks. Are health resources within countries utilized on a problem-solving basis, with appriate mixes of preventive, curative, promotive, and rehabilitative services? Which medical interventions are truly effective and specific? Can these be described so that the necessary skill and knowledge for their application can be assessed? Can health care systems be designed to carry out the tasks to reach the greatest proportion of persons at risk, as early as possible, at the least cost, and in an acceptable manner? These questions have been asked by the former Director General of the World Health Organization, who observed that persons outside the health establishment might

> even express astonishment at these questions because many fondly assume that their health services are designed to deal with problems; the interventions they pay for are known to be effective and appropriate; and the person who is responsible for the medical care they receive is the appropriate person in training and position for their needs. Such is not the case.[24]

The Effectiveness of Medical and Health Expenditures

Because all mortals are fallible, we should look for evidence to support or refute this rather gloomy opinion, even though it comes from an authority in world health. One place to look is in the correlation between the amounts of money spent on health care and the level of health in various countries. Several investigators have studied annual health expenditures per capita (or the percentage of GNP devoted to health services) and age- and sex-specific mortality rates in various countries. For large blocks of countries there is a general correlation (Table 11-3), but among the wealthier countries the correlation is poor. We recall Wilkinson's finding that beyond a certain level of health expenditures there is no predictable relationship be-

Table 11-3. Health Expenditure and Indicators, by Demographic Regions, 1990

Region	Population		Expenditure				Child Mortality[a]	Life Expectancy
	Million	%/ World	$Billion	%/ World	$ Per Capita	% of GNP		
Established market economies	798	15	1,483	87	1,860	9.2	11	76
Formerly socialist economies	346	7	49	3	142	3.6	22	72
Demo-graphically developing	4,123	78	170	10	41	4.7	106	63
Latin America[b]	444	8	47	3	105	4.0	60	70
Middle Eastern crescent	503	10	39	2	77	4.1	111	61
China	1,134	22	13	1	11	3.5	43	69
Other Asia and islands	683	13	42	2	61	4.5	97	62
India	850	16	18	1	21	6.0	127	58
Sub-Saharan Africa	510	10	12	1	24	4.5	175	52
World	5,267	100	1,702	100	329	8.0	96	65

Source: Adapted from World Bank (1993) Table 1, p. 2 and Table 3.1, p. 52.

[a]Probability of dying between birth and age 5, per thousand live births.

[b]And Caribbean.

tween improved health on the one hand and the additional amount or cost of resources devoted to health services on the other. In view of this apparent discrepancy we can ask whether in some countries health problems are simply more expensive than in others (which is possible), whether in some countries money is being
spent unproductively (which is likely), and whether there are other societal goals
being bought besides reduction of mortality and morbidity (which is highly probable).

In very poor countries where basic needs are unmet, money spent for promotive,
protective, and primary care services can result in relatively large and rapid improvements in health indicators and have significant external benefits (to the community at large). Poor people usually have inexpensive possessions, and this includes their illnesses. Hookworm, cholera, and amebiasis cost very little to get,
compared with a sports-car accident, a transplant rejection, or even ischemic heart
disease. Diseases cheaply acquired may also be relatively cheaply prevented (al-

though not always cheaply treated). Although capital investments in water supply and sewerage systems are high, their long service life and broad utility can make them very cost-beneficial to users from a health standpoint alone, not to mention the accompanying improvement in the standard of living. With advancing development and per capita income, most of the problems attributable to malnutrition, poor sanitation, and other manifestations of poverty will decline, and health dollars (or pesos or rupees) are increasingly spent to improve the quality, rather than the quantity, of life.

Why does the recognizable benefit derived from the health care enterprise correlate so poorly with the costs involved? Why do different individuals and different countries buy different amounts of health for the same amount of money? Part of the answer lies in distinguishing central from peripheral aspects of personal medical care.

We can identify a central cluster of practices and procedures essential to maintaining or restoring good health whose application is both cost-beneficial and cost-effective. This core of interventions, sometimes termed the *essential package*, is embedded within a far broader area replete with practices and procedures that cost more than their social value. These peripheral elements may be sought for a variety of purposes considered of value by the persons concerned but not really essential for health and providing no positive externalities to the community. As longevity in the United States has reached a high level, much of the attention of pharmaceutical companies and physicians is diverted to products and procedures to enhance appearance or performance rather than save lives. The distinction is becoming blurred between so-called *recreational drugs*, which are illegal, and *lifestyle-enhancing drugs*, which are merely expensive. Countries and regions are increasingly establishing priorities for public funding and classifying procedures into essential and nonessential, as discussed further in the next chapter.

There is another problem, and that is in local medical practices. Nobody would argue with the need for a hysterectomy in a woman with uterine cancer or certain other indications. Hysterectomy is therefore clearly an essential procedure *for those patients*. But what if hysterectomies were performed on women who did not "really need" them or did not benefit (or were even harmed) by them? In the United States, it was found that

> There are no data on what proportion of women, on the balance, are benefited by elective hysterectomy. While the benefits are unmeasured and uncertain, the costs are large. These costs are rarely paid by the patient. Society, if it is to pay the costs, must decide whether to allocate public funds for a procedure if it appears to be more of a convenience or luxury than a necessity. [25]

The same dilemma is true for many other medical procedures in the United States and elsewhere: Too many coronary bypass operations, too many caesarean sections, too few controls. Physicians are adamant that outsiders should not make such judgments, but over time clinical decision-making is slowly being infused with economic accountability.

Understanding the "Health Market"

Any consideration of a health market must deal with the specifics of place and time because these are so diverse in the real world. Persons in poor areas have limited access to medical facilities and even less choice about the care they may receive. Therefore there is little in the way of a "market" to discuss. In the western world numerous competing choices may be available to generate a complex marketplace for health-related products of all kinds. We need to consider here at least six interconnected factors. *First*, the "health market" uses money differently from the more familiar market of goods and services. For personal medical care in particular, the patient (i.e., the consumer) has very little control over how his or her money is spent. Whereas a television set or a theater ticket can be bought now or delayed with little consequence, an accident or illness may require (or may seem to require) immediate medical care. Once the decision has been made by, or for, a person to enter the medical system as a patient, someone else then takes charge of further expenditures. The medical profession, by special knowledge and legal privilege through licensure, maintains exclusive control of procedures, prescriptions, and facilities. Decisions about diagnostic tests, surgery, medicines, return visits, and many other costly "purchases" are made not by the consumer but by the physician. Moreover, the choice of grade, size, quality, and cost per item, usually available to the consumer, is also absent. The consumer is not only essentially powerless to control expenditures but often ignorant of the need for the particular item in the first place. Most importantly, however, it is generally impossible after the money has been spent to tell whether the expenditure was necessary, useful, or even harmful. The dissatisfied customer in wealthier countries may try to obtain a second opinion from another physician, but is likely to encounter much the same level of service. In attempting to cure or to satisfy the patient, a physician may not place first priority upon cost. In the United States, for example, the practice of "defensive medicine" to avoid potential accusations of malpractice often demands that all available diagnostic and therapeutic procedures be provided to the patient. Under various payment plans the provider may have an incentive to increase income by giving unneeded or questionable services. This traditional lack of professional concern with costs is changing in concert with health sector reforms around the world (Chapter 13).

The asymmetry of knowledge between patient and provider can work both ways because individuals may have special knowledge about their own health status. In insurance markets, a person who knows himself to be at higher risk, and more likely to consume costly services, can profit by concealing that information.

Second, the money spent or allocated by the physician is often third-party money, from an insurance company or a government program. Hence, neither the patient nor the physician may have an incentive to save. In fact, both may have strong motivations for overusage: the patient because it "doesn't cost me anything," and the physician "to provide the maximum level of services." The policies of the impersonal third-party payer therefore become very important in controlling expenditures, and the forces that determine those policies assume a decisive position. In many countries "physicians overprescribe drugs because of the profits they earn from directly dispensing them. In China, Japan, and Korea such incentives helped to drive drug spending up to 35 to 50 percent of total health spending."[26] In 1990, Japanese spent an average of $412 on prescription drugs; Germans, $222, Americans, $191, Norwegians, $89. Does an average Japanese person really need four and a half times as many drugs as a Norwegian, or are drugs that much more expensive in Japan?

Third, varying amounts of money charged to health services may go to purposes having no health benefit. Some medical procedures are clearly useless or peripheral (*placebo technology*). In addition, high incomes, beautiful buildings, premiums for malpractice insurance, corruption and "shrinkage" of commodities, error and inefficiency, and inordinate bureaucracies absorb substantial amounts of health sector funds in different countries. Overhead and administrative expenses may consume up to a quarter of total health expenditures in the United States.

Fourth, money is not the only resource to be considered. Where money is not limiting, time may be. Many people in the United States and elsewhere do not hesitate to pay money in exchange for convenience. The use of preprocessed food products, for instance, instead of preparation "from scratch" is justified on the basis of saved time. So is spending more money to have more readily available doctors and nearby facilities, rather than spending time waiting or traveling.

Fifth, health services reflect the characteristics and values of the societies of which they are a part, and the use made of health resources has been determined ultimately by cultural and factors and the influence of political pressure groups, rather than by rational allocation based on cost-effectiveness. The decade of the 1990s may have witnessed the beginnings of a change in that situation.

Finally, as mentioned repeatedly in this book, the state of health is determined by many factors. Income, education, housing, and nutrition are at least as important medical care. Reductions or increases in the price of school fees, rents, and food, or the ability to pay for them through employment will rapidly affect health. That is why government subsidies in the form of food stamps or unemployment benefits may have a greater effect on health than health services themselves.

Defining Marginal Technology

It has been said that "the main cause of problems is solutions." Technology can be characterized as the application of human ingenuity to make things to satisfy human wants. But many solutions are serendipitous products of technology which was conceived for entirely different purposes. *In vitro* fertilization (IVF) is a commercial outgowth of basic research in reproductive biology and applied research in livestock production. A drug to treat high blood pressure was reported by some patients to help grow hair, and a market was created. A drug being tested to help men suffering from chest pains was found to have an odd side effect: Some men reported unexpected penile erections. As these novelties become available, some people want them, expect to get them as health benefits, and expect someone else to pay for them. Is infertility a "terrible disease," as one IVF physician described it? Is baldness, or impotence? Shall governments, through public taxes, or health insurance programs through the pooled funds of their members, pay for these things?

The effect of life-saving medical procedures is not to lengthen the total life span but to change the shape of survivorship curves of the type shown in Figure 11-2. The benefits of preventive health measures, sanitation, and education at early ages can add economically productive lives to a population at very low cost. Such services will yield an increase in the mean working life and pull the curve in the direction of the arrow. The total resource cost for proceeding from each curve to the next becomes progressively greater as appropriate expenditures on health come closer and closer to achieving attainable goals. The increase in appropriate resource costs may be compared to the decay of an isotope of a given half-life. A given investment of time (or expenditure) will see a certain reduction in activity (or mortality). A second identical investment will result in perhaps half the amount of reduction, a third investment, a quarter of the original effect, and so on in increasing diminution. While this analogy is imperfect, it does illustrate the kind of limits involved. The important question that any society must ask itself is: How much are we willing to spend for a given increment in the survivorship curve, and what is the quality of life in the years added?

Drawbacks to health investment

Flattening the survivorship curve brings with it all the problems that accompany the growth and aging of populations. The addition of potentially economically productive lives to a community is of little avail in the absence of employment or other opportunities to *be* economically productive. Developing economies under pressure may look with alarm upon further additions to the already underemployed work force. India has an annual population increase of about 16 million.

"The situation is very serious, and all our efforts to remove poverty and raise the standard of living are getting nullified" said Saroj Kharpade, the country's Minister of State for Health and Family Welfare . . . Miss Kharpade warned that India was moving toward a situation where 'there would be no houses, no water, no schools, no health facilities in adequate measure to take care of the increasing numbers."[27]

In addition to the burdens of providing services and employment for growing populations, increased survivorship invokes the epidemiological transition and changes the kinds of health problems to be faced. While conducting extensive child survival and primary health care programs, China is speaking of "the second health revolution," which entails care for the chronic and degenerative diseases of the growing proportion of elderly.

The Market for Physicians

Whether charged to the Ministry of Health, the Ministry of Education, or elsewhere, investment in the training of physicians is a major expense in many countries. Although the meaning of the term *physician* or *doctor* varies a bit from one country to another, it is used here to mean a person fully trained to modern biomedical standards and legally licensed to practice medicine. The term does not include chiropractors, naturopaths, traditional healers, folk practitioners, and the like, even though they provide substantial patient care, account for a large proportion of household medical expenditures in certain countries, and may be highly valued by their patients.

It seems to be commonly believed that a major cause of ill health and premature death in the poorer countries is lack of medical care, itself owing to insufficient investment. Conversely, it may seem self-evident that most health problems in developing countries would be overcome if only there were more physicians. The true situation is far more complex, in part because the relationship between physicians and health is not really well established. Certainly the treatment of illness by physicians does save lives and restore persons to productive activity. This is clearly true for individuals, but the amount of health added to a population by clinical activity is more difficult to demonstrate.

It is a truism that people are generally healthier in the wealthy countries where physicians are relatively abundant, but it might be argued that the density of physicians is a result (and not a cause) of a population with enough money to be healthy anyway and to support more doctors just as they have more cars, newspapers, and most everything else.

Most countries today, rich and poor, are producing more physicians than they can use. Does this mean that they have more physicians than they *need?* That is a difficult question: Certainly the perceived need varies greatly from one country to another. The determining factor is not how many doctors might ideally be used to care for every possible health care demand, but how many doctors the local economy can afford to maintain. Such physician surplus as there may be exists relative to the market, not relative to the "need," however defined. The bottom line on physician utilization in a population is determined by economics, not by health.

Acting on the impulse to increase physician production, many countries, including the United States, adopted policies in the past aimed at supporting medical schools. In the United States the Hill-Burton Act of 1946 among other laws mandated the construction of hospital facilities, and additional legislation was passed to send money to expand postgraduate training programs in those hospitals. Within a decade the number of hospital-based residencies quadrupled, far outpacing the number of American medical school graduates. Immigration of foreign medical graduates was encouraged by an official declaration that in issuing visas preference be given to aliens in occupations in short supply—including physicians and surgeons.

During the intervening years in the United States, the perceived physician shortage of the 1950s has been more than overcome. The number of physicians per capita increased by 51% between 1965 and 1986, with even greater growth in the proportion of specialists. During the same period, the number of general and family practitioners per capita declined by 25%. Federal aid to schools of health professions was sharply reduced in the 1980s. After years of reliance on "market forces" to regulate physician numbers, an American Medical Association report in 1986 called for downsizing of medical school classes and limitation of the number of foreign-trained doctors permitted to enter the system.

Research

Even the most sanctified of all health-related activities, medical research, has its detractors, often within the establishment. An unfortunate but deep cleavage exists between "basic" research which is pure and prestigious, and "applied" research, which is practical and somehow tainted. With some diseases, such as AIDS, behavioral research and modification appears to provide the best hope of control. Nevertheless, work on behavioral or epidemiological aspects of health has not achieved sufficient status or legitimacy in the view of many basic medical scientists, who are concerned with the "how" of disease processes (i.e., basic biology) rather than the "why" of illness in the community. This is true even in many developing countries, where public health hazards are much more prominent. Both basic and applied research have historically been highly cost-beneficial, although future benefits of today's investigations are impossible to estimate. This does not mean, however, that expenditures for medical research, like any others, should not be evaluated against the best available standards of efficiency, effectiveness, and benefit.

Excessive expenditures for the elusive pursuit of quality are not just a phenomenon of the richer countries. Elaborate showpiece hospitals, with the latest medical instrumentation, have been built in Latin America, Africa, and Asia, frequently with foreign donor capital. Unfortunately, shortages of trained staffs and operating funds have too often resulted in underutilization and rapid deterioration both of buildings and equipment. Nor have medical schools in developing countries been immune from criticism, as they strive to emulate the philosophies of medical care and medical education adopted directly from the most advanced institutions in wealthy countries. Understandable, but inappropriate.

The title for this chapter is taken from that of a pioneering book on health economics by C.-E. A. Winslow (1951).

NOTES

1. While this analysis can be done with fair confidence for specifically defined conditions and interventions, it is exceedingly difficult to do for the health sector or health care system.

2. Mills (1997).

3. Acuña (1975).

4. Prescott and de Ferranti (1985).

5. Enke and Brown (1972).

6. Shmueli (1995).

7. Feachem *et al.* (1990).

8. Among the many publications that emphasize this point see the World Bank's World Development Report for 1993, especially pages 18, 40, 47, and 157.

9. Weisbrod (1983).

10. Barnum (1981).

11. Newhouse (1984).

12. Lane and Millar (1969); Lane et al. Although no case of smallpox has been reported in the world since 1978, U.S. military personnel are still vaccinated against this disease.

13. Jordan (1985).

14. Exposure to schistosomiasis occurs when persons are in contact with water containing larval parasites released by certain species of freshwater snails. The larvae penetrate the skin and adult worms eventually develop within the hepatic portal veins. Their eggs, which pass out of the body with the feces, can give rise to a different type of swimming larvae, which infect new snails and maintain the life cycle.

15. This is called secondary prevention.

16. Berk and Monheit (1992).

17. Cutler and Meara (1997).

18. Uniform premiums and benefits for a pool of asociated people regardless of health status is called "community rating." Premiums, or benefits, may be adjusted based on age, family size, and so on.

19. It is not unheard of for auto accidents to be staged or buildings to be burned down to collect insurance money.

20. See Chapter 12.

21. Fuchs (1974) .

22. Abel-Smith (1972) .

23. Enthoven (1997).

24. Mahler (1976).

25. Bunker *et al.* (1977).

26. World Bank (1993).

27. Hazarika (1988).

12

Inventing the Health Sector

Global spending on health is very large: the World Bank estimates that in 1990 about $1.7 trillion, or about 8% of all world income, was spent on health.[1] Some consider this to be the world's largest single industry. The term *health sector* has come into widespread use in recent years, in parallel with similar usages such as industrial sector, financial sector, and agricultural sector. Interpreted broadly, the health sector includes all activities concerned with the preservation and restoration of human health, so it incorporates more limited concepts such as *health care system, health services*, and *medical care system*. The health sector specifically includes both public and private enterprises—that is, government services and private markets. As we can not possibly describe all of the diverse health care systems of 200 countries, we look here at several important patterns, as archetypes, and compare the circumstances of their development.[2] Necessity, controversy, and ingenuity have generated many different strategies, but none is perfect; dissatisfaction with the current health care system is as common as faith in the existence, somewhere, of a superior one. The health sector is under universal scrutiny, as people hope to learn from the successes and mistakes of others. The next chapter will concentrate on the worldwide efforts at reform and rationalization of the health sector in various countries.

The principal factors that determine the state of health of a population such as income, education, agricultural production and marketing, transportation, and housing, are not a direct part of the health sector at all. Within the health sector the most important elements are *public health* activities such as water supply and sanitation, food inspection, vector insect control, disease surveillance, reduction of industrial pollution, and regulation of pharmaceuticals. Most people, who rarely come into direct contact with public health activities, do not think of these as health care functions. What the public regards as the health care system are the *personal clinical* or *medical care* services, which absorb the vast majority of money, facilities, and personnel but are less important in determining the level of health of a population.

We can view a *health care system* as an organized arrangement to provide specified promotive, preventive, curative, and rehabilitative services to designated persons, using resources allocated for that purpose. Health care systems come in a great variety of sizes, forms, and levels of comprehensiveness and effectiveness. Within the structure of every sovereign government there is some entity, usually a Ministry of Health (MOH), which is the official agency charged with certain responsibilities relating to the health of the population. The MOH may be the dominant provider of medical care in any particular country, or its main function may be to supervise and regulate the work of other organizations (Table 12-1).

Most countries have a formal written health policy, sometimes enshrined in the national constitution, specifying the responsibilities assumed by the state. Tables, charts, diagrams, and written descriptions of each system provide useful in-

Table 12-1. Categories of Medical Care Systems

Category	Funding	Role of the State
Universal and comprehensive, socialist and centrally planned	General revenues or taxation	Operator
Welfare-oriented social insurance	Specifically earmarked employer and employee and/or government contribution to social security or sickness insurance funds	Regulator
Prepaid voluntary member-supported health maintenance organizations	Employee and employer contributions and/or individual out-of-pocket payments	Regulator
The entrepreneurial private practice of medicine (including commercial health insurance companies)	Various: contracts, capitation, out-of-pocket payments, subscription fees	Regulator
Wholly owned private organizations such as mines, factories, and plantations, primarily for their own workers and their dependents	Employer with or without employee payments	Regulator or minimal
Charitable and altruistic organizations	Donations, some fees	Regulator or minimal
Indigenous, traditional, spiritual, empirical, or folk healers observing specific or stylized cultural practices	Fees, donations, payment in kind	Usually minimal or none

Source: Adapted from Basch (1990) Table 10-3.

sights into the means of implementing this policy. Two real MOH mission statements are:

> The overall mission of this Ministry is to promote and provide for the health care needs of the People, to develop appropriate service for those with special needs, and to provide social and psychological support to all members of the family. The main objective of the Ministry is to promote and ensure ongoing social well-being of the society, through the provision of care services needed to improve the health and welfare of all citizens, the provision of the necessary monitoring and control mechanism to ensure that ongoing services are encouraged and to enhance and promote sound family values.

and

> The mission of the Ministry of Public Health is to promote and improve the total health of the population through actions directed at prevention, protection, recuperation and rehabilitation of health, the provision of services of high quality, economically accessible to the people, and by control and regulation of risks to health.[3]

There seems to be a common misconception in the United States that most European countries have monolithic "socialized medicine" systems under which a person need only appear on a hospital doorstep to be showered with free services. Perhaps equally widespread is the idea, promoted by television pictures of starving hordes, that most developing countries have no health care systems at all. Neither of these extreme images is accurate.

While often useful, comparative studies have their limitations. On a superficial level, comparative health services research can uncover statistics on the numbers of facilities, physicians, hospital beds, and so on; on money and other resources put into the system; and on the number of patient visits or immunizations given over a certain period of time. It can also illustrate certain structural relationships within systems, such as the organization of divisions of a health ministry or the regionalization of hospitals, health centers, clinics, and dispensaries. Pages of tables and charts can be prepared in such studies, but skill and care are needed to draw correct conclusions from these data. There are two basic problems: (1) what the data show and (2) what they do not show.

Among the elements not shown on an organizational chart is, first, the historical context. Health care is a continuously evolving process impossible to describe adequately in an instantaneous snapshot, any more than a single frame can exemplify a long and complex motion picture. Second, the fact that a system for health care exists does not necessarily mean that it functions according to design or that it is used, or used appropriately, by the people whom it is intended to serve. The *official* health care system is not necessarily *the* health care system, because all countries have several parallel systems, such as those listed here. Persons may by necessity (= lack of access) or by intent (= distrust) circumvent the official system. Indeed, in some countries only a minority of the population may make use of official health services, preferring to consult pharmacists, healers, or others whose services are not recorded on government charts and tables. Third, whereas the elements of a system, and the resources put into it, can be counted and described, the *output* or product of the system, in terms of improved health, is impossible to measure and may even defy estimation. Fourth, attitudes, motivations, and policies cannot be indicated on an organizational chart. Government and professional leaders may be public-spirited, open, and responsive to the needs of the people, or dominated by self-serving interests so that special knowledge, ability, or association is carefully husbanded as a means for accumulating power or personal advancement. Nations vary greatly in demographics, diseases, and development. The degree to which the general public (the "consumers") is involved in the operation of the system also varies greatly in time and place.

Comparative anatomists can look at the skeletons of a chicken, dinosaur, fish, and man and make sense of the relationships between the various bones because they are guided by the principle of evolutionary homology of parts. They see in the unfolding of an embryo a recapitulation of the ancestral history of the species. Researchers in comparative health care systems are not so fortunate because they have little theoretical basis for comparing structural or functional elements in countries with different historical traditions, political systems, and population structures. As pointed out in this book, the patterns of demographic, epidemiologic, and fertility transitions of the poorer countries do not necessarily follow along the path previously taken by today's wealthier nations. Comparisons between countries are therefore analogies, not homologies, and their utility for making predictions is limited.

It may seem that comparison of health care systems is a fruitless academic exercise. It is not. For the advancement of scholarly knowledge it is just as valid to study the historical, functional, and structural characteristics of health care systems as of any other significant aspect of human society. And it is always possible that such examinations will turn up useful ways of doing things and point out potentially avoidable difficulties that have already been endured by someone else.

Medical care systems and subsystems, providing particular kinds of benefits (in cash or services) to specified segments of the population, are often linked, or interwoven, with programs offering other kinds of social assistance: retirement or survivorship pensions, unemployment insurance, funeral expenses, and the like. In the United States, the former Department of Health, Education and Welfare has been supplanted by the Department of Health and Human Services. It is difficult to disaggregate health from other aspects of well-being, and, within the health arena, to draw an unambiguous circle around medical care services. Prenatal supervision and hospital delivery are certainly included, but what about a cash maternity bonus? Rehabilitation of a worker permanently injured in an industrial accident usually would be considered medical care. Is his retraining for a simpler occupation so classified?

While recognizing such problems of definition, we shall follow the conventional idea of medical care as personal services rendered by trained individuals to others specifically for promotion of health and prevention, alleviation, and cure of illness.

For cultural, economic, and historical reasons every country has developed its unique system. Moreover, all systems are continually being modified under the dictates of politics, finances, and technology. The end of the 20th century has seen more rapid and more extensive changes than any other period in history.

Gradual evolutionary development of social structures is the norm, but sudden changes in form and direction also may occur. Successful revolutions create an immediate demand for remedies from former repression. The countries that achieved independence from colonialism (Table 3-2) needed to get their new governments established quickly. The breakup of the former Soviet Union led, almost overnight, to a number of new sovereign entities (Table 13-3) that faced similar problems. Health care systems quickly put in place face difficulties in functioning effectively, especially in an atmosphere of social upheaval.

Financiers, administrators, economists, and physicians may differ in their interpretation of medical care systems. We—scholars and students—may find useful the categories of medical care systems shown in Table 12-1. These systems are by no means mutually exclusive. All countries have some of the systems, some countries[4] have all of them, and there may be several subsystems in each category. For instance, different (or sometimes parallel) services may be provided by national, provincial, district, municipal, or other governments. (Note that the word *state* may be construed in two meanings: In most countries it means "from the central sovereign government"; e.g., as in state socialism, but in countries such as the United States, Mexico, and Brazil it refers to the major subnational jurisdictions elsewhere [e.g., Canada] called *provinces*.) Many countries have quasi-governmental (or *parastatal*) organizations, typically limited to provision of certain social services, and these are becoming more diverse in an age of health sector reform (next chapter). Where private practice exists there may be many alternative or competing kinds of providers offering similar services.

THE ORIGIN OF HEALTH CARE SYSTEMS

Although healers have treated patients for centuries and churches have long provided care for indigents, an organized system to oversee the health of a large population is a relatively recent development. A visiting Martian with superhuman intelligence and no knowledge of worldly affairs might design an ideal health care system. Lacking such ultimate wisdom, mere humans have invented several strategies to get the job done. The basic elements that make up a system are shown in Table 12-2.

An organization that we would accept as a credible modern health care system could not have developed until the necessary conditions were in place. It is useful to think of what these conditions might be:

- A stable and effective national government with strong leadership
- A supportive political and legal environment

Table 12-2. Building Blocks for Medical Care Systems[a]

By assembling blocks from each section, it is possible to describe in general terms any type of medical care service in any country. Items on this list are only examples and many more could be mentioned. For example, there are 700 recognized health care job classifications in the United States.

I. Usership
   A. *Eligibility*
      1. Age
      2. Citizenship
      3. Dependency status
      4. Diagnosis
      5. Employment
      6. Ethnicity; religion
      7. Income; wage level
      8. Residence
      9. Other
   B. *Choice*
      1. Compulsory
      2. Optional
      3. Voluntary
II. BENEFITS
   A. *Type*
      1. Ambulatory; outpatient
      2. Comprehensive
      3. Dental
      4. Drugs & appliances
      5. Education
      6. Emergency
      7. Eyeglasses
      8. Hospital
      9. Maternity
      10. Medical
      11. Mental health; psychiatry
      12. Prayer, healing ritual
      13. Preventive, checkups, immunization
      14. Primary health care
      15. Secondary health care
      16. Tertiary health care
      17. Sexually transmitted diseases; AIDS
      18. Surgical
   D. *Mode*
      1. Cash
      2. Service

III. Providers
   A. *Personnel*
      1. Vocation
         a. Community or village health worker/Auxiliary
         b. Dentist
         c. Midwife
         e. Nurse
         f. Optometrist
         g. Paramedic
         h. Pharmacist
         i. Physician
         j. Traditional healer, folk practitioner
      2. Remuneration
         a. Capitation
         b. Contract
         c. Fee-for-service
         d. None (volunteer)
         e. Salary
         f. Voluntary contribution
IV. Facilities
   A. *Locus*
      1. Clinic; dispensary
      2. Extended care facility
      3. Home of patient
      4. Hospital
      5. Mobile; community
      6. Office
      7. Church or shrine
      8. School
      9. Workplace
V. Financing
   A. *Source*
      1. Public sector
         a. from taxation at national, state, provincial or district level
         b. Through loans from Development

Banks to government
         c. Through direct support from multilateral or bilateral agency.
      2. From benefactors
         a. Religious/ethnic organizations
         b. Secular NGOs
      3. From individual and Household resources
         a. Personal assets
         b. Medical Savings Account
         c. Informal; in-kind and non-cash
      4. From mixed sources
         a. Employment-related earmarked contributions from employee, employer and government
            i. Compulsory
            ii. Voluntary/ optional
         b. Other
VI. Supervision
   A. *Regulation*
      1. Legislative
      2. Unofficial or traditional
      3. External agency
   B. *Administration*
      1. Bureaucrats
      2. Appointed Board
      3. Owners; Investors
      4. Providers
      5. Users; members
      6. Community
      7. Donor or external agency

Source: Adapted from Basch (1990) Table 10-4.

- Compatible social and historical values
- An organized medical profession willing to participate
- A sufficient level of scientific knowledge and clinical practice to make medical intervention useful and desirable
- An educated and compliant population accepting of the medical system
- An infrastructure of physical facilities
- An economy capable of financing the system
- Appropriate incentives to the various stakeholders[5]

On the following pages we will look at vignettes of the health systems of Germany, Great Britain, the former Soviet Union, Saudi Arabia, the Peoples' Republic of China, and Singapore. Each of these countries has approached the personal medical care imperative in a different way.

The Social Welfare Concept: Bismarck's Germany

The conditions just listed were met in Germany in the 1880s, where a comprehensive health care system was developed that has continued to the present time. But that system had its own antecedents. Voluntary insurance against sickness and death has a long history in Europe, arising from early guild organizations. The underlying idea of insurance is to reduce the risk to individuals of certain losses by pooling that risk among a group. The working class that developed during the industrial revolution formed many voluntary mutual-help groups, whose members agreed to make regular contributions to a common fund that would provide cash benefits in the event of sickness or unemployment.

Semiautonomous health funds or associations were often organized along occupational, ethnic or religious, political, geographic, or other bases, with eligibility for membership defined correspondingly. Over time hundreds of such local voluntary funds appeared in Germany and elsewhere in Europe. The Prussian Parliament formalized that system into law in 1854, requiring regular contributions from workers to be matched by their employers. Three decades later the German chancellor, Otto von Bismarck, motivated to suppress social unrest among industrial employees, introduced a series of social insurance programs to protect vulnerable urban workers from the hazards of dangerous factories and life in unsanitary environments. The 1883 Sickness Insurance Act required low-wage workers to be insured by such a fund and established guidelines and standards for the operation of the funds. A year later a second law covered workers in case of industrial accidents, with all contributions made by employers as a cost of doing business.

This was the birth of the concept of social security, which eventually spread throughout the world. In Germany and elsewhere it was soon extended to other risks—especially old age (pensions), invalidity, unemployment, death and widow's benefits, maternity, children's allowance, and more. Applied to medical care, usually with wage-loss compensation, the idea had spread to 70 countries by 1985.[6]

In the 1880s Germany had more than 20,000 small local sickness funds (*krankenkassen*), and more than a century later more than 1000 separate statutory funds were still in operation. Despite the disruption of two major wars and the drastic political changes during Hitler's Third Reich, this highly decentralized system has proved to be extremely durable. Existing funds are regional or employment-based. All employees earning less than a stipulated amount, and their employers, must each pay about 6.5% of wages into a fund. About 90% of Germans participate in these mandatory insurance schemes, while another 9% (wealthier citizens) maintain private funds.[7] Sickness funds must provide a minimum package of benefits including ambulatory, hospital, and dental care to members and their families. Other benefits include maternity and nursing care, drugs and appliances, cash payments for loss of income during illness, funeral benefits, and even visits to health spas.

The funds are nonprofit organizations. They do not provide medical care directly but function only as *financial intermediaries*. Physicians in Germany are separated into two classes: those who provide ambulatory care and those who work in hospitals. They do not work for the funds. A patient (fund member) may select any ambulatory care physician. Every three months the physician submits a bill for payment for all services to his or her own regional physicians' association. Hospital-based physicians are salaried by their hospitals, which get their operating income by billing the sickness funds for patient-days provided to fund members.

Once each year there is a major conference of representatives of the funds, the 19 regional associations of physicians, hospitals, and pharmaceutical companies, to work out the contribution rate and other details. The government does not provide any funding to the system but is very active in regulating and monitoring it.

The basic features of the social-insurance-based health system have been adopted in France, Japan, Austria, Belgium, Switzerland, the Netherlands, and other countries. In Canada and Australia welfare-oriented systems have been greatly modified.

As the social security movement developed, with sickness insurance as a general priority, a great variety of plans for indemnification, prepayment of costs, and contracts with providers has emerged, each a product of intense negotiations. Four parties emerged with major roles:

- Participants or fund members (often represented through a group such as a labor union)
- Employers and their organizations (usually when unions were involved)
- Providers, especially the medical profession but also including hospitals and therefore often religious and charitable organizations
- Governments at various levels

It is mainly because of the tugging and pulling of these diverse interests that few countries, at least in western Europe, have really been able to integrate or even to coordinate fully the diverse health programs accumulated over the decades. Nevertheless, a general consensus in Europe holds that health care is a community responsibility, and participation of all parties in these programs has broadened in various directions.

In Europe, strong political forces have often acted to maintain the independence of specific sickness funds. Most common among these are separate plans for government employees, postal, railroad, and communcations workers, miners, and seamen. Many countries maintain independent social security funds for agricultural workers and the self-employed, for whom membership is often voluntary, or for members of certain professions.

Some countries have merged existing insurance schemes into more comprehensive national programs. Nevertheless, private insurance and fee-for-service programs may continue to operate vigorously in these countries. Sometimes there are several parallel systems: In Denmark, 95% of inhabitants are classified as group I members with free access to the services provided, while the remaining 5% in group II can choose their physician freely but must pay a portion of the costs of benefits. The Danish system is highly decentralized: The central government makes policy and exercises general supervision; counties provide curative medical services, and municipalities take care of prevention, public health, nursing home, and old age services. About a thousand separate sickness funds in Denmark are based on the district of residence.

The complex Swedish system also bases its medical care services at the county government level. Counties levy their own income taxes for this purpose, with additional payments made by the national government and by the general insurance system. Belgium has a sickness and disability insurance program which covers almost everyone, but an important place is reserved for the private medical sector. In Austria, 99% of the population is eligible for comprehensive social security and sickness services. In Switzerland while all wage earners are insured against accidents, membership in sickness funds is compulsory in some cantons (= provinces) and certain municipalities for residents with income below a specified limit. More than 95% of Swiss citizens are members of one or another fund. In Israel, separate sickness funds for agricultural settlements and trade unions, established during the period of British mandate, have fused within the General Federation of Labor, whose unified sickness fund, the *Kupat Holim*, covers the great majority of the Jewish population and many Arabs in Gaza and the West Bank, while a few smaller funds plus social welfare agencies cover the remainder.

The National Health Service Concept: Beveridge's England

Great Britain has a long tradition of legislation regulating the practice of medicine and the welfare of the poor. In 1800 the Royal College of Surgeons was established;

15 years later the Apothecaries' Act recognized three kinds of doctors: physicians, surgeons, and apothecaries, who provided basic services to the poor. In 1804 there were one million members of "friendly societies" in England, growing to seven million by the turn of the 20th century. By the 1840s, these mutual aid societies were beginning to be supported by progressive employers interested in the welfare of their employees. The Poor Law Reform Bill of 1843 appointed poor law medical officers to be responsible for medical care for indigents. In 1858 Parliament passed the General Medical Act, which established minimal requirements for licensure, and set up the General Medical Council, responsible for preparing an annual list of all qualified medical practitioners and removing any guilty of unprofessional conduct. Many other laws and regulations recognized an obligation to provide welfare services of various kinds to the poor. In Britain "where provision for the acute sick by charitable effort was inadequate to provide for all who needed care, the acute sector of hospital care was, from 1870 onwards, gradually supplemented by public authorities."[8] It was not until 1881 that a major British hospital accommodated any paying patients at all.

By 1911 the British government under Lloyd George, determined to make medical care more generally available to the least well-off sectors of the population, passed the Health Insurance Act. The National Health Insurance scheme came into effect in 1912, mandating basic medical benefits for workers earning, at that time, under £160 per year. Workers were enrolled in approved mutual aid societies, which collected a portion of wages. Doctors were paid through locally based insurance committees made up of insured workers, doctors, and government officials. Unlike the German system, where doctors were paid for the amount of services provided, the British doctors usually chose to be reimbursed on a capitation basis—that is, a set fixed fee for each patient on that doctor's 'list' independent of the number of visits, The approved societies were also permitted to sell additional insurance (i.e., for dental coverage) to workers and could also sell health insurance to the general public on a voluntary basis.

The decades after1912 were hard on the British people. World War I and the Depression left large numbers unemployed and disheartened. World War II was a time of further stress and testing. As the buzz bombs and V-2 rockets rained destruction on British cities and the British endured severe rationing, the government set up a commission in June 1941 to survey unemployment and social insurance. Its findings, known as the *Beveridge Report* (1942), said that poverty came from two main causes: (1) interruption of earning power from unemployment, illness, or old age, and (2) the existence of large families. Accordingly, the report recommended the provision of (1) state insurance to cover unemployment, ill health, old age, and widowhood and (2) allowances to meet family needs.

Medical treatment covering all requirements will be provided for all citizens by a national health service organized under the health departments . . . and post-medical rehabilitation treatment will be provided for all persons capable of profiting by it . . . A comprehensive national health service will ensure that for every citizen there is available whatever medical treatment he requires, in whatever form he requires it, domiciliary or institutional, general, specialist, or consultant, and will ensure also the provision of dental, ophthalmic, and surgical applicances, nursing and midwifery and rehabilitation after accidents . . . *and to divorce the care of health from questions of personal means.* "[9]

During the war, in 1944, Churchill's conservative government issued four "white papers" on official policy toward social insurance, workmen's compensation, employment policy, and a national health service. Although a free health service was part of Beveridge's plan, there were few details in his report on how this should be achieved. The main focus of his report was on relieving poverty. A free health service was needed to prevent impoverishment from the cost of medical bills. Beveridge's biggest contribution was to unify social policy across class distinctions by proposing a social insurance scheme for the whole nation and redistributing risk among the entire British community. Basic protection against the hazards of illness and mortality, and the vagaries of the economy was, like the vote, to be every citizen's birthright.

The National Health Service Act was passed by Parliament in 1946, and after much discussion and negotiation the National Health Service (NHS) came into effect in 1948. Plans for the NHS were opposed by physicians who feared loss of autonomy and insisted on the right of private practice for fees. The government (led by Health Minister Aneurin Bevan) in turn insisted on public ownership for hospitals. In what was perhaps an echo of 1815, the NHS emerged with three categories of doctors: general practitioners, specialists, and public health physicians. As in the German system, community- and hospital-based specialists are clearly separated. Primary medical care is provided through general practitioners (GPs), with whom individuals register for general medical services. The organization of GPs is quite different: Although they contract with the NHS as self-employed professionals, they receive subsidies for their staff and for the cost of their premises, and they participate in NHS pension programs. Other health professionals such as dentists, optometrists, and pharmacists practice on a more independent commercial basis with few subsidies.

With the creation of the National Health Service in 1948, coverage was extended to the whole of the population, benefits were expanded, and hospitals were nationalized in order to control their size, location, and operation. Central councils and committees were established. Regional hospital boards were created, each centered in a university medical school, and hospital management committees oversaw nonteaching hospitals. County and borough councils were charged with community and environmental health services. The structure was criticized as soon as it was created.

Until about 1960 the system was dominated by medical professionals, mainly medical directors in hospitals and independent contractor GPs. In a 1960s modernization plan, numerous general hospitals were built for districts of about 250,000, designed to replace the Victorian infirmaries. Until the early 1970s community health and social services were run by local government under the direction of medical officers of health.

By 1968 the NHS was composed of "15 Regional Hospital Boards, 36 Boards of Governors, 336 Hospital Management Committees, and 134 Executive Councils administering the services of 20,000 general practitioners while 175 local health authorities ran the community services."[10]

The all-inclusive (polyvalent, comprehensive, horizontal) medical care system that these groups administered was described by the Department of Health and Social Security in 1971, in terms reminiscent of 1912:

> To provide for all who want it, a comprehensive service covering every branch of medical and allied activity, from care of minor ailments to major medicine and surgery which would include the care of mental as well as physical health, all specialist services, all general services (i.e. by family doctor, dentist, optician, midwife, nurse and health visitor) and all necessary drugs, medicines and a wide range of appliances.
>
> To ensure that everybody in the country—irrespective of means, age, sex or occupation—should have equal opportunity to benefit from the best and most up-to-date medical and allied services available ... To divorce the care of health from questions of personal means or other factors irrelevant to it and thus encourage the obtaining of early advice and the promotion of good health rather than only the treatment of ill health.

A major reorganization in 1974–1975 established a new tier of 90 Area Health Authorities (AHAs). Each AHA was responsible both for planning and for providing services to 250,000 to one million people. Owing to continued dissatisfaction the British NHS was further reorganized and streamlined in 1982 during the conservative regime of Margaret Thatcher. Although Mrs.Thatcher was zealous in reducing the role of government in Britain, she defended the principles of the NHS: "The principle that adequate health care should be provided for all, regardless of their ability to pay, must be the foundation of any arrangements for financing health care."[11]

The 1980s (the Thatcher years) saw tight NHS budgets and growing incentives for private health insurance. The 1982 reorganization of Britain's National Health Service retained private practice as a matter of policy both within and outside the NHS. The numbers of people privately insured increased from 5% in 1979 to 12% in 1994.

Further sweeping reforms were introduced in 1989, recognizing the influence of market forces in the Conservative party philosophy. These and other ongoing changes are extremely complex and beyond the limitations of this textbook. Briefly, improved efficiency was expected when newly formed Trusts, made up of NHS providers, would have to compete among themselves and with the private sector. The average length of hospital stay was greatly reduced and the number of beds halved from the 1960 level. Medical care continued its long transition from hospital to community. At the level of patient–physician interactions the changes were much less evident. The 1991 NHS and Community Care Act separated purchasers and providers and created the complexities of GP fundholding. While maintaining the principle of universal and comprehensive coverage the NHS became much more market and competition-driven, and that has made it very unpopular in some circles. At the time of writing, on the 50th anniversary of the NHS, its future is murky. The Labour prime minister, Tony Blair, was elected on a promise to "turn the clock back," sweep away the NHS internal market, and "renationalise the NHS." Conservatives argue against a return to the conditions that preceded Margaret Thatcher, when "the NHS was an under-managed muddle, fragmented not by a market but by feuding medical overlords."[12]

The Central Planning Concept: Semashko's Soviet Union

In contrast to the relatively deliberate steps toward health services in Germany and England, the Soviet system was born in calamity and mayhem. Although a rudimentary rural medical system, the Zemstvo, and a trace of industrial social insurance was created in rural czarist Russia, the close of World War I found Russia destitute and in shambles. The Bolshevik Revolution of 1917 had defeated the monarchy and created a new government with almost no resources. Soon after the proletariat siezed power the scattered medical activities of the individual departments were unified by the Council of Medical Boards. Local councils took charge of local health affairs and all private hospitals, clinics, and pharmacies were nationalized. In July 1918, the People's Commissariat of Health in the Russian Soviet Federative Socialist Republic was established as a central body in charge of the entire health work of the new nation. The first people's commissar of health was Nikolai Aleksandrovich Semashko, a close friend of V.I. Lenin. Born in 1874, he had been arrested and exiled in 1907 for carrying out revolutionary activities. In Geneva and Paris he worked side by side with Lenin, and returned to Russia after the February Revolution. In July 1918 Lenin authorized the organization of a People's Commissariat of Public Health to be in charge of all medical institutions and sanitation activities. Semashko was named to head the new People's Commissariat of Health, a post he held for 12 years.

The major issue in Russia was not the health of factory workers, for there were very few in the predominantly rural country, but the control of epidemic disease. Typhus infected tens of millions, and millions died. In 1919 the Russian Communist party (Bolsheviks) emphasized the importance of broad measures of health and sanitation, aiming at the prevention of disease as the principal activity in the field of public health. As Lenin declared in 1919, "Either socialism will defeat the louse, or the louse will defeat socialism." Accordingly the Russian Communist Party set as its immediate tasks:

1. The resolute implementation of broad sanitary measures in behalf of the workers, such as a) improvement of health conditions in residential areas (protection of soil, water, and air); b) establishment of communal feeding on scientific-hygienic principles; c) organization of measures to prevent the outbreak and spread of contagious disease; d) enactment of sanitation legislation
2. The control of social diseases (tuberculosis, venereal diseases, alcoholism, etc.)
3. The providing of accessible, free, efficient medical and pharmaceutical services[13]

On December 30, 1922, the Congress of Soviets proclaimed the establishment of the Soviet Union. The constitution, ratified in 1923, created Health Commissariats in all of the constituent republics in a necessarily decentralized arrangement because of the vastness of territory and uneven development of the various regions. Nevertheless, uniform principles of Soviet medicine were applied in all the republics. The constitution of 1923 gave the federal government the right to establish general rules for the protection of health. Comprehensive free medical care was guaranteed in the Soviet Constitution. Article 120 of the 1936 version stated:

> The Soviet state acknowledges the right of every citizen of the USSR to obtain not only full medical attention, but also material assistance during illness, in old age or in invalidism at the expense of the state. Soviet mothers have the right to obtain the material assistance of the state during pregnancy, childbirth, and the rearing of their children. These rights are guaranteed by the Constitution of the USSR.

The plan of Semashko was complete government control of all aspects of Soviet public health with identical tasks, forms, and operational methods in all medical establishments. All were interlinked and so designed as to achieve the same objectives—a reduction in the death rate of the population, continuous betterment of health, and an increase in the average life span by ameliorating working and living conditions. A distinctive feature of Soviet public health was rigid central planning. Under a strictly hierarchical system the apex of the health pyramid, the minister of health of the USSR, directed the ministers of each of the Union republics,[14] who in turn controlled regions, districts, local areas, and institutions, each of which had its own health administrative apparatus. Corresponding political councils shared responsibility at each level. The base of the health pyramid was formed by innumerable health committees organized in every factory and farm, wherever people work. Local facilities made requests for needed resources, which were combined at each level and forwarded up through the system, while allocations of funds and other resources came from the top down. Larger strategic planning was done in five-year cycles. The various local and state plans were consolidated into the All-Union Health Plan, the *Five-Year Plan* which established a definite quota for each of the five years.

The Soviet system was marked by extreme and narrow political orthodoxy, which extended into scientific and health matters. In a typical book by an operative of the Soviet health care system, the author found a need to display the official party line about the science of genetics:

> Relying on the Bourgeois idealistic genetics of Mendel, Morgan, and Weisman, the eugenists attempt to prove that it is not the living conditions of the people or their environment, but heredity, i.e., the innate properties acquired by an organism from its parents, that determines their physical development and health as well as the occurrence of various diseases. These pseudo-scientists maintain that heredity is affected not by the environment, but by genes inherited from parents. According to these "theories," the high death rate, wars, and epidemics are favorable factors actively conducive to "purging" mankind of physically and mentally inferior elements. It is quite apparent that this reactionary Bourgeois "science," invoked to defend the interests of capital, tries to justify capitalist exploitation, imperialistic wars, racial discrimination, and their pernicious effect on the health of workers.[15]

From the users' point of view the system began in his or her local polyclinic, a multifunction health center located primarily in urban areas and industrial installations. Adults, pregnant women, children, and workers attended distinct, specially staffed and equipped institutions. Rural areas had health posts staffed by paramedical personnel, generally midwives and *feldshers* (assistant doctors). Patients with complex conditions could be referred up the system to district or larger hospitals.

The Soviet system was strictly under bureaucratic control, and all personnel were full-time government employees. Although private practice was strictly banned, persistent complaints about inefficiency and lack of service led to unofficial "moonlighting" or paid private practice by physicians during their off hours. With the advent of *glasnost* (openness) and *perestroika* (restructuring) in the late 1980s a certain amount of private practice was officially tolerated in the USSR and a few private clinics with fee-for-service practices operated openly in the larger cities. The entire system collapsed around 1990 with the end of the Soviet Union.

The hierarchical polyclinic-based Soviet system was duplicated in USSR-influenced countries such Cuba, North Korea, and Vietnam. Until the breakup of the USSR the formerly communist countries of eastern Europe, including the former German Democratic Republic (East Germany), Poland, Czechoslovakia, Hungary, Bulgaria, and Albania, copied the Soviet model with greater or lesser fidelity in harmony with the prevailing economic and social conditions.

The breakup of the Soviet Union in the early 1990s necessitated the complete restructuring of health care systems in all of the former Soviet republics, a process discussed in the following chapter.

Free Health Care: The Kingdom of Saudi Arabia

The Kingdom of Saudi Arabia, whose population had grown from nine million in 1980 to 19 million in 1995, is unusual in how it provides health care to its citizens. Like the United Kingdom, it is the policy of the Saudi Arabian government that no one should be denied medical care for economic reasons. Government-funded health services are mostly free. Unlike Britain, however, Saudi Arabia has no income tax. Government revenues come directly from production and sale of petroleum. Free services are, therefore, really free to users, and Saudis have come to expect that the government will provide social services and utilities at no or very low cost. Nevertheless, the majority of physician visits and of hospital stays are paid for privately, through out-of-pocket payments or from private employers. Many persons eligible for free government services prefer to utilize the private sector because they can afford to and because they believe that the quality and convenience are greater. The large number of expatriate workers and their dependents receive their medical care through a private cooperative insurance program paid for by their employers. The great majority of health personnel in the kingdom are foreign workers, including 87% of physicians, 89% of nurses, and 65% of other health personnel. The kingdom also maintains a quasi-governmental payroll-funded social insurance agency for occupational hazards and annuities.[16]

The People's Republic of China—Another Special Situation[17]

China has been an object of fascination for the West since before the travels of Marco Polo in the 13th century. With more than a fifth of the world's population, China is an emerging giant of exceeding importance. Its history in the 20th century has been filled with turbulence and violent swings of policy. The Imperial period, which had lasted for millennia, ended in 1911, and was followed by the rule of the Kuomintang (KMT) government. Internal strife and the trauma of occupation in World War II left China, "the sick man of Asia," exhausted and impoverished. The successful revolution of Mao Zedong's forces and the establishment of the People's Republic of China (PRC) were accompanied by the flight of the KMT forces to Taiwan in 1949. The young PRC enjoyed a period of close cooperation with the Soviet Union from 1949 to 1960, during which time the health care system, among other things, was influenced by the USSR. Prior to the 1950s there had been essentially no medical care system in the vast rural areas, except for practitioners of traditional Chinese medicine. In the towns and cities there was only private practice, aside from some western missionary clinics and hospitals. In 1949 all private capital was confiscated by the state, including hospitals, and rural land was taken from landlords and distributed to collectives of peasants. These rural communes, which operated from the 1950s to 1970s, maintained a three-tier system of health facilities, with county hospitals, commune (township level) clinics, and brigade (village level) health centers. State control extended to all aspects of life. In 1950 Shanghai had 10,885 private physicians; this was reduced to 1514 in 1965 and to zero in 1966 when the Great Proletarian Cultural Revolution was under way. The decade-long turmoil of the Cultural Revolution was marked by extreme political orthodoxy. It was set off on June 26, 1965, by Chairman Mao's stinging denunciation of the then existing medical establishment, which was quoted in Chapter 7.

During the Cultural Revolution from about 1965 to 1975 formal medical education was halted, and physicians and professors were sent to do menial work in the countryside. Cooperative Medical Schemes (CMSs) grew up throughout the rural areas, based on grassroots insurance plans in which commune members decided on the benefits they could afford to provide, the amount of copayments needed for various services, and so on. Most of the primary medical care was given by barefoot doctors, who were local workers selected by their comrades to be given several months of medical training, usually at county level. These part-time low-tier medical workers then returned to their brigades and were awarded work points, donated by their comrades, for their health work in lieu of time spent in the fields. In this way, accessible, low cost basic medical services were extended to 90% of rural villages while the state conducted endless patriotic health campaigns to educate and motivate the peasantry.

After Chairman Mao's death in 1975 Chinese society changed radically. The constraints of the Cultural Revolution were criticized and repudiated. China officially adopted a "socialist market economy." Medical schools reopened. The private practice of medicine was sanctioned in 1980. The commune system was dismantled in favor of individual production. Village health workers were no longer paid collectively and many barefoot doctors either dropped out or upgraded their skills and opened private practices as rural doctors. Health stations were privatized. The *household responsibility system* meant private production of crops and private payment for medical services. The health care changes accompanying the responsibility system in rural China have been described dramatically:

> Under the new system, emphasis on preventive programs has decreased, because they are not as profitable as medical treatment. Private demand for preventive services is small, even at a very low price (for example, a vaccination costs only five cents) because peasants do not like to spend money without immediately visible results . . . The financing of health care has also changed drastically. The peasants are now richer and no longer use "risk pooling" schemes, which for 30 years had been the backbone of health care financing.[18]

By the early 1990s CMS's existed for about 5% of rural residents, while the others simply paid for services out of pocket, but coverage is increasing. The need for these plans is evident, particularly in poor rural areas where medical expenses could be ruinous to peasants with low incomes. Some programs were retooled and supported by profits from new nonagricultural enterprises, and new ones were developed, particularly in wealthier regions, although they still serve a small minority of rural residents. Generally termed *cooperative health care schemes*, these have the following general characteristics:

- They aim to ensure access at low cost to essential services to all including the poor.
- They are part of larger social welfare systems and are not for profit.
- They are based on insurance principles with strict budgets, risk sharing, and negotiation with providers and third-party payers.
- Funds are generated from households, collectives, and local governments, and used to reimburse certain defined health care expenses.
- They are administered by management committees representing the various interested parties.[19]

Urban residents who are eligible are served by two main programs. One is the publicly funded Government Insurance System (GIS or *gongfei yiliao*) for civil servants, college students, and disabled military officers. The GIS is financed by general revenues and serves about 29 million people. The other is the Labor Insurance System (LIS or *laobao yiliao*) for workers in state-owned and collective enterprises. The LIS is financed by employer contributions and serves about 144 million people. Persons who are not eligible for coverage under these systems, such as those in the private sector, pay privately for their medical care. A model of prepaid membership in health maintenance organization (HMO)-type plans is developing and may become prominent in the future of urban China.[20]

The solution to distribution of medical care developed by the Chinese differs greatly from the centralized, government-provided universal service adopted in the former USSR Medical care in China is in fact far less "socialized" than in many western countries. The system or systems in China still have many problems. For example:

The introduction of a market based economy into the health care system in China since the early 1980s has meant that health professionals and hospitals have to generate most of their income, including the salaries of staff in many cases. Central directives ensure that the cost of basic medical care . . . [is] kept low while profits are made almost entirely from charging for drugs and for the use of technology. Drugs can be charged at a mark up of 15%, which leads to massive overprescription and in particular to excessive use of injections and infusions. This results in two extremes . . . rich people are showered with often useless medicines, while many poor people are afraid to seek health care because of inability to pay for the drugs that will be prescribed.[21]

Individual Responsibility: The Case of Singapore

Singapore is a modern island nation of about 3.3 million mostly prosperous and well-educated people, primarily ethnic Chinese in origin. Life expectancy, infant mortality, and other vital statistics compare favorably with those of England, the United States, and other western countries. The government has given priority to reducing cigarette smoking, promoting healthy lifestyles, health education, and the school health service. Rising incomes from rapid economic growth have also led to improvements in health status. Singapore has the sixth highest per capita income in the world. Before a major reorganization in 1984, Singapore followed the British NHS system of providing medical care through the public sector, financed by general taxation. By 1980 the government realized that it needed to rethink the health sector, and did so along these lines:

- Consumers should have free choice.
- Self-accountability and self-reliance should be stressed.
- Free market competition should be deployed wherever possible.
- Government should be the provider of last resort, and offer minimal standards to those who cannot afford to pay.[22]

The solution arrived at in Singapore is a system of compulsory *medical savings accounts* (MSA's) and government subsidies. The government maintains control over facilities, medical manpower, and the overall operation of the system. Each citizen must place a percentage of his or her monthly income into an MSA (Medisave). The required payments, matched by employers, vary with age: 3% of income for those under 35, up to 4% for people over 45 years of age. Contributions are tax exempt, earn interest, and accumulate until a specified target amount has been reached. At retirement a certain amount must remain in the account, but any overage may be withdrawn for other uses. At death the account becomes part of the estate and can be transferred to relatives like any other asset. Persons who choose to pay extra can obtain a higher level of service. Singapore also has a thriving private sector, encouraged by the government, for those who elect to use it.

Although the collection of contributions from employees and employers sounds like a social security program, Medisave is very different. Under the Singapore system each individual has a separate, personally owned account, which is not pooled into a general fund. Medisave is a forced savings plan, not insurance. When medical care is needed, the person's account is drawn on to pay for the costs as far as possible. In case of catastrophic illness another fund called Medishield will pay additional costs. A third program called Medifund provides a safety net of last resort for people without resources who cannot afford medical care at all. Medifund comes entirely from the government. The combination of individual responsibility and government subsidies has limited the health sector expenditures to only 3% of Singapore's gross domestic product.

What we see here are three separate interlocking funding plans intended to ensure that no citizen is deprived of basic medical care. Medisave is an innovative plan of compulsory individual savings accounts usable only to pay for medical care. Medishield, funded by a proportion of money taken from individual Medisave accounts, is basically an insurance scheme, collecting small amounts as premiums against specified risks. In this way it is like social security. Medifund is like a national health service but limited to the poorest segment of the population. The MSA system is designed to limit demand, raising the public's awareness of costs by taking medical care expenses directly from individuals' own savings. The government describes it this way:

> We propose a hybrid approach to controlling health care costs: neither to create a totally regulated national health service, nor to give providers full freedom to organise and to price health services in a completely free market.[23]

Singapore has further reduced costs by paying only for a limited menu of services:

> We cannot avoid rationing medical care, implicitly or explicitly. Funding for health care will always be finite. There will always be competing demands for resources, whether the resources come from the State or from individual citizens. Using the latest in medical technology is expensive. Trade-offs among different areas of medical treatments, equipment, training and research are unavoidable. When public funds are involved, doctors have to decide which patients will benefit most from an expensive treatment. To get the most from a limited health budget, we need to exclude treatments which are not sufficiently cost-effective to belong to the basic health package available to all. We must allocate resources according to rational priorities so that they can do the most good for the largest number of people.[24]

Specifically excluded are in vitro fertilization; gender reassignment operations; heart, lung, liver, and bone marrow transplants; purely cosmetic procedures;[25] unproven drugs and techniques; and "extravagant efforts to keep gravely ill patients alive using high technology equipment, regardless of their quality of life and prospects for recovery." Those patients who can afford to pay for these treatments can obtain them from private physicians.

Medisave is part of a national system for pensions, health care, and education,[26] which takes a healthy 22% of wages, plus an additional 18% from employers.

PUTTING THE BLOCKS TOGETHER

We have now examined several different models for providing medical care to large numbers of people. However diverse, these systems and all others can be thought of as consisting of certain elements or building blocks. The primary functional elements to be examined are defined here under the six headings of Usership, Benefits, Providers, Facilities, Financing, and Supervision, as outlined in Table 12-2. All of these elements interact and none makes much sense without the others. By proper selection and combination of these modular units, the rudiments of any existing system can be assembled. Consider first those who use the system.

Usership

The term *usership* is employed here to indicate, for each medical care system, those persons who have a legal right to obtain benefits and who exercise that right. An individual may make use of any, several, all, or none of these systems, depending primarily on his or her eligibility, choice, access, and preference with respect to each.

Eligibility

As described, some governments have accepted full responsibility for the health of their citizenry and have medical care available to all at no or small charge to the user. More governments have enunciated this principle than have been able to bring it to reality. For instance, the Nkrumah administration in newly independent Ghana (1957–1966) tried to provide free medical care for all, but personnel, facilites, and money available were only a fraction of those needed and the program collapsed. In India, the *Bhore Report* of 1946, clearly influenced by Beveridge, specified that following independence, "medical services should be free to all without distinction and the contribution from those who can afford to pay should be through general and local taxation." Although several thousand primary health care centers were built during the first and second Five-Year Plans (1951–1960), reality fell short of the ambitious goal and universal coverage has never been achieved in India.

More commonly, full medical care supported directly by the central government is provided only for specific segments of the population. Almost everywhere, members of the military services are in this category, usually with their immediate families. After World War I the United States and many European countries established veterans hospitals, first for treatment of war-related disabilites, then for general medical care, extending in some cases to dependents of veterans. Other groups eligible for central-government-supported medical care often include pensioners, inmates of prisons, and members of aboriginal or tribal populations.

Along with general public health services, the health of pregnant women, mothers, and young children is ususally considered a community responsibility. Direct government support of these groups, connected with maternity benefits, may exist independently of other programs. Developing countries, subscribing to the principles of the Primary Health Care, Child Survival, and Safe Motherhood initiatives (Chapter 7), have often established programs in these areas. Many industrialized countries also have special programs. In the United States many federal, state, and municipal AFDC (Aid to Families With Dependent Children) programs exist, particularly for young children from poor and single-parent homes.

Not only are certain groups of people usually eligible for government-sponsored general medical care, but frequently all persons are eligible for specific kinds of care. Most commonly these are extensions of public health functions. In Israel, for instance, personal preventive (but not curative) services are provided free to all inhabitants directly through the Ministry of Health. In many countries certain diseases are the subjects of specified services (sometimes called vertical, categorical, or monovalent) in which preventive, diagnostic, and curative care is offered, typically free of charge. Tuberculosis, leprosy, and sexually transmitted diseases often fall into this category. For example, publicly funded programs for education, identification, and counseling of HIV positive individuals and AIDS patients have been set up in many countries. Ambulance and emergency services are also commonly provided to all by local governments, sometimes followed by bills for reimbursement of costs.

A distinction must be made between one government's policy decision to provide medical care, as a right, to all or part of its population, and another government's assumption of the burden of medical care for the indigent, considered as charity and performed with graceless reluctance. Unfortunately, the situation in several countries may resemble that described in prerevolutionary Cuba:

> Only people in extreme hardship used the government services. Indeed when someone already beyond his first youth was not given to saving or providing for his own future or was unemployed or unmarried, it was frequently said that this unhappy person would end his days in a government hospital, as if that were the worst thing that could happen to anyone.[27]

Choice

As we have seen, membership in some national health services is compulsory: Insofar as use is made of any medical care services, it must be those offered by the government. Other systems offer options. In Canada, for example, health insurance is compulsory throughout the provinces, but some opting out is permitted in Ontario and Alberta. Persons of means can legally circumvent the system in Britain and in most countries with compulsory insurance.

Access is a key to the actual utilization of medical care services. In the United States the annual number of physician visits per capita is about five; in some European countries people see their doctor on average every month; and in many poor areas the average is much less than once per year—often never. Much of the difference can be explained by variations in the availability of, and access to, the appropriate facilities. The dilemma arises in large part from the geographic distribution of existing personnel and facilities. Most countries exhibit the well-known concentration of physicians relative to population in urban areas, particularly in the national capital. In developed countries the ratio of physicians to population is roughly two to three times greater in high-income than in low-income jurisdictions; in developing countries the imbalance is typically much more extreme (Tables 12-3 and 12-4). Other categories of health personnel, laboratories, and equipment

Table 12-3. Distribution of Physicians in Rural and Urban Areas, Selected Developing Countries, Recent Years

Country	Percent Rural	Physicians per 10,000 Population			Rate Ratio, Rural/Urban
		Total	Urban	Rural	
Least developed countries					
Afghanistan	82	1.56	5.94	0.08	0.01
Benin	61	0.62	1.41	0.29	0.21
Burkina Faso	92	0.17	2.55	0.08	0.03
Burundi	94	0.47	5.36	0.29	0.05
Central African Republic	56	0.43	0.67	0.09	0.13
Djibouti	21	2.40	2.73	0.52	0.19
Guinea	76	0.17	4.89	0.10	0.02
Malawi	85	0.86	1.51	0.03	0.02
Mali	81	0.43	2.84	0.02	0.01
Myanmar	83	2.67	3.15	0.06	0.02
Nepal	96	0.33	6.57	0.06	0.01
Niger	82	0.26	1.58	0.04	0.02
Other developing countries					
China	53	10.0	14.6	5.9	0.41
India	73	3.97	9.09	1.11	0.12
Indonesia	78	1.06	1.75	0.69	0.40
Iran	47	3.60	6.41	0.53	0.08
Korea, Republic of	29	8.58	9.20	3.07	0.33
Madagascar	77	1.00	3.58	0.52	0.15
Morocco	53	0.76	4.07	0.29	0.07
Namibia	46	2.54	4.24	0.54	0.13
Papua New Guinea	85	1.62	4.91	0.06	0.01
Peru	31	9.60	22.94	4.07	0.18
Philippines	58	1.49	5.69	1.69	0.30
Thailand	83	1.59	8.54	0.35	0.04
Vietnam	89	10.05	11.75	1.25	0.11

Source: Adapted from Blumenthal (1994). Table 1.

such as x-ray machines and operating theatres are usually far more disproportionately distributed than are physicians. The situation has been described graphically:

> Although three-quarters of the population in most developing countries live in rural areas, three-quarters of the spending on medical care is in urban areas, where three-quarters of the doctors live. Three-quarters of the deaths are caused by conditions that

Table 12-4. Geographic Imbalances of Physician Distribution, Selected Developed Countries, Recent Years

| Country | Percent Rural | Physicians/10,000 Population by District[a] | | | Ratio Low/High |
		Total	Highest	Lowest	
Austria	43	22.0	37.2	14.9	0.4
Belgium	3	33.0	49.9	22.0	0.44
Canada	24	20.9	22.4	9.0	0.4
Denmark	14	25.1	26.1	14.5	0.48
Finland	40	22.6	31.1	12.8	0.41
France	26	26.2	34.3	19.6	0.57
Germany	14	28.9	45.0	19.9	0.44
Greece	39	24.8	45.8	7.4	0.16
Japan	22	16.4	22.4	9.7	0.43
Italy	32	42.7	53.0	26.0	0.49
Norway	26	28.8	51.1	16.0	0.31
Sweden	16	22.0	35.0	14.0	0.40
Spain	23	38.2	54.1	28.3	0.52
Switzerland	39	15.3	27.2	8.7	0.32
United States	26	21.1	31.5	12.5	0.40

[a]Rates are for the province or other administrative subdivision with the highest and lowest such rates in the country.

Source: Adapted from Blumenthal (1994). Table 2.

can be prevented at low cost, but three-quarters of the medical budget is spent on curative services, many of them provided for the elite at high cost.[28]

People often do not use health services even when they appear to be easily accessible. There are often subtle barriers to public access other than distance. The hours of operation may be more convenient for the clinic staff than for potential users, who must often work during most daylight hours. The cost, in money or in time lost from other activities, may be prohibitive or be considered excessive. Some persons may be too ill or too weak to get to the clinic or hospital. There are also the more complex sociocultural barriers. In many countries relationships between the government and the people are hardly cordial. Mistrust and negative reactions are common, the more so when people feel themselves to be treated with disdain or insensitivity. In Europe early social insurance funds of working people organized separate ambulatory care centers when patients did not want to go to the hospital outpatient departments because such places were identified with charity services.

Underutilization of primary health care facilities was studied at the Companiganj Health Project in Bangladesh.[29] The study district, population 120,000, had two hospitals and seven satellite clinics plus community health workers. Although PHC services were free and were staffed by trained professionals, many rural people preferred private, semitrained "western" practitioners *(Daktars)* or traditional healers for their care. The major correlates of utilization were found to be age of the patient, socioeconomic status of the family, season, and the total number of health care providers in the community. Although 42% of persons surveyed said that they preferred to use PHC services, only 25% actually did so. Due to their easy availability, place of treatment, lack of travel and waiting time, and type of medications given, the daktars' services were more attractive to most villagers than were those of hospitals and clinics.

Benefits

Just as the usership of medical care systems is diverse and complex, so is their benefit structure.

Type

Some medical care systems are established for a specific, limited purpose. Sometimes referred to as monovalent, selective, or vertical, these may strive to control particular diseases or problems such as malaria, trachoma, AIDS, or domestic violence. A specially constituted service may combine activities such as immunization or case finding with medical care benefits—for example, diagnosis and chemotherapy of tuberculosis. Somewhat broader systems function in areas such as maternal and child health. A monovalent system may be temporary, activated by a special threat, such as when yellow fever is reported in Latin America or Africa, and then become relatively dormant. Many such systems are permanent, having large establishments. Tuberculosis, leprosy, mental health, sexually transmitted disease, and maternal and child health services may operate networks of diagnostic and treatment centers. Monovalent systems are extensions of public health functions: Often largely preventive in nature, they may target persons who are not ill and who have little immediate incentive to come in to receive the benefit. Certain forms of therapy may be available as benefits in particular medical care systems where users share a certain cultural background. In India, Ayurvedic hospitals operate in tandem with western ones; in China acupuncture and moxibustion are available to those desiring them.

At the other extreme is the all-inclusive (polyvalent, comprehensive, horizontal) medical care system exemplified by the British National Health Service, described earlier.

Primary care is offered to the population at the point of entry into the health system, ideally combining the preventive and curative, personal and community, individual and environmental aspects. Primary care services are provided by health workers alone or in teams, at work sites, schools, homes, dispensaries,[30] clinics, or other health facilities. General and family practitioners provide primary care in industrialized countries. In less developed countries the measures undertaken should be simple, effective, accessible, and ongoing, and they should also be an integral part of community development. These programs are described in detail in Chapter 7.

An existing comprehensive primary care network is often used as a platform from which to launch a monovalent system. Sometimes the reverse is true—for example, in francophone West Africa where the *Service Prophylactique de la Maladie du Sommeil*, the antisleeping sickness service founded in 1931, developed into the *Service Générale d'Hygiene Mobile et de Prophylaxie*. After independence, this service formed the basis for the health care systems in Upper Volta, Mali, Senegal, Mauritania, and Niger.[31]

Secondary care comprises the standard inpatient services and specialist consultations, often on referral from primary care providers, and in less developed countries commonly organized at municipal, county, district, or provincial levels. In industrialized countries, particularly in western Europe where social insurance mechanisms are highly developed, benefits are generally divided into ambulatory or general physician care, and specialist and hospital care. *Tertiary care* includes highly specialized services such as neurosurgery or neonatal intensive care, available in advanced hospitals. In poorer areas such services, if available, may be limited to university teaching hospitals or national-level institutions.

Mode

The underlying philosophy of insurance schemes is different from that of national health services. The former spells out predetermined levels of compensation or indemnification for specific contingencies under a contractual arrangement, while the latter assumes responsibility for all risks. In nationalized medical care programs short-term sickness benefits are provided directly as *services*, while in other countries they may be provided as services or as *cash* (also sometimes called indemnity) through a variety of reimbursement schemes. Medical benefits paid as cash reimbursements must be distinguished from sickness benefits intended to replace lost wages, which may come from a different agency. Where health insurance is compulsory, as in Scandinavia, these two types of systems may blend. In Norway, for example, citizens are entitled to free care in public hospitals, in obstetric clinics, and in sanatoria for treatment, convalescence, and rehabilitation. If they choose to enter a private hospital, monetary reimbursement is provided according to a specified schedule. Because of the scattered population in Norway, free transportation to a hospital is a specific benefit. In Sweden free hospitalization in general wards is limited to a specific number of days. In France, where there is no limitation of access to any physician, patients are charged in a fee-for-service scheme and then reimbursed directly by the Social Security Administration. Although a standard schedule of fee reimbursements established by an annual convention exists, certain physicians officially considered more prestigious may exceed these charges. The combinations and differences in detail are virtually infinite.

Early European health insurance funds provided for service benefits to the patient and direct payment on his behalf by the sickness fund to the physician. This arrangement was resisted by physicians' groups as they became more organized. The doctors' incomes, as well as their control of the system, was greater under cash-benefit schemes in which the patient paid the physician's fee and then presented the bill to his insurance fund for recoupment of expenses up to a specified amount. Physicians could then charge more than the stipulated reimbursement level and the patient would make up the difference out of pocket.[32] France, New Zealand, Finland, Sweden, and parts of Canada, for example, follow this practice. In some countries higher charges are permitted only to patients from higher-income families. In countries such as Austria, Greece, Germany, Israel, Italy, and Japan that have multiple sickness funds, benefits very greatly depending upon the political strength and negotiating skill of the various parties involved. The same is true in the United States, where specific benefit schedules may be negotiated in labor–management contracts. Where commercial health insurance is available, policyholders may be permitted to purchase separate coverages for ambulatory, hospital, surgical, indemnity, or other types of benefits.

Sometimes considered an invisible benefit is the "free choice" of a physician by the patient. Even though the actual selection of a doctor is always limited by the realities of geography and economics, many people resent arbitrary assignment in this regard. Both patients and physicians may be adamant about maintaining at least nominal free choice. The handling of issues such as pharmaceutical benefits varies greatly and is not always predictable. In many countries, drugs given in hospital are paid for through the hospital coverage plan, while those for use at home are bought by the patient. In Australia, Sweden, and Norway life-saving drugs are free and others must be paid for. In Britain there is a small flat charge for any prescription. The common practice in poorer countries of issuing very small amounts of drugs, free or at minimal cost, has both good and bad features. Wastage is prevented, overdosage is minimized, and patients are discouraged from selling their drugs to others. However, repeated visits are annoying, inconvenient, expensive to the patient, and wasteful of staff time. Insufficient dosages of drugs may lead to resistance by microorganisms. Whereas many medical benefits have upper use limits, some countries have made special provisions for catastrophic illness. In the United States patients with particular conditions, such as chronic kidney disease, have special government funding or receive help from disease- or organ-related voluntary agencies.

Providers

Just as we could not discuss users without also describing their manner of use (i.e., benefits), we cannot divorce the medical care personnel from the contexts in which they function (i.e., facilities).

Churches, through religious orders, still control a substantial part of institutional care in some countries. Their ownership and management of hospitals is declining, however, and the orders are concentrating on care for the retarded, handicapped, and disabled. In Latin America from the earliest days, the *beneficencia, santa casa,* and *casa de socorro* were operated by local charitable welfare boards of leading citizens (the J*unta de Beneficencia*) with heavy involvement of the Catholic Church. As time passed, government subsidies were needed to assist with the high costs of these institutions, which are still a primary source of medical care for the poor. In Africa and India, the demise of colonialism, coupled with rising nationalism and increasing numbers of local professionals, has sharply reduced the role of the medical missionary. In many nations, such as Tanzania, some former mission hospitals have been absorbed into the national network, sometimes with their staffs placed on salary or contract. Nevertheless, mission hospitals still provide the only curative medical care services in many remote areas.

Indigenous and traditional healers

Despite the many systems described above, most of the world's people receive no modern medical care, and vast numbers get no care at all. Among those receiving some modern medical care, many also consult traditional healers at times. The combined populations of North America, Europe, Japan, and Oceania together constitute less than 30% of the world's people, and various forms of "nonofficial" healing are practiced even in these regions. Thus, the usership of traditional medical care systems exceeds that of scientific or western medicine by a factor of at least two to one.

Only a few countries, most notably India and the People's Republic of China, have made conspicuous efforts to integrate their indigenous medical practices with modern "western" medicine. In China, persons may elect to receive treatment by traditional (herbal, acupuncture, moxibustion, etc.) or modern medicine or by a blend of both. The acceptance and integration of the traditional sector were resisted by the Chinese medical establishment following independence in 1949 and required well over a decade to achieve. It is interesting that in Cuba, another Marxist state, medical care is organized along strictly scientific lines and folk medicine has been banned. In less developed countries in general, attitudes vary toward traditional medical practitioners. Following the Alma-Ata conference in 1978, a number of countries have integrated traditional midwives into their maternal and child health programs.

The private practice of medicine

The prevailing free enterprise system in the United States is reflected in its predominant system of private medical practice and in the large number of independent, profit-making, voluntary health insurance companies. However, private fee-for-service medical practice also exists in countries where the numbers of poor are proportionately much larger. An abundance of physicians is often available in the large cities of developing countries for those who can afford to pay for their services. In Brazil, for example, the private sector, including hospitals and clinics, prepaid health plans, pharmacies, and physicians in private practice, accounts for two-thirds of the total national health expenditures but is really available only to a small portion of the total population. However, where a very large number of physicians in private practice compete for patients, as in urban areas of the Philippines, their fees may be relatively low. Many of the more ambitious physicians emigrate from such conditions, and more marginal ones are forced to seek work in other sectors of the economy.

In many countries, persons already covered by compulsory health insurance can buy additional private policies to obtain better coverage or amenities such as private or semiprivate hospital rooms. Physicians or specialists not on the approved list of a health insurance fund may be consulted privately and simply be paid out of pocket.

Physicians

The keystone of medical care in all countries is the physician, a graduate of a medical school with professional responsibility for all aspects of patient care. In more developed countries, and for the wealthier segment of the population elsewhere, the physician is normally the initial point of contact for all curative and some personal preventive services such as immunization. Whereas different physicians may use the same technology for diagnosis, the same surgical procedures, or the same drugs, the form of medical practice varies greatly between and often within countries.

A physician may be paid in either (or both) of two ways: a specified fee for a certain unit of service, or a fixed salary. In the United States, the individual entrepreneurial ("solo") practice of medicine has been the rule, in what has been called America's last great cottage industry. However, group practice under many arrangements has been developing in the United States since the brothers Mayo established their multispecialty clinic in Minnesota in 1887. In recent years there has been a rapid growth of group practices in which three or more physicians work together and pool their incomes. Some large private prepaid insurance schemes, notably the Kaiser-Permanente system, contract with physicians groups and also distribute bonus payments to them according to a predetermined schedule. Small group practices, with a handful of physicians, are becoming increasingly common in many countries of western Europe.

Salaried physicians have long existed in Europe. In the late 19th century, salaried community (general practice) doctors were engaged on a large scale to supervise public health and provide medical care to the poor. In the *Zemstvo* system of Poland and czarist Russia physicians worked in regional polyclinics in order to save the time and cost of the home visits enjoyed by a wealthier clientele. This system was adopted by the sick funds of Jewish immigrants to Palestine and is still used in the polyclinics of the Kupat Holim in Israel.

In developing countries the government medical services, and usually the social security hospitals and clinics, are based on salaried physicians. In many countries all new physicians must undertake a period of full-time government service,[33] generally in rural areas, and sometimes all physicians must spend a proportion of their time working for the government, although this can be done where the doctor wishes, usually in a city. Because of the low wages in Latin America and elsewhere (e.g., Indonesia, Egypt, Thailand), some physicians devote part of the day to government service and maintain their private practice at other times. Government service may consist of medical school teaching, directing diagnostic laboratories, research, or administration, but most commonly it involves extensive patient contact in government clinics. In some European countries a system of split practice finds many physicians dividing their time between government service, service under a private medical insurance plan, and their own personal practice.

Remuneration

General practice physicians may function under a variety of payment mechanisms. In Australia the doctor can bill the patient (who then claims reimbursement from the health insurance commission) or may bill the government directly at a 15% discount. The system by which the patient pays the doctor and then seeks full or partial reimbursement is popular with physicians in many countries such as Belgium, France, Sweden, Switzerland, and (in part) Japan. In Canada the same idea is used in some provinces; in others, physicians bill directly to the health plan, which then collects the amount from the provincial and federal governments. Often the patient pays the full bill and is then reimbursed by the government, again simplifying life for the physician. A feature common to all of the reimbursement schemes is that a certain predetermined percentage or amount is paid by the insurance scheme or government, and the patient must pay the difference, if any, up to the amount requested by the doctor.

Two other types of payment mechanisms must be mentioned. The first is the capitation method mentioned earlier, used by the British National Health Service and in Spain, the Netherlands, and to some extent in Italy and Denmark. In this plan a patient selects a general physician and becomes enrolled in his or her panel. The physician is then paid by the government according to the size of the panel, not by the number of service units performed. There is a clear incentive to minimize return visits and unneeded patient contact under this plan, and this is true also for salaried physicians. At least in theory, however, doctors paid through a capitation system have an incentive, by increasing their panel, to see more patients than those who receive a salary regardless of their productivity. Also mentioned previously is the complex system of sickness funds used in Germany (*krankenkassen*) and some other countries, in which regional physicians' associations contract on a quarterly basis to provide care for fund members. Sickness insurance funds pay a negotiated lump sum to the physicians' associations, which pass on to each participating physician a share of the total that depends on the services provided and is weighted according to standard fee schedules. Both the capitation and negotiated-sum systems retain a measure of selection by both practitioner and patient, and more importantly they preserve the private entrepreneurial status of the doctor who does not wish to be regarded as anyone's employee.

The foregoing descriptions have dealt primarily with general medical practitioners—who in western Europe cherish their independence as private contractors—undertaking ambulatory care of patients. The physicians's day often includes both office practice and home visits in a proportion that varies among countries. In Belgium, for example, the general practice physician spends a large part of his or her time on home visits and even hospital-based specialists may make house calls to patients. In some other countries, home visits may be made on private time during off-duty hours. In the United States, house calls are essentially a thing of the past but may become more common in proportion to an increasing surplus of physicians.

The number of medical schools in Asia, Africa, and Latin America has been increasing greatly in recent years. Yet many people remain critical and unconvinced of the overall usefulness of this effort to produce more physicians in developing countries. Those who wish to maintain international standards favor the training of more doctors by scientific medical faculties on the western model. This will permit graduates to obtain advanced specialty training and experience abroad so they may practice the most modern medicine upon their return. In this view, all patients deserve first-class care, which can only be delivered by a thoroughly educated physician. Advocating this position is a large proportion of the existing medical establishment, whose prospects for career advancement may depend to a large extent on the prestige of association with London, Paris, or Boston. Another argument for training physicians in developing countries is that medical curricula and textbooks are well established and known by local and expatriate faculty. New instructional pathways perceived as leading to "substandard" practitioners do not appeal to many students, who resist being labeled second-class doctors. A third argument is that even in poor countries some people are able and willing to pay for private medial care by physicians who speak their language and understand their problems and that these people deserve to receive such treatment.

Opposing the production of larger numbers of conventionally trained physicians in developing countries are the following arguments:

- It is economically impossible to produce enough physicians. The actual cost of training a doctor to international standards is often higher in poor countries than in wealthier ones, because maintenance of faculties, libraries, and physical facilities is extremely expensive.
- After physicians are trained it is often difficult, if not impossible, to employ them properly in their home countries and large numbers join the "brain drain" and migrate, often permanently, to developed countries. It seems paradoxical that where the proportion of doctors in the population is very low by world standards, there may still be an excess relative to the nation's economic capacity to absorb them. This is true to a greater or lesser extent in the major de-

veloping countries of origin of physician migrants, such as India, Iran, Pakistan, the Philippines, and South Korea. In part this problem stems from the realities of income distribution in developing countries. The emigration of medical graduates from poor countries is often referred to as "reverse aid," or a subsidy from poor to wealthy nations. It has been suggested that the "export" of physicians is encouraged by some governments so that they will send back remittances of hard currencies. Some authors suggest that increasing the number of conventional physicians trained in developing countries would only increase this attrition by emigration.

- The conventional medical school curriculum in more advanced countries is simply not applicable to local needs.

Other professionals

Medical care naturally involves many more people than just patients and physicians. Extreme variations are found from one country to another in the use of various kinds of medical and health workers. In the United States the great majority of physicians are male, and of nurses are female—with a ratio of 1.4 nurses per MD. Despite the fact there is about one nurse per 300 inhabitants, the United States has a severe shortage of nurses. Thousands of foreign nurses have come to the United States to work, particularly from the Philippines, where there is one nurse for approximately 2500 people.

In a great many countries in the developing world there are fewer nurses (and other nursing persons) than physicians: India has about 1.3 doctors per nurse, and in Bangladesh the ratio is two to one. The number of nurses is very low in Latin America, where nursing is often looked down upon as a low-prestige occupation, not to be followed by refined women. The restricted educational and vocational opportunities for women in most developing countries have kept the number of nurses low in many developing countries. In Europe the relative number of nurses is much higher: Sweden and Finland have more than four RNs per MD. Considering the variety of forms of medical practice, it is difficult to specify the role of a nurse as distinct from that of a physician. Certainly some nurses are better trained and assume more responsibility for patient care than some doctors, particularly in medically underserved areas.

Medical auxiliaries (see Chapter 7) are well established in many areas.[34] In contrast to the long and extensive use of feldshers in the former Soviet Union, the use of physician's assistants and nurse practitioners in the United States is still not so common.

Facilities

In the United States a community-based physician can admit a patient to a hospital (at which he or she has "hospital privileges") and continue management of that patient, dividing practice time between office-based ambulatory care and hospital-based inpatient care. In western Europe, however, these roles are generally divided to the extent that the general practitioner relinquishes care of the hospitalized patient to the separate full-time specialist medical staff of the hospital. The patterns of hospital ownership and usage vary widely. The Scandinavian countries in particular have tried to rationalize their hospital systems. Sweden, for example, has a strongly institution-based medical care system with a hierarchy of municipal health centers providing primary ambulatory care for about 15,000 people, local district hospitals of about 300 beds for secondary care (60,000–90,000 people), county hospitals (*lasarett*) of 800 to 1000 beds (250,000–300,000 people), and regional hospitals for tertiary subspecialty care for about a million persons each. In Sweden there is little development of general family practice and the public has direct access to specialists via hospital outpatient departments. Norway has a similar system of hospital organization and also operates numerous "cottage hospitals" of eight to 20 beds in remote areas, often under the charge of the district health officer. In Scandinavia generally hospitals are operated by local authorities, although there are some privately operated facilities. The hospital-based tradition may be softening: Finland has passed legislation (The Primary Health Care Act of 1972) to strengthen PHC services and integrate them with existing hospitals. Elsewhere practices vary. Italy has both public *enti ospiedalieri* belonging to the state, region, province, or commune and many private *cliniche* or *case di cura*.

In Japan, 15% of hospitals are operated by local governments and 5% by the national government, while 80% of facilities are private, operated by one or a few physicians. There are more than 76,000 clinics of from two to 19 beds (certain licensing regulations change with 20 or more beds). In a country with poorly developed nursing homes and other extended care facilities, it is the practice to maintain both "acute" and "chronic" patients in hospitals. Therefore long stays, averaging 37 days, are the norm in Japan.[35] In contrast to the extensive commercialization of privately operated facilities in Japan, the Netherlands prohibits for-profit private hospitals. Some 75% of Dutch hospitals are voluntary, operated largely by religious groups, with the other 25% run by the government. The variety of arrangements is nearly endless, and these few examples should suffice to show the range.

The various facilities in which health and medical services are provided have been discussed in this and previous chapters. Table 12-2 lists some categories of patient care institutions.

Financing

The question of paying for health and medical care services is a universal lightning rod for comment and criticism (see Chapter 13). As a (perhaps *the*) crucial element, this topic merits close scrutiny everywhere. Many financing systems have been mentioned above and in preceding chapters. And all are subject to continual tinkering in line with changes in world and local economies, social and political thinking, programmatic needs, technologic advances, and the demographic and epidemiological picture.

The proportion of GNP spent on the health sector continues to spiral upward in industrialized countries, passing 14% in the United States. In typical developing countries, health services generally account for about 5% of all public spending and 2% to 4% of GNP.

An admittedly rough estimate of typical developing country proportionate expenditures in the health sector may be:[36]

- *Curative care* (personal outpatient and inpatient services and sales of medicines, 70% to 87%)
- *Patient-related preventive services* (immunization, maternal and child health, health promoter visits, 10% to 20%)
- *Other preventive services* (disease control, e.g., antimalarial spraying, vector control, sanitation, surveillance, health education and promotion, 3% to 10%)

The proportion of total health expenditures paid privately (rather than from governmental sources), while imprecisely defined, constitutes an important element in the financing equation. Current figures are hard to find, but estimates of private payment as a percent of total health expenditures among industrialized countries in the decade of the 1980s range from 4% in Norway to 7% in the United Kingdom, 36% in Australia, and 57% in the United States. Proportionate private expenditures are also highly variable among developing countries—for example, Lesotho, 12%; Colombia, 33%; Sudan, 41%; Venezuela, 58%; Ghana, 73%; India, 84%; Bangladesh, 87%; Afghanistan, 88%. These percentages may change quickly with changes in economic conditions and government policies. Although part of the variations arises from differences in definition of "health expenditures" and "private," it would be difficult to predict *a priori* the ratio for any particular country.

Discussions of cost containment are everywhere centered around issues of revenue enhancement, operating efficiency, appropriate use of technology, social equity, and societal benefit, which are the basis for the following chapter. Especially in developing countries, problems are compounded because available funds, already insufficient, are often spent ineffectively. Community-based primary health care posts sit idle while hospital waiting rooms are overcrowded. Costly medicines and other supplies are purchased, stored, distributed, and dispensed unwisely. Preventive maintenance for faciities and vehicles is neglected. Pilferage and corruption dishearten staff and user alike. Most commentators agree that drastic changes are necessary, but there is little consensus about what to do.

An exemplary study of health care financing on a national basis was carried out in Thailand by Myers *et al.* (1985). Existing innovative financing mechanisms include drug funds, established in one-third of all villages in Thailand. Usually launched with an inventory of products supplied by the Ministry of Public Health (MOPH), drug funds are managed by local committees and maintained with capital raised from households by sales of shares. Nutrition and sanitation funds are found also in many villages. Health card funds are an initiative of the MOPH. The inexpensive cards entitle household members to treatment of eight illness episodes a year at local health centers, plus MCH and immunization service and expedited attention at district or provincial hospitals. The program is designed to encourage the use of local facilities and preventive services, reduce congestion in hospitals, and raise revenues.

Well-conceived, innovative experiments such as these are urgently needed not only in developing countries but throughout the world.

Supervision

Regulation

The issue of control over health and medical services is crucial, complex, and dependent on the particular political and economic context of each country. Much of the preceding discussion has been concerned with the relative roles of the public and private sectors, users, providers, employers, and third-party payers such as insurance companies. Further definition of the specific place of each in the power structure is in the province of a treatise of medical sociology.

MANAGED CARE ORGANIZATIONS (MCOS) AND HEALTH MAINTENANCE ORGANIZATIONS (HMOS)

In 1960 the health sector in the United States consumed about 6% of GNP. Decades of political pressure from the physician and hospital lobbies were supported by legislators eager to please a trusting public, which led to wasteful oversupply of personnel and facilities. These efforts were based on the pervasive assumption that more is almost always better; more hospitals offering more intense services, more professionals with more training, and more research and research workers to do it. As a result, by the 1980s there were too many acute hospitals, each at 60% of capacity, and medical specialists outnumbered generalists by 3 to1. A huge research establishment devised expensive new treatments but few cures, and life expectancy had stopped increasing. Many commentators were frustrated and alarmed by the excessive costs and gross inefficiency of the health sector in the U.S. Efforts in the early 1990s to control the health care behemoth, including a major initative by President Clinton, were unsuccessful. By 1997 nearly 15% of GNP was spent on health, which had become the largest industry in the U.S., employing 1 of every 7 Americans. "These problems were . . . the results of what most Americans had once regarded as enormous success."[37]

One response to the system just described is *managed care*.[38]

The drive to control explosive growth in health care costs has propelled managed health care from a novel alternative to the cornerstone of the health care delivery system . . . The term *managed care organization* has become a wastebasket expression to describe organizations that have overall accountability for the health of an enrolled population. These organizations integrate financing or insurance functions with management of health care delivery. They manage both access to provider networks and the quality of health outcomes.[39]

Such a system exerts control over patients, who may utilize only a limited range of contracted providers and are discouraged from going to others whose charges are not covered by the plan. The MCO exerts control over providers by "utilization management" to contain costs, assure access to members, and maximize quality of care.

Some form of managed care has existed in the United States for more than a century. Early forms of prepaid health services were provided by employers for immigrant workers, and group practices in various forms emerged to fill the demand for services. Modern HMOs had their early origin in the early 1930s in a clinic in the Mojave Desert of California that served workers building a water aqueduct to Los Angeles. The clinic contracted with the project's insurance company, which agreed to pay a specified level of compensation in advance for each worker. Prepayment covered total medical care for each covered worker and avoided the need for fee-for-service billing on a case by case basis;[40] it placed the hospital on a predictable financial footing and also saved money for the employers. Similar arrangements followed at other construction sites, including the Grand Coulee Dam in Washington State. The contractor at Grand Coulee was the industrialist Henry J. Kaiser, who was impressed by the hospital's effciency and emulated the idea in his operations. A few years later World War II had started and Kaiser began building cargo ships. By 1944 prepaid group health plans covered thousands of steel- and shipworkers in California and Washington. A hospital was purchased in Oakland, California, and established as a nonprofit charitable trust[41] to finance medical care for the prepaid health plan. At the close of the war in 1945 the group's physicians extended coverage to the general public. The plan grew rapidly but retained a social purpose: "to demonstrate a new way of delivering medical care to the American people."[42] As of 1998 the plan enrolled more than nine million members in 17 states and the District of Columbia, with a staff of 100,000 and an annual budget of more than $12 billion.[43] The 28 medical centers and more than 300 medical offices used the services of 10,500 physicians, 57% of whom provided primary care. The medical staff are not direct employees but are organized into partnerships or professional corporations of physicians who take responsibility for providing and arranging necessary medical care at all Kaiser-Permanente facilities.

By the late 1990s there were almost 600 HMOs in the United States, plus many other types of managed fee-for-service plans with a bewildering variety of structures. Some are for-profit companies; others (such as Kaiser-Permanente) are not-for-profit organizations. The distinctions between independent prepaid health plans, traditional insurance companies, and other types of funders and providers are breaking down in a maze of mergers, acquisitions, and joint ventures.

NOTES

1. World Bank (1993).

2. Our knowledge of this subject has been greatly enriched by the publication of *National Health Systems of the World* by Milton Roemer. Volume 1 (The Countries) and Volume 2 (The Issues). 1991 and 1993, respectively.

3. Mission statements such as these may be found on some of the web pages of Ministries of Health listed in the Appendix to Chapter 5.

4. The United States, for example.

5. The jargon term *stakeholder* is widely used to designate those individuals and groups having a claim or interest in the health care system.

6. Roemer (1991).

7. Roy (1993); Jackson (1997) and Warner-Roedler *et al.* (1997) have useful reviews of the German system.

8. Abel-Smith (1965).

9. Italics added for emphasis. See Beveridge (1942).

10. Levitt and Wall (1984).

11. Cited by Maynard and Bloor (1995).

12. Jones (1996).

13. For early history see Sigerist (1951) and Roemer (1991).

14. Russian Soviet Federative Socialist Republic, Ukrainian Soviet Socialist Republic (SSR), Byelorussian SSR, Azerbaidzhan SSR, Georgian SSR, Armenian SSR, Turkmen SSR, Uzbek SSR, Tadzhik SSR, Kazakh SSR, Kirgiz SSR, Karelo-Finnish SSR, Moldavian SSR, Lithuanian SSR, Latvian SSR, Estonian SSR.

15. Maystrakh (1956).

16. Umeh (1996).

17. See Bloom and Gu (1997); Feng *et al.* (1995); Grogan (1995); Gu *et al.* (1993); Ho (1995); Liu et al. (1994, 1995); Liu and Hsiao (1995); Roemer (1991); Shi (1993); Yang et al. (1991); Young (1989); Xu (1995); Zhang et al. (1996); Zheng and Hillier (1995); and Zhu et al. (1989).

18. Young (1989).

19. Feng *et al.* (1995)

20. Ho (1995).

21. Hesketh and Zhu (1994).

22. Hsiao (1995).

23. Singapore Ministry of Health (1993).

24. *Ibid.*

25. Liposuction, face-lifts, mammoplasty, and cosmetic dentistry are not covered.

26. The Central Provident Fund .

27. Tejeiro Fernandez (1975).

28. Morley (1976).

29. PRICOR (1987).

30. In the British system, primary care physicians' offices are called *surgeries.*

31. Imperato (1974).

32. Abel-Smith (1965).

33. See Blumenthal (1994).

34. World Health Organization (1976a).

35. Hashimoto (1984).

36. de Ferranti (1985).

37. Fox (1998).

38. Loosely defined as "any system of delivering health services in which care is delivered by a specified network of providers who agree to comply with the care approaches established through a case management process." Block (1997).

39. Behnke (1997).

40. Sometimes called, "one ill, one pill, one bill."

41. Named the Permanente Foundation after the Permanente Creek in California, much admired by Mr. Kaiser; named by Spanish settlers because it never ran dry.

42. Greenlick (1997). See also Anon. (1997).

43. Private sector employee groups account for 59% of Kaiser-Permanente membership; state and local governments, 18%; federal government, 9%; education, 4%; and individual members, 10%. The percentage of the general population who are Kaiser-Permanente members varies by geographic area: about 40% of people in the northern California division, to less than 5% in some other areas.

13

Reforming the Health Sector

ANTECEDENTS: BACKGROUND AND CONTEXT

It is easy to make a picture of a building. We find little difficulty in describing its appearance: walls and windows; roof tiles; kitchen and parlor. Looking more deeply we can study blueprints that reveal the details of construction: hidden beams, pipes, and wires. Greater scrutiny takes us down to the foundation, and then beyond, to the underlying soft soil or bedrock, the neighborhood, and broader environment. A full description embraces the work of carpenters and plumbers, architects and engineers, planners and regulators. But understanding the *significance* of a structure demands attention to the historical and stylistic contexts by which we recognize its heritage, and to the dynamics of human relationships with the structure, its furnishings, and its surroundings.

It is costly and disruptive to remodel an existing building. As more modern materials become available, the kitchen slowly declines into obsolescence, but there may be little day-to-day pressure for a refurbishing. Although the neighbors modernize, the dictum, "If it ain't broke, don't fix it," can apply for a very long time. Cosmetic changes can maintain appearances, but when systems fail or a hurricane hits, the need for rebuilding becomes indisputable. Even so, it is almost impossible to install a foundation under an existing house except when circumstances absolutely demand it. And the same is true of the health sector.

As we saw in the previous chapter, the existence of a complex system implies that there are reasons why that particular system developed as it did. To the extent that the original forces—structural, political, economic—are still in place a system cannot change easily. Altered power relationships, pressures, and incentives provide conditions for renovation. When revolution displaces evolution the impetus and opportunity are in place for rapid and fundamental restructuring.

In seeking the roots of the current movements to reform the health sector, most commentators have rounded up the usual suspects: dissatisfaction with existing systems, excessive costs, inefficiency, misallocation of resources, poor management, perceived unfairness in access to services. Some nominate alleged villains such as multinational corporations or the IMF. In truth the pressures for reform originate in part within health sectors and in part from other internal forces within each nation, but they really represent broad transnational secular trends. The universality of the movement toward reform has its roots in landmark social and political events that on their surface seem unrelated to the inner workings of health systems.

There is a story, perhaps apocryphal, that someone asked Chairman Mao Zedong for his estimation of the French Revolution. He is reputed to have answered, "I don't know. It's too soon to tell." In that vein, it is not stretching too far to begin this discussion in the mid-19th century. In 1848 Karl Marx, with Friedrich Engels, issued the *Manifesto of the Communist Party*. There, and in *Das Kapital* two decades later, Marx considered the free enterprise system of the time to be seriously flawed. The accumulation and concentration of wealth through exploitation of the working classes by the *bourgeoisie* was seen as the root cause of human misery. Private ownership of the means of production was at the heart of the class system. Therefore, he argued, for people to be truly free, societies must evolve to a classless condition in which the means of production are publicly owned by the community as a whole. The 19th century revealed the worst excesses of the Industrial Revolution, which continued throughout Marx's lifetime. When the first volume of *Das Kapital* was published in 1876 the employment of children under the age of ten in factories was still legal in England. But in England and elsewhere in Europe state control was already eroding the uninhibited latitude of the private sector. Whether from social reformers or from competing politicians (recall the paternalistic German state under Otto von Bismarck) comprehensive social welfare legislation became the norm. Because of the excesses of unfettered markets, governments felt compelled to impose their muscle.

As related in Chapter 10, knowledge in chemistry, biology, and engineering has yielded an abundance of health-related technologic products from diagnostic drugs to whole-body irradiators to in vitro fertilization and genetic analysis.[1] Revolutions in production and transportation have generated vast markets served by immense industrial enterprises. Chairmen and CEOs may reign over enterprises that dwarf the resources available to many presidents and prime ministers, as consolidations and mergers make some corporations larger than most sovereign governments.

Thanks in large part to technology, the world has undergone demographic and epidemiologic transitions tied to economic development. Greater prosperity leads to more and more people with rising expectations, whose demands may outstrip the easy supply of amenities, including health care. The ceaseless demand and a declining marginal product of health expenditures have put immense pressure on the public purse. "Very few governments want to accept what is virtually a law: that it is impossible to satisfy the population's demand for health care. Moreover, anxiety over meeting those demands always leads to an increase in costs."[2]

> Until about the early 1980s, the decision of those who provide health care and its related product tended to drive the health system. The rest of society more or less passively accepted these decisions and paid for them. Since the 1980s, the balance of power of health care has shifted from the supply side to those who write the final checks in health care: governments and employers. Their decisions now tend to drive the health system, forcing the providers to accept whatever payments are forced down their throat. So far, however, this demand-driven health policy has proceeded blindfolded. Few of these decisions emanating from the demand side are based on reliable information on what works and what does not work in health care, that is, on what is and what is not worth paying for. It is a safe bet that in the next century, decisions in health care increasingly will be driven by sophisticated information systems available to both sides of the market.[3]

The roots of health sector reform are anchored in these struggles; indeed, their political nature has kept health services in the vanguard of the persistent public/private battles that represent a much wider process of social and political restructuring.

GOVERNMENTS AND MARKETS[4]

The Bolshevik Revolution of 1917, which launched a rigid, centrally planned Soviet Union, was a landmark event. It started an impoverished backwater on the road to becoming an industrial superpower. In the west, the growing power of business trusts and the economic turbulence and market failures of the 1920s and 1930s forced many governments to play an increasing role in regulating, and often operating, markets. Social welfare programs of various kinds led to a variety of mix-and-match recipes involving the public and private sectors. In Britain, Europe, Latin America, and elsewhere, state planning, with nationalized and parastatal[5] companies, were common features of the political and economic scene over most of the 20th century.

In the United States increasing government involvement in the form of Social Security and other social programs distinguished Franklin Roosevelt's New Deal of the late 1930s. Prosperity returned, helped not a little by the full economy stimulated by World War II. Public sector regulation of industries from broadcasting to transportation to securities trading continued for half a century and became respectable to all but the most ardent libertarians and conservatives. But the "liberal" President Clinton, in his 1996 State of the Union speech, declared that "The era of big government is over." How did this change in attitude come about?[6]

The decades that saw government activities grow and consolidate also witnessed increasing criticism of the public sector for inefficiency and poor performance.

Disapproval of interventionist governments led around 1980 to Reaganism and Thatcherism, with downsizing of bureaucracies and deregulation in the United States and divestiture of state-owned companies in the United Kingdom. Echoes of these policies reverberated widely. "Less government and more individual responsbility" became a mantra. Domestic private sectors expanded in size and power, accompanied by the growing influence of many multinational corporations. Technology and telecommunications allowed commerce to leapfrog over national borders and controls—by the mid-1990s more than a trillion private dollars flew around the world each day. Demographics played a role. Lack of faith in the stability of Social Security in the United States led to an intense accumulation of private financial assets by citizens concerned about their impending decades of retirement.

Undoubtedly, the key landmark in the ascendancy of "the market" over central state control was the collapse of the Soviet Union at the end of the 1980s. The USSR had finally succumbed to the fatal flaw of centrally planned economies: structural rigidity and inability to innovate and evolve. Only slightly less dramatic was the vast and truly revolutionary set of economic reforms undertaken in China under Deng Xiao-ping. Not so sensational but no less important are the steady moves toward market reforms in more or less closed and protectionist economies such as India, whose strong central government was planned by the Soviet-influenced Jawaharlal Nehru in the 1940s. At that time many countries now termed *developing* or *Third World* needed a strong government because there was little in the way of an indigenous private sector beyond petty traders.

Partly from political orientation, partly from necessity, many newly independent countries of the 1960s adopted free health care (at least in principle) as the basis of their public sector health policy. The ability of the population to pay was extremely low, the elite and middle classes were very small, and large sections of the population in the rural areas practiced a barter economy. It was felt also that health should not be regarded as an ordinary commodity. The predominant welfare state philosophy dictated that health, education, and social services were the prerogatives and responsibilities of the state. The fervent hope and optimistic expectation was that economic growth would strengthen governments, release resources for internal development, and build a country in which people became better educated, had higher incomes, and would approach an optimum level of health as enshrined in the Constitution of the WHO.

As inexperienced political leaders tried to stimulate industrialization and address poverty, their economic development was largely underwritten by loans from multilateral banks and bilateral support from OECD countries. This external development assistance was called upon to build infrastructure and obtain equipment for vertical programs to combat major diseases, to support maternal and child health projects, and to provide technical assistance until national staff could be trained to take over. Those funds were available directly, and exclusively, to sovereign governments.[7] Frequent instability in fledgling countries with coups and insurrections

spurred the concentration of government power, often in totalitarian directions that
were tolerated or even promoted as the United States and USSR both sought stability above all in their client states. That geopolitical incentive toward maintaining
strong central governments crumbled with the Berlin Wall and the explosion of international trade in the 1990s. Foreign aid has declined in the 1990s in part because
of the end of the Cold War, and also because of a growing perception that it really
hasn't accomplished its goals. As securities markets have matured around the world,
the flow of official development assistance has been eclipsed by transfers of private
investment capital despite frequent upheavals in various "emerging markets." The
trend toward private sector activities is strong even in centrally planned economies
such as China and Vietnam, but not (yet) in Cuba or North Korea.

Through these trends toward market economies, governments have generally (and
sometimes reluctantly) retained custody over programs for the general welfare. Once
launched, popular entitlements such as the Social Security and Medicare programs
in the United States and the British National Health Service (NHS) are essentially
irreversible. But even well-entrenched public benefits such as these are subject to
tinkering by conservative governments. The NHS has been periodically reconfig-
ured (chapter 12) to introduce greater market competition. New Zealand and other
countries have followed suit.

The countries of Europe and North America have a long history of enacting an-
titrust legislation, securities and exchange regulations, sunshine laws, and the like,
all in response to abuses in the markets and all over the opposition of those who
profited from the prior situation. Many western political leaders have been relentless in pushing for free markets, open trade, lower tariffs, and an end to protec-
tionism. The global system has suffered from imbalances and failures, such as the
debt crisis of the 1980s and the "Asian crisis" of the late 1990s in which many banks
failed and the value of currencies fell drastically. Growing globalization has been
discussed before, in connection with health and management information systems.
Commercial integration has tied all economies together, demanding uniform principles and practices in open markets.

Those nations in which governance and regulation were weak, where nepotism,
cronyism, and under-the-table deals were common,[8] were the hardest hit by the financial crisis. Conversely, those countries with the greatest transparency and
strongest accountability were the least affected. It is easy for westerners to dismiss
such deeply ingrained practices as mere corruption, but they must also be viewed
from the perspective of centuries of familial and ethnic loyalties, political and economic rivalries within the region, and established channels of trust and custom. Yet,
as in sports, all teams must play the game by the same fair rules or chaos will result. The problem is that the rules of the game at this point in world history are generally western ones and, like it or not, all teams that wish to compete must accept
them. The underlying conflict is largely cultural. By western standards, those who
gained the most by the unfairness of kleptocratic regimes and crony capitalism com-

plained the loudest when markets were made more transparent. The IMF sees its conditionalities as reinforcing market principles and assuring that uniform standards and procedures are followed in order to forestall or mitigate economic disasters. But many at the receiving end perceive them as draconian neocolonialist coercion enforced by a rapacious international conspiracy determined to exploit poor nations. The Visitor from Mars might view the conflicts as inevitable stresses and strains among diverse groups swept into the inevitability of global technologic and administrative homogenization.

The same principles of efficiency and transparency that underlie global commerce are being advocated for health care systems, whether operated by governments, the private for-profit sector, nonprofit organizations, or a combination of all. Clearly, the health sector is being influenced by global trends.

An inkling of the dramatic shift in outlook comes from two documents from the World Bank. A 1980 *Health Sector Policy Paper*[9] reflected the then prevailing world view. Its reference to the private sector was brief and unenthusiastic:

The private market cannot be expected to allocate to health either the amount or the composition of resources that is best from a social perspective. The most critical failure of the market derives from the inability of consumers of health services to make well-informed, rational choices. This inability is, in part, a consequence of the extraordinary complexity of medical problems, but also reflects the fact that consumers typically have little information or experience pertinent to specific health problems. Market failure also results from the presence of externalities. For example, procedures that halt the spread of communicable disease yield benefits to entire communities and, therefore, cannot be chosen properly by individuals acting in their own interest. Moreover, the health care system possesses many of the properties of public utilities. Often the unit producing services . . . must be large relative to the local service area in order to employ staff efficiently; thus, effective competition is not possible. For these and other reasons, governments have found it necessary to intervene in the health sector . . . In this case, the private market mechanism undeniably operates, but the distortions are very serious. Maldistribution of incomes in countries where average incomes are also very low means that the health needs of the poor are not translated into effective demand. While the distortion caused by income inequality applies to all sectors, the consequences for health are particularly tragic. Because of the emotional appeal of health issues, it may be politically attractive to redistribute welfare through government provision of health care.

. . . User charges are unpopular with governments because of the high cost of their administration and widespread problems of misappropriation of cash by health workers. User charges are also criticized for discouraging the use of preventive services and eary treatment of disease. Many countries have proclaimed the right to free health care, thereby limiting opportunities to impose charges.

. . . governments will have to spend substantially more on health. It is very difficult to reduce spending on most existing health care programs, and especially to cut those which are most costly and of lowest priority (e.g., large, urban referral hospitals and medical schools). Thus, new funds must be provided to cover most of the additional costs.

By 1987, the bank had changed its collective mind and proposed a new approach. "Simply stated, this approach would reduce government responsibility for paying for the kinds of health services that provide few benefits to society as a whole (as opposed to direct benefits to users of the service)."[10] In other words, the classical public health services of general benefit to the population (i.e., *public goods*) were considered to be reasonable responsibilities of governments. For medical services to individuals, four policy reforms were suggested:

- *Charge users of government health facilities.* Institute charges at government facilities, especially for drugs and curative care . . . Use differential charges to protect the poor. The poor should be the major beneficiaries of expanding resources for and improved efficiency in the government sector.
- *Provide insurance or other risk coverage.* Encourage well-designed health insurance programs to help mobilize resources for the health sector while protecting households from large financial losses . . . in the long run, insurance is necessary to relieve the government budget of the high costs of expensive curative care.
- *Use nongovernment resources effectively.* Encourage the nongovernment sector (including nonprofit groups, private physicians, pharmacists, and other health practitioners) to provide services for which consumers are willing to pay. This will allow governments to focus resources on programs that benefit whole communities rather than particular individuals.
- *Decentralize government health services.* Decentralize planning, budgeting and purchasing for government health services, particularly the services offering private health benefits for which users are charged . . . use market incentives where possible to better motivate staff and allocate resources. Allow revenues to be collected and retained as close as possible to the point of service delivery. This will improve both the collection of fees and the efficiency of the service.

GOALS AND PRINCIPLES OF REFORM

Health sector reform has been going on for decades with subtle shifts in the influence of the various players, underlain by powerful economic forces, but only in the 1990s was it named as a specific universal strategy. The discussion is not about the state of people's health or efforts to improve health *per se*. As we have pointed out repeatedly, the really cost-effective population-based interventions that matter most, such providing as safe water and food, nutrition education, smoking prevention, reduction of injury and accidents, and gun control, are not an issue. They are conceded to be the responsibility of the state. Rather, attention is riveted on purchasing and transferring the commodity called *health care* (that is, the entire panoply of clinical medicine, including diagnostics, procedures, pharmaceuticals, and the like) from providers to consumers. At the most basic level is the people's perception of the value of health—their confidence that the health establishment can protect and preserve health and, when necessary, make appropriate repairs—and their willingness to pay for it in the face of competing priorities.

Pressures for reform, mainly economic, exist no less in wealthy than in poor countries. In the European Community, for example, the proportion of GDP devoted to health services has risen (Table 13-1), financial support from central governments for health services has met greater resistance, and the demand for cost containment continues to grow. The health sector is forced to seek other sources of funds and to increase its productivity. As the conflict between state and market receives greater scrutiny from health economists, attention to market failures has led to an increasing realization that unhindered free enterprise in health will not yield a socially optimal or economically efficient result. For many developing countries, declining economic fortunes in the lost decade of the 1980s led to a decrease in government support for health services and a crisis in the health sector.

Table 13-1. Total Health Expenditure as a Percentage of GDP, European Union Member States and United States, 1970, 1980, 1988, and 1993

Country	1970	1980	1988	1993
Austria	5.4	7.9	8.4	9.3
Belgium	4.1	6.6	7.7	8.3
Denmark	6.1	6.8	6.5	6.7
Finland	5.7	6.5	7.3	8.8
France	5.8	7.6	8.6	9.8
Germany	5.9	8.4	8.8	8.6
Greece	4.0	4.3	5.0	5.7
Ireland	5.3	8.7	7.1	6.7
Italy	5.2	6.9	7.6	8.5
Luxembourg	3.8	6.3	6.8	6.9
Netherlands	5.9	7.9	8.1	8.7
Portugal	2.8	5.8	7.2	7.3
Spain	3.7	5.7	6.3	7.3
Sweden	7.1	9.4	8.6	7.5
United Kingdom	4.5	5.6	5.8	7.1
United States	7.3	9.3	11.6	14.1

Source: Mossialos et al. (1997) Table II. From OECD data.

The policy goals of the primary health care movement from the late 1970s through the 1980s were directed toward providing broad, basic services to the most underserved people.[11] Equity was foremost, with little research on efficiency or cost-effectiveness. Although a concern with equity is retained, the center of gravity has now shifted from social interventionism in the community to evidence-based planning in the Ministry of Health.

Health sector reform has been defined as "sustained, purposeful change to improve the efficiency, equity, and effectiveness of the health sector" with emphasis on:

- The important connections between health, the health sector, and the broader goals of sustainable human development. Health improvement and health sector reform have important externalities affecting social well-being.
- A vision of the health sector as a whole, not just of one or another of the parts. Specifically, there is growing awareness of the importance of non-government health care providers in many developing countries.
- A changing role for government in the health sector. In many developing countries, state efforts have gone almost exclusively into paying for government-provided health care. Governments increasingly need to redefine their role from one of service provider to one of financier and manager of growth and change in the health sector.
- New tools for both public and private action. Governments must develop their capacities in managing a broader array of fiscal tools: fees, taxes, subsidies, and incentives to bring about desired change. Legal and administrative tools, such as regulation, licensing, and quality control will also play a larger role. Governments can also increase their provision of information to both providers and consumers to improve health sector functions. Private financiers and providers must also develop new skills, as they may be required to increase their provision of public and merit goods.
- A wide range of specific reform strategies. These have been proposed based on analysis by international organizations and recent national experience in the richer and poorer countries. These strategies include strengthening public management, explicit priority setting for a universal package of assured interventions; decentralization; new methods of generating and managing finances for health and enhancing the role of private providers in national health systems.[12]

More succinctly, Joseph Kutzin[13] has listed specific goals of health sector reform:

- To improve health status and consumer satisfaction by increasing the effectiveness and quality of services
- To obtain greater equity by improving the access of disadvantaged groups to quality health care

- To obtain greater value for money (cost-effectiveness) from health spending, considering improvements in both the distribution of resources to priority activities (allocational efficiency) and the management of resources that have been allocated (technical efficiency)

The WDR93 hinted at the breadth of changes needed for fundamental reforms, but the recommendations in group 1 in Table 13-2 have been overshadowed by the attention given to the group 2 and group 3 recommendations. A very large number

Table 13-2. Relevance of Policy Changes for Reform of the Health Sector in Three Groups of Countries

Government Objectives and Policies	Type of Economy[a]		
	Low Income	Middle Income	Formerly Socialist
1. Foster an enabling environment for households to improve health			
a. Pursue economic growth policies that benefit the poor	++	+	+
b. Expand investment in education, especially for females	+++	++	—
c. Promote the rights and status of women through political and economic empowerment and legal protection against abuse	++	+	+
2. Improve government investments in health			
a. Reduce government expenditures for tertiary care facilities, specialist training, and discretionary services	++	+++	++
b. Finance and ensure delivery of a public health package, including AIDS prevention	+++	++	++
c. Finance and ensure delivery of essential clinical services, at least to the poor	++	++	+
d. Improve the management of public health services	+	++	+++
3. Facilitate involvement by the private sector			
a. Encourage private finance and provision of insurance (with incentives to contain costs) for all discretionary clinical services	+	+++	+++
b. Encourage private sector delivery of clinical services, including those that are publicly financed	++	+	++
c. Provide information on performance and cost	+	++	++

[a]— not relevant; + somewhat relevant; ++ relevant; +++ very relevant.

Source: Adapted from World Bank (1993), Table 7.1.

of analyses, commentaries, and recommendations have condensed around a relatively small menu of goals and approaches:

- Reorient Ministries of Health.
    Make ministries smaller and less hierarchical.
    Emphasize management of performance and resources.
    Shift away from technical and clinical issues to management, finance and planning.
    Separate the provision of services from the financing of services.
    Introduce competition into public and private sectors.
- Institute user charges for publicly provided services.
- Establish or expand health insurance schemes.
- Decentralize to regional/district government levels.
- Contract out or privatize publicly provided services.

During the early 1990s health sector reform was a prominent issue everywhere, not only in the poor countries. It was the first major initiative of President Clinton, and although his reforms were not approved, national attention was focused on the subject. As the president learned, political conflicts are inevitable as familiar channels are disrupted and vested interests are challenged. At the same time, other countries were undergoing similar soul-searching, and the World Bank was preparing the WDR93, *Investing in Health.* Although it is common shorthand to speak of "the bank's" report, many persons from outside the bank participated in preparatory consultations, including a Steering Committee from the World Health Organization, officials of many governments, academicians, foundation staffers, and others. *Investing in Health* did not create health sector reform, but its thoroughness and prestige quickly made it the manifesto for health sector reform throughout the world. Priorities given to specific health problems were based on DALYs and the Global Burden of Disease, described in Chapter 4. The WDR93 contained an indictment of business as usual in health systems of developing countries. It specified four pervasive defects that hamper progress in reducing the burden of disease and frustrate efforts to respond to new health challenges and threats:

- *Misallocation.* Public money is spent on health interventions of low cost-effectiveness, such as surgery for most cancers, at the same time that critical and highly cost-effective interventions such as treatment of tuberculosis and sexually transmitted diseases (STDs) remain underfunded. In some countries a single teaching hospital can absorb 20 percent or more of the budget of the Ministry of Health, even though almost all cost-effective interventions are best delivered at lower-level facilities.
- *Inequity.* The poor lack access to basic health services and receive low-quality care. Government spending for health goes disproportionately to the affluent in

the form of free or low-cost care in sophisticated public tertiary-care hospitals and subsidies to private and public insurance. Further inequities are based, for example, on urban/rural residence, ethnicity, or gender.

- *Inefficiency.* Much of the money spent on health is wasted: brand-name pharmaceuticals are purchased instead of generic drugs, health workers are badly deployed and supervised, and hospital beds are underutilized.
- *Exploding costs.* In some middle-income developing countries health care expenditures are growing much faster than income. Increasing numbers of general physicians and specialists, the availability of new medical technologies, and expanding health insurance linked to fee-for-service payments together generate a rapidly growing demand for costly tests, procedures, and treatments.

The prescription to correct these deficiencies (they call it "Agenda for Action") is summarized in Table 13-2. The blend of recommended policy changes differs for low-income, middle-income, and formerly socialist economies.[14] Many other institutions have been active in health sector reform, not least of which is the WHO.[15]

Scarcity of Resources

The cardinal law of economics, that resources are scarce relative to wants, is as true for health services as for other aspects of life. Regardless of political system or national income, no country possesses the personnel, facilities, material, knowledge, and resolution to resolve every health problem. But even if resources were unlimited and money grew on trees, someone would have to make decisions about what needs to be done, how to do it, which people so serve, and how to evaluate and improve the outcome.

SETTING POLICIES

The jocular comment, "There's no reason for it, it's just our policy," illustrates a common conception of a policy as an arbitrary rule mindlessly applied. Each of us has encountered some situations in which that seems to be the case. Nevertheless, the determination and implementation of policies is a necessary and even critical element in any public enterprise, including health.

Policy and Planning

Process versus outcome

Most people would view a policy as correct or flawed if the results do or do not meet expectations. But there is a more important way to look at policies, independent of the outcome. United States Treasury Secretary Robert Rubin emphasized

this difference in a discussion of a program in which a large amount of money was
sent to support the Mexican government during a financial crisis:

> He points not to the happy result—that Mexico paid us back ahead of schedule, with a
> tidy profit for the Treasury—but to the sound decision. "If the Mexican support pro-
> gram had gone bad, I would still have said that it was the right thing to do," he says.
> "But it was judged successful because it worked. I don't think that's actually the way
> it should have been judged. It should have been judged based on whether it was the
> right judgment for our national interest in terms of everything that could be known at
> the time." Rubin says that focusing on the result rather than the decision is what's wrong
> with Washington, because it deters people from "acting optimally."[16]

Deliberately skewing policies to achieve one or another outcome compromises the
objectivity of information and the validity of the decision-making process. Nevertheless, policies are often based on short-term political advantage rather than sober
and scholarly analysis.

The status of policy and planning

Health policy and planning have been the subjects of great scrutiny in the era of
health sector reform. Several notable books on this subject, primarily from British
authors, have appeared in the 1990s.[17] Determining a national policy can be a rather
scary enterprise. Much is at stake. The future is unpredictable. Resources are scarce.
People fight over personal interests. Who gets to set the agenda, and who has to
pick up the pieces if it doesn't work as hoped? How does personal clinical medical
care fit into an overall health policy, and how does health policy fit into an overall
national economic or development policy? Always in the background is uncertainty
about the determinants of health; why people behave as they do; how to make health
care systems more efficient; and how to adapt health policy making to the realities
of globalization.

   As health systems developed through different paths, some aspects of policy were
emphasized depending on the political and pragmatic makeup at the time. Over the
decades a key set of major issues has become predominant, and the profession of
health service planner has arisen to wrestle with them. Health-related policies may
aim at specific problem-solving, but they are often grounded in fundamental issues
of social equity and resource allocation.

   The Executive Board of the WHO has defined a national health policy as "an expression of goals for improving the health situation, the priorities among those goals,
and the main directions for attaining them," commenting that:

> Health policy formulation and analysis has received insufficient attention. Many diffi-
> culties have been encountered in the past in defining country-wide programmes in terms
> of their national priority, and these difficulties have often arisen as late as during pro-

gramming and implementation. This serves to emphasize the need to establish firm links between governmental programme management levels and the national policy-making levels. Policy formulation is an ongoing governmental activity. Policies, formal as well as unwritten, emerge continuously from governmental processes. The problem is to ensure that planning, programming and implementation serve the national policies as pronounced by the highest authorities in the country.[18]

For our purposes we can view a policy as a guide for a course of action intended to further a particular interest or help attain a defined goal or objective. In general, goals may be stated in various terms, which are not always mutually exclusive. For example,

- *Mortality, morbidity, or demographics*—to reduce deaths among people aged 15 to 64 by at least 25% by 2010; to reduce incidence of measles among 1–5 year-olds by 80% within 1 year; to limit population growth to 1% per year within 5 years
- *Service*—to screen all newborns in the Southern Territory for phenylketonuria by 1994; to provide nutrition counseling to all pregnant women
- *Facilities or resources*—to establish a dental clinic in each town of 10,000 or more by 2010; to put a rural health center in every village of 1,000 by 2005.
- *Capabilities*—to manufacture measles and polio vaccine locally rather than importing them; to certify every traditional midwife in basic obstetrical care
- *Social welfare, ethics, and philosophy*—to expand services to residents of outlying islands or to slum-dwellers; to improve equity; to reduce poverty and stimulate self-reliance
- *Economics*—to increase (or to reduce) the proportion of GNP (or government budget) spent on health services to $n\%$ by 2005

Formal national health goals are desirable because they define commitments and tend to ensure that they will be met. As suggested by the WHO Executive Board, countries function to some extent on informal or unwritten policies. This may be necessary on an *ad hoc* basis to stay ahead of emerging situations, but it is done also in an ongoing way because of the difficulty of reaching consensus and to retain flexibility in making and funding commitments.

Examples of specific goals are those on health promotion and disease prevention stated by the United States Department of Health and Human Services in its *Healthy People 2000* program.[19] Here are some goals selected at random from 112 highly detailed pages :

- Reduce coronary heart disease deaths to no more than 100 per 100,000 people.
- Reduce overweight to a prevalence of no more than 20 percent among peo-

ple aged 20 and older and no more than 15 prcent among adolescents aged 12–19.

- Increase to at least 75 percent the proportion of mothers who breastfeed their babies in the early postpartum period and to at least 50 percent the proportion who continue breastfeeding until their babies are 5–6 months old.
- Reduce pregnancies among females aged 15–17 to no more than 50 per 1,000 adolescents.
- Reduce alcohol consumption by people aged 14 and older to an annual average of no more than 2 gallons of ethanol per person.
- Reduce drowning deaths to no more than 13 per 100,000 people.
- Reduce diabetes to an incidence of no more than 2.5 per 1,000 people and a prevalence of no more than 25 per 1,000 people.
- Increase to at least 50 percent the proportion of large businesses and to 10 percent the proportion of small businesses that implemented a comprehensive HIV/AIDS workplace program.

Levels of Policy Implementation

Julio Frenk has defined four policy levels:

- The *systemic* level deals with the structure and functions of the system, by specifying the institutional arrangements for regulation, financing and delivery of services.
- The *programmatic* level refers to the substantive content of the system, by specifying its priorities, for example through a universal package of health care interventions.
- The *organizational* level is concerned with the actual production of services, by focusing on issues of quality assurance and tecnical efficiency.
- The *instrumental* level generates the institutional intelligence for improving system performance through information, research, technological innovation, and human resource development.[20]

Strategies spelled out in policies are supported by tactical programs or plans of action. These may be general or focused, long term or short term, confined within the health sector or under broad intersectoral sponsorship, as the situation may demand. Within programs, specific projects will usually be carried out to make the programs work. Each project may be further broken down into specific activities or tasks. At Frenk's organizational level, organizations such as governments propose rules and regulations to help assure uniformity in carrying out the policy. Here is an example of two different approaches to help achieve a single goal in the area of child survival. *Goal*: improve infant and child health by reducing morbidity and mortality from infectious diseases:

	1	2
Policy	Immunize all children	Reduce mosquitoborne diseases
Program	Preschool polio vaccine	National malaria control program
Project	Village X health center immunizations	Village X domestic spraying
Regulation	Give each child oral trivalent polio vaccine at specified ages unless he is immunosuppressed, . . .	Spray all houses with four walls using a *n*% solution of DDT twice annually unless mosquitoes are numerous, in which case spray at bimonthly intervals, . . .

In these two examples the overall goal is the same, but policies, programs, projects, and regulations are increasingly different. One could cite a very long array of configurations and rearrangements of the basic elements. As a general rule, *projects* are relatively brief and have a limited purpose with a clear endpoint, such as the construction of a building or checking everyone in a town for infection with tuberculosis. Note that regulations, such as building codes, immunization or spraying protocols, or similar operational details may be constant for many separate but parallel projects. *Programs* come in all shapes and sizes and are usually of intermediate duration; *policies* tend to be long-lived; and, barring revolutions, *goals* are either delimited by an epidemiological or temporal target or are more or less permanent.

Some characteristics of policies

Goals, as enunciated ideals, may be utopian and admittedly unachieveable, but policies must have reasonable objectives. Thus one would probably not establish a goal to reduce neonatal mortality to zero, but might more reasonably establish a target level believed to be achievable through programs for improved prenatal care, genetic counseling, neonatal intensive case nurseries, maternal education, and the like. Note that some of these measures can serve also for other purposes, such as the promotion of family planning. Maintaining consistency among many diverse policies may be difficult, and implementation of one policy may have unexpected consequences with respect to others. For example, a requirement that unlicensed folk practitioners must take training in midwifery might conflict with another policy that supports the unhampered practice of traditional medicine.

Where policies come from

Policies may be imposed on a country by various intergovernmental organizations. As members, governments are bound to accept a range of policies which they may view with varying degrees of enthusiasm. These policies may cover an infinity of topics from disease reporting to adoption of major national campaigns. However, most of the pressures that determine fundamental policies exist internally. Major players have always included the state, through its leaders and bureaucracy, the medical profession, employers, and other commercial interests (where these exist, outside of socialist centrally planned economies), and, as far as their voice can be heard, the clients of the system. Advocacy groups of all kinds play a role. In the 19th century it was sanitary and humanitarian groups; the late 20th century finds many single-issue organizations with causes ranging from abortion to pesticide control. Barker has commented about AIDS policy:

> The reader will observe that there are many reasons for which an issue becomes seen as one demanding attention, and that these depend heavily on how the public—and particular sections and groups within society—see the issue. The arena in which an agenda such as this one is set is highly charged with emotion and conflicting political and ethical values.[21]

The term *policy gatekeepers* has been applied to the media because of their decisions about which events to cover and what issues are important.[22]

Health Planning

Planning is in essence the process by which one envisions a better future and charts a way to get there. The purpose of planning is to determine how, when and where to employ resources to achieve goals most effectively. In the classical approach there is first an analysis of problems, including a range of proposed solutions. Then priorities are set, decisions are made, and (where appropriate) details of programs and projects are spelled out with relevant procedures and regulations. "Many writers do not distinguish between policy and planning, but for me, planning follows policy: planners help to put policies into practice, although the planning process itself may help to develop and refine health policies."[23]

In Zambia, the permanent secretary of the Ministry of Health has subjected any plans for health sector reform to four simple questions: What do we want? What do we have? What do we need? What can we afford?[24]

In the wealthier countries the profession of planner or administrator has evolved through necessity only in recent decades; in many less developed countries these functions are no less necessary but do not yet represent an established career path. Among the many kinds of planners more commonly employed are agricultural, city (urban), defense, development, economic, educational, energy, environmental, financial, health, industrial, manpower (human resource), public sector, recreational, regional, resource, rural, and transport planners. All of these specialists must coordinate through some mechanism, such as a planning ministry or consultative group, agency, or department, often in the prime minister's office. Health planning may be the responsibility of a Ministry of Planning or similar body which may not know very much about health. Worse yet is the rather glum assertion that

> Most health care service organizations in developing countries produce what they think should be produced . . . They are usually dominated by physicians who want large sophisticated hospitals that meet their own needs (and the needs of the politicians) but do not provide simple, basic services. Such planning frequently results in services and facilities that neither respond to actual health needs nor integrate with health-related activities of the non-health sectors. What we have then is a situation in which neither health planning nor health care services planning seems to fit the needs.[25]

Needs in health planning

Successful planning requires a clear view of objectives at each level, including the means for measuring progress toward achieving them. Schedules and forecasts are an integral part of planning. Also to be determined are needs for personnel, their proper training, conditions of service, responsibilities and relationships (chains of command), evaluation, incentives, promotion, and discharge. Material resources to be planned for include facilities, equipment and its maintenance (including vehicles), and supplies of all kinds, including communications. Logistic support must be arranged for the actual production and delivery of services. Liaison should be established with various agencies or other parties within or outside the government, or with international agencies that may have an interest in the program. And of course sources of capital and operating funds must be identified, and budgeting, financial management and auditing procedures must be standardized.

Planning procedures may sound tedious, mundane, and unexciting to those scientists accustomed to working on a higher intellectual plane, but the failure of any element can destroy important current programs and jeopardize future ones, waste valuable resources (including time), and lead to disillusionment and loss of faith in the health establishment. The work of the public health planner is no less difficult or important, and should be no less prestigious, than that of the researcher or clinician.

Because health programs cannot function in a vacuum, a high degree of intersectoral cooperation is needed. However, in countries with a decentralized political structure, where decision-making is spread among overlapping and competing authorities, perceived threats to power bases may hamper collaboration. Programs and projects should normally have a predetermined life span, with a built-in schedule for periodic review and evaluation. It is easier to begin projects than to end them, because emotions and livelihoods are involved. Experienced administrators often find that it is far simpler to solve the technical questions than to deal with the human relations issues.

Despite the best intentions, impediments may be expected in the planning and execution of any health program.

In developing countries where many aspects of life are uncertain, there persists an understandable lack of a sense of need for planning. The cynic asks: Why plan when it is impossible to get delivery of materials to complete our constructional works? Why plan when the top decision-makers overturn our recommendations with ad hoc politically-based decisions? Why plan when we can't ensure that we will get the needed staff? Why plan when we can't rely on the timely delivery of drugs and supplies? Why plan when it will be impossible to get the transport to carry out the survey? These are hard questions to answer. But they reflect the realities of life. Perhaps the only answer is that when we are faced with such uncertainties, it becomes all the more important to plan, and to know in advance what our alternatives can be. That is, to build flexibility into our actions and be prepared for whatever may come. And regarding those political decisions continually overriding the planning process—a well-done plan based on sound policy is the best defence against *ad hoc* political action.[26]

EQUITY AND THE QUESTION OF PRIORITIES[27]

Is health a "right?" The preamble to the Constitution of the World Health Organization (1946) stated the general case: "The enjoyment of the highest attainable standard of health is one of the fundamental rights of every human being without distinction of race, religion, political belief, economic or social condition."

This statement was followed (1948) by the Universal Declaration of Human Rights, which said in Article 25.1: "Everyone has the right to a standard of living adequate for the health and well-being of himself and of his family, including food, clothing, housing and medical care and necessary social services."[28]

These declarations fall short of stating that everyone deserves to be "given" good health *per se*, but both refer to an undefined "standard." Clearly each citizen cannot demand from society unlimited efforts to reverse the effects of advancing years or to undo every bodily defect. There must be some baseline that reflects the community standard of adequacy, and the degree of responsibility accepted by society to achieve and maintain that standard. Some governments have not accepted this obligation: In the mid-1990s the United States still had about 40 million citizens without any form of health insurance.

If there exists a right to health, or to health care, there must be someone from whom its fulfillment may be demanded. Therefore an adversary relationship is implicit in the idea of health as a right, whose claiming is viewed by the left as a manifestation of class struggle. The practice of public health involves the political process and the challenging of some powerful interests in society, which will not readily yield their influence.[29]

Clearly, whenever "health" is mentioned, clinical medical care is foremost in the minds of administrators and public alike. Although many factors are more important than medical care in determining the state of health, resources are rarely given to other sectors (such as education) in order to improve health. Similarly, little attention is given to public health functions, which may be considered by budget authorities merely as a necessary cost of doing some routine business. When "equity" is mentioned, it is taken to mean an acceptable way to apportion medical care services among the population. Then how should medical care services be allocated?

- *Equally to all citizens.* But if services are to be offered equally to everyone, then it will inevitably cost more to provide them to some than to others. Physical distance, social distance, and many other factors destabilize equal distribution based on expenditure per capita. The cost of providing services to a thinly dispersed rural population may be far more than that for town dwellers.
- *According to their medical need*—that is, the state of their health. But here again we are caught in a dilemma. The greater the need, as in the case of gravely or terminally ill patients, the less may be the likelihood of recovery despite the consumption of substantial resources. Is it fair to the majority to devote to the already hopelessly ill an amount of effort and money that could permit many less serious illnesses to be treated (or better yet, prevented) before they progress to an intractable stage?

Medical care is in fact often rationed by ability to pay. Since ancient times this has seemed to some unjust, so the very poorest in many societies have received services from private charities or public funds, but in the past century governments in general have underwritten an increasing proportion of medical care expenses, often intermixed with personal payments.

It is often suggested that health care resources should be distributed on the basis of *optimal social value*—to improve population-based health indicators and provide the greatest good for the greatest number.

"Priorities" is the more politically correct inverse of the nasty word "rationing." Under either banner, choices are made so that some people and not others receive certain interventions. Robert Maxwell has said, "How to use our healthcare resources wisely and justly is a wicked, not a tame, problem. That means the puzzle has no permanent solution." He posits five related axioms:

- No country, however rich, is going to be able to pay for all the health care that could benefit its citizens and they would like to have.
- We have an urgent and inescapable duty to minimize the harm that will be done in rationing of health care by avoiding expenditure that offers little benefit.
- Managing demand offers opportunities, as well as managing supply. This means taking health promotion and disease prevention seriously.
- Rationing should be based firmly on principle and the fundamental criterion should be capacity to benefit from the intervention. No citizen should be given lower or higher priority on the basis of *who* they are.

- Rationing is not new, but its methods are largely arcane. We need more understanding of how it works in any system, and a willingness to learn to do it better.[30]

Resources can be rationed according to any of three principles:

- Political preference or other imposed means of selection
- Willingness and ability to pay
- "Need" and the likelihood of benefit

The first principle has often been applied in countries with authoritarian regimes. The second, the conservative view, is much the simpler, as all decisions are made by the market. The third, held by liberals or egalitarians, is more complex as it requires many, often difficult, decisions to be made, but it is the current principle of choice. One basis for establishing priorities is to evaluate health benefits and drawbacks according to objective criteria within a cost-effectiveness environment.

> Remarkably . . . few key decision-makers anywhere in the industrialized world seem to rely on these types of analysis in their daily operations. The occasional use of economic evaluations so far has been almost experimental and sporadic. To date, most decisions concerning treatment methods are still driven by untested or only crudely tested medical theories.[31]

The usual criteria for determining priorities for action include the number of people affected and their age; the extent of individual suffering; the interventions available to improve quality of life of those affected; the cost per case of the intervention; and the total cost of helping everyone affected by the problem.[32] These criteria reflect back to the emotional content of health care decisions, particularly those related to the margins of life and death, and help explain the widespread reluctance to rely on dispassionate rules. Although public policy must take account of these cultural sensitivities, a willingness to recognize priorities and set limits seems to be proportional to the level of frustration with ever-increasing costs. A much-cited example of rational priorities for medical care comes from the state of Oregon, where a commission was appointed in 1989 to make recommendations to the state legislature on how to expand coverage and set priorities in the Medicaid program. Uninsured people were to be added to the Medicaid list to cover every resident whose income was below a certain level, but this could be afforded only by reductions in the benefit package. After much consultation with health professionals and public hearings and community meetings held throughout the state, the commission produced a list of almost 700 condition–treatment pairs grouped in 17 categories and ranked according to priority.[33] According to the plan the Medicaid program would pay only for items above a certain cutoff point on the list, to be determined from time to time by the legislature. The plan was implemented in 1994 and has been politically popular among the general public and with Medicare recipients. As of 1998 it is limited to relatively poorer persons eligible for the state Medicaid program, and has not been extended to the general public.

Because of continually rising costs, several countries have set priorities for coverage of medical interventions. Singapore has already been mentioned (Chapters 11, 12). The government of New Zealand appointed a Core Services Committee in 1992 to advise on the specific procedures that should be included in their publicly funded health system. Rather than preparing an Oregon-style list, the committee focused on currently provided services and specified a process to determine more specific priorities. They organized consensus conferences and workshops, conducted reviews of published research, consulted experts on contemporary practice, and held public hearings. Their purpose was to draw up guidelines, based on therapeutic effectiveness and on cost-effectiveness, to help the Ministry of Health to determine which people were most likely to benefit from receiving a particular service so that resources could be targeted to achieve the greatest health gain.

In 1990 the Dutch state secretary for welfare, health and sport set up a Committee on Choices in Health Care (the Dunning Committee) whose report was published in 1992. Although they did not specify the items, they proposed a basic package of health care available to all Dutch citizens through their compulsory social insurance plans. As in Oregon, condition–treatment pairs would be arranged in priority order, determined by a community-based process and considerations of cost-effectiveness. The basic social insurance package would be limited to necessary care. Inclusion or removal is based on four criteria—two medical (whether a treatment is effective and whether it can be efficiently done) and two judgmental (whether the treatment is necessary and whether the patient can pay for it). Under those criteria dental care and physiotherapy, for example, have been removed from the basic package.

Priorities may be stated in positive or negative terms. The simplest case is pharmaceuticals. A positive priority list will display the names of all products for which a program will pay. A negative list will specify those items for which a program will *not* pay, assuming that all others are covered.

The most highly promoted example of a specific priority is the *package of essential health services* (PEHS) recommended by the WDR93 and based on the burden of disease estimates in that publication. The package is reminiscent of the "selective primary health care" approach advocated 14 years earlier (see Chapter 7).[34] The WDR93 actually recommended two subsets of packages:

- A *public health package* consisting of the augmented Expanded Program on Immunization; school health including deworming, micronutrient supplemen-

tation, and health education; information on health, nutrition, and family planning; tobacco and alcohol control programs, monitoring and surveillance; vector control programs for prevention of AIDs.
* A *clinical services package* consisting of short-course chemotherapy for tuberculosis; management of the sick child; prenatal and delivery care; family planning; treatment of sexually transmitted diseases; and limited clinical care

A combination of the public health and clinical packages was calculated to cost about $12 (U.S.) per person per year in low-income countries and about $22 in middle-income countries. It is estimated that the package could eliminate 21% to 38% of the burden of premature mortality and disability in children under 15, and 10% to 18% of the burden in adults.

> The cost would exceed what governments now spend on health in the poorest countries but would be easily affordable in middle-income countries. Governments should assure that at the least, poor populations have access to these services. Additional public expenditure should then go either to extending coverage to the non-poor or to expansion beyond the minimum collection of services to an essential national package of health care including somewhat less cost-effective interventions against a larger number of diseases and conditions.[35]

QUALITY

Quality is more difficult to define than equity, but no less prominent as a determinant of health service utilization and productivity. Persons who are denied equity may lack access to services, but those who are dissatisfied with quality may refuse to use them. The other side of the quality picture is tied up with effectiveness and outcome in terms of improved health.

Many health facilities in developing countries provide service that is both inequitable and of low quality. In one study of drug-dispensing practices in rural Bangladeshp[36] the average consulting time per patient was 54 seconds, and not more than 37% of examinations were considered adequate. Only 41% of drugs were prescribed according to standard treatment guidelines. A quarter of all patients were treated with antibiotics, and 17% with metronidazole, irrespective of diagnosis, and only 55% of patients correctly understood the dosage.

In settings of this kind where the provision of minimal services is a struggle, the quality of health care has not been foremost in the minds of health planners and providers. Policy priority has gone to extending coverage. The prevailing view appears to be that improving quality is beyond the financial means of many countries. Nevertheless, many authorities are coming to realize that *errors are costly* and *good quality is cost-effective.* With the support of USAID and other agencies, quality assurance (QA) programs have been launched in many developing countries. Health sector reform provides an opportunity to reformulate services with a vew to quality built in. Comprehensive quality indicators can be designed to account for input, process, and outcome variables that allow comparison of quality of care in various situations. Studies are also needed on the relationship between quality and other health system variables, such as demand, costs, revenues, and equity.[37]

One way to assess quality is to ask users, who are the best source of information, about the degree to which their expectations are met by the available health services. Users do not think of cost-effectiveness or outcome but in more personal terms. In Santiago, Chile, women who received reproductive health services at a family planning and maternal and infant care clinic were asked about their concepts of quality. They defined high quality of care as "being treated like a human being" and identified the following elements: cleanliness, promptness and availability of service, time made available for consultation, learning opportunities for themselves and their partners, and cordial treatment. The client's view is determinant if improvements are to result in greater acceptance and sustained use of the services offered. The issues mentioned are not technical or difficult and should be negligible in cost to the clinic. They are largely a matter of attitude and planning but make a large difference in acceptance of services.[38]

Using another strategy, the quality of care of family planning services was investigated in Haiti using trained Haitian housewives playing the role of "mystery clients." These women visited clinics without prior notice and made direct observations of family planning services and clinic conditions. These simulated clients ranked the interaction with the provider, the adequacy of information, and competence of the health promoter. They identified deficiencies in quality of care such as the paternalistic attitudes of the medical staff, the lack of competence of promoters, and the lack of informed choice.[39]

PRIVATIZATION

A private health sector of some sort has existed in most countries for a very long time. In poorer regions religious missions have operated health facilities, and a commercial private sector came into being quite early. Out-of-pocket expenditures went for drugs sold in private pharmacies, maternity clinics, and similar facilities, and on consultation fees for physicians and other health personnel in both the "modern" and "traditional" sectors. Such spontaneous growth of the private sector, where it is not specifically forbidden, has been called *passive privatization.*[40] Even where private enterprise was banned, as in the former Soviet Union, a substantial amount of money changed hands in a "gray market" where favors or even basic services were performed in exchange for a covert cash incentive.

In the developing world the economic and debt crises of the 1980s and late 1990s forced many governments to adopt restrictions and/or reforms of their public services as part of structural adjustment plans. In some countries health systems deteriorated, salary payments were delayed, services were reduced, and fewer drugs and suppplies were furnished to health facilities. Governments sought funding from sources other than the state budget. Some turned to donors of external aid. Some set up cost recovery systems to help cover the shortfall from state financing. In some countries certain NGOs (particularly religious missionaries), previously banned, were permitted to reopen.

> At the same time, people began to question the concept of the Welfare State and the role of the State in the health system, not only in the financing of health services but also in the organization and production of services. Discussion focussed on two areas: the involvement of the State in implementing health services; and the insufficient recognition of the existence of the private sector, and the importance of full integration of that sector into the national health system.[41]

Muschell (1995) defines privatization as "a process in which non-government actors become increasingly involved in the financing and/or provision of health care services." Privatization denotes real changes in public and private roles and responsibilities and generally includes changes in the actual ownership of the means of financing and/or producing health care. The private sector includes both for-profit and not-for-profit organizations. It is often assumed that being free from the red tape and hassles typical of public bureaucracies, the competition and incentives found in the private sector will lead to improvements in service quality and provide health services more efficiently and effectively. Remaining government resources will then be devoted to the poor who are unable to pay for health services outside the public sector.

Privatization often involves the actual divestiture of public assets through transfer of ownership to the private sector in order to reduce the scale of government commitments. In the People's Republic of China, for example, many of the formerly communally owned barefoot doctor village health centers have been sold to individuals who operate them as private clinics. Similarly, some of the former Soviet "satellite" states in central Europe have transferred facilities to the private sector. It is hoped that competition and private initiative will improve the quality of care over the former government system, but the big danger of divestiture in the eyes of many social activists is the likelihood that private ownership, particularly by for-profit individuals or groups, will foster inequities and curtail care for those unable to pay. It is also possible that in an attempt to maximize revenue, private facilities will employ expensive or unnecessary procedures or skimp on essential care, sell unneeded drugs, and reduce overall quality.

The peril of inadequate regulation in a recently privatized system is shown in the drug situation in China. Hospitals are allowed to sell drugs at a profit. Although consultation fees remain low, drug costs are so high that in 1989 they accounted for 60 to 80 percent of hospital revenues. Since government subsidies to hospitals were terminated in 1997 health care institutions have come to depend on income from the sale of drugs to stay afloat. Chinese-made traditional and western medicines, whose prices are tightly controlled, are neglected in favor of profitable foreign products. Paying for western drugs and equipment has contributed greatly to a 35% annual increase in medical costs.

> Western drug companies have been aggressively courting China's doctors and hospitals not only with new pills, but also sometimes with gifts, money and even kickbacks, practices that are banned in the United States. . . . foreign drug and medical equipment companies at times pay for Chinese doctors to study overseas, buy hospitals new furniture and provide airline tickets and hotel vouchers for conferences. In an even more contentious practice, the companies commonly pay hospital administrators and individual doctors "commissions" for stocking and prescribing their drugs, though such payments are against corporate policies and are illegal in China.[42]

Incentives to private sector growth may include upgraded private for-pay beds in government hospitals, allowing public medical staff to run private clinics in government facilities outside normal hours; tax relief to private providers; or permission to collect user charges. These adjustments may be viewed as incentives designed to deter physicians and medical staff from leaving government service.

Contracting of Publicly Provided Services

Besides divestiture many governments have looked into setting up plans for contracting with the private sector. Under this plan, public funds are used to buy clinical or nonclinical services from private providers, intending to increase productivity through gains in quality, decentralized management, and greater transparency and accountability.

The most common way for monopolistic government health services (especially in lesser developed countries) to privatize is by contracting nonclinical hospital services such as security, laundry, food service, maintenance and cleaning, or bookkeeping. Great care must be taken to assure transparency in the contracting process— that tenders are written fairly; bidding is open; contracts are awarded without favoritism, fraud, abuse, or kickback; and that work is done according to the contract. Performance criteria need to be specified, with sanctions for poor performance. The administrative costs including management and monitoring may exceed any immediate cost savings from transferring services to the private sector, especially early on. However costly, this learning process appears to be a necessary step in the path toward privatization. Among the variations in contracting plans are programs in which costly or rarely needed services are purchased *ad hoc* from private providers. In Namibia, for example, surgical services are contracted to surgeons in the private sector, but in such arrangments there is a risk that surgeons may give priority to their own private patients.

Contracting can be a means of partial subsidization of non-profit-making non-governmental providers. In some countries, particularly in sub-Saharan Africa, the not-for-profit private sector is incorporated to varying degrees into the government health system. Support may range from tax-free import of equipment and drugs, the right to purchase commodities at discount from government stores, and benefits to NGO employees, to actual payment of staff salaries. The state may provide incentives for private providers to locate in areas with little or no government service. Zimbabwe, Lesotho, Swaziland, Zambia and Tanzania contract with mission hospitals to provide services at government expense. The public may prefer to be served at NGO facilities rather than at government clinics.

The use of social security funds to buy services from private providers is a mainstay of the German system and is found in many other countries where physicians want to retain their autonomy. In the revised British National Health Service fundholders (usually groups of general practitioners) contract for inpatient services with hospitals that compete for the patient population. In the United States some prison or military health services are conducted under contracts with private sector providers. In the Philippines and Chile the government may permit social security recipients to enroll in private HMOs which will provide better benefits at government rates.

Competition

Major trends occurring in western European countries include defined budgets for health services with priorities and limits on drugs and procedures; separation of purchasers from providers; and enhanced competition among providers. The broad movement toward market mechanisms is intended to increase productivity and reduce wastage of resources through economic incentives realized through competition. In the United States cost containment efforts from the early 1980s have given rise to a large number of private for-profit and not-for-profit[43] provider organizations which compete openly for members. In the United Kingdom, major reforms in the early 1990s reduced the dominance of the state as provider of services and stimulated the private sector through competition and market forces. Joint ventures between the government and the private sector are encouraged. In countries where nepotism and "tea money" are the norm, care must be taken to assure true competition among potential contractors, that contracts are fairly awarded and effectively managed, and that competition leads to efficiency and cost savings in the services provided.

Just as providers compete among themselves for public contracts, they must compete for members (that is, patients or potential patients) in a process sometimes called *consumer-led competition*. On a small scale this occurs in Britain and elsewhere where GPs compete to market themselves to consumers who choose their own physicians. In a competitive marketplace, the long-term prospects for health service providers will be tied to the perceived quality of their performance and service. They would therefore have effective incentives to produce maximum value for money, whether open to the public or catering to enrolled subscribers. In systems with per capita prepayment the providers become accountable and assume a greater financial risk when their cost of care is uncontrolled, or if their quality of care is poor and patients opt to go elsewhere. Governments are encouraging diversity and market competition as a strategy to improve quality and reduce costs, both in the private sector and within public systems.

Not everyone is thrilled with growing competition in the medical care field. Among the criticisms are:

- Market mechanisms are regressive, poor people are left out, and inequity increases unless governments provide close regulation to maintain availability and accessibility of services to all population groups.
- Unregulated competition can permit "cream-skimming" by insurers; preferred risk selection must be prohibited or minimized by close government regulation.
- The level of institutional development in low-income countries does not permit an efficient market or sufficient regulation of the private sector.
- Management and administrative costs increase, especially for management information systems.
- The cost of an intervention cannot be identified clearly, so cost recovery contracts may be unrealistic.
- Services are duplicated by various providers in a competitive system, so overall costs may not be reduced.
- Excessive and costly technology may be used mainly as a marketing lure to attract subscribers and maximize profit rather than to benefit patients.
- Capitation plans, where providers receive a fixed annual payment per patient, carry an incentive to skimp or cut corners in patient care.
- It is generally assumed that the market is more efficient than public services, but insufficient rigorous economic analyses have been done, and "the evidence is thin concerning the supposed merits of the private sector in health care settings."[44]

In the UK, where health care rationing debates currently abound, there has been no formal evaluation of the role of the market in allocating scarce health care resources. The market in health care has increased administration, fragmented services, eroded local accountability, and decreased choice. This fragmentation, and the associated competition between purchasers and providers, means that resource allocation can no longer be monitored and evaluated in a national context. The loss of a population focus has left a vacuum in planning.[45]

Among the shifts from social or collective responsibility for health in favor of greater individual responsibility is the medical savings account, most firmly developed in

Singapore and discussed in the previous chapter. An enthusiastic advocate of MSAs has emphasized their role as a lever to stimulate competition:

> With MSAs, therefore, workers effectively would be spending their own funds for non-catastrophic health care. As a result, they would have full market incentives to control the costs of such care. They would seek to avoid unnecessary care or tests and look for physicians and hospitals which would provide good quality care at the best prices. That, in turn, would stimulate true cost competition among physicians and hospitals. Since consumers would be choosing on the basis of cost as well as quality, providers would compete to minimize bills as well as maximize quality, as in a normal market. Accordingly, developers of innovations and new equipment would compete vigorously to produce new items that cut cost as well as improved quality . . . That would add up to an enormous reduction in spiraling health costs. MSAs are the sole means of controlling them consistent with consumer choice and people's control over their own health care. Other proposed reforms, such as managed competition, would force people into health maintenance organizations (HMOs), in which a bureaucracy working for the insurer ultimately decides what care patients will get, or include global budgets, under which the government dictates how much may be spent on health care, reducing resources and ultimately services for the middle class and the elderly.[46]

The Role of Managed Care in Health Sector Reform

Managed care organizations were described briefly in the previous chapter. Just as in the United States, many other countries are experimenting with various forms of membership-based prepaid health maintenance organizations. Managed supply-side market reforms are prominent in countries emerging from socialism and Semashko-type systems, and in limited regions of developing countries. In the People's Republic of China, a number of prepaid systems closely resemble western HMOs. In Taiching County near Shanghai, for example, a cooperative medical system has been extended from villages to employees of rural industries and townships, providing a larger risk pool, better financial stability, and an increased choice of providers for members. Annual fees are set as a percentage of household disposable income, "and consequently the total collected increases every year in line with economic growth." The plan also requires high copayments at time of use, which increase physicians' incomes, limit demand, and allow premiums to be set at affordable levels.[47] In other regions, such as Latin America, managed care plans are found in both private insurance and social insurance programs. Managed care models are found in Argentina, Brazil, Chile, Colombia, Costa Rica, the Dominican Republic, and Uruguay, constituting a significant share of the health insurance market in some countries.[48]

> The development of managed care is described as an unexpected product of competition between public and private purchasers of health care. Managed care is a series of

purchasing techniques that employers have applied to reduce the cost of their employees' health benefits. Its most significant use has been as a device for bargaining with individual health care providers by encouraging or requiring employees to purchase health care services from a select set of providers.[49]

FINANCING AND ORGANIZATION

[O]ne of the assumptions on which the British National Health Service was based, was a belief that there existed in any community a finite pool of ill-health, which, through the application of health services, could be reduced in such a fashion that the need for health care itself would in the long-term decline. Forty years later there are few health service managers who would adhere to that view . . . health demands will *always* outstrip the resources available, even in the (albeit untenable) extreme position in which *all* of a country's resources were devoted to health.[50]

The reference is to 1948, when Aneurin Bevan, architect of the NHS, believed that free treatment would cause the costs of running the NHS to decline because people would become healthier and demand less medical care. The intervening half century has seen myriad approaches to financing of the health sector but nirvana has nowhere been approached, much less achieved. Everyone agrees that true public health measures are the responsibility of governments, but the age-old debate over public *versus* private financing of personal clinical care remains to be resolved.

The main challenge in reform is to attain financial and institutional sustainability, whether the system is financed publicly, privately, or from a combination. Public financing can eliminate adverse selection and pool risks over the entire population, but will still face cost problems due to moral hazard. Private insurance can allow for greater consumer choice and preclude economic losses from coercive taxes, but it can be unaffordable for high risk groups unless heavily regulated.[51] Public financing is feasible in countries with a secure tax base. In middle- and upper-income countries the main objectives of reform are often cost containment, cost-effectiveness, quality, and acceptability to the public. The means of achieving these are changing organizational structures and offering incentives to service providers. In low-income countries the objective must be to increase revenue to rectify the inevitable shortfall in health sector funding while expanding efficiency and equity. Taxation in developing countries is limited by the following realities:

- Much of the population is widely dispersed in rural areas.
- Most of the population is self-employed in subsistence, small-scale agriculture where much of the income is in kind, transactions are hard to trace, and high rates of illiteracy and poor accounting and record-keeping on expenses limit the use of personal income or profits taxes.

- In urban areas there is a large informal sector of small and transient firms, and even individuals employed in the manufacturing sector work in small firms.
- Large firms tend to be government enterprises or extractive industries that are often owned by foreigners.
- Agricultural products and mineral resources face unstable and unpredictable world prices.
- The dualism of a modern urban sector and a traditional rural sector, and the market segmentation it creates, distorts commodity and labor markets, increasing tax burdens.
- High levels of income inequality tend to result in higher tax rates, greater tax avoidance, and higher efficiency losses.
- Trade distortions—import tariffs, quotas, export taxes, differential exchange rates, foreign exchange rationing—abound, resulting in resource misallocations and inequity.
- The influence of state-owned enterprises, coupled with nonoptimal user charge structures, often results in inefficient public investment decisions.
- Tax administration capacity is limited.[52]

User Charges

Among the measures proposed to fund health services in low-income countries are community financing, expanded social insurance, and user charges in the form of fees or copayments, which can be a source of revenue when it is not feasible to collect taxes. In addition, user charges can discourage excessive use of services. However,

> The argument that patients make unnecessary or frivolous use of services assumes that people can always tell whether use is necessary or not. Secondly, it assumes that charges will deter the unnecessary user. The two assumptions are very questionable. Many patients are in no position to know whether their symptoms are serious or not.[53]

The various stances of the World Bank on user charges have been mentioned, and the subject remains a source of controversy. One bone of contention is equity: The regressive nature of user fees is likely to exclude the poorest, who are most in need of the services. To compensate for this dilemma, many countries have experimented with means-tested exemptions so that the poor will remain eligible for services without charge. That plan also has difficulties: On the one hand, the truly poor can suffer social embarrassment, and on the other, some people may be tempted to hide income or assets so as to qualify unfairly for free services. And it is never clear just where the cutoff line should be set. In Kenya the main obstacle to implementing exemptions from fees is the inability to easily identify that minority of people who are truly unable to pay.[54] In Bangladesh, Stanton and Clemens found that "these fees may impede access of the most needy to medical care and thereby have a negative impact on the health of individuals. Indeed, while possibly economically rational, these fees may seriously undermine the effectiveness of the governmental health care system in improving the nation's health."[55] A lengthy review concluded that

> Unreserved faith in charges as a panacea in all contexts is clearly misguided but it is difficult to see an alternative for those countries whose health systems are most degraded, for which there is no prospect of improved public funding and in which the majority who may gain still suffer from the 'diseases of poverty' and must be regarded as poor by any objective standard.[56]

Another controversy over user fees is whether they are really useful in raising revenue. Some studies suggest that the administrative costs of collecting small amounts of cash in remote health centers and sending them to central locations are more than the fees are worth. Others see a tendency toward shrinkage as the coins pass from one hand to another with little effective oversight.

A plan to use user charges specifically for community-based financing of essential drugs was proposed in 1987 in Bamako, the capital of Mali. This plan, since known as the *Bamako Initiative*, has been strongly advocated by UNICEF but criticized by some others on the predictable grounds of equity and sustainablity. The program has had most success in francophone countries such as Cameroon and Guinea where revolving funds have helped to maintain drug supplies in local clinics and avoid the need for villagers to travel to other facilities. However,

> So far the experience with user fees as a source of finance for health care has been disappointing. Except in cases of vertical programs and community-based projects, user fees have failed to provide more than 5 percent of recurrent ministry of health costs— much less than the 20 percent anticipated. This potential is not realized because of management and organizational problems.[57]

In an interview survey of about 900 outpatients and 1800 households in Tanzania, it was found that the majority of users are willing to pay for improved services. "By far the most important improvement they are seeking is the ready availability of drugs. Failings in drug supply are a much more important consideration than waiting time." The authors concluded that "modest charges, with attempts to exempt the poor, would be less inequitable than the existing situation, if the revenue could be used to ensure that supplies were always adequate at government health services. The level of charges suggested was based on what the majority surveyed said they were willing to pay."[58]

REORGANIZING MINISTRIES OF HEALTH

The ministry of health is often described as the Cinderella among ministries. In the hierarchy it will usually come after the ministries of finance, defence, foreign affairs, industry, planning and education. Although the ministry of health, as with education, is a high-expenditure department, largely because of the salaries paid to its workers, it nevertheless has relatively low status in the departmental hierarchy.[59]

Cinderella or not, health ministries need to position themselves efficiently to make the best of the benefits and drawbacks of health sector reform. According to the statement above, the MOH typically has little clout within governments and may need to convince the power structure of the logic of reform. Following WDR93 recommendations, the ministry may decide to concentrate on public health and reduce its clinical role from provider of services to overseer and regulator. It will require long and careful planning and considerable persuasion in legislatures, professional groups, and the general public to carry out these far-reaching reforms. There must be numerous changes in governance, particularly in the legal position of the central government vis-à-vis regional authorities, aspects of financial responsibility, and regulations governing relationships with the private sector. Divestiture of government assets, if planned, will certainly be a thorny issue. Ideally, reforms should lead to a greater degree of transparency in all MOH transactions.

Decentralization

Decentralization of the health sector is a cornerstone of health sector reform, but its exact meaning is imprecise and variable. In general, the term refers to the transfer of resources, decision-making, planning, and management functions (i.e., authority, responsibility, and accountability) from the central government to units that are both smaller and more widely distributed. Three models of decentralization have been described:

- *Deconcentration*: transfer of administrative responsibility to subdivisions of the central government such as regional offices of the MOH.
- *Devolution*: transfer of significant decision-making or political power to regional, provincial, district, or municipal governments.
- *Delegation*: The state transfers managerial responsibility to organizations indirectly controlled or regulated by government—for example, provider institutions such as hospitals; parastatal companies,or social insurance funds.

Decentralization is promoted on the rationale that it:

- Supports public participation and the empowerment of communities
- Increases responsiveness to local needs—for example, in areas of ethnic minorities
- Helps to implement relevant primary health care; promotes equity by helping the poor to obtain access to public goods and services
- Helps to improve the competence, experience, flexibility, efficiency, and responsiveness of local managers and personnel

- Weakens the grip of uncaring centralized bureaucracies
- Might be part of the process of transferring assets from the public to the private sector and the introduction of market mechanisms

Many questions remain about decentralization, which at its essence involves a transfer of authority, or dispersal of power, from higher to lower levels. As a general rule those who have power are reluctant to cede it to others, so we must see just how such transfer can be arranged amicably. Authority may be transferred to local bureaucrats, elected officials, administrators, health providers, citizen groups, or to for-profit or non-profit organizations. Once a policy of decentralization has been adopted, decisions must be made as to the degree of autonomy and accountability to be given to (or acepted by) each level. The central government may devolve certain powers to regions or provinces, which in turn may transfer them to districts, communities, or even individual health centers.

What kinds of powers will be decentralized? A level of independence in planning, management, and decision-making seems necessary. Financial power is always crucial, and with it the ability to collect and retain fees and charges locally, and to plan and carry out separate budgets. The control of staffing and personnel is important because salaries are usually the largest budget items.

Although decentralization may seem quite rational and desirable, it is very difficult to design and implement. Before that can be done, a clear statement of policy objectives is needed. Will the decentralization plan be based on a needs assessment and an inventory of assets and capabilities? Will it account for issues such as civil service reform, equity as an explicit concern of the government, and the role of multilateral and bilateral agencies? Are structural adjustment conditionalities in force? The extent and form of public participation should be described, as well as any increased role and regulation of the private sector.

In addition to the dilution of power from central authorities, other interest groups may have incentives to resist change. In many countries labor unions of government workers are quite powerful, and long-term civil servants will be concerned about the prospects for revised work conditions, benefits, and retirement programs if their employer is suddenly changed from the central government to a poorer and perhaps less stable agency. Decentralization must conform to legal, administrative, and regulatory structures, which may spark arduous battles in national and regional legislatures. These confrontations may be beneficial if issues are ventilated and a truly improved system can be put in place. National and local priorities will most likely differ, and coordination will be more complex than in a single nationwide system. As the central government shifts away from delivering services directly, it must give proportionately more attention to policy, planning, and regulation of the entire health sector. Lines of authority and accountability must be clearly defined. As the periphery is given more independence in decision-making, it must have, or obtain, the managerial capacity and the technological resources to run programs efficiently. More money may be needed for increased administrative expenditures and more staff may be necessary to cope with additional responsibilities. Local authorities may be suspicious that their new-found independence is simply a way for the central government to unload a financial and administrative headache. They main gain nominal authority, which is not very useful unless the central government provides financial support or allows revenue to be raised locally. Duplication of equipment, facilities, administrative costs, and staff may arise, and economies of scale may be lost—for example, when purchases of supplies or drugs move from national to local levels.

The unit of decentralization must be internally consistent within the health sector in terms of levels of referral to hospitals or other facilities and should also be compatible with patterns of decentralization in other sectors of government.

More importantly, decentralization has the potential to reduce or to increase inequalities among regions. If services depend entirely on locally generated funds, the residents of wealthier areas will be better off than those in poorer districts. Adjacent districts should coordinate benfits and disincentives such as user fees. If different regions get different services the inequalities will generate not only resentment but may stimulate 'district hopping' or fraud in claiming eligibility for benefits. These issues must be tackled early on and decisions about allocation of resources must be made wisely to prevent an increase in regional disparities.

Decentralization cannot be introduced suddenly and completely. Pilot and experimental programs will be needed as well as a plan for phasing in changes while maintaining services. Training schedules and technical support must be built up and balanced to bring the capacity of all units up to an aceptable standard. As new structures are created old ones must be terminated, which may not be a simple matter where careers and assets are involved.

Decentralization of health services in developing countries has been criticized on various grounds.[60] Lack of trained staff and inadequate human resources in the periphery are blamed for severe problems of existing decentralization programs in Asia and Africa. The relative weakness of lower-level governments makes them vulnerable to the influence of local landowners, merchants, and industrialists whose interests may not coincide with those of the people. Decentralization to municipal government level may strengthen the dominant hold of regional and local politicians. And "so-called decentralization to what appears as local government is often nothing more than the extension of central government control over local government."[61]

Health Sector Reform in Central and Eastern Europe[62]

Central and eastern Europe is a region of roughly 350 million people in two to three dozen current or former countries, depending on how one wishes to count them. The 15 sovereign *newly independent states* of the former Soviet Union, the breakup states of the former Yugoslavia, and those that were independent but in the Soviet sphere (Table 13-3) followed the Semashko pattern of health services (Chapter 12)

Table 13-3. The Newly Independent States of the Former Soviet Union and Transition Economies of Central and Eastern Europe

Newly Independent States of The Former Soviet Union	The Countries of Central and Eastern Europe
Armenia	*The former Yugoslavia*
Azerbaijan	
Belarus	Bosnia and Herzogovina
Estonia	Croatia
Georgia	Former Yugoslav Republic of Macedonia
Kazakstan	Serbia and Montenegro Slovenia
Kyrgyz	
Latvia	*Previously independent states*
Lithuania	
Moldova	Albania
Russian Federation	Bulgaria
Tajikistan	Czech Republic[a]
Turkmenistan	Hungary
Ukraine	Poland
Uzbekistan	Romania
	Slovakia[a]

[a]Part of former Czechoslovakia.

with complete or moderate fidelity. Many descriptive acronyms have been coined for all or some these nations, including the following:

CCEE	Countries of Central and Eastern Europe
CEE	Central and Eastern Europe
CIS	Commonwealth of Independent States (former USSR)
ECA	East Europe and Central Asia
FSE	Formerly Socialist Economy
FSU	Former Soviet Union
NIS	Newly Independent States (former USSR)

The sovereign states can be categorized into three groupings based on the status of their health sector reforms:

- Those that began reforms as early as the mid-1980s and have made or are making major changes (Czech and Slovak Republics, Hungary, Lithuania, Estonia, Latvia, Poland).
- Those in which reforms are at various stages, often delayed because of political, civil, or military upheavals (Bulgaria, Belarus, Croatia, Romania, Russian Federation, Slovenia, Ukraine).

- Those suffering unrest, still implementing the Semashko type of health care, or just starting reforms (Transcaucsian and Central Asian countries).

The old system

In the classical Semashko model (Chapter 12) the state operated all health facilities and employed all personnel. Private practice was prohibited. Public health and curative medicine were rigidly separated, as were ambulatory, primary, and hospital care. Everything was centrally planned and health care was seen as a public good. The system was rigidly hierarchical and organized on a geographic basis equal to national, provincial, regional, district jurisdictions, each with specified facilties.[63] Health systems in socialist countries suffered from a number of weaknesses which limited their effectiveness. Among these were:

- A lack of incentives for efficiency, quality of care, and responsiveness to patients
- A lack of patient choice
- Limited managerial autonomy and management skills
- Narrowly trained health personnel
- Excess physical capacity
- Overemphasis on hospital and curative care
- Unsuccessful health education and promotion effforts
- Insuficient attention to environmental and occupational risks[64]

There was also a substantial amount of large- and a small-scale corruption and favoritism. Health care budgets in the USSR did not exceed 3% to 4% of GDP, but ironically in that classless society, as much as half of this amount was spent in the "fourth department" of the Health Ministry reserved exclusively for political elites, who accounted for less than 1% of the population.[65] On a small scale, informal but illegal payments called "gratitude money" or "thank-you money" were (and still are) given from patients to providers as cash tips for providing personal or clinical services, drugs, medical supplies, or tests. Without such incentives, the services might just not have been given in an environment of chronic shortage, where supplies and basic medications were sufficient to meet only 10% to 20% of need.

Challenges faced by the transition countries

The problems faced by the CEE countries, to a greater or lesser extent, include economic and political crises, high inflation rates, bankruptcies, and unaccustomed mass unemployment. The health consequences of economic collapse resemble other circumstances in which a population is subject to sudden extreme poverty—diminished nutrition; increased infectious diseases, often from contaminated water; epidemics of measles, tuberculosis, and sexually transmitted diseases; dilapidated and inadequate housing poorly heated in the harsh winter; increased domestic violence, murder, and suicide; deteriorated health and environmental services; and so on.

> The Soviet Union stressed the number of hospitals and polyclinics and not the quality of care or comprehensiveness of services. The more health facilities and doctors, the better. The results of this approach and the collapse of the country's infrastructure are profoundly disturbing. For example: In hospitals and clinics no more than 50 miles from Moscow, there is often no running hot water; and in facilities 100 miles away, there is often no water at all.[66]

In the FSEs the GNP per capita fell below $3000, economic growth rates became negative, and consumer prices soared. From 1990 to 1993 production declined by 32% in Hungary and Poland, by 54% in Romania and Bulgaria, and by 58% in Albania. The Russian Federation reached only 50% of its 1989 production level.[67] Fiscal revenues in these countries have dropped up to 60%. "Thus the need to do more with less has dominated the debate over health system reform."[68]

Beginning in the late 1970s and early 1980s improvements in health status had begun to stall, or even to decline. The "health gap" with the West became wider, at first slowly and then accelerating in the early 1990s. A boy born in Russia in 1993 had a life expecancy 5.3 years less than his brother born in 1989. Unhealthy lifestyles, despondency, unclean environments, and breakdowns in prevention and control efforts contributed to increases in disability and death from both acute and chronic diseases.

Health sector reform in the CEE/CIS countries

Since the late 1980s the CEE countries have been shifting from central planning toward market-based economies. After years of inadequate services, patients and providers want a fresh start with a minimum of government involvement. The public wants competent care at a reasonable cost and a free choice of doctors. Physicians want better working conditions and higher incomes. Politicians want a health care system that satisfies the citizenry and professionals and relieves government budgets. Each country is different and space does not permit detailed descriptions, but the health system reforms tend toward western Bismarckian models with these general objectives:

- Payroll-tax-financed, employment-based health insurance systems
- Separation of payers from providers
- Insurance companies or sickness funds under government regulation with varying degrees of independence from the state
- Specified benefit packages
- Supplementary health insurance available on a voluntary privately paid basis
- Reduced central government expenditures

- Government funding only for the elderly and the uninsured
- Establishment of new provider payment mechanisms
- Development of private, nongovernmental medical group practices
- Some degree of privatization and contracting of services
- Introduction of market competition
- Decentralization of public sector services
- Recognition of patient choice
- Introduction of out-of-pocket user charges
- Efficient organization and management of health services
- Public health activities, medical education, and research to be financed by central government

The changes in the health sector of course reflect general changes in all other aspects of these societies, guided by the general slogan of "Back to Europe," meaning a "return" to western European–style enterprises. There is a temptation to make a clean sweep to purge the negative aspects of the old system. However, some thought might be given to retaining the "positive bequests" (Table 13-4) in order to maximize equity and unversality. Reformers are warned to temper enthusiasm with reality:

> [T]he uncritical intention to implement the "Bismarck model" in the FSEs faces several problems and requires certain preconditions, which can be summarized in one main point: the relative stability of the German health care system, which may be attractive to the FSEs, is based on economic prosperity and on a strong ability to assert the will of the central state institutions . . . It is nearly impossible to adopt, ad hoc, this special relationship between purchasers, providers, and oversight by the state, which is the main structural feature of the German health care system that has developed over the last century. These preconditions are not present in the FSEs. Socioeconomic conditions, economic prosperity, and historical development are not exportable.[69]

In the late 1990s the CEE/CIS countries fell into two groups with respect to financing:

- Those that still rely on general revenue to finance health care, generally spending 3%–5% of GDP (Albania, Bulgaria, Latvia, Lithuania, Poland, Romania).
- Those that have had, or recently adopted, a national health insurance system financed by payroll taxes. These countries spend from 6% to 8% of GNP on health (Estonia, Croatia, Hungary, Slovakia, the former Yugoslav Republic of Macedonia, Czech Republic, Slovenia). In these countries insurance revenues have generally supplemented, not supplanted, government expenditures.[70]

In the Russian Federation, legislation for mandatory health insurance (MHI) was passed in 1991. In extreme contrast to the old Soviet system, MHI is highly de-

Table 13-4. The Newly Independent States of the Former Soviet Union and Transition Economies of Central and Eastern Europe: Legacies from the Socialist Regimes

	Positive bequests
Entitlement	Entire regional population
Burden of financing	Evenly distributed
Access	Few financial barriers
Range of services	Comprehensive
Network of facilities	Structurally integrated
Resource base	Extensive infrastucture

	Negative bequests
Health status	High mortality, especially in adult men High morbidity Unhealthy life styles and environment
Policy-making / management	Ineffective intersectoral coordination Low priority of health and good health care Lack of responsiveness to local needs Weak management, tracking, and evaluation
Structure	Rigid, overcentralized structure Overemphasis on institutional care Neglect of public health and primary care Distortions in public/private mix
Function	Lack of functional integration Ineffective, inefficient, and low quality
Resources	Arbitrary statistical norms (physical and human) Imbalances with surpluses and shortages Overutilization
Training; research and development	Narrow overspecialization and isolation Graduate education isolated from universities Research isolated from teaching Noncompetitive funding
Financing	Underfinancing compared with capitalization Adverse incentives

Source: Preker (1994) Tables 1 and 2.

centralized with each of the 88 regions designing its own system within limits set by federal guidelines. The MHI follows the usual plan in which employers make income-related contributions for their employees into a regional fund. The fund allocates resources to competing insurers, who pay local providers. Local authorities pay into the fund for the nonworking population.

Reforms have played differently in the various countries: A publicly sponsored private firm (national health insurance company or equivalent) overseeing many separate sickness funds is found in the Czech Republic, Estonia, Hungary, Slovakia, and Slovenia, while Albania has a single national social insurance fund. Employer and employee contributions are equal (50:50) in Slovenia, but in Estonia the employer pays 99% with 1% from the employee.

Problems with reforms in the CEE/CIS countries

The economic declines in CEE countries have resulted in a greater percentage of poor people in the population. Concerns about the inability of the poor and unemployed to pay formal (and "unofficial") user fees for access to health services has sparked the same controversies about equity that we saw in Africa and other regions. At the same time, the rise of entrepreneurial and middle classes has led to economic polarization of the population. In Russia

> many of the more affluent are turning to the increasing array of private health services, available only through cash payment. The picture that is emerging of contemporary Russian medical care is of a developing dual system: the old state system, facing chronic underfunding, and a second, poorly understood, loosely regulated system, of better equipped and staffed private practices available only to those with the cash to pay the doctor's bill . . . Throughout Russian health care, entrepreneurs and opportunists are looking for ways to capitalize on the developing reforms.[71]

Frequently the cost of providing medical care has been found to exceed revenues, leading to operating deficits that are passed on to the central government.

> The swift rise in the share of GDP for health also reflects the inadequate attention paid to the structure of financial incentives for health care providers and patients. This became apparent in the fiscal crises that followed dramatic increases in health insurance costs in the Czech Republic, Hungary and Slovakia. In the rush to introduce "western style" health insurance, insufficient thought was given to setting limits on basic insurance coverage, to defining actuarially appropriate premiums, or to establishing payment mechanisms with incentives for efficiency and cost containment.[72]

Alexander Preker has provided a valuable summary of a wide range of adverse consequences associated with the health sector transition in CEE countries (Table 13-5).

The Czech Republic: a case study

Medical care in the old Czechoslovakia was of a high European standard, but decades of inefficiency under the postwar communist regime caused the health care system to deteriorate badly. A year after the 1989 "velvet revolution" a new system of health care was created based on community participation, guaranteed access to all, ending the state monopoly on health care provision, and establishment of compulsory insurance. In 1992 a mandatory employment-based health insurance system was in-

Table 13-5. Problems During Economic Transition in the Former Socialist States of Central and Eastern Europe

Antecedent	Consequence
Effects Due to an Overshoot in Economic Liberalization	
Unregulated markets	Market failure
Unrestrained privatization	Profiteering with pillage of assets
Price/wage liberalization	Inflation, widening income distribution
Market-driven production	Decrease in output
Unrestrained demand	Collapse in supply network
Massive layoffs	Labor dislocations, housing shortages
Unbalanced incentives	Breakdown in expenditure controls
Economic disequilibrium	Recession, bankruptcies, unemployment
Effects Due to Rejection of Constraints on Freedom	
Overreliance on autonomy	Loss of collective protection
Excessive consensus seeking	Weak leadership and government
Distrust of totalitarian rule	Parliamentary/legislative overload
Effects Due to Collapse in Institutional Framework	
Abolition of centralized planning	Policy vacuum
Purged *nomenklatura*[a]	Lack of experienced senior staff
Excessive decentralization	Splintered/uncoordinated services
Breakdown in distribution system	Supply shortages
Fiscal crisis and underfunding	Deteriorating infrastructure

[a]In the former Soviet Union *nomenklatura* referred to influential senior posts in government and industry, to which members of the Communist party elites were appointed.

Source: Preker (1994) Tables 4, 5, 6.

troduced. In 1993 Czechoslovakia split into the Czech Repubic (CR) and Slovakia, which have opted for somewhat different policies. Slovakia has decided to retain greater state control, while the CR, with a population of about ten million, has moved rapidly toward the full set of market reforms.

Relatively advanced among CEE\CIS countries, the CR has aggressively encouraged competition and free-market reform. Twenty-two private insurance companies were quickly established with large bank loans to make fee-for-service payments to all physicians who cared for their policyholders. The insurance companies compete for subscribers by offering certain extra services, such as dentistry, within the standard payment. Market incentives encouraged newly privatized physicians to generate greater volume and consume more resources than those physicians who remained as state employees. After the change from state financing to the semicompetitive insurance system, government expenditure on health dropped considerably, but within two years after the introduction of the insurance-based system, overall health care spending increased by 50%. Nevertheless, doctors went on strike in 1995 and 1996 for higher rembursement rates. In February 1996 the biggest private insuror became insolvent and the government, as the legal guarantor, was forced to take over its debt.[73]

Another example of insufficiently regulated privatization in the Czech Republic is the private pharmacies, which proliferated rapidly with liberalization.

> Anybody was allowed to start and own a pharmacy—at a high price . . . The aim was to improve the availability of drugs, and to allow market forces and competition to influence prices . . . There is a tendency, however, to stock only the more expensive drugs. If a GP prescribes a cheaper drug, the pharmacies have a habit of changing this for a more expensive brand, and patients have to pay the difference. Prior to 1990 some 110–180 pharmaceuticals were registered annually. Following the deregulation of drug imports in 1990, the number of registrations increased drastically. In 1991, 1992 and 1993 there were 827, 1344 and 1356, respectively. Now there are more than 10 000 brand names on the drug market. Total spending on drugs approximately doubled between 1991 and 1993.[74]

Similar excesses, combined with deteriorating economic conditions, have caused extreme difficulties in financing health sector reforms in other CEE countries including Poland, Romania, and the Russian Federation.

Merging Systems: East and West Germany[75]

The situation in Germany is almost the inverse of that just discussed. Instead of one system fragmenting into a number of units, Germany faced the opposite problem of fusing or merging two distinct systems into one. The Bismarckian legacy had changed over the years, and the original system of sickness funds fell on hard times during the Nazi period.

> These funds were immensely unpopular with physicians, and the changing political climate during the rise of the Third Reich was seized as a means to institute drastic changes in the system. After 1933, physicians joined the Nazi party in greater proportion and sooner than did members of any other profession. By 1938 virtually all physicians sympathetic to autonomous sickness funds had been deported or killed. After World War II, West Germany was rebuilt, and its system of social insurance was restored.[76]

As the Federal Republic of Germany (West Germany) rebuilt the Bismarckian organization, the German Democratic Republic (East Germany) upon its creation on

October 7, 1949, converted to a Soviet-style system. As the occupying forces of the Soviet Union worked quickly to create a communist state they stood the Bismarckian health care system on its head. In a short time they converted a private decentralized system to a public hierarchical one in an approximation of that in the USSR. The East German system was not precisely like the Soviet one because 70 years of experience with sickness funds could not vanish without a trace. A remnant of the funds persisted as workers and employers both paid health insurance contributions. About 90% of East Germans were insured in this way through the Free German Trade Union and the other 11%, mainly the self-employed, state employees, and their dependents, were covered by the state. One difference from the Soviet system is that higher-income workers could buy extra benefits in exchange for higher payments. The keystone of the GDR health services was a network of company-based health clinics and health stations within which the majority of contacts with the health system occurred.

After the fall of the Berlin Wall the two Germanys, separated for 40 years, signed a Treaty of Reunification on August 31, 1990. Although there was some discussion of experimenting with other arrangements, the new system, with West German–style sickness funds and payment mechanisms, was in place by the beginning of 1991. Because it took some time to unravel all the details, the entire system was privatized within two years.

Although Germany is one country, vestiges remain from the period of separation. The area of the former GDR is still economically depressed in comparison with the western part of the country and this is reflected in the health system. For example, Germans who earn less than a certain amount (mainly retirees and low-paid workers) must join a statutory health insurance fund. In 1997 that amount was set at 6150 deutsch marks (DM) in the West but only DM 5350 in the East. Various payments are similarly adjusted: copayments for a hospital day are DM 17 in the West and DM 14 in the East. After a lifetime in poorly paid government service, physicians in the East lacked capital and experience to set up private practices. Hospitals in the East were so shabby in comparison with their West German counterparts that the federal government together with sickness funds and other sources must pay hundreds of millions of deutschmarks each year to bring them up to standard.

THE FUTURE OF HEALTH SECTOR REFORM

After the quick tour of health systems in this and the previous chapter it is evident that every country has developed a plan in accordance with its cultural values, economic capabilities, and domestic political pressures, overlain by the demands of world events. Yet regardless of the specific arrangement that has evolved, all health care systems face the same problems, which were listed at the beginning of this chapter: dissatisfaction with existing systems, excessive costs, inefficiency, misallocation of resources, poor management, and perceived unfairness in access to services. The compartmentalization of nations into separate sealed boxes is no longer tenable, if it ever was. Increased globalization in all aspects of life, like all other changes, is reflected in health systems. Governments, prodded from the outside by international agencies and internally by their own bureaucrats, health providers, and a better informed public, will be forced to confront these issues in a coherent and systematic way. Health professionals must share the stage with economists and managers as models of reform become increasingly broad and comprehensive.

NOTES

1. Many of these technologies were developed with publicly funded research support and have become expensive commercial products, but governments generally have not asked for a share in the profits.

2. Alleyne (1995).

3. Reinhardt (1997).

4. Strictly speaking we should distinguish between *states* and *governments*. Some countries have a *Head of State*, such as a hereditary monarch, and also a *Head of Government*— for example, a prime minister. In general we will consider the governmental or *public sector* as contrasted with the *private sector* which operates by *market mechanisms*.

5. Parastatal companies are wholly or partly owned by governments in a great variety of forms. They may have directors from both the public and the private sector and may act as monopolies or receive preferential treatment from governments.

6. For a lengthy discussion see Yergin and Stanislaw (1998).

7. As described in Chapter 3, the International Finance Corporation (founded in 1956) made loans to the private sector, but this was a very minor part of the World Bank Group's activities.

8. The system is sometimes termed *crony capitalism* and those countries that are dominated by corrupt ruling families or oligarchies are aptly referred to as *kleptocracies*.

9. World Bank (1980).

10. Akin et al. (1987).

11. Primary health care was nominally for everyone, including residents of wealthier countries, but in practice attention was concentrated on the poorer countries, and within those, on children and mothers. See Chapter 7.

12. Berman (1995).

13. Kutzin (1995).

14. Low-income economies are those with a per capita gross national product of $635 or less in 1991. Middle-income economies had a per capita GNP between $635 and $7911 in 1991. Formerly Socialist Economies of Europe include the European republics of the former Soviet Union and the formerly socialist economies of eastern and central Europe.

15. Among the WHO programs is the Forum on Health Sector Reform. The forum meets regularly and has issued a number of significant discussion papers.

16. Weisberg (1998).

17. See, for example, Walt (1994), Barker (1996), and Green (1992). See also the journal *Health Policy and Planning*, published by Oxford University Press.

18. World Health Organization (1980).

19. From *Healthy People 2000 Midcourse Review and 1995 Revisions.* "Appendix A: Summary List of Objectives." U. S. Department of Health and Human Services.

20. Frenk (1995).

21. Barker (1966).

22. Walt (1994).

23. *Ibid.*

24. Kamanga (1996).

25. Adizes and Zukin (1977).

26. Zukin (1987).

27. See Chapter 15 for further discussion of health and human rights.

28. The history and legal basis for a right to health are discussed in detail by Taylor (1992).

29. The World Bank, in a 1975 policy paper.

30. Maxwell (1995).

31. Reinhardt (1997).

32. For a thoughtful discussion of priorities and ethics see Musgrove (1995b).

33. Examples: acute conditions that could be fatal and for which treatment could provide complete recovery (ranked first); acute treatable conditions unlikely to be fatal; maternity and newborn services; preventive care of proven efficacy; those that yield minimal improvement in the quality of life (last). Among many studies see Bodenheimer (1997).

34. Walsh and Warren (1979).

35. Bobadilla *et al.* (1994).

36. Guyon *et al.* (1994).

37. Reerink and Sauerborn (1996).

38. Vera (1993).

39. Maynard-Tucker (1994).

40. Muschell (1995). By contrast, *active privatization* comes from a specific policy in which the government actively encourages changes in the public/private mix.

41. Perrot *et al.* (1997).

42. Rosenthal (1998).

43. Sometimes a close reading of the annual report is needed to distinguish between these two groups.

44. Collins *et al.* (1994b).

45. Pollock (1995).

46. Ferrara (1996).

47. See for example Khan *et al.* (1996) The many innovative membership-based health insurance plans in China are described in numerous studies and reports.

48. Medici *et al.* (1997).

49. Drake (1997).

50. Green and Barker (1988).

51. Schieber and Maeda (1997). See Chapter 11 for explanation of terms.

52. Schieber and Maeda (1997) Box 2, p. 20.

53. Abel-Smith and Rawal (1992).

54. Huber (1993).

55. Stanton and Clemens (1989).

56. McPake (1993).

57. Wang'ombe (1997).

58. Abel-Smith and Rawal (1992).

59. Walt (1994).

60. See for example Collins and Green (1994) and Green (1995).

61. Collins and Green (1994).

62. This section was prepared with the aid of several key publications that review the status of health systems in eastern Europe in the late 1990s. These include Barr and Field (1996),

Cichon and Normand (1994), Deppe and Oreskovic (1996), Preker (1994), Preker and Feachem (1995), Saltman and Figueras (1997), and Vienonen and Wlodarczyk (1993).

63. In the USSR these were roughly Republic, Oblast, Rayon, and Uchastok.
64. Goldstein *et al.* (1996).
65. Barr and Field (1996).
66. Davidow (1996).
67. Deppe and Oreskovic (1996).
68. Preker *et al.* (1996).
69. Deppe and Oreskovic (1996).
70. Saltman and Figueras (1997).
71. Barr and Field (1996).
72. Saltman and Figueras (1997).
73. Earl-Slater (1996), Massaro *et al.* (1994), and Robbins (1995).
74. Saltman and Figueras (1997).
75. See especially Knox (1993), Deppe (1992), Jackson (1997), and Kamke (1998).
76. Jackson (1997).

14

Infectious Diseases: Submerging and Emerging

The popular notion that the world is teeming with pathogens has been fostered by sensationalist books and movies and by the evening news. Even so, some believe, erroneously, that the great epidemics are a thing of the past. In this chapter we look at a variety of infectious diseases and describe and contrast three: smallpox, malaria, and AIDS (Table 14-1). For two of these, worldwide eradication programs have been undertaken, one successfully, one not; for the third, the idea of eradication is only a fantasy.

On October 26, 1979, the Director-General of the World Health Organization participated in a ceremony in Nairobi, Kenya, to mark a significant anniversary. Exactly two years earlier, the world's last known case of natural infection with smallpox virus had been diagnosed in a remote area of Somalia, bringing down the curtain on the most daring and successful public health campaign in human history. The day of the ceremony, declared "Smallpox Zero Day," preceded by a few months the official declaration by the Global Commission for Certification of Smallpox Eradication that the disease was indeed a thing of the past.

It is ironic that, unsuspected by the Director-General, an unknown, perhaps recently evolved virus was on that October day spreading quietly and relentlessly around the world, perhaps having touched the very audience that witnessed the self-congratulations of the international health authorities. That virus is now generally known as HIV (human inmmunodeficiency virus), the causative agent of acquired immune deficiency syndrome, or AIDS.

Table 14-1. Some Comparisons Among Smallpox, Malaria, and AIDS

	Smallpox	Malaria	AIDS
Agent	The smallpox virus, *Variola*	Any of four species of *Plasmodium*, each with local variants.	Variants of the human immunodeficiency virus (HIV)
Transmission	Direct, by contact with a case	Passage through a female *Anopheles* mosquito; transplacentally to child; blood inoculation	Sexual contact; blood inoculation; congenitally; via milk
Incubation period	8 to 17 days	1 week to many months	5 to 10 years?
Visibility of the infection	Pox are usually obvious	Not evident by appearance	Not evident by appearance
Period of infectiousness	About 3 weeks. Highest the first week	May be prolonged; weeks to years	Prolonged; years or lifetime
Immunity after natural infection	Usually solid and lifelong	Partial and temporary	Unknown
Seasonality	Usually pronounced	Often pronounced; sometimes none	None
Nonhuman reservoir	No	Unimportant	None
Prevention and control	Safe & effective vaccine; isolation of cases	Screens, bednets; environmental changes; insecticides; prophylactic drugs	Control of blood products; control of intravenous drug paraphernalia; elimination of sexual exposure
Specific treatment	None	Effective chemotherapy	Various; prolonged and expensive

DISEASE ERADICATION: BASIC CONCEPTS

The word *eradication* has, at its root, a root: the Latin *radix*, which serves us well also in *radical*, *radish*, and other familiar words. To eradicate a disease or agent means to extinguish it (i.e., make extinct), to cause it to disappear utterly and entirely from the world. By contrast, the word *elimination* indicates a halt to transmission of an infectious organism from a defined area. A country or continent ultimately becomes free from new cases although importation or reintroduction will always be a concern.

It seems certain that many potential pathogens of mankind have become extinct through natural selection over geological time, but the list of diseases intentionally and successfully eradicated by mankind is modest, containing exactly two entries: vesicular exanthema of swine and smallpox of humans.

How was the world able to eradicate smallpox when it has been unable to do so for any other human disease? Granted that triumph, why does the world still tolerate the spread of cholera, malaria, infant diarrheas, AIDS, and so many other great diseases of mankind? In answer, we can say that eradication is an extraordinary achievement. We will never really know whether it is possible with any of these diseases until it is done. The enormous commitment of resources and effort necessary to achieve eradication must be maintained until it is accomplished and for some time afterward, because we may not recognze the zero moment even when it is reached. Moreover, unsuccessful eradication programs are not without risk. Abandoning an effort after 99% reduction of transmission may be equivalent to never having started, or it may be worse. Consider the situation in which natural infection with an agent of disease produces some immunity in humans. Following a strenuous and successful control effort over several years, a large part of the public, particularly small children, has no experience with the disease and therefore no immunity. Resurgence of the agent after a prolonged absence might then be more damaging to the health of a newly susceptible population than if the disease had been present all along.

Some diseases are simply not candidates for eradication. This is especially true for those infections, such as tetanus, coccidioidomycosis, and histoplasmosis, that arise from spores in the soil and do not spread from person to person. Others, such as yellow fever, African sleeping sickness, Chagas' disease, leishmaniasis, and plague are primarily infections of wildlife and firmly established in nature. There is, however, some good news. It is likely that poliomyelitis and dracunculiasis will be gone very soon (see below). Moreover, measles, epidemic typhus, and yaws have been nominated as potential future members of the exclusive eradication club.

It is possible that the first pathogen for which a specific, purposeful global eradication program was announced was hookworm, the subject of an early program of the Rockefeller Foundation in the early decades of this century. Despite intensive efforts, hookworm is still with us, but we learned a lot in the process.

Choosing Between Control and Eradication

Benefits of eradication include:

- Avoidance of all future pain and suffering from the disease
- Cost savings from termination of control programs and specific medical expenses
- Availability of that money for other public health uses (we hope!)
- Creation of coalitions of partners ready to tackle other public health problems
- Greater community interest and support of public health efforts
- Increased equity because rich and poor are permanently protected

Every human effort has its critics, and those who dislike eradication programs contend that:

- Eradication programs can weaken health services by diverting people and re-sources from routine work.
- Concentration on one disease can leave people unprotected from others.
- Money saved will likely be taken away from public health and used for other purposes.
- Failure to achieve eradication can demoralize health workers and the public and inhibit further attempts.

Over-enthusiastic and optimistic conceptions have led governments and international health agencies into costly eradication ventures in situations where a more critical and cautious approach might have foreseen the formidable obstacles that eventually thwarted their success; in other instances, fears engendered by gloomy theories on the utopian nature of the concept of eradication have prevented or delayed perfectly feasible ac-tions for eradication.[1]

A successful time-limited eradication program, however capital and labor intensive, is bound to be a bargain in the long run, because the long run is forever. Never-theless, ongoing control efforts may have beneficial spillover effects on diseases other than the primary target. For example, the marginal cost of adding another vac-cine to an existing immunization program would probably be quite small, and a pro-tected water supply installed for cholera control would reduce illnesses from other waterborne pathogens.

SMALLPOX

The smallpox story has been related several times, with variations,[2] but it bears sum-marizing in the context of this textbook. It must be examined closely and searched for lessons, generalizable strategies, or tactics that could be applied to other dis-eases with any prospect of similarly spectacular results.

The concept of eradicating smallpox through *vaccination* was stated clearly by Edward Jenner (1749–1823), inventor of the very word (from *vaca*, Latin for cow, from which *vaccine* was also derived). In his little book *The Origin of Vaccine In-oculation* he said prophetically that "It now becomes too manifest to admit of con-troversy that the annihilation of the smallpox, the most dreadful scourge of the hu-man species, must be the result of this practice." Jenner had not, however, invented the idea of immunization by prophylactic inoculation. That honor must go to di-verse ancient peoples who observed (as did Jenner) that an early intimate exposure to certain biological materials helped to prevent later illness.

Smallpox immunization was practiced in ancient China, where the idea of preventive medicine was well entrenched. According to Ho Kung (about AD 320): "Thus the adept disperses suffering (physical or mental) before they have begun and cures disesases before they have made their appearance. He practices his therapy before any untoward signs have manifested themselves, and does not have to pursue what has already happened."[3]

The idea of inoculation against smallpox arose, at least in China, through the observation that any person had the disease but once. The actual method for inducing protection seems to have been a closely held professional secret among medical practitioners so that there is little written documentation before about AD 1500. Old documents reveal that an inoculum was prepared by grinding up pustules and administering the powdered material in a wad of cotton or silk fibers put into the nose—an efficient route for immunization. It is likely that naturally attenuated strains of smallpox virus, probably from patients with the clinically less severe form *variola minor*, were carefully selected and nurtured, by the best of the doctors, through passage from person to person. Grinding up pustule scabs from active cases of severe smallpox (*variola major*) was known to be a dangerous practice with substantial mortality. Although the derivative process of variolation was eventually adopted in many countries (including the American colonies in 1791), such dangerous measures would not be acceptable today.

Jenner's big contribution to the vaccinee was a dramatic reduction in the health risk posed by the first (immunizing) infection with cowpox, which protected against a later challenge, exposure to virulent smallpox virus. Jenner knew nothing about viruses, of course, and little of immunology, but he was an astute observer and daring experimenter, and luck was on his side.

The realization of Jenner's prediction had to wait for the occurrence of several things—each necessary, none by itself sufficient. First, worldwide programs need worldwide coordination, which demands an organizational framework. This was supplied by the World Health Organization, which adopted the general goal of smallpox eradication in 1958 and established an intensified global smallpox eradication program in 1966. At that time the second element, money, entered the picture with a budget of $440,000 (U.S.), a pitifully small amount to launch a program intended to vaccinate 1.2 billion people in some 33 countries where the disease was then still endemic. Little could have been accomplished without the goodwill and enthusiasm of individuals and laboratories all over the world who collaborated in preparing guides and handbooks, in offering expert advice, and in many other ways. The initial budget was increased later and many expenses were met by the affected countries themselves (Table 14-2). The grand total expenditure of $313 million over ten years was certainly the best health investment ever made. It has saved the world much more than that amount each year since 1977, and will do so forever.

Table 14-2. Cost of the Smallpox Eradication Program

Source of Funds	Amount (U.S. dollars)
WHO regular budget	37,930,000
WHO voluntary fund for health promotion	43,168,946
Bilateral aid	32,246,898
Estimated national expenditures	200,000,000
Total (approximate)	313,000,000

Source: World Health Organization, 1980.

As originally planned, the program was divided into phases in an echo of the malaria eradication program established a decade earlier (see following section):

- *Attack phase.* Where smallpox was endemic with a substantial number of unvaccinated persons, the aim was for 100% vaccine coverage. When documented coverage reached 80% and the incidence of smallpox fell below five cases per 100,000 inhbitants, the program was considered ready to move into the
- *Consolidation phase.* At this point mass vaccination was to terminate and it was considered necessary to vaccinate only new arrivals and newborns. Surveillance activities were to be augmented, case detection improved, and an effort made at concentrated local vaccination of case contacts. Where no new cases occurred over two years, the program went to the
- *Maintenance phase.* Surveillance and reporting were normally shifted to the national or regional health service, and any cases detected would receive intensive investigation.

Clearly, nothing could be done without a safe and effective vaccine. Some changes were obviously necessary before Jenner's "variolous matter from a fresh pustule" could be utilized on a mass scale. Over the centuries a mutated virus, now known as vaccinia, appeared. Most likely derived from cowpox, its origin is a mystery. Active vaccinia virus induces solid protection against smallpox with a relatively small risk of harmful side effects. However, tropical temperatures cause a rapid decrease in potency of this and other "live virus" vaccines. The technology of lyophilizing (freeze-drying) the liquid vaccine for later reconstitution, developed in England in the early 1950s, maintains potency at body temperatures for weeks and proved to be critical for its use in the field.

A massive program of vaccine production was started, and by 1967 some 64 laboratories in 62 countries were producing freeze-dried vaccine, often of questionable quality. Seed vaccine of specified strains was soon produced by a few major collaborating laboratories for distribution, with expert advice, to the smaller ones. The primary donor of vaccine to the WHO program was the USSR, which contributed 140 million doses annually totalling about $15 million. The largest financial supporters of the program were the United States, which contributed more than $26 million, and Sweden, which contributed more than $15 million. Together with other donors and with domestic production in the affected countries, vaccine needs were eventually met by the eradication program without any direct cost to the WHO.

These doses needed to be administered and an appropriate methodology had to be devised for the billions of vaccinations originally contemplated. Smallpox vaccine is not injected by syringe as with most inoculations, nor eaten on a sugar cube like live oral polio vaccine. Rather, it is scratched into the skin. Originally a simple sewing needle was used for this purpose in most countries. Some countries promoted the use of the Ped-o-Jet injector, an apparatus something like a miniature sprayer that blows a dose of vaccine into the skin by means of air pressure produced with a foot-pedal-operated compressor. This device was invented by an alert physician called to treat a diesel engine technician injected with vaporized diesel fuel by accidental contact with a diesel engine fuel injector. Millions of people were vaccinated by this method in West Africa in a program operated by the U.S. Public Health Service and the Agency for International Development. However, the machine is expensive, cumbersome to use, difficult to keep clean, and requires a lot of vaccine. A better method of administration was needed and this was found in the form of a bifurcated needle, a device invented by Dr. Bernard Rubin in 1961. The needle is simply a tiny fork with two sharp prongs which hold exactly 0.0025 milliliters of vaccine between them by capillarity. Gentle jabbing with the needle causes the vaccine to spill out and enter the skin. The needle can be sterilized simply by heating in a flame, and reused immediately. A quick dip of the needle "fork" into a vial of vaccine refills it with the correct amount of liquid. Cost and weight are minimal, there are no moving parts, vaccinators are quickly trained, and vaccine consumption per person is a quarter of the previously used dose. The world's vaccine supply was suddenly quadrupled. A stroke of genius.

The final element necessary for smallpox eradication was in some ways both the simplest and the most complex. This was the epidemiological basis upon which the vaccine was to be administered—the strategic and tactical principles that underlay actual implementation in the field. The three-phase strategy has been described above. The early hope had been simply to vaccinate everyone in the world, with a target of at least 80% of the population (atack phase). This was done effectively in many localities. However, as the program got under way it became clear that in some areas smallpox cases continued to appear despite high levels of vaccination. Comprehensive surveillance and reporting was needed to understand the situation, and intensive efforts were made to identify cases in areas where conventional reporting at the time missed up to 99% of the infections.

When it was realized that smallpox was not broadly or sporadically distributed in populations but occurred in relatively slow-growing focal clusters, attention was centered on identifying cases and locating and vaccinating their immediate contacts in a plan that came to be known as *surveillance and containment*. As employed in India, this strategy involved a myriad of health workers known as "searchers" who went to schools, markets, public places, and households with pictures of smallpox victims and requests for information about any similar cases. A program of cash rewards encouraged reporting. Early results of the surveillance and containment strategy were spectacularly successful. India was declared free of smallpox in May 1975 and some other highly endemic countries such as Sierra Leone were made smallpox-free within months.

Early in this century, during the lifetime of people now living, smallpox affected every continent and almost every country on earth. By the 1940s the disease had been essentially banished from most of Europe, North America, Australia, and New Zealand, but there was a constant danger of reimportation from the remaining endemic areas. Within five years of the start of the Global Programme on Smallpox Eradication in 1967, the disease had been eliminated from South America, Indonesia, and most of tropical Africa; another three years saw its disappearance from the Indian subcontinent, leaving the Horn of Africa as the final battleground in the war against smallpox. The consequence of this intense activity over the minimal span of a single decade was the identification in Somalia, on October 26, 1977, of the world's last case of smallpox.

OTHER CANDIDATES FOR ERADICATION

Two candidates are on the brink of joining smallpox in the elite group of eradicated diseases. These are poliomyelitis and dracunculiasis (guinea worm disease).

Polio

The almost universal use of polio vaccines since the 1960s has eliminated paralytic poliomyelitis caused by wild viruses[4] in many countries. In 1988 a Global Advisory Group of the WHO set a target for worldwide eradication of poliomyelitis by the year 2000. The last case of wild-acquired paralytic polio in the Western Hemisphere occurred in Peru in 1991 and the WHO certified the region of the Americas free from polio in 1994. Globally, the incidence of paralytic polio dropped by 90% in the decade after 1988, but an estimated 40,000 cases still occurred in the world in 1997.

The situation with polio vaccines is more complicated than with smallpox vaccine. There are two quite different vaccines designed to prevent cases of paralytic polio. These are:

- The injectable original (Salk) inactivated polio vaccine, or IPV (sometimes called KPV, for killed polio vaccine)
- The live oral (Sabin) vaccine or OPV

The IPV was introduced in the mid-1950s, was rapidly adopted throughout the developed world, and as quickly replaced in many countries by OPV when it became available in the 1960s. Some advantages and disadvantages of these two vaccines are shown in Table 14-3. Note that OPV consists of living attenuated polio viruses, which can reproduce within the intestine and even immunize other people through fecal contamination. Because the viruses are alive there is some statistical risk of reverse mutation to become virulent, and all recent cases of paralytic polio in the Americas have occurred in OPV recipients or their contacts. Critics point to this as evidence that immunization is harmful, but they fail to acknowledge the tremendous number of cases of paralysis that were averted by polio vaccines. There are two ways to prevent *all* cases of vaccine-associated polio:

- Give IPV, which cannot cause paralysis, as the first dose. Then when some immunity is induced, use OPV for boosters.[5]
- When polio is truly eradicated, cease all polio immunizations, as was done with smallpox.

Table 14-3. Poliomyelitis Vaccines: Advantages and Disadvantages

Live (Sabin) poliomyelitis vaccine

Advantages

- Confers both humoral and intestinal (= mucosal) immunity, like natural infection, and does not require continued booster doses
- Rapidly infects the alimentary tract, blocking spread of wild virus
- Antibody is induced very quickly in a large proportion of vaccinees
- Oral administration is more acceptable to vaccinees than injection, easier to accomplish, and avoids the risk of AIDS transmission from reused needles and syringes
- Administration does not require the use of highly trained personnel
- When stabilized, OPV can retain potency under field conditions with little refrigeration
- Immunity induced may be lifelong
- Is relatively inexpensive to produce and to administer
- Vaccine progeny virus spreads to others (Note: Some people consider this spread to be an advantage, but the progeny virus spread by vaccinees may have mutated, with unknown characteristics)

Disadvantages

- The vaccine viruses can mutate, revert to neurovirulence, and (rarely) cause paralytic poliomyelitis in recipients or their contacts
- Vaccine progeny virus may spread to persons in the community who have not agreed to be vaccinated
- The vaccine has been very successful in the industrialized countries but induction of antibodies has been relatively difficult to accomplish in the tropics unless repeated doses are administered
- Contraindicated in those with immunodeficiency diseases and their household associates, as well as in persons undergoing immunosuppressive therapy
- The virus is relatively stable at refrigerator temperatures, but loses its efficacy if exposed to heat. A continuous cold chain is still needed from manufacture through use, to prevent inactivation of the viruses

(*continued*)

Table 14-3. Poliomyelitis Vaccines: Advantages and Disadvantages (*continued*)

- The three serotypes interfere with each other and all may not "take" after the first dose. The vaccine may also interfere with other live viral vaccines
- Type 2 vaccine virus may interfere with responses to types 1 and 3, and the absolute and relative dosages of the three components may need to be adjusted locally from time to time

Inactivated (Salk) poliomyelitis vaccine

Advantages

- Confers humoral immunity in a satisfactory proportion of vaccinees if a sufficient number of doses is given
- Can be given together with live viral vaccines
- Absence of living virus precludes potential mutation and reversion to virulence. Therefore this vaccine may be used in the final stages of an eradication campaign in which a small number of cases might be caused by reversion of the attenuated viruses in OPV
- Absence of living virus permits its use in immunodeficient or immunosuppressed individuals and households
- Appears to have greatly reduced the spread of polioviruses in small countries where it has been properly used (wide and frequent coverage)
- May prove useful in certain tropical areas where live vaccine has failed to take in young infants

Disadvantages

- Does not induce local (intestinal or mucosal) immunity in the vaccinee
- More costly than live vaccine
- Use of virulent polioviruses as vaccine seed could lead to a tragedy if a failure in virus inactivation were to occur during production of the vaccine

Source: Basch (1994) Table 5-4.

The polio eradication effort has been greatly assisted by the PolioPlus campaign of the service organization Rotary International. Through its 28,000 clubs and 1.2 million members Rotary International has collected and donated hundreds of millions of dollars to this effort. In 1996 alone, Rotary's financial commitment represented up to 40% of the funds provided to support mass immunization campaigns in 29 African countries. In addition to Rotary International, the eradication effort in the Americas was supported by a coalition of donors including UNICEF, USAID, World Bank, Inter–American Development Bank, the Pan American Health Organization (PAHO), and the Rockefeller Foundation. Still, more than 80% of the cost was provided by the countries.[6]

A cost–benefit analysis of polio eradication that examined net costs and savings during the period 1986 to 2040 projected a saving of *$13.6 billion* by the year 2040 in addition to the avoidance of suffering and paralysis.[7]

Guinea Worm Disease

The guinea worm is a roundworm parasite that causes a painful, disfiguring disease affecting the legs of rural residents so that people are unable to work in their fields or perform normal tasks. The parasite, found in parts of Asia and Africa, is transmitted through an intermediate host, a tiny freshwater crustacean found in open ponds and reservoirs. The "water flea" carries the larva of the worm. When a person swallows the crustacean in unfiltered pond water, the parasite emerges, migrates to the legs, and grows. When a person who harbors a mature worm stands in fresh water, the worm releases larvae that find and enter the intermediate host to complete the cycle. Control should be relatively simple and depends entirely on education, as there is no vaccine or practical treatment. People in endemic areas need to filter their drinking water through a cloth and must not enter water used for drinking when they are infectious. An intensive campaign supported by national and local leaders has reduced transmission to low levels in many formerly endemic areas, and some public health authorities envision the eradication of this disease. The World Bank has estimated that the return on investment for guinea worm eradication will be about 29% per year.

MALARIA

Malaria is without doubt the most important vector-transmitted disease complex in the world. As far back as records extend, malaria has been endemic in much of tropical Asia, Africa, and Latin America, and has caused millions of deaths annually. It is not so well appreciated that malaria was a serious threat in much of Europe and North America until recent decades. For many people still living in the southeastern United States, malaria was a frequent summer childhood companion.

Although a worldwide program to eradicate malaria was launched in 1955, a decade before the smallpox eradication program was begun, more people are dying of malaria now than in the 1950s. Today it is estimated that about 300 to 500 million cases occur in the world each year, with about 1.5 to 2.7 million annual deaths, 90% of which are in sub-Saharan Africa. Perhaps one million children a year, mainly under five years of age, die of malaria in Africa alone, roughly 3000 every day. Malaria is estimated to account for 2.3% of the global disease burden (and 9% in Africa), surpassed only by pneumococcal pneumonia and tuberculosis. The continuing importance of malaria was highlighted by Dr. Gro Harlem Brundtland, who announced an initiative to "Roll Back Malaria" in May 1998, when she was still Director-General-elect of WHO. Details of this initiative are described below.

It is necessary first to understand the nature of malaria. In humans, distinct diseases arise from infection with each of four species of protozoan parasites of the genus *Plasmodium*. These are: *P. malariae*, which causes quartan malaria; *P. ovale*

(ovale malaria); *P. vivax* (benign tertian); and *P. falciparum*, the cause of malignant tertian malaria and practically all the mortality from this group of diseases.

Human involvement begins with the injection into a capillary of single-celled *sporozoites* during the act of feeding by a female *Anopheles* mosquito. The sporozoites circulate briefly in the blood and then enter a host liver cell where they undergo numerous divisions, culminating in the rupture of the host cell and release of hundreds or thousands of daughter cells into the bloodstream. The parasites enter red blood cells. There they again multiply and initiate a cascade of red blood cell infections and destructions that in the case of malignant tertian infections may lead to the death of the host. In benign tertian malaria infection of liver cells may persist for a few years, and in quartan malaria a small number of parasites may remain alive but undetected in the blood for years or even for decades.

From their inception early in this century until World War II, scientific malaria control efforts were based on killing *Anopheles* mosquito larvae in their natural aquatic habitats. This was accomplished through engineering programs such as swamp drainage and by the spraying of larvicidal oils. Although quinine had been used for malaria treatment and prevention for centuries, the development of synthetic antimalarials in the 1930s made chemoprophylaxis a more practical method of control. The availability of the sensational new insecticide DDT in the mid-1940s made possible the residual spraying of houses, which was intended to kill adult female *Anopheles* mosquitoes which rested on the walls. Great reductions in malaria morbidity and mortality were reported by control programs in many countries. Malaria was eliminated from North America and much of Europe in the first decade after World War II. Emboldened by these early successes, the eighth World Health Assembly, meeting in Mexico City in 1955, passed a resolution urging member states to adopt malaria eradication as a national policy despite misgivings of some delegates. Among these was the Liberian representative, who stated that:

> Large-scale malaria control might present no difficulties in a relatively well-developed country . . . but the magnitude of the task of spraying residual insecticides in every village of Liberia, in the face of bad communication and adverse weather conditions, could hardly be imagined unless it had been experienced . . . it would be ill advised to arouse the hopes of governments and run the risk of censure when results failed to come up to expectations.[8]

Nevertheless, enthusiasm prevailed and within a year the strategy and tactics of malaria eradication had been codified by committees of international authorities, and the worldwide program was launched. It was presumed in principle that, if transmission could be interrupted for three consecutive years, the great majority of cases would either undergo spontaneous cure or would be effectively treated. The remaining parasite reservoir could then be eliminated by active case detection and treatment of those found infected. Typical of the top–down hierarchical global campaigns of the day, the eradication plan was divided into a series of universally recognized phases.

- *Preplanning phase*: administrative, organizational, financial, and technical preparation; intra- and intercountry coordination.
- *Preparatory phase*: geographical reconnaisance and detailed logistical planning; training of personnel; setting up the organization and physical facilities; collecting parasitologic, entomologic, ecologic, and social information.
- *Attack phase*: Spraying of residual insecticide on walls was the primary means of interrupting transmission, supplemented by case-finding and chemotherapy to reduce the total parasite reservoir and shorten the duration of the attack phase. When the malaria infection rate reached 5% or less of the population, more vigorous case-finding and treatment were to be done by active house-to-house visits as well as in hospitals, clinics, and health centers. Community participation was considered essential. As the parasite rate continued to fall, full surveillance was to begin, including epidemiologic investigations of fever cases to determine the source of infection of each case and subsequent spread, with specific focal control measures such as augmented spraying or local mass distribution of drugs.
- *Consolidation phase*: When the annual malaria incidence was below 0.1 per thousand population, spraying was to be discontinued unless importation of malaria was a problem. Rely on comprehensive surveillance, immediate antimalarial treatment of those found positive; epidemiologic investigation and follow-up of each case or focus until there are no more indigenous cases for three years, confirmed by adequate surveillance.
- *Maintenance phase*: Maintenance of malaria eradication becomes the responsibility of the general health services as part of their normal communicable disease control activities, making certain that sufficient attention is given to surveillance and vigilance work.
- *Certification of eradication*: to be issued by the WHO after application by the local government and inspection by a WHO team.

Early Successes

The malaria eradication program was never lavishly funded. From 1956 to 1963, $20.33 million was donated, of which $17.5 million was from the United States. Commitments of money and effort were made also by the WHO, UNICEF, and national governments in endemic areas. Many countries in sub-Saharan Africa were excluded from malaria eradication because of the intensity of transmission and the limited health infrastructure available for the program.[9]

Initial successes in southern Europe, the USSR, the Middle East, India, Sri Lanka, Southeast Asia, Mexico, Venezuela, and the Caribbean were spectacular. By 1968 nearly one billion people in previously endemic areas were freed from the threat of malaria, which had been eliminated from 36 of 140 formerly malarious countries.[10] Although these included temperate areas in Europe and the Americas where elimination was relatively easy, in the warmer zones of the eastern Mediterranean, Southeast Asia, the Americas and the western Pacific, the "eradication umbrella" saved at least several hundred thousand lives each year.[11]

By the end of the 1960s a combination of technical, economic, and political issues contributed to a slowing of progress. Technical issues included emerging DDT resistance of vector mosquitoes and also increasing resistance by concerned environmentalists to the widespread application of DDT. Attitudes of some donor organizations changed as the likelihood of achieving eradication began to recede. Political issues in some countries centered around the relative independence or integration of malaria eradication programs vis-à-vis general health services. In 1969 the World Health Assembly decided on a revised strategy in which countries should continue to work toward malaria eradication as an ultimate goal but should continue control programs until eradication appears feasible. According to Farid (1980), this resolution "gracefully laid a wreath on the tomb of the global malaria eradication programme." Moreover, it was suggested that malaria control should become part of general health and development programs, a recommendation echoed by the 38th World Health Assembly in 1984 and thereafter. Unlike malaria eradication programs, malaria control is willing to accept some transmission provided that malaria is not permitted to become a major public health problem or to interfere with national development.

The demise of the worldwide malaria eradication program was complex and many-faceted. A respected malariologist saw it this way:

> How often one reads or hears that malaria eradication failed because the vectors became resistant to insecticides and the parasites reistant to chloroquine. This is a nice "scientific explanation" that appeals to hard scientists whereas the main reasons for failure have to be sought in the soft sciences—human behaviour, politics, economics—which are not seen as having scientific reality.[12]

Malaria in the 1990s

Through the 1970s and into the 1980s the malaria situation deteriorated in some countries, especially in South and Southeast Asia and some parts of Latin America. In much of Africa, where in general little improvement had ever occurred, the situation remains grim.

A WHO conference on malaria in Amsterdam in 1992 produced a *World Declaration on the Control of Malaria* and a new *Global Malaria Control Strategy* that were later confirmed by the full membership of WHO and even by the United Nations General Assembly. The familiar elements of the "new" 1992 strategy are to:

- Provide early diagnosis and prompt treatment
- Plan and implement selective and sustainable preventive measures, including vector control
- Detect, contain, or prevent epidemics
- Strengthen local capacities in basic and applied research to permit and promote the regular assessment of a country's malaria situation, in particular, the ecological, social, and economic determinants of the disease[13]

As the word "eradication" is still anathema, there are two fairly modest but nevertheless challenging objectives:

- To have appropriate malaria control programs implemented in at least 90% of malaria endemic countries by 1997
- To reduce malaria mortality by at least 20% below 1995 levels in at least 75% of affected countries by the year 2000

In tune with the times, this strategy is designed to be decentralized, flexible, collaborative, cost-effective, and sustainable as opposed to the rigid and normative design of the earlier eradication program. More importantly, the plan gives priority to sub-Saharan Africa, which was essentially written off by the earlier strategy. By mid-1997, 47 of the 49 countries of sub-Saharan Africa had completed national plans of action for malaria control and more than 10,000 persons had been trained, but lack of funds remained a great impediment.

The basic mechanics of prevention of smallpox and of malaria are radically different. In the former it is vaccination; in the latter, an armamentarium of environmental and personal measures. Yet because these are both exclusively human diseases the underlying necessity in both is case-finding and diagnosis. It may be argued that measures such as swamp drainage are effective in reducing malaria, which may be true, but case-finding and diagnosis are still necessary to determine the extent of malaria in a community, to assess the effectiveness of control, and to estimate the degree of future transmission.

The twin prongs of malaria control are transmission reduction and chemotherapy. Leaving aside engineering projects, vector control directed at larval mosqitoes includes biological methods such as the introduction of predatory *Tilapia* fish, and larviciding with oils or insecticidal sprays or chemicals. All of these measures have certain environmental side effects. Vector control directed at adult mosquitoes has meant residual spraying of walls with DDT until resistance in some regions forced agencies to turn to other insecticides which have other adverse effects and are far more expensive than DDT. In addition, multiple insecticide resistance has appeared in many regions, leading to further logistic and financial problems. Much attention has been given recently to *integrated vector control*, in which environmental management, source reduction, and adulticiding are all done together, but to date no generally applicable magic formula has been found.

One aspect of malaria control sometimes considered trivial is human protection with screens, nets, clothing, repellents, mosquito coils, and the like, which can be quite effective in reducing transmission. Bednets soaked with the insecticide permethrin have been used with excellent results in many countries and can save many lives if used consistently. However, these tend to be costly and require periodic retreatment. All means for control require education, motivation, and long-term appropriate behavior, as well as a certain economic level to stimulate their utilization. Here again is a contrast with smallpox control, in which an individual need be willing only to be immunized once, usually at no personal cost, and with no need for change in subsequent behavior or activity.

The other major strategy of malaria control is the use of drugs, both for prophylaxis and for treatment. Here also there are problems of cost and possible side effects, and the major issue of parasite resistance to the drugs. The reduced effectiveness of chloroquine in treating malignant falciparum malaria was reported independently in Colombia and in Thailand in 1960 and has since become widespread throughout almost all endemic areas. Chloroquine resistant malaria became commonplace in East Africa in the early 1980s. Resistance was reported from scattered sites in Central and West Africa in the middle of the decade, and it will be a significant factor throughout the continent for the foreseeable future. As in the case of multiply insecticide-resistant mosquitoes, strains of *Plasmodium* are now known that are resistant to virtually every drug, including quinine, further compounding the therapeutic dilemma. Drug resistance is increasing much faster than the ability of the pharmaceutical chemists to produce and test new compounds.

Smallpox was eradicated by a vaccine, and the possibility of an antimalarial vaccine has raised considerable interest as potentially the first really new element in malaria control for many decades. Work on malaria vaccine development has been supported for many years by USAID. Several candidate vaccines have been made, but despite herculean efforts and optimistic predictions, the practical application of such materials remains in doubt. Between 1994 and 1998 approximately 16 clinical trials of various candidate vaccines were conducted at phase I, II, and III[14] FDA levels, including field trials of a synthetic peptide-based antimalarial vaccine in Colombia, the Gambia, Kenya, Tanzania, and Thailand—without great success. Other vaccines have undergone preliminary trials in Sri Lanka and Papua New Guinea.[15]

Epidemiologically, a malaria vaccine can be employed to protect

- Populations living in endemic areas, particularly small children, to make them immunologically equivalent to older persons in the community who after a lifetime of exposure are "semi-immune" to infection with local strains of malaria

- Nonendemic populations, such as tourists, travelers, and especially the military, such as American soldiers who have no natural resistance to malaria that they might encounter in a tropical setting

Possible targets of a malaria vaccine include the following:

- *The sporozoite* injected by the mosquito—to prevent the establishment of parasites by blocking entry to liver cells. If effective this would abort infections entirely.
- *The early liver stage*—to prevent dissemination of parasites from the liver cells into the blood
- *Stages in the red blood cells*—to restrict replication of the parasite's asexual stages
- *The sexual stages taken up by the mosquito*—to block further development within the mosquito vector

In comparison with a viral vaccine, such as that used for smallpox or yellow fever, the potential malaria vaccine presents many difficulties, including:

- A complex target organism (*Plasmodium*) thousands of times larger than a virus and consisting of several different species with genetically diverse geographic strains and many biologically distinct stages.
- Uncertainty about the specificity, strength, and duration of natural and vaccine-induced immunity in humans.
- Need for 100% effectiveness and very quick action by an antisporozoite vaccine. Sporozoites circulate in the blood only for perhaps 30 minutes, and if a single one escapes, a fatal infection may ensue. A continuous high level of appropriate antibody may need to be maintained.

Whether successful or not, it is certain that the effort to make antimalarial vaccines will result in increased knowledge about the parasites and also about the human immune system. In the long run, some unanticipated spinoff from vaccine research may prove to be more important in malaria control than a vaccine itself. Progress toward a malaria vaccine would have been unthinkable without a number of biomedical advances made since the mid-1970s, including development of a method for artificial cultivation of *Plasmodium* in the laboratory, the technology for making monoclonal antibodies, and advances in the techniques of molecular biology and immunology.

Roll Back Malaria (RBM). This program was established by the cabinet of WHO as a priority project, intended to attack all aspects of the disease by:

- Assisting countries to strengthen their health sectors to enable effective responses to the health care needs of malaria, including its prevention, and to for-

mulate implementation plans based on sound evidence at the community and
district levels
- Building and sustaining a strong global partnership of stakeholders and donors
  to act in a concerted manner to assist countries in implementing their plans, and
- Supporting global research and development on cost effective tools with which
  to combat malaria.

The objectives of RBM are a 50% reduction in malaria-associated mortality by 2010
and another 50% reduction by 2015. Although an African Initiative on Malaria was
set up in 1996 among the African Regional Office of WHO, the World Bank and
several African nations, the focus of RBM is sub-Saharan Africa, where malaria
constitutes more than 10% of the total disease burden and is a frequent cause of
death of children. Specific program elements include

- formulation and implementation of country-specific malaria control plans
- Needs assessment and intervention at district and country level
- Access to and quality of anti-malaria drugs at the local level
- Improving quality of care in the home
- Sector-wide approaches and financing
- Malaria control in complex emergencies and war-torn zones
- Developing and maintaining a relational database to include information on
  malaria and related health systems activities including health financing in en-
  demic countries, RBM partners, RBM Resource Networks and individual ex-
  perts who may support country level activities.
- Developing a Geographic Information System for malaria and health care.
- Fast track development of drug combinations for the treatment of malaria to
  reduce the impact of drug resistance, increase the life of existing anti-malarial
  drugs and provide alternatives to currently used first line drugs.

Predictions about malaria control range from gloomy to optimistic. The primary
strategies available for this purpose are well established, but local differences in the
parasites, vectors, epidemiologic situation, national capacity and interest, community
participation and the like may argue against a universal plan of action. It is clear that
the talents of many kinds of specialists will be needed. The RBM approach will integrate WHO expertise in tropical diseases, child health, environmental health, pharmaceuticals, and national health systems. It intends to build new partnerships with
other parts of the UN family, the private sector, the research community and NGOs.[17]

AIDS

Acquired immune deficiency syndrome was first recognized as a distinct clinical
entity in 1981, although in retrospect a few cases, puzzling to physicians, had been

seen earlier. By 1987, more than 100 countries had reported cases. The World Health Organization estimated that by June 1998, a cumulative total of 11.7 million people had died from AIDS, 9.7 million of these in sub-Saharan Africa. There were 5.8 million new infections (10% in children) and 2.3 million deaths (440,000 in children) per year. Approximately 16,000 new infections occurred each day, about 10% of which were in children under 15 and half of the remainder in people from 15 to 24. Despite the fact that two-thirds of cases were in Africa, the country with the largest number of infected persons was India, with approximately four million. A total of 30.6 million people had become infected, distributed as follows:

Sub-Saharan Africa	20,800,000
South and Southeast Asia	5,800,000
Latin America	1,300,000
North America	860,000
Western Europe	530,000
East Asia and Pacific	440,000
Caribbean	310,000
North Africa and Middle East	210,000
Eastern Europe & Central Asia	150,000
Australia and New Zealand	12,000

The disruption of family life owing to AIDS in parts of sub-Saharan Africa is extreme. In 1998 the UN estimated that up to 1997, 470,000 children in Zambia and 1.7 million children in Uganda had lost one or both parents to this infection. It was not unusual for grandmothers in these and neighboring countries to care for a dozen or more children orphaned by AIDS.

HIV constantly evolves into new strains. Globally there are two simultaneous epidemics—of infection with HIV-1 and HIV-2. Most strains of HIV-1 are are designated as M, or major; others, particularly in West Africa, are designated as O. HIV-2 occurs mainly in Asia and West Africa. The origin of HIV remains undetermined, but it has affinities to certain simian retroviruses that occur in primates in Central Africa. A new strain of HIV-1 found in Cameroon in 1998, called N strain, closely resembles retroviruses in chimpanzees and other nonhuman primates. The primate origin of HIV is plausible when it is recalled that other viruses such as monkey herpes B and Ebola are known to be transmissible to humans. HIV-2 in Guinea-Bissau is closely related to Simian Immunodeficiency Virus (SIV) in mangabey monkeys. In Cameroon, HIV-O, a rare strain, resembles a local SIV. Although there is evidence that HIV existed in humans in Africa as early as 1959, infection and disease did not become epidemic until the late 1970s. Population movements, increased urbanization, changes in sexual behavior, common use of needles by intravenous drug addicts, and improvements in highway and air travel have all played a role in its dissemination.

Infection with HIV is lifelong, with no symptoms perhaps for years, but steadily increasing risk of immune breakdown and consequent severe infection with any of a large number of opportunistic pathogens including viruses, bacteria, fungi, and parasites. These agents form part of the background of infectious organisms that are common to human experience everywhere but normally held in check by the uncompromised immune system. The opportunistic infections that are found in one geographic area may not be the same as those found elsewhere, so the clinical presentation may differ although the underlying cause (HIV infection) is the same.

One example of the dangerous infections that follow AIDS and HIV infection is the increased risk of mycobacterial disease, caused especially by bacteria of the *Mycobacterium avium* complex and by *M. tuberculosis*. Entirely new epidemiologic and clinical patterns of mycobacteriosis exist in patients with AIDS, with severe disseminated disease and very large numbers of organisms in tissues and blood. Even clinical tuberculosis often takes unusual form in these patients. Classical lung disease is rarely seen, replaced by varied extrapulmonary pathology. The interaction of tuberculosis and HIV infection has created new categories of disease. In developing countries where tuberculosis is relatively frequent, HIV infection often activates a formerly silent or quiescent infection so that it becomes a life-threatening illness. It has even been suggested that some HIV-infected children immunized with BCG, a live bacterial vaccine, to protect against tuberculosis have instead suffered overwhelming and sometimes fatal infections from the BCG organisms themselves!

Spread of HIV is accomplished in the following ways:

- Sexual activity with transfer or exchange of fluids
- Blood inoculation by transfusion, intentional sharing of intravenous needles by drug abusers, contaminated dental tools, or accidental needle stick (laboratory personnel, doctors, nurses)
- Medical injection with a contaminated needle or syringe
- Injection of prepared blood fractions and products such as clotting factors used by hemophiliacs
- Organ or tissue transplantation such as kidney, heart, or bone marrow
- Semen donation for artificial insemination
- From mother to child in utero, at birth, or through breast milk (see Chapter 7)

There is no evidence that HIV is spread like smallpox, through normal contact or by inhalation of room air. And although the virus has been shown to survive in the mosquito stomach for a few days, there is no evidence of transmission by these or other biting insects. The transmission of HIV does share characteristics with certain other infectious agents. As a sexually transmitted microorganism it is like herpes virus, *Chlamydia*, and the agents of syphilis or gonorrhea. Its transmission by contaminated needle stick is like that of hepatitis virus, and in its passage through blood transfusion it resembles hepatitis, malaria, and Chagas' disease. A number of viruses as well as malaria can be transmitted transplacentally to the fetus, and donated organs have been known to carry toxoplasmosis to the recipient. Therefore, although HIV has its own epidemiologic constellation, it has no patent on any unique route of transmission.

Control of AIDS

If AIDS is such a serious hazard, why has nobody seriously suggested a worldwide AIDS eradication program? Probably because nobody knows how to do it. It might be possible to identify a drug that would render persons resistant to infection, prevent replication of the virus, or stop the shedding of virus particles. However, such a compound has not yet been developed for HIV—nor, indeed, for any virus. Prospects for control of AIDS by antiviral drugs are therefore not bright.

Many believe that, as with smallpox, the only long-term solution to the control of AIDS will lie in a vaccine. However, this presents many special problems. The AIDS virus is composed of a core containing RNA and proteins, surrounded by an envelope. This outer coat, derived from host cell membrane, has certain attached proteins that help determine the host cell specificity of the virus. It is to these complex envelope proteins that immune responses can be directed in order to neutralize viruses. Technical problems are formidable. First, the virus mutates readily, even more so than some other changeable viruses such as influenza. Therefore antibodies against one form may not recognize another. Second, the antibodies present in HIV-infected people (as found in the serologic test) do not appear to be effective in neutralizing the virus. An attenuated form of live HIV might be developed that would induce protection but would not cause disease. But how could one be certain that there is not the remotest possibility of reversion to virulence, such as occurs with live polio vaccine; and with a five- or perhaps ten-year prepatent period, who would be willing to take that chance?

In a strange irony, it has been suggested that the gene(s) from HIV that codes for envelope protein could be spliced into the much larger vaccinia virus (i.e., smallpox vaccine), which could then be administered as a vaccine against AIDS. The recombinant vaccinia would infect the host and induce antibodies against the HIV envelope proteins as well as against itself, protecting additionally against the now nonexistent smallpox. This may in fact be accomplishable, but in the event that the vaccinee is already infected with HIV, the live vaccinia might induce severe adverse reactions. And the presence of vaccine-induced antibodies might compromise AIDS testing by serologic methods causing uninfected vaccinees to test positive. Clearly the issue is extremely complex. Nevertheless, an important spinoff from a successful vaccine against the retroviruses causing AIDS may be knowledge helpful in designing vaccines against at least some of the human leukemia and lymphomas now known or suspected to be caused by related viruses.

In the absence of an AIDS vaccine, or any means of eradication in the foreseeable future, the only approach to control is through prevention. A United Nations program (UNAIDS) to accomplish this on a global basis has involved all collaborating national governments in three ways:

- Furnishing AIDS-related information and education to the population
- Helping to insure safe blood transfusion and injections
- Providing care to those already infected

The willingness and ability to undertake these efforts vary among governments. For example, after the *New York Times* reported on November 8, 1985, that many African leaders had been reluctant to acknowledge the existence of AIDS within their borders, at least one African government seized copies of newspapers containing that very article. Such early hostility and denial were short-lived, because countries have had to come to grips with the seriousness of the epidemic. In the former Zaire (now the Democratic Republic of the Congo), policies regarding public discussion of AIDS changed from secrecy to openness when it was found that 15 new cases were detected daily in the Mama Yemo hospital in Kinshasa alone and that an estimated 5% to 8% of the adult population (and 25% of female sex workers) in the city were infected. As a result, a program of public information on prime time television helped to raise public awareness and knowledge about AIDS, and mothers began to demand new needles for their childrens' immunizations. In Brazil, the Ministry of Health has sponsored educational radio and television spots about AIDS and foreign travelers to the *carnaval* in Rio de Janeiro have been warned about sexual promiscuity through leaflets distributed on incoming aircraft. In some other countries, government officials have decided against similar actions, stating either that "people would panic," or more frankly, that "No one wants to interfere with tourism."

Most European governments have undertaken educational programs for their populations. In Switzerland an informative brochure about AIDS has been mailed to every household in the country, as was also done in the United States. In the Netherlands and France intravenous drug addicts are supplied with clean new syringes and needles in exchange for used ones and in several countries syringes are now for sale over the counter. As in the United states, these programs have not been without their critics: Some allege moral objections; others allege ineffectiveness.

The distribution of condoms, a cornerstone of AIDS prevention, has met with a variety of responses from the public. These have included bewilderment, amusement, and derision, particularly in developing countries where these devices were essentially unknown or simply unavailable. Moreover, the cost of condoms is prohibitive to many poor people in developing countries. The United States Agency for International Development has supplied about 500 million condoms annually worldwide, primarily for purposes of family planning, and other donor agencies have contributed smaller numbers. However, moralistic and religious condemnation has centered on their contraceptive function and on their presumed role in encouraging "immoral" behavior. As difficult as it has been to promote the widespread use of condoms, it has been an even more complex matter to change ingrained patterns of sexual behavior in some countries.

In comparison with other infectious diseases, AIDS presents special problems in its prevention and control. These include the following:

- Most people infected with HIV have no symptoms but are infectious to others. They must be persuaded not to spread an infection that they may not even know they have.
- People at high risk, such as intravenous drug users, sex workers and their clients, and homosexual men in some areas, are difficult to reach through conventional channels of communication. They may be separated from most community institutions by social and legal barriers. They may distrust doctors and other sources of information and consider themselves victims or scapegoats.
- AIDS is often associated with practices considered immoral and illegal in many places. Consequently, some authorities have not supported educational or preventive programs on the grounds that these encourage unsanctioned behaviors, and others may consider HIV infection as appropriate punishment.
- Some consider discussion of risk factors and preventive measures to be offensive and socially unacceptable, thereby inhibiting public education programs— in some cases, particularly in schools.
- The cost of case detection is very high. One ELISA test costs more than the total per capita health budget in some countries. One confirmatory immunoblot (western blot) costs the equivalent of six months' total income in some poor African countries.
- The possibility of infection through blood transfusions and used hypodermic needles places an additional burden of expense on health services least able to cope. This may lead to distrust and lack of use by the population and consequent increase in other diseases.
- The cost of medical care for AIDS cases is very high and diverts funds from other preventive, curative, and rehabilitative activities of national, local, and voluntary health services.

If all of these facts about AIDS appear overwhelming and discouraging, it should be remembered that at one time the control of other great epidemic diseases such as plague, cholera, and malaria was considered equally formidable and mysterious. However daunting those diseases were at the time, a combination of scientific knowledge, socioeconomic improvement, and public education has by now made each of them controllable. The acquisition of HIV follows the same epidemiological laws as that of other sexually transmitted or blood-induced pathogens. Even in an area of high transmission, it is an easier matter for an adult to avoid getting AIDS than to avoid getting malaria. It need not be argued whether the key to AIDS control lies basically in the medical or in the educational arena; if the known means of prevention are universally applied, one day AIDS may go the way of smallpox.

EMERGING INFECTIOUS DISEASES

Scientists do not always get it right. A rash of misplaced enthusiasm in the 1960s suggested that infectious diseases had become a thing of the past. Nobel Laureate Sir McFarland Burnet wrote, "One can think of the middle of the 20th century as the end of one of the most important social revolutions in history—the virtual elimination of the infectious disease as a significant factor in social life."[18] Even the then Surgeon General (1964–69) of the United States, William Stewart, opined that "The time has come to close the book on infectious diseases."[19] Despite these optimistic statements, interest in the threat of infectious diseases is now higher than ever. The term *emerging infections* or *emerging infectious diseases* (EIDs) has become part of the official lexicon and the basis of a thriving growth industry. In the United States many official and semiofficial agencies have been involved, including:

- Institute of Medicine of the National Academy of Sciences—panels, committees, publications, and the *Forum on Emerging Infections*
- Centers for Disease Control and Prevention—numerous official contacts and publications, including the *Emerging Infectious Diseases Journal*, whose full text is available online (www.cdc.gov/eid/) and *Strategic Plan for Addressing Emerging Infections in the United States* (1994 and 1998); training and fellowship programs
- Food and Drug Administration—*FoodNet*, a surveillance system for foodborne infections
- National Institute of Allergy and Infectious Diseases—*Research Agenda for Emerging Infectious Diseases*
- State Department—Emerging infectious disease and HIV/AIDS programs
- Department of Defense—study of vulnerability to global epidemics and bioterrorism
- National Security Council—study of preparedness to respond to global epidemics

International agencies are also involved, such as the WHO through its Communicable Diseases cluster.

Definition of Emerging Infectious Diseases

In general these are "infections that have newly appeared in a population or have existed but are rapidly increasing in incidence or geographic range."[20] Table 14-4 lists a number of commonly cited EIDs. Emerging diseases can be viewed as falling into one of three groups:

- Truly new diseases, such as hanta virus pulmonary syndrome, or HIV/AIDS in the late 1970s and early 1980s
- Newly recognized entities, such as amebic infection of the sinuses and brain, which has always occurred but was never recognized until recent decades
- Diseases that are increasing greatly in atypical areas, such as cholera in Africa and Latin America

Most emerging infections are caused by organisms already present in the environment which become prominent through some change in conditions such as those shown in Table 14-5. A good example is Legionnaire's disease.

> Legionnaires' disease can be traced to more subtle differences in human behavior and social conventions that have an effect on the microbial world. Thus, the aerosolization of water, now so prominent in the Western world from the widespread use of showers instead of baths to the spraying of produce in large markets to air conditioning, likely has played an important role in the emergence of Legionnaires' disease and also of *Mycobacterium avium* infection in both healthy and immunocompromised persons. *Legionella pneumophila*, the Legionnaires' bacillus, is found in nature as an infectious agent of predatory protozoa. Introduction of this organism, often as part of an aerosol of potable water into the alveolus of the lung, results in the microorganism's finding a new niche in the macrophage instead of in its usual host *Acanthamoeba* or *Hartmannella*.[21]

Many diseases once prominent, then in decline, are being recycled as emerging infections. Tuberculosis is in this cateory, as is cholera. The recent pandemic of cholera was introduced to Africa in 1970, spreading from Guinea up and down the coast and into the interior. Some localities in Africa have reported the highest incidence rates of cholera in the world:

> Rwandan refugee camps in Goma, Zaire had the highest number of cases ever recorded in such camps with very high case-fatality rates. It was estimated that around 700,000 refugees from Rwanda entered Goma in 1994, living in areas with poor sanitation, inadequate infrastructure, overcrowding, lack of safe water and food, resulting in conditions favourable to the spread of *V. cholerae*. A total of 58,057 cases with 4,181 deaths were reported.[22]

In Latin America cholera was unknown in recent times until 1991 when a raging epidemic hit the Pacific Coast of Peru, with 30,000 cases and 114 deaths in three weeks. By the end of 1991 approximately 400,000 cases were reported. By 1994 about a million people had been infected, but the epidemic waned and in 1997 only 18,000 cases were reported. In Peru 3500 cases of cholera were noted in all of 1997,

Table 14-4. Some Emerging Infections and Probable Factors in Their Emergence

Infection or Agent	Factor(s) Contributing to Emergence
Bovine spongiform encephalopathy (cattle)	Changes in rendering processes

Viral agents

Argentine, Bolivian hemorrhagic fever	Changes in agriculture favoring rodent host
Dengue, dengue hemorrhagic fever	Transportation, travel, and migration; urbanization
Ebola, Marburg	Unknown (in Europe and the United States, importation of monkeys)
Hanta viruses	Ecological or environmental changes increasing contact with rodent hosts
Hepatitis B, C	Transfusions, organ transplants, contaminated hypodermic apparatus, sexual transmission, vertical spread from infected mother to child
Human Immunodeficiency Virus (HIV)	Migration to cities and travel; after introduction, sexual transmission, vertical spread from infected mother to child, contaminated hypodermic apparatus (including during intravenous drug use), transfusions, organ transplants
Human T-cell lymphotropic virus (HTLV)	Contaminated hypodermic apparatus, other
Influenza (pandemic)	Possibly pig–duck agriculture, facilitating reassortment of avian and mammalian influenza viruses[a]
Lassa fever	Urbanization favoring rodent host, increasing exposure (usually in homes)
Rift Valley fever	Dam building, agriculture, irrigation; possibly change in virulence or pathogenicity of virus
Yellow fever (in "new" areas)	Conditions favoring mosquito vector

Bacterial agents

Brazilian purpuric fever	Probably new strain (*Haemophilus influenzae*, biotype *aegyptius*)
Cholera	In recent epidemic in South America, probably introduced from Asia by ship, with spread facilitated by reduced water chlorination; a new strain (type O139) from Asia recently disseminated by travel (similar to past introductions of classic cholera)
Helicobacter pylori	Probably long widespread, now recognized (associated with gastric ulcers, possibly other gastrointestinal disease)
Hemolytic uremic syndrome	Mass food processing technology allowing *Escherichia coli* O157:H7 contamination of meat

(continued)

Table 14-4. Some Emerging Infections and Probable Factors in Their Emergence (*continued*)

Infection or Agent	Factor(s) Contributing to Emergence
Legionella (Legionnaires' disease)	Cooling and plumbing systems (organism grows in biofilms that form on water storage tanks and in stagnant plumbing)
Lyme borreliosis (*Borrelia burgdorferi*)	Reforestation around homes and other conditions favoring tick vector and deer (a secondary reservoir host)
Streptococcus, group A (invasive; necrotizing, "flesh-eating")	Uncertain
Toxic shock syndrome (*Staphylococcus aureus*)	Ultra-absorbency tampons
Parasitic agents	
Cryptosporidium, Cyclospora, other waterborne pathogens	Contaminated surface water, faulty water purification
Malaria (in "new" areas)	Travel or migration
Schistosomiasis	Dam building

[a]Reappearances of influenza are due to two distinct mechanisms: annual or biennial epidemics involving new variants due to antigenic drift (point mutations, primarily in the gene for the surface protein, hemagglutinin) and pandemic strains, arising from antigenic shift (genetic reassortment, generally between avian and mammalian influenza strains.).
Source: Adapted from Morse (1995) Table 1.

but there were 2863 cases in one month of 1998, most likely because of weather changes caused by El Niño.

Another waterborne disease with a different means of dispersal is infection with the protozoan *Cryptosporidium parvum* (Table 14-4). Contamination of the municipal water supply of Milwaukee, Wisconsin, led to more than 400,000 cases and 4000 hospitalizations in 1993.

Some diseases, such as typhoid, gonorrhea, syphilis, and tuberculosis, are found only in humans, but people have always shared an enormous number of infectious agents with other animal species. In some cases pathogens can jump from their natural avian and mammalian hosts into the human population, as happens regularly with influenza strains. Many such *zoonoses* are known, possibly including HIV-2 in West Africa, which strongly resembles viruses isolated from the sooty mangabey monkey, an animal widely hunted for food in rural areas.

Foodborne Diseases

In the United States alone, foodborne illnesses affect up to 80 million persons, cause perhaps 9000 deaths, and cost an estimated $5 billion annually. Recently described

Table 14-5. Some Factors in Emergence of Infectious Diseases

Category[a]	Factors	Examples of Diseases[b]
Ecological changes (including those due to economic development and land use)	Agriculture; dams, changes in water ecosystems; deforestation/reforestation; flood/drought; famine; climate changes	Schistosomiasis (D); Rift Valley fever (D,I); Argentine hemorrhagic fever (A); Hantaan (Korean hemorrhagic fever) (A); Hantavirus pulmonary syndrome (W)
Human demographics, behavior	Societal events: population growth and migration (movement from rural areas to cities); war or civil conflict; urban decay; sexual behavior; intravenous drug use; use of high-density facilities	Introduction of HIV; spread of dengue; spread of HIV and other sexually transmitted diseases
International travel/ commerce	Worldwide movement of goods and people; air travel	"Airport" malaria; dissemination of mosquito vectors; ratborne hanta viruses; introduction of cholera into South America; dissemination of O139 *V. cholerae*
Technology and industry	Globalization of food supplies; changes in food processing and packaging; organ or tissue transplantation; drugs causing immunosuppression; widespread use of antibiotics	Hemolytic uremic syndrome (*E. coli* contamination of hamburger meat); bovine spongiform encephalopathy; transfusion-associated hepatitis (B, C); opportunistic infections in immunosuppressed patients; Creutzfeldt-Jakob disease from contaminated batches of human growth hormone (medical technology)
Microbial adaptation and change	Microbial evolution, response to selection in environment	Antibiotic-resistant bacteria, "antigenic drift" in influenza virus
Breakdown in public health measures	Curtailment or reduction in prevention programs; inadequate sanitation and vector control measures	Resurgence of tuberculosis in the U.S.; cholera in refugee camps in Africa; resurgence of diphtheria in the former Soviet Union

[a]Categories are not mutually exclusive; several factors may contribute to emergence of a disease.

[b]A = agriculture; D = dams; I = irrigation; W = weather.

Source: Morse (1995) Table 2.

organisms such as *Escherichia coli O157:H7*[23] and drug-resistant *Salmonella ty-phimurium* Type 104 have become important public health problems in the United States. Other foodborne diseases include salmonellosis, listeriosis, toxoplasmosis, and campylobacteriosis. *Cyclospora* infection from imported berries from Central America has caused considerable anxiety about importation of contaminated foods from overseas. Other outbreaks in the United States from imported foods include cholera from coconut milk from Thailand, shigellosis from Mexican green onions, and salmonellosis from an Israeli snack food. Similar importations are reported from around the world, illustrating the growth of globalization and another aspect of international health.

Drug Resistance

The action of natural selection never stops. Bacteria, like all other living things, are constantly reacting to their environment. When overuse of antimicrobial drugs causes that environment to become an antibiotic soup, the result will be the emergence of antibiotic-resistant bacteria.[24] Antibiotic abuse arises from overprescription by physicians or ready availability without a prescription to the self-medicating public, as occurs in many countries with lax laws and ineffective supervision. Bacteria can also acquire new antibiotic resistance genes from other, often nonpathogenic species.

Travel

International travel has grown dramatically. In the late 1990s more than 500 million annual trips across international borders were made on commercial aircraft. Virtually any place in the world can be reached within the incubation period for most infectious diseases. Rapid air travel, together with population movements of refugees and displaced persons, has facilitated the global spread of new and reemerging infectious diseases. Infectious diseases do not respect international boundaries. An outbreak of disease anywhere may be a threat anywhere else, especially in countries that are major hubs of international travel.

Bioterrorism

The use of pathogens as weapons against military or civilian targets is perceived by many as a plausible threat, fed by revelations that one or another rogue nation may have, or covet, a biological warfare capability. There have been suggestions from some quarters in recent years that the dengue hemorrhagic fever epidemics in Cuba and Nicaragua and the 1994 plague outbreak in India were due to biological attacks. Many people are convinced that HIV was intentionally designed, produced, and disseminated as an instrument of genocide.

Control of Emerging Infectious Diseases

One lesson is clear. Humans are potentially vulnerable to infection by an infinity of agents that are continually being generated and modified in the great laboratory of nature. However sophisticated we may consider ourselves to be, we cannot really distance ourselves from our biological heritage as part of the natural world, nor can we find refuge within the arbitrary borders of any nation. The keys to addressing outbreaks or threats of infectious diseases, emerging or not, are knowledge, continuous surveillance, and the capacity to respond quickly. Everything depends on accurate and timely information, which is the foundation of disease control. The EID problem is global and requires global leadership and organization. The WHO is responsible for collecting and publishing epidemiological data from around the world and implementing the international health regulations. The WHO also interacts with collaborating centers around the world, particularly the CDC in Atlanta, Georgia, to mobilize scientific and medical information and respond to outbreaks.

Several specific targets have been identified for early action: influenza, exotic virus diseases, antimicrobial resistance, and foodborne pathogens. Some of these networks are already well developed and have proven their worth. For example, the influenza network, comprising more than 200 laboratories around the world, serves to isolate and characterize influenza viruses in circulation. These results are then forwarded to one of three WHO collaborating centers (located in Atlanta, London, and Melbourne) where isolates are further characterized genetically and antigenically and the global results summarized. Each February, representatives of the three centers meet at WHO headquarters in Geneva to decide on the composition of the influenza vaccine. This system has proven to be quite successful in matching the vaccine produced to the major influenza strains in circulation each year.[25]

NOTES

1. Yekutiel (1980).
2. See for example Shurkin (1979), Yekutiel (1980), Fenner (1982), Behbehani (1983), Hopkins (1983).
3. Cited by Needham (1980).
4. A *wild virus* is one obtained in the community by natural exposure, as opposed to a living attenuated *vaccine virus* that is intentionally administered as oral polio vaccine.
5. The IPV/OPV strategy has been officially adopted in the United States, at an added cost of $230 million per year, to further reduce the small risk (usually about five to ten cases annually) of vaccine-associated paralytic polio in the United States.
6. Hull *et al.* (1994).
7. Bart *et al.* (1996).
8. Cited by Trigg and Kondrachine (1998).
9. Trigg and Kondrachine (1998). Ethiopia, South Africa, and Zimbabwe (then Southern Rhodesia) were the only sub-Saharan countries included.
10. Bruce-Chwatt (1987).
11. Farid (1980).
12. Black (1980).
13. Trigg and Kondrachine (1998).
14. See Basch (1994) for explanation of clinical trial phases.
15. Engers and Godal (1998).
16. Brooke (1987).
17. Nabarro and Tayler (1998).
18. Burnet and White (1972).
19. Stewart (1967).
20. Morse (1995).

21. Falkow (1998).

22. *Weekly Epidemiological Record* (1997).

23. *Escherichia coli* O157:H7 infection is the most common cause of acute kidney failure in children in the United States. Hamburgers contaminated with this organism and served in a fast-food restaurant chain caused more than 600 illnesses including 56 cases of kidney failure and 4 deaths in 1993.

24. Some parasites, including most strains of *P. falciparum* malaria, have become drug-resistant for the same reason.

25. LeDuc (1996).

15

The Practice of International Health

As we approach the end of this journey into international health, you may find that your interest has been satisfied by the pages to your left; or you may be stimulated to learn more, or even to become involved in some aspect of world health.

AN EXPERIENCE IN INTERNATIONAL HEALTH

Professionals in international health often receive inquiries from persons who want to obtain some sort of health-related experience abroad, generally in a developing country. Such a goal may be valuable for cultural, professional, and personal development. Candidates generally fall into one of the following groups: active health professionals; students of medicine, public health, and other health professions; undergraduate students, often premeds; and members of the general public. Motivations and goals are equally variable: training and experience in tropical diseases, humanitarianism, response to a specific disaster, intellectual curiosity, and escape from some vexing life situation. Those in the last category are well advised to reconsider their plans.

Attitudes for the Latitudes

Travel is broadening and should be encouraged. There is nothing wrong with wanting to go abroad "merely" to see, experience, and learn something. That is the passion of a scholar of any age or occupation. The desire to be of service is a laudable motivation, but an overseas experience need not be justified on the grounds of "helping" people, especially when they have not asked for the help. Indeed, most people who undertake a health-related experience overseas find that the greatest benefit is received by themselves. We need to recognize, perhaps reward, idealism without promoting cultural naïveté, or romantic notions of tropical adventure.

> The traditional view of skills and knowledge as a one-way transfer from developed to developing countries is now out of date—particularly for long-term development. In addition, the need for the high tech skills of Western medicine and nursing learnt in this country have virtually disappeared ... There are two main areas of international humanitarian assistance for which certain clinical and managerial skills are sought: emergency relief after man made or natural disasters, and long term development aid. In addition, a few but a decreasing number of basic medical posts are needed.[1]

The key attitude must be respect for the people in the host country and community. In the past it was commonplace for citizens of the more privileged nations to display paternalism or condescension toward non-European peoples. This attitude can be seen in a paper, published in a prestigious psychiatric journal, on "Frontal Lobe Function and the African," that dealt with Africans of "all degrees of sophistication and education ... not feeble-minded or evil, but fair samples of their race." The African, it was said,

> is in any case not used to looking very far ahead, but if he does it is merely to think that the European is all-powerful and can doubtless produce firewood somehow when he needs it and it is even possible that the sky might rain firewood at any moment ... a shoe is something to be cleaned and put in a particular place, a completely incomprehensible ritual anyway, and so to be memorized by rote and performed unquestioningly ... "The house-boys cannot put furniture back level with the wall, put the table at right angles to the wall, hang pictures straight, etc." This requires a type of spatial perception that is foreign to the African; it can be learned in regard to specific positions for particular items, but a general geometric orderliness is hardly attainable. His attempts to solve, for instance, the Cube Imitation performance test, which requires some spatial apperception, would be pitiful in a European child of eight.

Such remarks might have been written in the 1750s as justification for the slave trade, but in fact these lines date from the second half of the twentieth century.[2] They underscore the degree of prejudice that still may be found in an inappropriately overeducated mind and the crucial need to control arrogance and build respect for the dignity of other people.

A humble villager can do many things beyond the ability of most foreign "experts": he or she can communicate freely in their own language, and often in several; make practical and attractive objects from local materials; and survive in an often hostile environment. The untutored person may be skilled in historical tradition, agriculture, hunting or fishing, animal husbandry, music, or navigation. There is no great vaccuum in their consciousness, waiting to be filled with knowledge from foreigners who may comprehend little of local problems. A reluctance to change may be based not on mulish obstinancy but on a lifetime of experience at the margin with the ever-present threat of disaster following an incorrect decision.

Conditioned by the experiences of centuries, people in developing countries are wary of further exploitation and may be understandably suspicious of the motives of outsiders. Through the entire six-year period of a pilot project on family planning in the Indian Punjab, the villagers searched for a clue to what the program was "really" about, never believing that anyone would devote such masses of money and personnel to its professed purpose.[3] The reported use of health and social programs as vehicles for accomplishing other goals such as surveillance, political indoctrination, or evangelizing has helped to foster such suspicions (see Chapter 7). Note that evangelizing need not be religious. The targets of environmental messages, for example, may perceive that their livelihood is threatened by some restriction proposed by strangers with questionable objectives. Despite all this, most people in developing countries are genuinely and unfailingly polite, hospitable, and gracious in the presence of strangers, even foreign experts.

Arranging an Experience

Many organizations can assign medical professionals to short- or long-term placements. These groups can often be located through professional societies and organizations, many of which have websites on the Internet. Medical and other graduate students may follow the same paths of inquiry and also work through the student affairs offices at their schools.[4] But caution is the watchword. Unfamiliar groups that claim to provide relief services or to offer exciting educational experiences abroad should be checked out thoroughly before any commitment is made.

Studies on the overseas experiences of medical students are few. In the mid-1990s, 93% of American medical schools permitted overseas electives, but one study found that only 15% of students who participate receive *any* formal training before departure.[5] In 1992 a reported 2500 U.S. medical students took an overseas elective, mostly in developing countries. Of 120 American medical schools responding to a survey, 32 said that they provide some training in international health, mainly in primary health care, public/community health, or tropical medicine. An organization consisting of faculty and administrators interested in this field is the *International Health Medical Education Consortium* (IHMEC), which has established a data bank to facilitate overseas experiences for medical students.[6]

Undergraduate students will need to search more intensely to identify a suitable site through personal contacts, church groups, or other sources. Experience over the years has shown that embassies, consulates, and other official representatives of foreign governments provide little useful information. Financial or other support from a foundation, private voluntary organization, professional group, business, or national or international agency should not be counted upon. Some students express interest in working for the World Health Organization or other international body.

The WHO does not operate any clinics or hospitals and does not provide direct medical care. Their work is largely advisory and administrative. However, students may be accepted from time to time as interns, primarily with programs at WHO headquarters in Geneva or perhaps at the six regional offices.

Every country has laws and regulations governing the practice of medicine. Students interested in clinical settings must not expect to examine patients, prescribe medicines, or engage in any other clinical activity that they would not legally be allowed to do at home. Moreover, there is usually no shortage of hands in developing countries. Many western students assume that they can provide some benefit to a community without understanding the problems, the political or social dynamics, the language, or the technical solutions. To reduce the likelihood of frustration on all sides, the applicant must have some relevant skill or ability that can be put to fairly immediate use. Nonmedical skills are often the most beneficial: a knowledge of how to set up a computer database, perform statistical analysis, write a report, teach a procedure, direct an educational campaign, or some similar capability may provide immediate and welcome support to a health facility in a developing country. Good intentions, an interest in people, and a willingness to work hard are necessary, but not sufficient, to secure a satisfactory experience. Professional personnel in government, mission or other hospitals, and clinics in developing countries are typically overworked and underpaid, and the burden lies with the applicant to prove that he or she will provide a real benefit to the local staff in the field.

Persons interested in engaging in research rather than patient- or community-centered activities must be knowledgeable about the technical issues, must have relevant skills, and usually should have experience in research work. Potential projects and destinations might be identified by asking knowledgeable professionals or by perusing current journal articles that report studies of interest to the applicant. Such publications can be identified through MEDLINE or similar databases. An approach can be made directly to the authors, whose address is given in the article. Some journals even provide e-mail addresses of authors. Where an institutional affiliation is listed in a publication, it might be possible to locate it through the Internet.

Any research to be carried out should be of a professional standard and likely to produce information of value. Simple observation or undisciplined data gathering should not be rationalized as "research." As an example, an American undergraduate's questionnaire intended to study women's health in an Indian village asked among other things, "Do you have a job?" The student had not thought through the meaning of "a job" in an environment where formal employment for women is an unfamiliar concept. Such poorly drafted questionnaires take the time of local people without providing them with any benefit and are ultimately unproductive to all concerned. Any research in communities must be approved by local authorities, including public health officials if appropriate, and the possible misgivings of local people must be kept in mind.

Applicants who have identified a potential host or field situation should correspond by airmail or, when possible, by fax or e-mail. An accompanying résumé should specify the applicant's background and skills; what he or she can contribute to the host's work or program; the time and duration of the proposed visit, goals from the applicant's point of view, and what is expected in return (payment, housing, local travel, etc.). The résumé should be sensitive to the context of the host country. For example, mention of summer work as a waitress, not unusual even for wealthy young Americans, may be viewed in some developing countries as an activity of the servant class and may unwittingly depict the applicant in an unfavorable way. Although the résumé must be completely accurate, such irrelevant information may be better omitted.

Americans seeking experience in voluntary work in the health field in developing countries should consider the Peace Corps or similar agencies. Nationals of other countries, primarily OECD members, should investigate whether analogous opportunities are available to them.

A Career in International Health

Students often ask about the necessary qualifications, and training opportunities, for workers in the international health field. As is true with volunteers, the motivations of the various individuals who identify themselves as international health professionals may include any combination of: genuine humanitarianism, scientific interest, political influence, nationalism, financial gain, professional advancement, religious passion, curiosity, and adventurousness. There is in fact "no real international health career pattern in this country, in the sense that such a career existed (and to some degree still exists) in the colonial powers who have had vast overseas administrative responsibilities."[7] A laboratory researcher, an entomologist in a vector control program, a computer expert setting up a health information data system, an administrator of a maternal and child health program, an economist, or a teacher each may make a significant contribution to international health. It is certainly not necessary to have an MD degree, but that is undeniably helpful and always provides added prestige, even when medical training is irrelevant to the work at hand. Competence as a physician is of course essential for anyone proposing to do clinical work with patients. Any person interested in short- or long-term engagement in international health needs to be patient and tolerant, a good listener, sensitive to the culture and needs of others, able to work with people in diverse fields and with varied backgrounds, and have technical expertise that is relevant within the work context.

Most international health professionals are employed in multilateral agencies (such as WHO, PAHO, or the World Bank), government agencies (such as USAID or CIDA), nongovernmental organizations (NGOs) of all types, private for-profit or nonprofit consulting firms or groups, and academic settings. Consulting is a special category with a flexible and imprecise definition. A consultant must have special knowledge or skill to sell that is needed on a temporary basis by someone who is willing and able to purchase it. Many professionals who do not work for consulting firms may accept occasional consulting assignments while maintaining employment elsewhere; i.e., in an academic or research position. Indeed, the consulting work may be an expected or even integral part of the job, for example of a civil engineer who designs water supply or sanitary sewer systems, or of a development economist. Consultants may participate individually or as members of a team in planning, designing, implementing, and evalauting projects of all kinds. Assignments may range in duration from days to years. Consultants may be able to work from their home or office, or may need to spend months in remote areas in the field. Depending on the subject of interest, potential employers might be found through the internet. Many consulting company websites include information for applicants. Conversely, agencies may issue requests for proposals that describe projects for which they seek contractors and/or consultants. Many organizations, such as the various development banks, maintain consultant rosters on which interested persons can request to be listed. Persons who believe themselves to be good candidates to undertake such assignments should, if possible, identify others who have already done so to learn about the opportunities, benefits, and drawbacks of this kind of work. Only the hardiest earn a living as a full-time individual consultant, being subject to the vagaries of funding cycles, competitive bidding for contracts, language requirements, geopolitical instabilities, arduous travel, unexplained delays, and seemingly endless report writing.

Formal training in international health, usually obtained from a School of Public Health, seems relatively rare. Most people who consider themselves international health professionals entered the field sideways, through unique and nonstandard pathways. Where, then, do people get their knowledge? Worldwide, training in international health does not seem strong. In 1990 a survey was sent to 100 randomly selected medical schools in 25 developed countries inquiring about the teaching of this subject. Of the 70 schools that responded, 43 claimed to provide some coverage of this topic, but only 26% listed it as a separate item in the curriculum. Generally a few hours per year were devoted to international issues as part of classes in nutrition, epidemiology, travel medicine, or tropical diseases.[8]

The fact is that, as in any other enterprise, the majority of workers in this field have limited responsibilities and horizons. The job description may call for expertise and skill in vital statistics, health economics, program administration, family planning, or any of the specific topics covered in this book. Twenty years of experience will develop great proficiency in, say, organizing immunization or family planning programs, but will not necessarily impart knowledge about anything else. If you have read this book up to this point, you may claim to know much more about international health than the majority of international health professionals. Dogged effort is needed to stay abreast of developments in the broader field. The job is made a bit easier by periodic updates of current literature searches on MED-

LINE and the profusion of websites, some of which are listed in the appendix to Chapter 5. The usual caveats apply in evaluating the credibility of all sources.

The total number of persons whose primary professional focus is international health is difficult to determine, mostly because the boundaries of the field tend to be so elastic. In 1984 it was estimated that there were approximately 9000 health professionals in the international health field in the United States. Of these, 3,800 were "long term"—that is, employed for one year or more; 1700 were short term, usually consultants; and 3200 were volunteers. Of the total, the largest category was nurses, then physicians, then administrators. Most professionals do not follow life-long careers in this field but devote an average of about 12 years beyond professional training.[9]

When all the NGOs and bilateral and multilateral aid agencies are viewed together, it may seem that their purposes and functions are not easily distinguishable. The precise mission of each group is often unclear not only to outside observers but also to the host government, to the people for whose benefit the services or advice is presumably intended, and perhaps even to the helping agency itself. The number of such groups in the more popular countries can grow almost without limit. Some years ago Claire Stirling described the aid scene in Kathmandu:

> At last count when I was there, about 700 missionaries of progress were rocketing around the town in their Land Rovers and Toyota jeeps, representing some fifty donor-states and agencies, all urging assorted projects on a nation the size of Arkansas. Among the foreign benefactors are USAID, the Indian Cooperation Mission, the Chinese, Russians, British, Canadians, Australians, New Zealanders, Pakistanis, and Swiss, the Japanese Overseas Cooperation Volunteers, the German Volunteer service, the Ford Foundation, the Rockefeller Foundation, the Dooley Foundation (using volunteer airline hostesses who take six months off for good works), Anglia University, Cornell University, the World Bank, the Asian Development Bank, the International Monetary Fund, the UN's Save the Children Fund, UNICEF (also for children), UNDP (development), UNIDO (international development), UNESCO (education and science), FAO (food and agriculture), WFP (food), ITU (Telecommunications), UPU (postal), UNIC (informational), and IMCO (maritime), this last of the opinion that landlocked Nepal ought to own a cargo vessel moored across India, in Calcutta.[10]

Given this profusion, it is appropriate to inquire as to the proper role for a foreign health-related agency (and its personnel) in the less developed countries of the world. Granting that every situation is different, are there any general principles to guide international health work?

Some Guiding Principles

The cardinal rule for international health work should be the same as it is for medicine: *primum non nocere*—first do no harm. A second guiding principle ought to be this: Health is not unitary or monolithic, nor is it the province of any one special interest. In a kind of Cinderella syndrome, each organization may believe that it alone is the one to wear the glass slipper, and that the application of operations research, or social marketing, or biotechnology, or family planning or whatever, will provide the only true solution. Perhaps so, but in the long run, parochialism by discipline may be just as inhibiting to success as parochialism by any other dogma.

The effectiveness of international health workers, and by extension, of their programs, depends as much on understanding broad issues as on possessing narrow technical skills. The sociopolitical roles of health workers discussed in Chapter 7 are also relevant to foreign workers and must be kept in mind. The international health worker should develop a keen awareness of:

- The place of health among other factors in the total scheme of national development
- The relationship of health services to health status
- The place of curative medicine within health services
- The likely epidemiologic and economic consequences of establishing, or of not establishing, a particular health program under consideration.

Inconsistencies and contradictions abound. The most advanced creations of science and technology must be weighed and, if need be, rejected, even as a gift. While the demand is manifest for grassroots, community-based primary care, attention must also be devoted to the apex of the national health services pyramid where the crucial process of planning must be made to take place. This is not to say that focused technical skills are not needed. They are.

As with any other career, international health has benefits and drawbacks. The work is challenging and satisfying, but openings for full-time professionals are not abundant, and sometimes are reserved for nationals of certain countries. Travel is stimulating but living abroad may be hard on family life. In the real workaday world, people in international health as in any other field must make a living, educate their children, and pay their bills. Organizations also want to survive. Therefore individuals, institutions, and businesses will write grant proposals and bid on contracts for things that they know how to do, or hope to be able to learn to do, and funding agencies will define and award projects in the best way they can to suit their own needs, purposes, and missions.

Undertaking Research in Developing Countries

There are many reasons for conducting investigations among populations in the poorer countries. Perhaps the strongest case is for learning to control diseases such as schistosomiasis, trachoma, and malaria, which can be done only in endemic areas. Clearly, research on functioning and financing of programs, such as rural primary health care, may appropriately be done only where such programs exist. Humanitarian considerations may also dictate certain health support programs in regions of human deprivation.

Host country professionals may be disturbed, with good reason, by well-funded overseas experts on short investigational assignments, sometimes termed "scientific safaris." Foreign researchers may gather material or collect data for their own publications, gaining personal advancement perhaps with little acknowledgement of the efforts of local colleagues. If there was ever any excuse for such behavior, that day is now long past. In developing countries today, resident scientists may be as well trained as their foreign guests, and they are certainly more knowledgeable about the local situation. Collaboration, not exploitation, is the key to scientific work anywhere, and particularly so in developing countries.

Increasing costs and restriction of research and development in industrialized countries may make it attractive to conduct trials for efficacy of drugs or vaccines in countries where expenses are low and administrative oversight may be relatively lax. More stringent justification is therefore needed for community-based trials in developing countries of pharmaceuticals, such as contraceptives, that have general applicability. It must also be demonstrated in such cases that findings from one population can be transferred to others without loss of validity.

It is often difficult to define "human experimentation." Trials of new drugs, vaccines, contraceptives, or invasive procedures clearly qualify, but certain other studies pose problems. What of a request for stool samples to validate a new laboratory diagnostic technique for which the stool donor is not even present? Is anthropological observation on certain health-related behaviors in this category? Is it human experimentation if a health clinic or water supply is established in one village, with another kept as control? The Council for International Organizations of Medical Sciences (CIOMS) in Geneva has defined research involving human subjects as any study (1) involving human subjects, and (2) directed to the advancement of biomedical knowledge, that (3) cannot be regarded as an element in established clinical management or public health practice, and that involves either (4) physical or psychological intervention or assessment or (5) generation, storage, and analysis of records containing biomedical information referrable to identifiable individuals. Such studies include not only planned interventions on human subjects but research in which environmental factors are manipulated in a way that could place incidentally exposed individuals at risk.[11]

The CIOMS has sponsored a number of conferences dealing with ethical issues in biomedicine. Their publication *Ethics and Epidemiology: International Guidelines*[12] includes sections on drug and vaccine trials and other epidemiologic investigations in developing countries.

To reduce uncertainty, funding agencies within the U.S. federal government have required all grantee institutions to establish an *Institutional Review Board* (IRB) to evaluate protocols for investigations dealing with human subjects, including fetuses, tissues, body fluids, and so on. Many countries and health ministries have mandated analogous review panels to consider outside requests to conduct investigations within their jurisdictions. Written experimental protocols should in general contain at least the following: the aim of the research; the reasons for proposing that it should be undertaken on human subjects, the nature and degree of known risks, the sources from which it is proposed that subjects should be recruited, and the means for ensuring that their consent is adequately informed. The protocol should be scientifically and ethically appraised by a suitably constituted body independent of the investigators.

Informed Consent[13]

In the years just after World War II, the Nuremberg War Crimes trials demonstrated the need to define standards for judging physicians and scientists who had conducted biomedical research on prisoners in concentration camps. The Nuremberg Code of 1947 established the requirement for voluntary consent of all human subjects. Following this prototype, many codes of research ethics have been promoted by various national and professional groups, all based on the principle of informed consent and the notion of individuals as autonomous agents. In the United States the basic document is found in the Code of Federal Regulations, Title 45, Part 46. This act (Public Law 93-348) also established a National Commission for the Protection of Human Subjects of Biomedical and Behavioral Research. The report of this commission, known as the Belmont Report (April 1979), states the basic ethical principles and guidelines for research involving human subjects. In sum, these are:

- *Respect for persons*. Individuals should be treated as autonomous agents. Persons with diminished capacity are entitled to protection.
- *Beneficence*. Persons are treated in an ethical manner not only by protecting their decisions and protecting them from harm, but also by making efforts to secure their well-being.
- *Justice*. Who ought to receive the benefits of research and bear its burdens? This is a question of justice, in the sense of "fairness in distribution" or "what is deserved."

According to U.S. law and practice, each research subject must be provided with the following information, subject to certain exceptions:

- A statement that the study involves research, an explanation of the purposes of the research and the expected duration of the subject's participation, a description of the procedures to be followed, and identification of any procedures which are experimental
- A description of any reasonably foreseeable risks or discomforts to the subject

- A description of any benefits to the subject or to others which may reasonably be expected from the research
- A disclosure of appropriate alternative procedures or courses of treatment, if any, that might be advantageous to the subject
- A statement concerning the extent, if any, to which confidentiality of records identifying the subject will be maintained
- For research involving more than minimal risk, an explanation as to whether any compensation and an explanation as to whether any medical treatments are available and, if so, what they consist of, or where further information may be obtained
- An explanation of whom to contact for answers to pertinent questions about the research and research subjects' rights, and whom to contact in the event of a research-related injury to the subject
- A statement that participation is voluntary, that refusal to participate will involve no penalty or loss of benefits to which the subject is otherwise entitled, and that the subject may discontinue participation at any time without penalty or loss of benefits to which the subject is otherwise entitled

Normally the subject's informed consent is documented on a written consent form signed by the subject or the subject's representative (e.g., a parent), who retains a copy of the document.

Surprisingly, the concept of informed consent is not welcomed in all industrialized countries. In Japan the traditionally paternalistic doctor–patient relationship has not provided patients with much information or autonomy. The cultural paternalism of traditional Japanese medicine is shown in practices such as concealing from patients the diagnosis of cancer, withholding from patients information about drugs, requiring patients to sign waivers of rights, and refusing patients access to their own medical records. However, pressures to modernize have caused the medical profession to incorporate "infomudo konsento" into medical practice, but in a minimal form which preserves professional autonomy.[14]

Informed consent in developing countries

The informed consent document designed for use in the United States contains idealized language that may be neither appropriate nor practical in many developing country settings. Special conditions apply for persons who for reasons of age, education, or world experience may not be in a position to evaluate potential benefits and risks of experimental procedure. Special efforts must be made to inform nonliterate subjects about the purpose of the study, the need for their consent, and their freedom to withdraw. Where signatures cannot be obtained, statements can be read to the subjects, or to their parents or guardians, who may question any aspect of the study. Thumbprints, witnessed written marks ("X"), or oral consent may be substituted for signatures. The situation is often more complex, particularly for persons living in very traditional communitites. Where the concepts underlying clinical trials are inconsistent with local tradition, informed consent in the western model may be simply unobtainable and essentially meaningless whether or not a signature or witnessed mark is obtained.

Doctor Ebun Ekunwe of Nigeria has introduced the term "reverse ethics" for the situation in which too much explanation and trying too hard can keep patients away. He has used the term "uninformed consent" for situations where the germ theory of disease causation is still not accepted. "People are afraid to sign or thumbprint any document. They feel, rightly, that the writer of the document has a hold, usually sinister, on them once they have signed."[15]

Similarly, in India it has been stated that:

> mere signatures would not ensure the requirements of informed consent. In many instances such a process serves only a ritual function, leaving the patient no more informed or autonomous than he or she would have been if no information had been disclosed . . . In some communities the very concept of experimental evaluation of therapy is alien and inconsistent with cultural precepts . . . [the] "doctor knows best" attitude is commonly prevalent in developing countries.[16]

Some societies put greater stress on the embeddedness of the individual within the community and define a person by his or her relations to others.[17] Where the notion of persons as individuals is not dominant, the consent process may shift from the individual to the family or to the community.[18] However, consent through a community leader "proxy" could be susceptible to inducement or fraud, and individuals could be reluctant to disagree with the declaration of the selected community leader, even if they have grave reservations about participation in the trial.

Where several different codes of informed consent may be applicable, investigators as a rule should adhere to the most stringent.

The AIDS/AZT trial controversy

It has been well established that a substantial proportion of infants of HIV-infected mothers were born with the infection and that the drug AZT is routinely given to pregnant women in the United States to reduce this risk to infants. In 1995 a series of experiments was undertaken with support from the U.S. Public Health Service[19] and collaboration of the WHO and health oficials of the countries involved to determine whether there may be less expensive ways to achieve the same benefit in developing countries. About 12,000 pregnant women in seven countries participated as subjects. According to the project design, half of the women received AZT in varying dosages and half received an inert placebo. Critics of this study pointed out that under this protocol hundreds of infants would needlessly have contracted HIV, and demanded that it be halted on ethical grounds. An editorial in the *New England Journal of Medicine* agreed and compared the study to the infamous

Tuskegee Study of untreated syphilis.[20] The editorial touched off an intense debate about the ethics of placebo-controlled randomized clinical trials in developing countries. Federal officials including the directors of the NIH and CDC[21] countered that the use of placebos was the only way to get quick, reliable results, and that the women in the study were not deprived of any therapy that they would otherwise have received. In the end, the use of placebos was abandoned and all women were given the drug.

Compensation to participants

The issue of payment presents many difficulties in developing countries, not only for clinical trials but also for other types of studies with local people. Any substantial material reward to subjects could easily influence individuals to participate primarily for that reason, negating all pretense of informed consent. The poorest individuals might be the most influenced, bringing a systematic bias into the study and exposing the investigator to a charge of exploitation. Similarly, a community leader or intermediary should not be presented with more than a symbolic token for his or her part in the project. Most experimenters consider the payment of compensation to subjects as inevitably corrupting. Some think that a modest *quid pro quo* should be provided to poor people who participate in a study. Doctor Adityanjee[16] has suggested principles along the following lines:

- If monetary compensation is to be given it should not be mentioned until informed consent has been freely obtained.
- The money should never be of a magnitude as to be an inducement to join the project.
- Costs of transportation, food, and loss of wages can be reimbursed if appropriate, and some compensation given for the biological samples taken; and there is no waiver of rights to later compensation for damages.

A reasonable alternative to compensation of individuals is to present something to the community for the benefit of all members, both subjects and nonparticipants. Athletic equipment, or items for the local school, religious center, or meeting hall might be presented as a thank-you gesture at the conclusion of the project, provided that the gift was not a precondition for participation. In one community in which a diarrheal disease study was conducted, the project directors established a community clinic. Families enrolled in the study, who had to provide frequent stool samples, complained that their nonparticpant neighbors also had access to the clinic. The project manager then started a raffle with prizes of household items such as blankets and pots, giving a ticket in exchange for each stool sample.

There are other interesting ethical issues in epidemiologic investigations. We can consider vaccine trials, although the same principles hold for other means of risk reduction such as drugs. In a classical double-blinded placebo-controlled randomized clinical trial a vaccine is tested against an inert substance (placebo) to compare their relative efficacy in preventing the disease among participants. The trials of the Salk polio vaccine in the mid-1950s, and of the first measles vaccine in the early 1960s, were of this type. At the time of those trials there was no other available means of prevention of polio or measles. But once a safe and effective vaccine becomes available, a simple placebo-controlled trial is no longer ethically acceptable. The reason for this is that an effective vaccine cannot be withheld just to see if a new product might be in some way better, because that would expose subjects unnecessarily to the risk of what has become a preventable disease. All subjects in the next generation trial would normally be randomized to receive either the new candidate vaccine or the existing one, without any placebo. Such a trial using what is called an "active control" is rational and ethical but far more costly than the original one that tested the existing vacine. We can see why if we assume that the existing vaccine protects 90% of those who receive it. In the second-generation trial, control subjects will be 90% protected because they are given the existing vaccine (active control) rather than a placebo. Therefore, other things being equal, the new trial must enroll roughly ten times more control subjects than the original trial to yield the number of cases that would have occurred if those individuals had been given a placebo.

There are some exceptions to this principle, such as a recent trial of a new pertussis vaccine.[22] So many people thought that the old DPT injection caused neurological damage in infants that in 1979 the government of Sweden decided to stop using the old DPT vaccine altogether (see Chapter 11). When a new and supposedly safer pertussis vaccine was developed in Japan, a field trial was set up in Sweden. The Japanese pertussis vaccine was tested against an inert placebo precisely to avoid the adverse effects of the existing vaccine. The Swedish government was willing to forgo the demonstrated protection of the existing vaccine against pertussis in exchange for the expectation of increased safety. That experimental design could not have been used in any country in which standard DPT was used routinely.

Immunization programs would seem to be morally unassailable, but even the eradication of a feared disease poses ethical dilemmas to some observers. An example is polio eradication, about which the following arguments have been made:

- Countries are pressured to defer their own priorities and to divert resources and efforts at the expense of other health activities.
- Financial benefits are greatest to wealthier countries.
- Poor countries bear the major costs and negative effects.

In rebuttal, the benefits of eradication are cited:

- Eradication is endorsed by all WHO member states and developing countries are enthusiastic in their support.

- Polio has a considerable economic cost to poor countries.
- Polio eradication attracts funds that otherwise would not be used for health.
- Eradication programs help build a "culture of prevention" with health infrastructure and intersectoral cooperation.
- Polio declined 89% between 1988 and 1996 and the world is approaching eradication of polio, which is a precondition for a campaign to eradicate measles.[23]

Community-based research without individual informed consent

In addition to studies on individiuals, research may be undertaken on a community basis. For experimental treatment of water supplies, health services research, environmental pesticides, nutritional supplementation of everyday foods, and similar broad-scale interventions, individual consent may not be feasible. Entire communities may be randomized to experimental or control status. The decision to undertake the research must be made by responsible authorities on behalf of the community.

Other Ethical Issues

Much of bioethics in wealthy countries is driven by technology, as new procedures such as *in vitro* fertilization, "fertility drugs," surrogate parenting, DNA fingerprinting, gene therapy, and pediatric intensive care generate novel dilemmas. As science advances, researchers are increasingly accused of "playing God," and a cohort of newly minted bioethicists is kept busy pondering the implications. These problems are of little importance to the developing countries.

Many observers have noted that the disparity between rich and poor is growing steadily. "Consider, for example, that in the 1960s the richest quintile of the world's population was 30 times richer than the poorest 20% and that this gap had increased to over 60 times by the 1990s."[24] The 77% of the world who live in developing countries receive about 15% of the global GNP, and economic exploitation is seen as increasing while development aid is shrinking. A group of advisors who are sensitive to ethical concerns have questioned the primacy of economic analysis in making health decisions and, by not so subtle implication, the approach of the World Bank, citing:

the pressure of macroeconomic policies on health policies, the increasing intervention of financial agencies in the health field, the links between health services, technology and money, the enormous weight of health expenditure in the economies of the rich countries, the effect of the aging of populations on such expenditure, and the need to rethink the organization and financing of health services in terms of societal choices. Here the first ethical demand is to avoid getting trapped, whether defensively or aggressively, within the confines of narrowly economic thinking. For example, to present health as a means of improving economic productivity quickly leads to the question of whether it is "worth" treating the unemployed and the old, given that they are, willingly or unwillingly, unproductive.[25]

In a similar vein is a comment by the architect of the Alma-Ata Declaration, the former Director-General of the WHO:

> I see a frightening global laissez-faire mentality in our increasingly amoral world, which is allowing global casino economics to ride roughshod over political, civil, social, economic, and cultural rights. In turn, this laissez-faire approach has removed a good deal of the solidarity, a good deal of the caring attitudes, that existed in the wake of World War II ... the central issue in the present health crisis of global concerns, in my opinion, is the ethical basis of health development. Equity in access to health and health-promoting care is at the very heart of WHO's Constitution ... Without equity, promoting health as a part of development just does not make sense.[26]

All aspects of international health are riddled with ethical dilemmas, many of which revolve around essential asymmetries both between and within countries, such as:

- *Unequal power, expressed as knowledge, technical capacity, political authority, money, and other resources.* Contentious issues of health-related trade policies with developing countries include charges of unfairness concerning the price and real value of primary goods; transfer of inappropriate advanced medical technologies; inequitable regulations concerning patents and drug marketing policies; exploitative trade in infant formulas and tobacco products; the migration of health professionals from poor to wealthy countries; the shipment of toxic wastes in the reverse direction; and many similar matters.
- *Cultural and religious differences in societal goals, moral teachings, the meaning of justice, and perceptions of individual autonomy.* Attitudes vary among human populations about the treatment of children, women, the handicapped, the elderly, and members of certain ethnic minorities and societal subgroups. The activities of international workers may conflict with locally established attitudes and cultural practices regarding abortion, family planning, the position of women, or a host of other conventions. In such cases the terms of reference of any bilateral agreement must be spelled out in particular detail and the scope of work of specific project activities of foreign workers must be carefully described and monitored to maintain respect for the ethical precepts of the host country. In extreme situations, official policy or habitual practice results in systematic abuse of groups of people ethically unacceptable to international health workers who must cancel or terminate their programs.

The growth of modern biomedical science has led to increasing pressure for sites for studies such as clinical trials of new pharmaceutical products and vaccines. As these studies and trials are conducted among local populations with varying cultural norms, the question has arisen whether it is ever justifiable to apply different ethical standards to different populations. For research conducted by investigators of one country on subjects of another, the ethical standards applied should be no less exacting than they would be for research carried out within the initiating country).[27] Approval from research or human subjects review boards of local participating institutions should be obtained; if such boards do not exist, their establishment should be enouraged. Formal authorities should sign off on any study, and it would be well to coordinate with local medical societies or similar groups.

• *Varying concepts of the significance of health and the causality of disease.* These are discussed in Chapter 6.

• *Wariness of exploitation on the one hand, and the potential for forcing unwanted or ill-advised beneficence on the other.* Especially since the end of World War II, there has been a conventionally accepted view that wealthier governments have a moral responsibility to provide aid to poor countries. The moral obligation to provide aid relates to three issues: the needs of extremely poor people in extremely poor countries; the large and growing inequalities between those with excess resources and those with insufficient resources; and historical relationships considered unjust and requiring restitution and/or compensation.[28] The force of this moral argument is diminished to the extent that foreign aid is viewed as a politically motivated transfer of funds to encourage favorable behaviors or to reward friendly governments for services rendered. The ethical basis of military assistance programs has often been challenged, as have the moral underpinnings of commercial transactions and investments in developing countries made with the goal of repatriating financial profits. Charitable donations, freely given by individuals or groups motivated by beneficence, equity, and distributive justice, are channelled through private voluntary organizations, religious or secular. These have also not been free of criticism (Chapter 9).

Some Official Development Assistance (ODA) funds flow from industrialized country governments through multilateral organizations such as the development banks, commonly in the form of loans at market or near-market rates. Other ODA, more altruistic in nature, is furnished directly from the donor government to the recipient government, under bilateral agreements, as grants or low-interest loans, which may account for a significant proportion of the net capital inflow of very poor nations. Donor country motivations and policies regarding ODA vary widely. In many instances the procurement of commodities is "tied," or restricted, to those originating in the donor country. The same may hold true for recruitment of expert technical assistance in project design or implementation. In some instances bilateral ODA is limited to certain sectors, or even to specific programs or projects that would not have been the first priority of the recipient country's government and people. The pursuit of donor country foreign policy objectives and restrictions on procurement of commodities and personnel may be in conflict with ethical principles or economic development goals, but may be necessary to obtain popular and legislative support for

ODA programs. Areas such as family planning are particularly sensitive among certain groups in both recipient and donor countries, the former fearing unwarranted interference or even genocidal intentions, the latter, as in the case of official U.S. policy, refusing to fund some kinds of activities such as abortion. Conflicts in goals and values become more apparent when the donor nations insist on pursuing their own policy objectives with little priority given to the recipient's needs.

- *Potential competition with local providers.* Food aid is often criticized because the transferred products may disrupt normal markets for local producers, create a preference for imported foods, or cause a shift in agricultural production away from local foods and toward export products. Moreover, the foods shipped may represent those in surplus in the donor country, produced under price support programs, and may not be those requested or desired by the recipients.
- *The accountability of science, technology, and commerce for their impact on society.* On a small scale, foreign projects and expatriate workers often have a relatively brief time commitment in country, leaving residents to bear the long-term consequences, for good or harm, of the trials or procedures. On a larger scale is the question of longer-term impact on population, resources, and environment, which was brought up in Chapter 8.
- *The potential for creating economic and political dependency through long-continued assistance.*

Among general areas of concern are the lack of a broad framework of philosophical models to govern relationships between aid donors and recipients, the process of decision making and priority setting, tensions between priorities established by local self-determination and the values of the international scientific community, and the resolution of conflict between the values of donors and recipients. An ethical model with features implicit in most current discussions of international health aid might cover the following (rather optimistic) points:

- It is fundamentally wrong that so much avoidable illness exists in the world.
- A much larger sum should be spent on international health, and if it were, it could do enormous good.
- A relatively small investment in basic research would bring a large return.
- A world health plan should be formulated.
- International justice, not national self-interest, is the only acceptable moral foundation for international health assistance.
- Since national self-interest so often corrupts unilateral health assistance programs, aid should be channelled through multilateral organizations, which are able to act in a wholly disinterested way.
- All decision-making on international health should be a joint partnership between those giving and those receiving aid.[29]

Individual and Collective Good

Efforts to reduce infant and child mortality, largely under the banners of the WHO, UNICEF, the USAID, and other organizations, have centered around universal immunization, the control of diarrheal and acute respiratory diseases, maternal and child health, and similar themes. Such programs are justified both on humanitarian and utilitarian grounds. One common moral consideration engendered by these activities is whether the lives of infants are saved, only to have them die at an age when they will appreciate their own death.[30]

In Chapter 8 we looked at recent discussions in the international health literature about the quality of the increment of life added by a postponement of early death, and particularly whether child survival efforts have led in some cases to an increase in total suffering. The more Malthusian argument cites unrelenting environmental pressure from increasing population growth, with resultant degradation of fragile tropical ecosystems. Maurice King has questioned whether there may be ethical differences between the collective activities of public health and the individual activities of clinicians, so that it might be acceptable for a large international agency to be much more ecological and long term-oriented in its decisions than a single doctor or even a mission society. He discusses the need to strike a moral balance between the sanctity of individual human life and the need to sustain the common environment, between the present and the future, and between the utilitarian "greatest good" and the deontological "absolute duty."[31] These arguments are countered on socioeconomic, ethical, and humanitarian grounds by those who believe that King merely shifts the burden of responsibility from the "haves" to the "have nots" and who urge the developed world to support better financed and technically improved voluntary family planning programs.[32]

Sometimes there is a conflict between individual and public priorities in establishing policies for health interventions. Assume that an immunization program can protect against a serious disease, but at the cost of frequent minor and occasional severe adverse effects. Can the damage to individuals be absolved because a greater, though rarer, evil is being protected against? Can individuals be expected, or even *compelled*, to accept a small risk in the name of a larger benefit for a collectivity such as the community or mankind in general? What of those individuals or families who for religious or other reasons refuse to accept immunization?

Each nation has the primary responsibility for its own development, including policies to assure adequacy, equity, and justice regarding the health care of its citizens. Governments should encourage individuals and communities to become informed and participate actively in protecting their own health. All nations have an obligation to exchange significant information about health conditions and work cooperatively to minimize local and international threats to health. The wealthier countries must not apply their superior resources to exploit the governments or inhabitants of poorer regions in the hope of commercial profit, scientific knowledge, or political advantage.

A model code of "ethics for an international health profession" was proposed a generation ago, emphasizing the need to develop concepts different from those of the conventional physician: a community and environmental focus, consideration of the underlying causes of social pathology, the sharing of information and skills with foreign colleagues, and a great breadth of interest. "Needs are so obvious that the temptation is great to rush in with programs that seem reasonable; but international health work is full of surprises. Each new activity needs to be carefully tested."[33]

Health and Human Rights[34]

In 1959 the World Health Organization adopted the Declaration of the Rights of Children. This is of importance in international health because roughly half the population in the developing world is young people, and because most nutritional deficiencies and infectious and parasitic diseases exert a disproportionate effect on the health of children. More explicit than its predecessors, the 1959 declaration specified that children need special protection from neglect, cruelty, or exploitation; have a right to adequate feeding, housing, leisure activities, education, and medical care; and should not be separated from their parents.

Many issues have been brought into the broad tent of "Human Rights," including access to education; economic and social protection; environmental sustainability; fair employment and labor rights; access to credit; equitable marriage, divorce, and custody laws; ownership of property; political freedom and choice; and right to adequate food, physical integrity, secure housing and living conditions, religious observance, and social justice. More specifically, health-related human rights issues are subjects of intense and often irresolvable debate, such as the abortion rights of a woman *versus* the rights of the fetus. Human rights issues as depicted in current publications can be categorized under many headings, including:

- *Environmental*: carcinogens, pollution, landmines, major disasters such as at Bhopal or Chernobyl, safe working conditions, finite resources and overburdened ecosystems, protection from tobacco products
- *Human conflicts and disasters*: domestic violence; rape as a systematic means of terror; torture of detainees; civil disturbances resulting in population displacement, widespread starvation, and the spread of epidemic diseases; intentional destruction of homes and means of livelihood in military, political, or ethnic disputes; participation of physicians in torture and capital punishment; forced exposure of military populations to atomic bomb testing, Agent Orange, and other harmful experiences
- *Exploitation of a research population*: use of prisoners for research, research on unwitting human subjects, failure to obtain informed consent, withholding of available beneficial treatment for study purposes
- *Enforced medical procedures*: forced or coerced abortion or sterilization; mandatory screening for HIV or other conditions; mandatory drug testing; im-

posed blood transfusions or imunizations to those morally or religiously opposed; compulsory detention, commitment, and administration of medication; psychiatric hospitalization for political dissidents; circumcision, female and male; punishment for pregnancy or birth of a child

- *Access to health services*: right to receive wanted medical services regardless of age, ability to pay, or medical condition; right to emergency care; appropriate referral; fair conflict resolution; availability of contraception, safe and legal abortion, and related information; right to be informed about one's clinical condition, prognosis, and options; rights of HIV- and TB-infected persons to receive counseling and to notify contacts
- *Privacy*: confidentiality of medical records and information; freedom from discrimination based on genetic predisposition and susceptibility; ownership of genetic materials, cells, organs, and body parts
- *Behavior*: right to sexual preference, reproductive choice; right to refuse treatment; right to die

Myths and Preconceptions in International Health

Myths, metaphors, biases and preconceptions are instilled in everyone from family, school, church, and community. Nevin Scrimshaw has written that

> We are all limited in our responses to health problems by a variety of myths, misconceptions, and, inevitably, cultural blind spots . . . Myths represent man's effort to explain environmental forces that he does not understand, to develop a rationale and guidelines for living in an uncertain and confusing world. They organize the chaotic into an apparently rational system and thus may serve a very useful purpose at a given point in time. However, in a world where values and conditions are changing, people may cling to them tenaciously long after this has become disadvantageous.[35]

To obtain an accurate and objective view of the health conditions of mankind, we must be willing to cast aside these myths. Scrimshaw named some of them:

- Knowledge of the agent of a disease is sufficient to understand its causation and to design programs for its prevention.
- The first need of populations in unfavorable circumstances is medical care or, expressed another way: programs of preventive medicine and public health are a luxury until medical care has been provided for the acute conditions.
- Modern health care is the priority need of all societies and has been responsible for the marked drop in mortality rates and the population explosion of recent decades.
- Population growth is such a major threat to the world that family planning should have absolute priority over the other expenditures for health in developing countries.

- The poorer a person is and the greater his need, the more time he will have to wait in clinics, bring children to health centers, make repeated visits, or attend lectures and demonstrations.
- A program is justified by good intentions.

After the publication of Scrimshaw's "myths," other authors followed the same track and published myth lists of their own. England[36] (1978) provided the following, more antiestablishmentarian list that questioned the basic precepts of primary health care:

- The myth of "put the rural areas first"
- The myths of simple prevention and easy treatment
- The myth of the referral system of health care delivery
- The myth of one doctor or thirty medical aides
- The myth of compulsory rural service

Space does not permit a discussion of these points nor of the controversy that ensued after their publication, but clearly these and similar depictions jangled some nerves.

WHERE IS INTERNATIONAL HEALTH GOING?

It is very difficult to enter so much uncharted territory all at once, to rank priorities, to balance among factions, and to benefit the greatest number. Urgent needs and strident demands leave too few moments for contemplation, and strict application of the scientific method with its randomized controlled trials costs both time and money when these are rarely made available for the purpose.

> For anyone who will function in the international health of the future, the basic principles of public health will remain the same as they are now. Similarly, the fundamentals of biostatistics and epidemiology are invariant. A solid grounding in these essentials will always be necessary and must be relearned by each generation of scholars. On the other hand, investigational and presentational technology will provide ever greater capabilities as more focused and specific laboratory techniques and statistical software packages appear without letup. While this is generally beneficial, there is the danger that individuals may become seduced by the tools and begin to believe that the gel or the computer is the subject of their investigation, rather than the control of transmission of *Plasmodium* and the improvement of health in the community.[37]

How then are choices to be made, and what suggestions may be given? One hundred fifty experiences are better than one, and the international health professional must know and be able to interpret the global scene to those whose responsibilities end at their respective national border. By observing the successes and noting the failures in other countries, by adapting and refining to local conditions, through imagination, practice, evaluation, and comparison, the international health worker can become a true collaborator for the benefit of all peoples. The world is indeed full of paradoxes, but it is these that provide our most exciting challenges.

As this book began with a quiz, so will it end:

1. Is it right to save lives by immunization, nutrition, ORT, or chemotherapy when those who are saved may face a life of despair?
2. What are our true motivations in advocating or performing international health work?
3. When are we justified in conducting drug or vaccine trials in developing countries?
4. If we conduct a diagnostic survey, have we any obligation to those we find positive?
5. What rights do we have to use resources taken from other people's countries?
6. Do the richer countries have any moral obligation towards the less developed ones? If so, what are the limits?
7. What should be our attitude towards physicians, nurses, researchers or other trained people from poorer countries who want to immigrate permanently to the wealthy nations?
8. When should external support for a beneficial program be terminated?
9. In the face of limited funds, who should receive benefits—infants? children? mothers? working people? old people? Why?
10. How can the present rate of military versus social expenditures be justified? Does improved health contribute to "national security"?
11. To what extent should we provide humanitarian help to countries with unfriendly political systems?
12. Should health aid be used as a tool to promulgate religious or political views?
13. Are we justified in withholding official contributions to any group advocating abortion or having other opinions with which we may disagree?
14. What are the ethical limits to activities of multinational corporations, especially in developing countries?
15. What is the meaning of informed consent of an illiterate person?
16. Are there any grounds for favoring one ethnic group over another?
17. Are we justified in altering people's customs and traditions when we know that they are not conducive to improved health?
18. How much corruption should we tolerate?
19. Should we introduce high-technology medicine such as cardiac transplantation into developing countries?
20. Why should we worry about other people's problems when there are plenty of problems here at home?

NOTES

1. Johnstone (1995). This brief paper contains general advice for physicians thinking of an overseas assignment.
2. Carothers (1951).
3. Mamdani (1974).
4. Those interested in an overseas experience should read the paper by Taylor (1994).
5. Bissonette and Routé (1994).
6. Heck and Wedemeyer (1995). See the appendix to Chapter 5 for the IHMEC website.
7. Koch-Weser (1984).
8. Bandaranayke (1993).
9. Baker *et al.* (1984) .
10. Stirling (1976).
11. CIOMS (1982).
12. Bankowski *et al.* (1991).
13. See Basch (1994).
14. Leflar (1998).
15. Ekunwe (1984).
16. Adityanjee (1984).
17. Christakis (1988).
18. LaVertu and Linares (1990).
19. Specifically, the National Institutes of Health (NIH) and the Centers for Disease Control and Prevention (CDC).
20. Lurie and Wolfe (1997); Angell (1997).
21. Varmus and Satcher (1997).
22. Pertussis is the *P* of the DPT vaccine, the other diseases protected against being diphtheria and tetanus.
23. Taylor et al. (1997), Sutter and Cochi (1997), Lee *et al.* (1998), and Hyder (1998).
24. Benatar (1998).
25. World Health Forum (1996).
26. Mahler (1997).
27. CIOMS (1982).
28. Riddell (1986).
29. Callahan (1976).
30. Woolley (1990).
31. King (1990).
32. See for example Claeson *et al.* (1994) and the response by King and Elliott (1995).
33. Taylor (1966).
34. See also Chapter 13 for discussion of equity in allocation of medical care.
35. Scrimshaw (1974).
36. England (1978).
37. Basch (1992).

References

Abel-Smith B. 1965. The major patterns of financing and organization of medical services that have emerged in other countries. Medical Care 3:33–40.

Abel-Smith B. 1972. Health priorities in developing countries: the economist's contribution. International Journal of Health Services 2:5–12.

Abel-Smith B and Rawal P. 1992. Can the poor afford "free" health services? A case study of Tanzania. Health Policy and Planning 7:329–341.

Acuña HR. 1975. Teaming up for health. Pan American Health 7:4–5.

Ada G. 1995. Global aspects of vaccination. International Archives of Allergy and Immunology 108:304–308.

Adams NA. 1993. Worlds Apart: The North–South Divide and the International System. London. Zed Books.

Adewunmi OA. 1993. Funds squeezed and stretched: the predicament of health care. World Health Forum 14:346–348.

Adityanjee. 1986. Informed consent: issues involved for developing countries. Medicine Science and the Law 26:305–307.

Adizes I and Zukin P. 1977. A management approach to health planning in developing countries. Health Care Management Review 2:19–28.

Adlakha A. and Banister J. 1995. Demographic perspectives on India and China. Journal of Biosocial Science 27:163–178.

Agarwal A. 1980. Mahler's revolutionary study. Nature 24:206–209.

Akin J, Birdsall N and de Ferranti D. 1987. Financing Health Services in Developing Countries. An Agenda for Reform. A World Bank Policy Study. 93 p.

Albala C and Vio F. 1995. Epidemiological transition in Latin America: the case of Chile. Public Health 109:431–442.

Alleyne G. 1995. Prospects and challenges for health in the Americas. Bulletin of the Pan American Health Organization 29:264–271.

Anand S and Hanson K. 1995. Disability-Adjusted Life Years: A Critical Review. Harvard Center for Population and Development Studies Working Paper Series 95.06. 33 p.

Anand S and Hanson K. 1997. Disability-adjusted life years: a critical review. Journal of Health Economics 16:685–702.

Angell M. 1997. The ethics of clinical research in the Third World (Editorial). New England Journal of Medicine 337:847–849.

Annet H and Rifkin SB. 1995. Guidelines for Rapid Participatory Appraisals to Assess Community Health Needs. Geneva. Publication WHO/SHS/DHS/95.8. p. 3.

Anon. 1995a. Different roads to development. The Economist 336(7928):35–36.

Anon. 1995b. The rise of international cooperation in health. World Health Forum 16:388–393.

Anon. 1997. Kaiser Permanente: a grand experiment. Inside Managed Care February:6–8.

Arnold D. 1997. The place of "the tropics" in Western medical ideas since 1750. Tropical Medicine and International Health 2:303–313.

Ashford RW, Desjeux P and de Raadt P. 1992. Estimation of population at risk of infection and number of cases of leishmaniasis. Parasitology Today 8:104–105.

Asthana S. 1994. Economic crisis, adjustment and the impact on health. Pp. 50–64. In Phillips DR. and Verhasselt V., Editors. Health and Economic Development. London. Routledge.

Azevedo MJ, Prater GS and Lantum DN. 1995. Culture, biomedicine and child mortality in Cameroon. Social Science and Medicine 32:1341–1349.

Backett M. 1989. The first forty years: a personal view. World Health Forum 10:48–57.

Badran A. 1995. Global overview: state of health and education in the world. Medical Education 29 (Suppl. 1):16–23.

Bähr J and Wehrhahn R. 1993. Life expectancy and infant mortality in Latin America. Social Science and Medicine 36:1373–1382.

Bailar JC. 1990. Deaths from all cancers. Trends in sixteen countries. Annals of the New York Academy of Sciences 609:49–57.

Baker TD, Weisman C and Piwoz E. 1984. United States health professionals in international health work. American Journal of Public Health 74:938–941.

Bandaranayake DR. 1993. International health teaching: a survey of 100 medical schools in developed countries. Medical Education 27:360–362.

Banerji D. 1990. Crash of the immunzation program: consequences of a totalitarian approach. International Journal of Health Services 20:501–510.

Bankowski Z, Bryant JH and Last J, Editors. 1991. Ethics and Epidemiology: International Guidelines. Geneva. Council of International Organizations of Medical Sciences. 163 p.

Banta D and Andreasen PB. 1990. The political dimension in health care technology assessment programs. International Journal of Technology Assessment in Health Care 6:115–123.

Barker C. 1995. Research and the health services manager in the the developing world. Social Science and Medicine 41:1655–1665.

Barker C. 1996. The Health Care Policy Process. London. SAGE Books. 187 p.

Barnum HN. 1981. The Economic Costs and Benefits of an Immunization Program in Indonesia. Ann Arbor. University of Michigan Center for Research on Economic Development. Discussion Paper 89.

Barnum H. 1987. Evaluating healthy days of life gained from health projects. Social Science and Medicine 24:833–841.

Barr DA and Field MG. 1996. The current state of health care in the former Soviet Union: implications for health care policy reform. American Journal of Public Health 86:307–312.

Bart KJ, Foulds J and Patriarca P. 1996. Global eradiction of poliomyelitis: benefit–cost analysis. Bulletin of the World Health Organization 74:35–45.

Basch PF. 1978. International Health. New York. Oxford University Press. 380 p.

Basch PF. 1990. Textbook of International Health. New York. Oxford University Press. 423 p.

Basch PF. 1991a. Technology Transfer and the Delivery of Health Care. Presented at Workshop on Science Policy for Developing Countries. Universidad Nacional Autónoma de México. Coordinación de La Investigación Científica. Hacienda de Cocoyoc, Mexico February 5–8, 1991.

Basch PF. 1991b. Policy Making in Health Technology. Prepared for Seminar on Rationality and Use of Health Technology in Mexico. at Centro Interamericano de Estudios en Seguridad Social. November 4–5, 1991.

Basch PF. 1992. Technology transfer and the international health profession. Pp. 249–259. In Pan American Health Organization. International Health A North South Debate. Washington, DC. Pan American Health Organization.

Basch, PF. 1993a. Technology transfer and the delivery of health care. Pp. 79–91. In Baldu JL and de la Fuente JR, Editors. Science Policy in Developing Countries. The Case of Mexico. Mexico City. Fondo de Cultura Económica.

Basch PF. 1993b. Technology transfer to the developing world: does new technology have any relevance for developing countries? Tubercle and Lung Disease 74:353–358.

Basch PF. 1994. Vaccines and World Health. New York. Oxford University Press. 274 p.

Bassett MT, Levy L, Chokunonga E, Mauchaza B, Ferlay J and Parkin DM. 1995a. Cancer in the European population of Harare, Zimbabwe, 1990–1992. International Journal of Cancer 63:24–28.

Bassett MT, Chokunonga E, Mauchaza B, Levy L, Ferlay J and Parkin DM. 1995b. Cancer in the African population of Harare, Zimbabwe, 1990–1992. International Journal of Cancer 63:29–36.

Batson A, Evans P and Milstein JB. 1994. The crisis in vaccine supply: a framework for action. Vaccine 12:963–965.

Bauman KE. 1997. The effectiveness of family planning programs evaluated with true experimental designs. American Journal of Public Health 87:666–669.

Behbehani AM. 1983. The smallpox story: life and death of an old disease. Microbiological Reviews 47:455–509.

Behnke LM. 1997. Managed care organizations and products. Gastroenterology Clinics of North America 26(4):725–740.

Bellagio Statement on Tobacco and Sustainable Development. 1995. Bulletin of the Pan American Health Organization 23:281–283.

Belloc NB. 1973. Relationship of health practices and mortality. Preventive Medicine 2:67–81.

Belloc NB and Breslow L. 1972. Relationship of physical health status and health practices. Preventive Medicine 1:409–421.

Benatar SR. 1998. Global disparities in health and human rights: a critical commentary. American Journal of Public Health 88:295–300.

Berg A. 1973. The Nutrition Factor: Its Role in National Development. Washington, DC. The Brookings Institution. 290 p.

Berk ML and Monheit AC. 1992. The concentration of health expenditures: an update. Health Affairs 11:145–149.

Berlinguer G. 1993. The interchange of disease and health between the Old and New Worlds. International Journal of Health Services 23:703–715.

Berman PA. 1984. Village health workers in Java, Indonesia: coverage and equity. Social Science and Medicine 19:411–422.

Berman P. 1995. Health sector reform: making health development sustainable. Health Policy 32:13–28.

Bevan G. 1991. Equity in the Use of Health Care Resources. Geneva. World Health Organization. Publication WHO/SHS/CC/91.1. 34 p.

Beveridge W. 1942. Inter-departmental Committee on Social Insurance and Allied Services.

Social Insurance and Allied Services. American Edition. Published by arrangement with His Majesty's Stationery Office. New York. The Macmillan Co.

Bicego GT and Boerma JT. 1993. Maternal education and child survival: a comparative study of survey data from 17 countries. Social Science and Medicine 36:1207–1227.

Bissonette R and Routé C. 1994. The educational effect of clinical rotations in nonindustrialized countries. Family Medicine 26:226–231.

Black RH. 1980. Farid is right (Commentary). World Health Forum 1:22–23.

Bloom G and Gu X. 1997. Health sector reform: lessons from China. Social Science and Medicine 45:351–360.

Blumenthal DS. 1994. Geographic imbalances in physician supply: an international comparison. Journal of Rural Health 10:109–118.

Bobadilla J-L, Cowley P, Musgrove P and Saxenian H. 1994. The Essential Package of Health Services in Developing Countries. World Bank. World Development Report 1993: Investing in Health Background Papers Series No. 1. 110 p.

Bodenheimer T. 1997. The Oregon health plan—Lessons for the Nation. New England Journal of Medicine 337:651–655; 720–723.

Boulding KE. 1970. Fun and games with the gross national product—the role of misleading indicators in social policy. Pp. 156–170. In Helfrich HW Jr, Editor. The Environmental Crisis. New Haven. Yale University Pres.

Bowman JA, Sanson-Fisher R and Redman S. 1997. The accuracy of self-reported Pap smear utilisation. Social Science and Medicine 44:969–976.

Brentlinger PE. 1996. Health sector responses to security threats during the civil war in El Salvador. British Medical Journal 313:1470–1474.

Brenzel L and Claquin P. 1994. Immunization programs and their costs. Social Science and Medicine 39:527–536.

Brinkmann UK. 1994. Economic development and tropical disease. Annals of the New York Academy of Sciences 740:303–311.

Briscoe J.1984. Water supply and health in developing countries. American Journal of Public Health 74:1009–1013.

Brockington CF. 1966. A Short History of Public Health. Second Edition. London. Churchill. 240 p.

Brockington F. 1975. World Health. Third Edition. Edinburgh. Churchill Livingstone. 534 p.

Brooke J. 1987. Zaire, ending secrecy, attacks AIDS openly. New York Times. February 8.

Brown P. 1991. How refugees survive. New Scientist 131(1780):21–26.

Bruce-Chwatt LJ. 1987. Malaria and its control: present situation and future prospects. Annual Review of Public Health 8:75–110.

Bunker JP, McPherson K and Henneman PL. 1977. Elective hysterectomy. Pp. 262–276. In Bunker JP, Barnes BA and Mosteller F, Editors. Costs, Risks and Benefits of Surgery. New York. Oxford University Press.

Burkholder BT. 1996. Rapid assessments in complex emergencies. Pp. 47–60. In Kita E, Editor. Final Report of the Research Project on a Study on the Health and Prospective Medical Assistance for Affected Persons. Tokyo. Ministry of Health and Welfare.

Burkholder BT and Toole MJ. 1995. Evolution of complex disasters. Lancet 346:1012–1015.

Burnet M, White DO. 1972. Natural History of Infectious Diseases, 4th Ed. Cambridge, Cambridge University Press. 310 p.

Buse K and Walt G. 1996. Aid coordination for health sector reform: a conceptual framework for analysis and assessment. Health Policy 38:173–187.

Buse K and Walt G. 1997. An unruly mélange? Coordinating external resources to the health sector: a review. Social Science and Medicine 45:449–463.

Bynum WF. 1993. Policing hearts of darkness: aspects of the international sanitary conferences. History and Philosophy of the Life Sciences 15:421–434.

Callahan D. 1976. Remarks at a conference on Ethical Issues in International Health. Cited by Levine C. 1977. Ethics, justice, and international health. Hastings Center Report 7(2):5–7.

Callahan D. 1985. What Kind of Life? New York. Simon and Shuster. 318 p.

Calman KC. 1997. Equity, poverty and health for all. BMJ—British Medical Journal 314:1187–1191.

Campbell O, Koblinsky M and Taylor P. 1995. Off to a rapid start: appraising maternal mortality and services. International Journal of Gynecology and Obstetrics 48 (Suppl.):S33–S52.

Carothers JC. 1951. Frontal lobe function and the African. Journal of Mental Science 97:12–48.

Carr-Hill R. 1990. The measurement of inequities in health: lessons from the British experience. Social Science and Medicine 31:393–405.

Cassels A. 1995. Health Sector Reform: Key Issues in Less Developed Countries. Geneva. World Health Organization. Publication WHO/SHS/NHP/95.4. 23 p.

Cassels A. 1996. Aid instruments and health systems development: an analysis of curent practice. Health Policy and Planning 11:354–368.

Cassels A. and Janovsky K. 1997. Sectoral investment in health: prescription or principles? Social Science and Medicine 44:1073–1076.

CDC. 1998. Recommended childhood immunization schedule—United States, 1998. Morbidity and Mortality Weekly Report 47:8–12.

Cebu Study Team. 1991. Underlying and proximate determinants of child health: the Cebu Longitudinal Health and Nutrition Study. American Journal of Epidemiology 133:185–201.

Charlton R and May R. 1995. NGOs, politics, projects and probity: a policy implementation perspective. Third World Quarterly 16:237–255.

Chen LC. 1986. Primary health care in developing coutnries: overcoming operational, technical, and social barriers. Lancet II:1260–1265.

Christakis A. 1988. The ethical design of an AIDS vaccine trial in Africa. Hastings Center Report 18:31–37.

Cichon M and Normand C. 1994. Between Beveridge and Bismarck—options for health care financing in central and eastern Europe. World Health Forum 15:323–328.

CIOMS—Council for International Organizations of Medical Sciences. 1982. Proposed International Guidelines for Biomedical Research on Human Subjects. Geneva. CIOMS. 49 p.

Claeson M, Hogan RC, Torres A and Waldman RJ. 1994. Double think and double talk. World Health Forum 15:382–386.

Collins C and Green A. 1994. Decentralization and primary health care: some negative implications in developing countries. International Journal of Health Services 24:459–475.

Collins CD, Green AT and Hunter DJ. 1994a. International transfers of National Health Service reforms: problems and issues. Lancet 344(8917):248–250.

Collins C, Hunter DJ, and Green A. 1994b. The market and health sector reform. Journal of Management in Medicine 8:42–55.

Cooper RN. 1986. International Cooperation in Public Health as a Prologue to Macroeconomic Cooperation. Brookings Institution Discussion Papers in International Economics No. 44. 103 p.

Cornia G, Jolly R and Stewart F. 1987. Adjustment with a Human Face. Oxford. Clarendon Press. 2 volumes.

Corteguera RLR. 1995. Strategies and causes of reduced infant and young child diarrheal disease mortality in Cuba, 1962–1993. Bulletin of the Pan American Health Organization 29:70–80.

Creese A and Kutzin J. 1995. Lessons From Cost-Recovery in Health. Geneva. World Health Organization. Publication WHO/SHS/NHP/95.5. 28 p.

Croner CM, Sperling J and Broome FR. 1996. Geographic information systems (GIS): new perspectives in understanding human health and environmental relationships. Statistics in Medicine 15:1961–1977.

Crozier RC. 1972. Traditional medicine as a basis for Chinese medical practice. Pp. 3–21. In Quinn JR, Editor. Medicine and Public Health in the People's Republic of China. US Department of Health Education and Welfare. Publication No. (NIH) 72–67.

Cruickshank R. 1976. Streptococcal infections and sequelae. Pp. 50–56. In Cruickshank R, Standard KL and Russell HBL, Editors. Epidemiology and Community Health in Warm Climate Countries. Edinburgh. Churchill Livingstone.

Curtin PD. 1968. Epidemiology and the slave trade. Political Science Quarterly 83:190–216.

Cutler DM and Meara E. 1997. The Medical Costs of the Young and Old: A Forty Year Perspective. National Bureau of Economic Research Working Paper 6114. 28 p.

Dall JLC. 1994. The greying of Europe. BMJ—British Medical Journal 309:1282–1285.

Darras C. 1997. Local health services: some lessons from their evolution in Bolivia. Tropical Medicine and International Health 2:356–362.

DaVanzo J and Adamson DM. 1998. Family planning in developing countries. An unfinished success story. Population Matters Issue Paper 176. Santa Monica, California. Rand. 6p.

Davidow SL. 1996. Observations on health care issues in the former Soviet Union. Journal of Community Health 21:51–59.

de Ferranti D. 1985. Paying for Health Services in Developing Countries. World Bank Staff Working Paper 721. 111 p.

Defoe D. 1722. A Journal of the Plague Year; Being Observations or Memorials of the Most Remarkable Occurrences, as Well Public as Private, Which Happened in London During the Last Great Visitation in 1665 . . . London. Penguin Books (Reprint, 1986). 255 p.

Denton FT, Gafni A and Spencer BG. 1993. The SHARP computer system—a tool for resource planning in the health care sector. Pp. 46–56. In Malek M, Rasquinha J and Vacani P, Editors. Strategic Isues in Health Care Management. New York. John Wiley.

de Onís M, Monteiro C, Akre J and Clugston G. 1993. The worldwide magnitude of protein-energy malnutrition: an overview from the WHO Global Database on Child Growth. Bulletin of the World Health Organization 71:703–712.

Deppe H-U. 1992. German unification and European integration. Health/PAC Bulletin Spring 1992:22–27.

Deppe H-U and Oreskovic S. 1996. Back to Europe: back to Bismarck? International Journal of Health Services 26:777–802.

de Savigny D and Wijeyaratne P, Editors. 1995. GIS for Health and the Environment. Proceedings of an International Workshop held in Colombo, Sri Lanka, 5–10 September, 1994. Ottawa. International Development Research Centre.

Desenclos J-C, Bijkerk H and Huisman J. 1993. Variations in infectious diseases surveillance in Europe. Lancet 341:1003–1006.

Diallo I, Molouba R and Sarr LC. 1993. Primary health care: from aspiration to achievement. World Health Forum 14:349–356.

Dirie M and Lindmark G. 1991. Female circumcision in Somalia and women's motives. Acta Obstetrica Gynecologica Scandinavica 70:581–584.

Disraeli B. 1845. Sybil, or The Two Nations. Reprinted 1939. London. Oxford University Press. 431 p.

Domschke E and Goyer DS. 1986. The Handbook of National Population Censuses: Africa and Asia. New York. Greenwood Press. 1032 p.

Drake DF. 1997. Managed care. A product of market dynamics. JAMA 277(7):560–563

D'Souza F. 1981. Who is a refugee? definitions and assistance. Disasters 5:173–177.

Dubin MD. 1995. The League of Nations Health Organization. Pp. 56–80. In Weindling P, Editor. International Health Organisations and Movements, 1918–1939. Cambridge. Cambridge University Press.

Earl-Slater A. 1996. Health-care reforms in the Czech Republic. Journal of Management in Medicine 10:13–22.

Eaton RDP. 1968. Amebiasis in northern Saskatchewan: epidemiological considerations. Canadian Medical Association Journal 99:706–711.

Eckholm E. 1985. Iodine deficiency in India seen to disable millions; health experts in Himalayas alarmed by recent findings. New York Times, April 2.

Economist. 1995. Good intentions, road to hell? October 7:91–92.

Edmonston B and Schultze C, Editors. 1995. Modernizing the U.S. Census. Washington, DC. National Academy Press. 468 p.

Ehrlich PR. 1968.The Population Bomb; ——. 1971. The Population Bomb, Revised and expanded edition. New York. Sierra Club/Ballantine Books.

Ekunwe EO. 1984. Expanding immunization coverage through improved clinic procedures. World Health Forum 5:361–363.

Elchal U, Ben-Ami B, Gillis R and Brzezinski A. 1997. Ritualistic female genital mutilation: current status and future outlook. Obstetrical and Gynecological Survey 52:643–651.

Engers HD and Godal T. 1998. Malaria vaccine development: current status. Parasitology Today 14:56–64.

England R. 1978. More myths in international health planning. American Journal of Public Health 68:153–159.

Enke S and Brown RA. 1972. Economic worth of preventing death at different ages in developing countries. Journal of Biosocial Science 4:299–306.

Enthoven A. 1997. Market-based reform of U.S. health care financing and delivery: managed care and managed competition. Pp. 195–214. In Schieber GJ, Editor. Innovations in Health Care Financing. Proceedings of a World Bank Conference March 10–11, 1997. World Bank Discussion Paper 365.

Epstein M, Moreno R and Bacchetti P. 1997. The underreporting of deaths of American Indian children in California, 1979 through 1993. American Journal of Public Health 87:1363–1366.

Erwin DO and Hackler C. 1998. Female circumcision: a cross-cultural conundrum. Health Care Analysis 6:35–39.

Faggiano F, Partanen T, Kogevinas M and Boffetta P. 1997. Socioeconomic differences in cancer incidence and mortality. Pp. 65–176. In Kogevinas M, Pearce N, Susser M and Boffetta P, Editors. Social Inequalities and Cancer. IARC Scientific Publications 138.

Falkow S. 1998. Who speaks for the microbes? Emerging Infectious Diseases 4:495–497.

Farid MA. 1980. The malaria programme—from euphoria to anarchy. World Health Forum 1:8–33.

Farley J. 1995. The International Health Division of the Rockefeller Foundation: the Russell years, 1920–1934. Pp. 203–221. In Weindling P, Editor. International Health Organisations and Movements, 1918–1939. Cambridge. Cambridge University Press.

Fauveau V, Yunus M, Islam MS, Briend A and Bennish ML. 1992. Does ORT reduce diarrhoeal mortality? Health Policy and Planning 7:243–250.

Fawzi WW, Herrera MG, Willett WC, Nestel P, El Amin A and Mohamed KA. 1997. The effect of vitamin A supplementation on the growth of preschool children in the Sudan. American Journal of Public Health 87:1359–1362.

Feachem R, Kjellstrom T, Murray CJL, Over M and Philips MA. 1990. The Health of Adults in the Developing World. Washington, DC. Published by Oxford University Press for the World Bank. 350 p.

Feeney G. 1994. Fertility decline in East Asia. Science 266:1518–1523.

Fendall R. 1985. Myths and misconceptions in public health care: lessons from experience. Third World Planning 7:307–322.

Feng X, Tang S, Bloom G, Segall M and Gu X. 1995. Cooperative medical schemes in rural China. Social Science and Medicine 41:1111–1118.

Fenner F. 1982. A successful eradication campaign. Global eradication of smallpox. Reviews of Infectious Diseases 4:916–922.

Ferguson EW, Doarn CR and Scott JC. 1995. Survey of global telemedicine. Journal of Medical Systems 19:35–46.

Ferrara PJ. 1996. A new prescription (medical savings accounts). Wilson Quarterly 20(3):25–27.

Fitzpatrick R. 1996. A pragmatic defence of health status measures. Health Care Analysis 4:265–272.

Foltz A-M. 1993. Modeling technology transfer in health information systems. International Journal of Technology Assesment in Health Care 9:346–359.

Fonseca W, Kirkwood BR, Victoria CG, Fuchs SR, Flores J and Misago C. 1996. Risk factors for childhood pneumonia among the urban poor in Fortaleza, Brazil: a case-control study. Bulletin of the World Health Organization 74:199–108.

Fowler B. 1995. World of ancient iceman comes into focus. New York Times. December 19.

Fox DM. 1998. Managed care: the third reorganization of health care. Journal of the American Geriatrics Society 46:314–317.

Fox RC. 1995. Medical humanitarianism and human rights: reflections on Doctors Without Borders and Doctors of the World. Social Science and Medicine 41:1607–1616.

Frazer JG, Sir. 1950. The Golden Bough. A Study in magic and Religion. Abridged Edition. New York. Macmillan. 864 p.

Freedman R and Berelson B. 1976. The record of family planning programs. Studies in Family Planning 7:1–40.

Frenk J. 1995. Comprehensive policy analysis for health system reform. Health Policy 32:257–277.

Frenk J, Bobadilla J-L, Sepúlveda J and López-Cervantes M. 1989. Health transition in middle-income countries: new challenges for health care. Health Policy and Planning 4:29–39.

Frenk J, Bobadilla J-L, Stern C, Frejka T and Lozano R. 1991. Elements for a theory of the health transition. Health Transition Review 1:21–38.

Frerichs RR. 1991. Epidemiologic surveillance in developing countries. Annual Review of Public Health 12:257–280.

Freund PJ and Kalumba K. 1986. Information for health development. World Health Forum 7:185–190.

Friedman M and Rosenman RH. 1974. Type A Behavior and Your Heart. New York. Knopf. 266 p.

Friedman TL. 1987. A forecast for Israel: more Arabs than Jews. New York Times. October 19.

Fuchs VR. 1974. Who Shall Live? New York. Basic Books. 168 p.

Garcia-Moreno C and Türmen T. 1995. International perspectives on women's reproductive health. Science 269:790–792.

Gardner JW and Sanborn JS. 1990. Years of potential life lost (YPLL)—what does it mean? Epidemiology 1:322–329.

Gelfand M. 1964. Rivers of Death in Africa. London. Oxford University Press. 100 p.

Gelfand HM. 1971. The patterns of disease in Africa. Central African Journal of Medicine 17:69–78.

Gelfand M. 1976. The pattern of disease in Africa and the Western way of life. Tropical Doctor 6:173–179.

Gellert GA. 1995. Humanitarian responses to mass violence perpetrated against vulnerable populations. BMJ British Medical Journal 311:995–1001.

Ghana Health Assessment Team. 1981. A quantitative method of assessing the health impact of different diseases in less developed countries. International Journal of Epidemiology 10:73–80.

Goldman N. and Pebley AR. 1994. Health cards, maternal reports and the measurement of immunization coverage: the example of Guatemala. Social Science and Medicine 38:1075–1089.

Goldsmith MF. 1993. Ancestors may provide clinical answers, say 'Darwinian' medical evolutionists. JAMA 269:1477–1478, 1480.

Goldsmith SB. 1972. The status of health status indicators. Health Services Reports 87:212–220.

Goldstein E, Preker AS, Adeyi O and Chellaraj G. 1996. Trends in Health Status, Health Services and Health Finance: The Transition in Central and Eastern Europe. Volume 1. World Bank Technical Paper 341. 56 Pp.

Goodman NM. 1971. International Health Organizations and Their Work. Edinburgh. Churchill Livingstone. 480 p.

Gourou P. 1980. The Tropical World. Fifth Edition. London. Longmans. 190 p.

Goyer DS and Domschke E. 1983. The Handbook of National Population Censuses: Latin America and the Caribbean, North America, and Oceania. Westport, CT. Greenwood Press. 711 p.

Graham WJ. 1986. Health Status Indicators in Developing Countries. A Selective Review. A Report Prepared for the Commonwealth Secretariat. 48 p.

Green A. 1992. An Introduction to Health planning in Developing Countries. Oxford. Oxford University Press. 351 p.

Green A. 1995. The state of health planning in the '90s. Health Policy and Planning 10:22–28.

Green A and Barker C. 1988. Priority setting and economic appraisal: whose priorities—the community or the economist? Social Science and Medicine 26:919–929.

Green RH. 1991. Politics, power and poverty: Health for all in 2000 in the Third World? Social Science and Medicine 32:745–755.

Greenaway D and Morrisey O. 1993. Structural adjustment and liberalisation in developing countries: what lessons have we learned? Kyklos 46:241–261.

Greenlick MR. 1997. The development of the social mission of Kaiser Permanente. The Permanente Journal 1:63–64.

Greenwood BM, Greenwood AM, Bradley AK, Tulloch S, Hayes R and Oldfield FSJ. 1987. Deaths in infancy and early childhood in a well-vaccinated, rural, West African population. Annals of Tropical Paediatrics 7:91–99.

Grenholm GG. 1983. The paradigms of health care delivery systems: Implications for the Third World. Pp. 97–109. In Morgan JH, Editor. Third World Medicine and Social Change. Boston. University Press of America.

Grogan CM. 1995. Urban economic reform and access to health care coverage in the People's Republic of China. Social Science and Medicine 41:1073–1084.

Gu X, Bloom G, Tang S, Zhu Y, Zhou S and Chen X. 1993. Financing health care in rural China: preliminary report of a nationwide study. Social Science and Medicine 36:385–391.

Guerra F. 1993. The European-American exchange. History and Philosophy of the Life Sciences 15:313–327.

Guerrant R. 1994. Twelve messages from enteric infections for science and society. American Journal of Tropical Medicine and Hygiene 51:26–35.

Gunatilleke G. 1995. Poverty and Health in Developing Countries. Geneva. World Health Organization. Publication WHO/ICO/MESD.16.

Guyon AB, Barman A, Ahmed JU, Ahmed AU and Alam MS. 1994. A baseline survey on use of drugs at the primary health care level in Bangladesh. Bulletin of the World Health Organization 72:265–271.

Harrold P and Associates. 1995. The Broad Sector Approach to Investment Lending. World Bank Discussion Papers. Africa Technical Department Series No. 302. 50 p.

Hashimoto M. 1984. Health services in Japan. Pp.335–370. In Raffel MW, Editor. Comparative Health Systems. University Park, PA. Pennsylvania State University Press.

Hazarika S. 1988. India's population tops 800 million. New York Times. June 2.

Heck JE and Wedermeyer D. 1995. International health education in U.S. medical schools: trends in curriculum focus, student interest, and funding sources. Family Medicine 27:636–640.

Helgason T. 1992. Epidemiological research needs access to data. Scandinavian Journal of Social Medicine 20:129–133.

Henderson RH. 1989. World Health Organization's Expanded Programme on Immunization: progress and evaluation report. Annals of the New York Academy of Sciences 569:45–68.

Hertz E, Hebert JR and Landon J. 1994. Social and environmental factors and life expectancy, infant mortality, and maternal mortality rates: results of a cross-national comparison. Social Science and Medicine 39:105–114.

Hesketh T and Zhu WX. 1994. Excessive expenditure of income on treatments in developing countries (Letter). BMJ—British Medical Journal 309:1441.

Heywood AB and Campbell BC. 1997. Development of a primary health care information system in Ghana: lessons learned. Methods of Information in Medicine 36:63–68.

Hilsum L. 1995. Save us from our saviours. The Observer (London). December 31.

Ho LS. 1995. Market reforms and China's health care system. Social Science and Medicine 41:1065–1072.

Hobbes T. 1651. Leviathan, or The Matter, Forme and Power of a Commonwealth, Ecclesiasticall and Civil. Baltimore. Penguin Books Reprint, 1968. 728 p.

Hoeppli R. 1959. Parasites and Parasitic Diseases in Early Medicine and Science. Singapore. University of Malaya Press. 526 p.

Hogerzeil HV, Couper MR and Gray R. 1997. Guidelines for drug donations. BMJ—British Medical Journal 314:737–740.

Holden C. 1995. "Ice man" markings seen as medical tattoos. Science 268:33.

Holden C. 1996. Ebola: ancient history of "new" disease. Science 271:1591.

Hookham H. 1972. A Short History of China. New York. New American Library (Mentor Books). 381 p.

Hopkins DR. 1983. Princes and Peasants: Smallpox in History. Chicago. University of Chicago Press. 380 p.

Horiuchi S. 1992. Stagnation in the decline of the world population growth rate during the 1980s. Science 257:761–765.

Horn J. 1969. Away With All Pests. An English Surgeon in People's China. London. Hamlyn. 192 p.

Horwitt E. 1977. Global warming to the 'net (Special Supplement: The Network 25). Computerworld 31(39):SA16–SA19.

Houtchens BA, Allen A, Clemmer TP, Lindberg DA and Pedersen S. 1995. Telemedicine protocols and standards: development and implementation. Journal of Medical Systems 19:93–119.

Howard-Jones N. 1975. The Scientific Background of the International Sanitary Conferences, 1851–1938. Geneva. World Health Organization. 110 p.

Hsiao WCL. 1995. The Chinese health care system: lessons for other nations. Social Science and Medicine 41:1047–1055.

Huber JH. 1993. Ensuring access to health care with the introduction of user fees: a Kenyan example. Social Science and Medicine 36:485–494.

Hughes CC and Hunter JM. 1970. Disease and "development" in Africa. Social Science and Medicine 3:443–493.

Hull C. 1994. Observations on health information systems in developing countries. Methods of Information in Medicine 33:304–305.

Hull HF, Ward NA, Hull BP, Milstein JB and de Quadros C. 1994. Paralytic poliomyelitis: seasoned strategies, disappearing disease. Lancet 343:1331–1336.

Hung R. 1996. The great U-turn in Taiwan: economic restructuring and a surge in inequality. Journal of Contemporary Asia 26:151–163.

Hyder AA, Rotllant G and Morrow RH. 1998. Measuring the burden of disease: healthy life-years. American Journal of Public Health 88:196–202.

Ibrahim MM, Omar HM, Persson LÅ and Wall S. 1996. Child mortality in a collapsing African society. Bulletin of the World Health Organization 74:547–552.

Imperato PJ. 1974. Nomads of the west African Sahel and the delivery of health services to them. Social Science and Medicine 8:443–457.

Imperato PJ. 1975. A wind in Africa. St. Louis. WH Green. 363 p.

Jackson JL. 1997. The German health system. Lessons for reform in the United States. Archives of Internal Medicine 157:155–160.

Jaffar S, Leach A, Greenwood AM, Jepson A, Muller O, Ota MOC, Bojang K, Obaro S and Greenwood BM. 1997. Changes in the pattern of infant and childhood mortality in Upper River Division, The Gambia, from 1989 to 1993. Tropical Medicine and International Health 2:28–37.

Janovsky K, Editor. 1996. Health Policy and systems Development. An Agenda for Research. Geneva. World Health Organization. Publication WHO/SHS/NHP/96.1. 245 p.

Jaravaza JE, McCoy MC, Dando BS and Kangano FD. 1982. Unified national health information system. Parts 1, 2, 3, 4. Central African Journal of Medicine 28:25–28; 57–64; 136–145; 167–171.

Johannesson M. 1994. QUALYs, HYEs and individual prefrences—a graphical illustration. Social Science and Medicine 39:1623–1632.

Johnstone P. 1995. Work in a developing country. BMJ—British Medical Journal 311:113–115.

Jolly J. 1951. Indian Medicine. Translated from German by Kashikar CG. Poona. CG. Kashikar. 238 p.

Jolly R. 1991. Adjustment with a human face: a UNICEF record and perspective on the 1980s. World Development 19:1807–1821.

Jones J. 1996. In sickness and health: restoring the NHS was one of Labour's pre-election promises, but how easy or desirable is it? New Statesman 126(4338):20–22.

Jordan P. 1985. Schistosomiasis. The St. Lucia Project. Cambridge. Cambridge University Press. 442 p.

Kacapyr E. 1996. Are you middle class? American Demographics 18:30–35.

Kahen B and Sayers BM. 1997. Health-care technology transfer: expert and information systems for developing countries. Methods of Information in Medicine 36:69–78.

Kahn H, Brown W and Martel L. 1976. The Next 200 Years. A Scenario for America and the World. New York. Morrow. 241 p.

Kamanga K. 1996. Can health system reform in Africa be driven by improving the efficiency of public hospitals? The case of Zambia. World Hospitals and Health Services 32:19–24.

Kamke K. 1998. The German health care system and health care reform. Health Policy 43:171–194.

Keirse MJ. 1984. Perinatal mortality rates do not contain what they purport to contain. Lancet 1:1166–1169.

Kent G. 1991. The Politics of Children's Survival. New York. Prager. 204 p.

Kessler II and Aurelian L. 1975. Uterine cervix. Pp. 263–317 In Schottenfeld D, Editor. Cancer Epidemiology and Prevention. Springfield, IL. CC Thomas.

Keys A. 1979. Coronary heart disease in seven countries. Circulation 41(Suppl 1):1–211.

Khan MM, Zhu N, Ling JC. 1996. Community-based health insurance in China: bending to the wind of change. World Health Forum 17:58–62.

King M. 1990. Health is a sustainable state. Lancet 336:664–667.

King M. 1993. Demographic entrapment. Transactions of the Royal Society of Tropical Medicine and Hygiene 87 (Suppl.):23–28.

King M and Elliott C. 1993. Legitimate double think. Lancet 341:669–672.

King M and Elliott C. 1995. Double think—a reply. World Health Forum 16:293–298.

Kinsella K and Taeuber MC. 1993. An Aging World II. U.S. Bureau of the Census International Population Reports P95/92–3. 160 p.

Knox RA. 1993. Germany: One Nation With Health Care for All. New York. Faulkner and Gray. 329 p.

Koch-Weser D. 1984. International health: academic specialty or humanitarian service? American Journal of Public Health 74:430–431.

Kranczer S. 1994. International cancer mortality comparisons. Statistical Bulletin, Met Life 75(1):2–11.

Kulczycki A, Motts M and Rosenfield A. 1996. Abortion and fertility regulation. Lancet 347:1663–1668.

Kunst AE, Groenhof F, Mackenbach JP and the EU Working Group on Socioeconomic Inequalities in Health. 1998. Mortality by occupational class among men 30–64 years in 11 European countries. Social Science and Medicine 46:1459–1476.

Kutzin J. 1995. Experience With Organizational and Financing Reform of the Health Sector. Geneva. World Health Organization. Publication WHO/SHS/CC/94.3. 59 p.

Ladipo OA. 1989. Preventing and managing complications of induced abortion in Third World countries. International Journal of Obstetrics and Gynecology 1989 (Suppl. 3):21–28.

Lancet. 1978. Water with sugar and salt (Editorial). Lancet II:30–301.

Lancet. 1992. Pressure on the eco-seams. Lancet 339:1265–1267.

Lancet. 1996. The World Bank, listening and learning (Editorial). Lancet 347:411.

Landis SH, Murray T, Bolden S and Wingo PA. Cancer statistics. 1998. CA—A Cancer Journal for Clinicians 48:6–30.

Lane JM and Millar JD. 1969. Routine childhhood vaccination against smallpox reconsidered. New England Journal of Medicine 281:1220–1224.

Lane JM, Ruben FL, Neff JM and Millar JD. 1970. Complications of smallpox vaccination, 1968: results of ten statewide surveys. Journal of Infectious Diseases 122:303–309.

Lane SD and Rubinstein RA. 1996. Judging the other. Responding to traditional female genital surgeries. Hastings Center Report 26(3):31–40.

LaVertu DS and Linares AM. 1990. Ethical principles of biomedical research on human subjects: their application and limitations in Latin America and the Caribbean. Bulletin of the Pan American Health Organization 24:469–479.

Leaning J. 1996. Human security and ethical lissues in disasters and complex humanitarian emergencies. Pp. 63–78. In Kita E, Editor. Final Report of the Research Project on a Study on the Health and Prospective Medical Assistance for Affected Persons. Tokyo. Ministry of Health and Welfare.

LeDuc JW. 1996.World Health Organization strategy for emerging infectious diseases. JAMA 275:318–320.

Lee PN. 1994. Comparison of autopsy, clinical and death certificate diagnosis with particular reference to lung cancer. A review of the published data. APMIS 102 (Suppl. 45): 42 p.

Lee JW, Melgaard B, Hull HF, Barakamfitiye D and Okwo-Bele JM. 1998. Ethical dilemmas in polio eradication. American Journal of Public Health 88:130–131.

Leff S and Leff V. 1957. From Witchcraft to World Health. New York. Macmillan. 236 p.

Leflar RB. 1998. The cautious acceptance of informed consent in Japan. Medicine and Law 16:705–720.

Leonard L. 1996. Female circumcision in southern Chad: origins, meaning, and current practice. Social Science and Medicine 43:255–263.

Lesthaeghe R and Jolly C. 1994. The start of the sub-Saharan fertility transitions: some answers and many questions. Annals of the New York Academy of Sciences 709:349–395.

Levine RE and Gaw AC. 1995. Culture-bound syndromes. Psychiatric Clinics of North America 18(3):523–536.

Levitt R and Wall A. 1984. The Reorganised National Health Service. Berkenham, UK. Croom Helm. 295 p.

Lewis O. 1968. A Study of Slum Culture. New York. Random House. 240 p.

Li C. 1974. A brief outline of Chinese medical history with particular reference to acupuncture. Perspectives in Biology and Medicine 18:132–143.

Lie KJ, Rukmono B, Oemijati S, Sahab K, Newell KW, Sie TH and Talogo RW. 1966. Diarrhoea among infants in a crowded area of Djakarta, Indonesia. Bulletin of the World Health Organization 34:197–210.

Lima Guimarães JJ and Fischmann A. 1985. Inequalities in 1980 infant mortality among shantytown residents and nonshantytown residents in the municipality of Pôrto Alegre, Rio Grande do Sul, Brazil. PAHO Bulletin 19:235–251.

Liu G, Liu X and Meng Q. 1994. Privatization of the medical market in socialist China: a historical approach. Health Policy 27:157–174.

Liu X and Hsiao WCL. 1995. The cost escalation of social health insurance plans in China: its implication for public policy. Social Science and Medicine 41:1095–1101.

Liu Y, Hsiao WCL, Li Q, Liu X and Ren M. 1995. Transformation of China's rural health care financing. Social Science and Medicine 41:1085–1093.

Loewenson R. 1993. Structural adjustment and health policy in Africa. International Journal of Health Services 23:717–730.

Loos GP. 1996. Field Guide for International Health Project Planners and Managers. London. Janus. 81 p.

Lumbignanon P, Panamonta M, Laopaibiin M, Pothinam S and Patithat N. 1990. Why are

Thai official perinatal and infant mortality rates so low? International Journal of Epidemiology 19:997–1000.

Lurie P and Wolfe SM. 1997. Unethical trials of intervention to reduce perinatal transmission of the human immunodeficiency virus in developing countries. New England Journal of Medicine 337:853–856.

Lwanga SK and Sapirie SA. 1995. Rapid Assessment of National Health Information Systems (HIS) Including Epidemiological Surveillance (ES) Strengthening Country Health Information Unit (SCI), Division of Epidemiological Surveillance and Health Situation and Trend Assessment (HST) World Health Organization Geneva. Available at www.who.int/programmes/hst/sci/a/objmaina.htm.

MacIntyre S. 1997. The Black Report and beyond—what are the issues? Social Science and Medicine 44:723–745.

Mahler H. 1976. Social Perspectives in Health. Address to the 29th World Health Assembly. May 4, 1976.

Mahler H. 1978. Bringing down the medical empire. Pan American Health 10:10–15.

Mahler H.1997. The challenge of global health: how can we do better? Health and Human Rights 2:71–75.

Malé S. 1996. Refugees: do not forget the basics. World Health Statistics Quarterly 49:221–225.

Mamdani M. 1974. The myth of population control. Development Digest 12:13–28.

Mandil SH. 1995. Telematics in health care in developing countries. Journal of Medical systems 19:195–203.

Maren M. 1997.The Road to Hell: The Ravaging Effects of Foreign Aid and International Charity. New York. Free Press. 287 p.

Markos A. 1983. The effect of culture, local traditions, and religious beliefs on the health behaviour in different African countries and tribes. Pp. 27–33. In Oberender P, Diesfeld JH and Gitter W, Editors. Health and Development in Africa. Frankfurt. Verlag Peter Lang. 432 p.

Marks G and Beatty WK. 1976. Epidemics. New York. Scribner. 323 p.

Marmot M and Feeney A. 1997a. General explanations for social inequalities in health. Pp. 207–228. In Kogevinas M, Pearce N, Susser M and Boffetta P, Editors. Social Inequalities and Cancer. IARC Scientific Publications 138.

Marmot M and Feeney A. 1997b. General explanations for social inequalities in health. IARC Scientific Publication 138:207–228.

Martorell R. 1996. The role of nutrition in economic development. Nutrition Reviews 54(4):S66–S71.

Massaro TA, Nemec J and Kalman I. 1994. Health system reform in the Czech Republic. JAMA 271:1870–1874.

Matthias AR and Green AT. 1994. The comparative advantage of NGOs in the health sector—a look at the evidence. World Hospitals 30:10–15.

Maxwell RJ. 1995. A puzzle for our times: using healthcare resources wisely and justly. World Hospitals 30:30–35.

Maynard A and Bloor K. 1995. Primary care and health care reform: the need to reflect before reforming. Health Policy 31:171–181.

Maynard-Tucker G. 1994. Indigenous perceptions and quality of care of family planning services in Haiti. Health Policy and Planning 9:306–317.

Mburu FM. 1989. Non-government organizations in the health field: collaboration, integration and contrasting aims in Africa. Social Science and Medicine 29:591–597.

Mburu FM. 1994. Whither community health workers in the age of structural adjustment? Social Science and Medicine 39:883–885.

McCaw-Binns AM, Fox K, Foster-Williams KE, Ashley DE and Irons B. 1996. Registration of births, stillbirths and infant deaths in Jamaica. International Journal of Epidemiology 25:807–813.

McKay D. 1981. Editorial. Journal of Tropical Medicine and Hygiene 84:93–94.

McKelvey JJ Jr. 1973. Man Against Tsetse. Ithaca. Cornell University Press. 306 p.

McKeown T.1988. The Origins of Human Disease. Oxford. Basil Blackwell. 233 p.

McKeown T and Lowe CR, Editors. 1974. An Introduction to Social Medicine. Second Edition. Oxford. Blackwell Scientific. 356 p.

McPake B. 1993. User charges for health services in developing countries: a review of the economic literature. Social Science and Medicine 36:1397–1405.

Meadows DH, Editor. 1974. The Limits to Growth: a Report for the Club of Rome's Project on the Predicament of Mankind. Second Edition. New York. Universe Books.

Mechanic D. 1972. Public Expectations and Health Care. New York. John Wiley. 314 p.

Medici AC, Londoño JL, Coelho O and Saxenian H. 1997. Managed care and managed competition in Latin America and the Caribbean. Pp. 215–231. In Schieber GJ, Editor. Innovations in Health Care Financing. World Bank Discussion Paper 365.

Merbs CF. 1992. A New World of infectious diseases. Yearbook of Physical Anthropology 35:3–42.

Merrick TW. 1993. Social Policy and Fertility Transitions. World Bank HCO Working Papers HROWP3. 9 p.

Michaud C and Murray JL. 1994. External assistance to the health sector in developing countries: a detailed analysis, 1972–90. Bulletin of the World Health Organization 72:639–651.

Mill JS. 1859. On Liberty. (Reprint 1956). Indianapolis. Bobbs-Merrill. 141 p.

Millard AV. 1994. A causal model of high rates of child mortality. Social Science and Medicine 38:253–268.

Miller CA. 1985. Infant mortality in the U.S. Scientific American 253:31–37.

Mills A. 1997. Leopard or chameleon? The changing character of international health economics. Tropical Medicine and International Health 2:963–977.

Mock N, Setzer J, Sliney I, Hadziatou G and Bertrand W. 1993. Development of information-based planning in Niger. International Journal of Technology Assessment in Health Care 9:360–368.

Modelmog D, Rahlenbeck S and Trichopoulos D. 1994. Accuracy of death certificates: a population-based complete-coverage one-year autopsy study in East Germany. Cancer Causes and Control 3:541–546.

Moodley D, Payne AJ and Moodley J. 1996. Maternal mortality in Kwazulu/Natal: need for an information database system and confidential enquiry into maternal deaths in developing countries. Tropical Doctor 26:50–54.

Moorehead A. 1966. The Fatal Impact. An Account of the Invasion of the South Pacific 1767–1840. New York. Harper and Row. 230 p.

Mootz M. 1986. Health indicators. Social Science and Medicine 22:255–263.

Morley D. 1976. Paediatric priorities in evolving community programmes for developing countries. Lancet II:1012–1014.

Morse SS. 1995. Factors in the emergence of infectious diseases. Emerging Infectious Diseases 1:7–15.

Mosley WH. 1994. Population change, health planning and human resource development in the health sector. World Health Statistics Quarterly 47:26–30.

Mossialos E, Kanavos P and Abel-Smith B. 1997. Will managed care work in Europe? Pharmacoeconomics 11:297–305.

Moulin AM. 1995. The Pasteur Institute between the two world wars. The transformation of the international sanitary order. Pp. 244–265. In Weindling P, Editor. International Health Organisations and Movements, 1918–1939. Cambridge. Cambridge University Press.

Muhuri PK, Anker M and Bryce J. 1996. Treatment patterns for childhood diarrhoea: evidence from demographic and health surveys. Bulletin of the World Health Organization 74:135–146.

Mull DS. 1992. Mother's milk and pseudoscientific breastmilk testing in Pakistan. Social Science and Medicine 34:1277–1290.

Murdock GP. 1980. Theories of Illness. A World Survey. Pittsburgh. University of Pittsburgh Press. 127 p.

Murray CJL. 1994. Quantifying the burden of disease: the technical basis for disability-adjusted life years. Bulletin of the World Health Organization 72:429–445.

Murray CJL. 1995. Towards an analytical approach to health sector reform. Health Policy 32:93–109.

Murray CJL and Acharya AK. 1997. Understanding DALYs. Journal of Health Economics 16:703–730.

Murray CJL and Chen LC. 1993. In search of a contemporary theory for understanding mortality change. Social Science and Medicine 36:143–155.

Murray CJL, Govindaraj R and Musgrove P. 1994. National health expenditures: a global analysis. Bulletin of the World Health Organization 74:23–637.

Murray CJL and Lopez AD. 1994. Global and regional cause-of-death patterns in 1990. Bulletin of the World Health Organization 72:447–480.

Murray CJL and Lopez AD. 1996. Evidence-based health policy—lessons from the Global Burden of Disease study. Science 274:740–743.

Murray CJL and Lopez AD. 1997a. Mortality by cause for eight regions of the world: Global Burden of Disease Study. Lancet 349:1269–1276.

Murray CJL and Lopez AD. 1997b. Regional patterns of disability-free life expectancy and disability-adjusted life expectancy: Global Burden of Disease Study. Lancet 349:1347–1352.

Murray CJL and Lopez AD. 1997c. Global mortality, disability, and the contribution of risk factors: Global Burden of Disease Study. Lancet 349:1436–1442.

Murray CJL and Lopez AD. 1997d. Alternative projections of mortality and disability by cause 1990–2020: Global Burden of Disease Study. Lancet 349:1498–1504.

Muschell J. 1995. Privatization in Health. WHO Technical Briefing Note. Task Force on Health Economics. Geneva. World Health Organization. Publication WHO/TFHE/TBN/95.1.

Musgrove P. 1995a. Mismatch of Need, Demand and Supply of Services: Picturing Different Ways Health Systems Can Go Wrong. World Bank. HCO Working Papers HCOWP 59. 6 p.

Musgrove P. 1995b. Cost-Effectiveness and Health Sector Reform. World Bank. HRO Working Papers, HROWP 48. 19 p.

Musgrove P. 1996. Public and Private Roles in Health. World Bank. Discussion Paper 339. 79 p.

Myers CN, Mongkolsmai D and Causino N. 1985. Financing Health Services and Medical Care in Thailand. Cambrdige, MA. Harvard Institute for International Development. Development Discussion Paper 209. 144 p.

Nabarro DN and Tayler EM. 1998. The "Roll Back Malaria" campaign. Science 280:2067–2068.

National Center for Health Statistics. 1981. Data Systems of the NCHS. Vital and Health Statistics Series 1 #16. 37 p.

Nations MK and Monte CMG. 1996. "I'm not dog, no!": cries of resistance against cholera control campaigns. Social Science and Medicine 43:1007–1024.

Ndong I, Gloyd S and Gale J. 1994. An evaluation of vital registers as sources of data for infant mortality rates in Cameroon. International Journal of Epidemiology 23:536–539.

Needham J. 1980. China and the Origins of Immunology. Hong Kong. University of Hong Kong. Centre of Asian Studies Occasional Papers and Monographs No. 41. 33 p.

Newhouse JP. 1984. The application of economics to problems of public health and the delivery of medical services. Pp. 219–232. In Holland WW, Detels R and Knox G, Editors. Oxford Textbook of Public Health. Volume 1. Oxford. Oxford University Press.

Nielsen GP, Björnsson J and Jonasson JG. 1991. The accuracy of death certificates. Virchows Archiv A Pathology and Anatomy 419:143–146.

Northrop FSC. 1959. Cultural mentalities and medical science. In Galdston I, Editor. Medicine and Anthropology. New York. New York International Universities Press.

Notestein FW. 1945. Population—the long view. Pp. 36–57 In Schultz TW, Editor. Food for the World. Chicago. University of Chicago Press.

Odero W, Garner P and Zwi A. 1997. Road traffic injuries in developing countries: a comprehensive review of epidemiological studies. Tropical Medicine and International Health 2:445–460.

OECD. 1996. Development Cooperation: 1996 Report. Paris. Organization for Economic Cooperation and Development.

OECD. 1997. Geographical Distribution of Financial Flows to Aid Recipients. Disbursements, Commitments, Country Indicators 1991–1995. Paris. Organization for Economic Cooperation and Development. 256 p.

Omran AR. 1971. The epidemiologic transition. A theory of the epidemiology of population change. Milbank Memorial Fund Quarterly 49:509–538.

Omran AR. 1982. Epidemiologic transition 1. Theory. Pp. 172–175 In Ross JA., Editor. International Encyclopedia of Population. New York. The Free Press.

Oppenheimer SJ, Gibson FD, Macfarlane SB. 1986. Iron supplementation increases prevalence and effects of malaria: report on clinical studies in Papua New Guinea. Transactions of The Royal Society of Tropical Medicine and Hygiene 80:603–612.

Orenstein WA, Bernier RH and Hinman AR. 1984. Assessing vaccine efficacy in the field. Further observations. Epidemiological Reviews 10:212–241.

Paddock W. 1967. FAMINE, 1975! Boston. Little, Brown.

Pan American Health Organization. 1988, Health profiles Brazil, 1984. Epidemiological Bulletin of the Pan American Health Organization 9(2):6–12.

Pan American Health Organization. 1993. Maternal mortality in the Americas. Epidemiological Bulletin of the Pan American Health Organization 14(1):1–9.

Pan American Health Organization. 1994. Demographic transition in the Americas. Epidemiological Bulletin of the Pan American Health Organization 15(1):1–12.

Pannenborg CO. 1991. Shifting paradigms of international health. Asia-Pacific Journal of Public Health 5:176–184.

Patel T. 1994. Eastern Europe heads for smoking catastrophe. New Scientist 22:12.

Paul BD. 1955. Health Culture and Community: Case Studies of Public Reactions to Health Programs. New York. Russell Sage Foundation. 493 p.

Peabody JW. 1996. Economic reform and health sector policy: lessons from structural adjustment programs. Social Science and Medicine 43:823–835.

Peabody JW, Lee S-W and Bickel SR. 1995. Health for all in the Republic of Korea: one country's experience with implementing universal health care. Health Policy 31:29–42.

Perrot J, Carrin G and Sergent F. 1977. The Contractual Approach: New Partnerships for Health in Developing Countries. Geneva. World Health Organization. WHO/ICO/MESD/24.

Pettenkofer M von. 1873. The Value of Health to a City. Translated from German by Sigerist HE. 1941. Baltimore. Johns Hopkins Press. 52 p.

Phillips M, Feachem RGA, Murray CJL, Over M and Kjellstrom T. 1993. Adult health: a legitimate concern for developing countries. American Journal of Public Health 83:1527–1530.

Phoon WO. 1975. The impact of industrial growth on health in South-East Asia. In Ciba Foundation symposium 32 (new series). Health and Industrial Growth. Amsterdam. Associated Scientific. pp. 107–126.

Pollitzer R. 1959. Cholera. World Health Organization Monograph Series No. 43. 1019 p.

Pollock AM. 1995. Rationing health care: from needs to markets? The politics of destruction: rationing in the UK health care market. Health Care Analysis 3:299–308.

Potts M. 1997. Sex and the birth rate: human biology, demographic change, and access to fertility-regulation methods. Population and Development Review 23:1–39.

Preker AS. 1994. Meeting the challenge: policymaking and management during economic transition. Journal of Health Administration Education 12:433–447.

Preker AS and Feachem RGA. 1995. Market Mechanisms and the Health Sector in Central and Eastern Europe. World Bank Technical Paper 293. 48 p.

Prescott N and de Ferranti D. 1985. The analysis and assessment of health programs. Social Science and Medicine 20:1235–1240.

PRICOR. 1987. Determinants of Health Care Utilization in Rural Bangladesh. Study Summary. Chevy Chase MD. PRICOR. 12 p.

Prins A. 1984. Community participation in health action through structural problem solving: lessons learned in the socio-health program of the Togo rural water project. Public Health Reviews 12:322–339.

Quigley MA, Armstrong Schellenberg JRM and Snow RW. 1996. Algorithms for verbal autopsies: a validation study in Kenyan children. Bulletin of the World Health Organization 74:147–154.

Rahmathullah L, Underwood BA, Thulasiraj RD, Milton RC, Ramaswamy K, Rahmathullah R and Babu G. 1990. Reduced mortality among children in southern India receiving a small weekly dose of vitamin A. New England Journal of Medicine 323:929–935.

Reerink IH and Sauerborn R. 1996. Quality of primary health care in developing countries: recent experiences and future directions. International Journal for Quality in Health Care 8:131–139.

Reinhardt UE. 1997. Making economic evaluations respectable. Social Science and Medicine 45:555–562.

Rice DP. 1992. Data needs for health policy in an aging population. World Health Statistics Quarterly 45:61–67.

Riddell RC. 1986. The ethics of foreign aid. Development Policy Review 4:24–43.

Rifkin SB and Walt G. 1986. Why health improves. Defining the issues concerning "comprehensive primary health care" and "selective" primary health care. Social Science and Medicine 23:559–566.

Rischard J-F. 1996. Connecting developing countries to the information technology revolution. SAIS Review 16:93–107.

Robbins A. 1995. A Prague winter for public health. Public Health Reports 110:295–297.

Robey B, Rutstein SO and Morris L. 1993. The fertility decline in developing countries. Scientific American 269(6):60–70.

Roemer MI. 1991. National Health Systems of the World. Volume 1. The Countries. New York. Oxford University Press. 993 p.

Roemer MI. 1993. National Health Systems of the World. Volume 2. The Issues. New York. Oxford University Press. 356 p.

Rosen G. 1958. A History of Public Health. New York. M.D. Publications. 551 p.

Rosenberg CE. 1962. The Cholera Years: The United States in 1832, 1849, and 1866. Chicago. University of Chicago Press. 257 p. Simon and Hughes. 1985.

Rosenthal E. 1998. West's medicine is raising bills for China's sick. New York Times. November 19.

Roy MJ. 1993. The German health care system: model or mirage? Southern Medical Journal 86:1384–1394.

Royston E and Lopez AD. 1987. On the assessment of maternal mortality. World Health Statistics Quarterly 40:214–224.

Sadik N. 1992. Public policy and private decisions: world population and world health in the 21st century (Editorial). Journal of Public Health Policy 13:133–139.

Salamon R, Leroy V, Maurice-Tison S and Le Blanc B. 1997. Health informatics: handle with caution. Methods of Information in Medicine 36:79–81.

Saltman RB and Figueras J. 1997. European Health Care Reform. Analysis of Current Strategies. Copenhagen. WHO Regional Office for Europe. WHO Regional Publications, European Series 72. 308 p.

Sandosham AA. 1959. Malariology. Singapore. University of Malaya Press. 327 p.

Savitt TL. 1977. Filariasis in the United States. Journal of the History of Medicine 32:140–150.

Savitt TL. 1978. Medicine and Slavery. Chicago. University of Illinois Press. 332 p.

Schieber G and Maeda A. 1997. A curmudgeon's guide to financing health care in developing countries. Pp. 1–40. In Schieber GJ, Editor. Innovations in Health Care Financing. World Bank Discussion Paper 365.

Schofield C. and Ashworth A. 1996. Why have mortality rates for severe malnutrition remained so high? Bulletin of the World Health Organization 74:223–229.

Schumacher EF. 1973. Small Is Beautiful. New York. Harper & Row (Perennial Library Edition). 305 p.

Scott HH. 1939. A History of Tropical Medicine. Baltimore. Williams and Wilkins. 1165 p.

Scrimshaw NJ. 1974. Myths and realities in international health planning. American Journal of Public Health 64:792–798

Selzer R. 1975. Twelve spheres of influence, eight bodily forces, and good old yin and yang. Harper's Magazine. January 1975: pp. 40–44.

Senewiratne B and Uragoda CG. 1973. Betel chewing in Ceylon. American Journal of Tropical Medicine and Hygiene 22:418–422.

Shaplen R. 1964. Toward the Well-Being of Mankind. Garden City, NY. Doubleday. 214 p.

Shi L. 1993. Health care in China: a rural-urban comparison after the socioeconomic reforms. Bulletin of the World Health Organization 71:723–736.

Shmueli A. 1995. Cost-effective outlays for better health outcomes. World Health Forum 16:287–291.

Shurkin JN. 1979. The Invisible Fire. The Story of Mankind's Victory Over the Ancient Scourge of Smallpox, New York, GP Putnam's Sons. 447 p.

Siegfried A. 1965. Germs and Ideas: Routes of Epidemics and Ideologies. English Edition. Edinburgh. Oliver and Boyd. 98 p.

Sigerist HE. 1951. A History of Medicine. Volume 1. Primitive and Archaic Medicine. New York. Oxford University Press. 564 p.

Simons RC and Hughes CC, Editors. 1985. The Culture-Bound Syndromes: Folk Illnesses and Anthropological Interest. Dordrecht, Netherlands. D. Reidel. 516 p.

Singapore Ministry of Health. 1997. Affordable Health Care. A White Paper. Singapore. SNP for the Ministry of Health. 60 p.

Sköld M. 1998. Poverty and Health: Who Lives, Who Dies, Who Cares? Geneva. World Health Organization. Publication WHO/ICO/MESD.28.

Social Security Administration. 1998. Social Security Programs Throughout the World. On the Internet at http://www.ssa.gov/statistics/ssptw97.html.

Söderlund N and Zwi AB. 1995. Traffic-related mortality in industrialized and less developed countries. Bulletin of the World Health Organization 73:175–182.

Specter M. 1998. Breast-feeding and HIV: weighing the risks. New York Times. August 19.

Spengler O. 1926–1928. The Decline of the West. New York. Knopf. 2 volumes.

Stanton B and Clemens J. 1989. User fees for health care in developing countries: a case study in Bangladesh. Social Science and Medicine 29:119–1205.

Stark R. 1985. Lay workers in primary health care: victims in the process of social transition. Social Science and Medicine 20:269–275.

Steadman DW. 1995. Prehistoric extinctions of Pacific island birds: biodiversity meets archaeology. Science 267:1123–1131.

Stefanini A. 1995. Sustainability: the role of NGOs. World Health Forum 16:42–46.

Stewart WH. 1967. A Mandate for State Action. Association of State and Territorial Health Officers. Washington, DC.

Stirling C. 1976. Atlantic report—Nepal. Atlantic Monthly October:14–25.

Stolnitz GJ. 1982. Mortality Trends 2. Post-World War II Trends. Pp. 461–469. In Ross JA, Editor. International Encyclopedia of Population. New York. The Free Press.

Sutter RW and Cochi SL. 1997. Comment: ethical dilemmas in worldwide polio eradication programs. American Journal of Public Health 87:913–915.

Tanner JM. 1968. Earlier maturation in man. Scientific American 218:21–27.

Tarimo E and Webster EG. 1994. Primary Health Care Concepts and Challenges in a Changing World. Alma Ata Revisited. Geneva. World Health Organization. Publication WHO/SHS/CC/94.2. 118p.

Task Force on International Development. 1970. U.S. foreign assistance in the 1970's: a new approach. Pp. 460–502. In U.S. Congress Joint Economic Committee. Subcommittee on Foreign Economic Policy. A Foreign Economic Policy for the 1970's. Part 3—U.S. Policies Toward Developing Countries. Hearings of May 13, 14, 18 and 19, 1970.

Taylor AL. 1992. Making the World Health Organization work: a legal framework for universal access to the conditions for health. American Journal of Law and Medicine 18:301–346.

Taylor CE. 1966. Ethics for an international health profession. Science 153:716–720.

Taylor CE. 1994. International experience and idealism in medical education. Academic Medicine 69:631–634.

Taylor CE, Cutts F and Taylor ME. 1997. Ethical dilemmas in current planning for polio eradication. American Journal of Public Health 87:922–925.

Tejeiro Fernandez AF. 1975. The national health system in Cuba. Pp. 13–29. In Newell KW, Editor. Health by the People. Geneva. World Health Organization.

Teutsch SM and Thacker SB. 1995. Planning a public health surveillance system. Epidemiological Bulletin of the Pan American Health Organization 16(1):1–6.

Tinker A. 1992. Women, Health, and Development. Presented at a conference on Women's Health and Nutrition, Rockefeller Conference Center, Bellagio, Italy, May, 1992.

Tolmie CJ and du Plessis JP. 1997. The use of knowledge-based systems in medicine in developing countries: a luxury or a necessity? Methods of Information in Medicine 36:154–159.

Toole MJ. 1995. Mass population displacement. A global public health challenge. Infectious Disease Clinics of North America 9(2):353–365.

Toole MJ. 1996. Humanitarian relief as a global health issue. Pp. 3–10. In Kita E, Editor. Final Report of the Research Project on a Study on the Health and Prospective Medical Assistance for Affected Persons. Tokyo. Ministry of Health and Welfare.

Toubia N. 1994. Female circumcision as a public health issue. New England Journal of Medicine 331:712–716.

Trigg PI and Kondrachine AV. 1998. Commentary: malaria control in the 1990s. Bulletin of the World Health Organization 76:11–14.

Trostle J and Simon J. 1992. Building applied health research capacity in less-developed countries: problems encountered by the ADDR Project. Social Science and Medicine 35:1379–1387.

Tulchinsky TH and Varavikova EA.1996. Addressing the epidemiologic transition in the former Soviet Union: strategies for health system and public health reform in Russia. American Journal of Public Health 86:313–320.

Tupasi TE, Lucero MG, Magdangal DM, Mangubat NV, Sunico ME, Torres CU, de Leon LE, Paladin JF, Baes L, and Javato MC. 1990a. Etiology of acute lower respiratory tract infection in children from Alabang, Metro Manila. Reviews of Infectious Diseases 12 (Suppl. 8):S929–S939.

Tupasi TE, de Leon LE, Lupisan S, Torres CU, Leonor ZA, Sunico ES, Mangubat NV, Miguel CA, Medalla F, Tan ST, and Dayrit M. 1990b. Patterns of acute respiratory tract infection in children: a longitudinal study in a depressed community in Metro Manila. Reviews of Infectious Diseases 12 (Suppl. 8):S940–S949.

Türmen T. 1995. Is child survival enough? Journal of Tropical Pediatrics 41:321–324.

Umeh JC. 1996. Healthcare financing in the Kingdom of Saudi Arabia: a review of the options. World Hospitals 31:3–8.

UNDP 1996. Human Development Report 1996. Published for the United Nations Development Programme. New York. Oxford University Press,

UNICEF. 1996. Women: maternal mortality. The Progress of Nations 1996:2–9.

United Nations. 1955. Methods of Appraisal of Quality of Basic Data for Population Estimates. Population Studies. No. 23. Document ST/SOA/Ser.A/23. 67 p.

United Nations. 1973. The Determinants and Consequences of Population Trends, Volume 1. UN Department of Economic and Social Affairs. Population Studies, No. 50. Document ST/STOA/Ser. A/50. 115 p.

United Nations. 1985. World Population Trends. Population and Development Interrelations and Population Policies. 1983 Monitoring Report. Volume 1. Population Trends. New York. United Nations ST/SER/SER.A/93.

United Nations. 1996. World Population Monitoring 1993. New York. United Nations ST/ESA/SER.A/126/1993.

USAID. 1986. Health Policy Statement. Washington, DC. United States Agency for International Development.

van der Geest S. 1982. The secondary importance of public health care in South Cameroon. Culture Medicine and Psychiatry 6:365–383.

Varmus H and Satcher D. 1997. Ethical complexities of conducting research in developing countries. New England Journal of medicine 337:1003–1005.

Vera H. 1993. The client's view of high-quality care in Santiago, Chile. Studies in Family Planning 24:40–49.

Victoria CG, Vaughan JP and Barrios FC. 1985. The seasonality of infant deaths due to diarrheal and respiratory diseases in southern Brazil, 1974–1978. Bulletin of the Pan American Health Organization 19:29–39.

Vienonen MA and Wlodarczyk C. 1993. Health care reforms on the European scene: evolution, revolution or seesaw? World Health Statistics Quarterly 46:166–169.

Vijayaraghavan K, Radhaiah G, Surya Prakasam B, Rameshwar Sarma KV and Reddy V. 1990. Effect of massive dose of vitamin A on morbidity and mortality in Indian children. Lancet 336:1342–1345.

Wain A. 1970. A History of Preventive Medicine. Springfield, IL. Thomas. 407p.

Walsh JA and Warren KS. 1979. Selective public health care. An interim strategy for disease control in developing countries. New England Journal of Medicine 301:967–974.

Walt G. 1994. Health Policy. An Introduction to Process and Power. London. Zed Books. 226 p.

Walus YE, Ittmann HW and Hanmer L. 1997. Decision support systems in health care. Methods of Information in Medicine 36:82–91.

Wang D, Zhang Z and Zheng S. 1993. Computers Against disease. World Health Forum 14:298–300.

Wang'ombe JK. 1995. The "permanent project syndrome": a counter productive consequence of philanthropy. Social Science and Medicine 41:603–604.

Wang'ombe JK. 1997. Cost-recovery strategies in sub-Saharan Africa. Pp.155–160. In Schieber GJ, Editor. Innovations in Health Care Financing. World Bank Discussion Paper 365.

Warner-Roedler DL, Knuth P and Juchems R-H. 1997. The German health-care system. Mayo Clinic Proceedings 72:1061–1068.

Weekly Epidemiological Record. 1997. Cholera in Africa. Summary background (1970–1990). WHO Weekly Epidemiolgical Record 72:89–93.

Weindling P, Editor. 1995. International Health Organizations and Movements, 1918–1939. Cambridge. Cambridge Universitry Press.

Weisberg J. 1998. Keeping the Boom From Busting. New York Times Magazine. July 19.

Weisbrod BA. 1983. Economics and Medical Research. Washington, DC. American Enterprise Institute for Public Policy. 171 p.

Whiting VR. 1984. The Politics of Technology Transfer in Mexico. University of California San Diego: Center for US–Mexican Studies. Research Report Series No. 37. 57p.

WHOQOL Group. 1995. The World Health Organization Quality of Life Assessment (WHOOL): position paper from the WHO. Social Science and Medicine 41:1403–1409.

Wilkinson RG. 1992. Income distribution and life expectancy. British Medical Journal 304:165–168.

Wilkinson RG. 1994. The epidemiological transition: from material scarcity to social disadvantage. Daedalus 123:61–77.

Williams CD and Jelliffe DB. 1972. Mother and Child Health. London. Oxford University Press. 164 p.

Williams G. 1969. The Plague Killers. New York. Charles Scribner. 345 p.

Winner L. 1993. The road from Rio. Technology Review (Massachusetts Institute of Technology) 96:60–64.

Winslow C-E A. 1951. The Cost of Sickness and the Price of Health. Geneva. World Health Organization, Monograph series No. 7. 106 p.

Woelk GB and Moyo IM. 1995. Development of a computerized information system in the Harare City Health Department. Methods of Information in Medicine 34:297–301.

Wohl AS. 1983. Endangered Lives. Public Health in Victorian Britain. Cambridge, MA. Harvard University Press. 440 p.

Wolff RJ. 1965. Modern medicine and traditional culture: confrontation on the Malay Peninsula. Human Organization 24:339–345.

Woolley FR. 1990. Medical ethics, technology and public health. Asia-Pacific Journal of Public Health 4:228–233.

Woolsey TD. 1979. Needed developmental research for measuring the health of populations in the less developed countries. US Public Health Service. Office of International Health. International Health Planning Methods Series 10:58–86.

World Bank. 1975. Health Sector Policy Paper. Washington, DC. World Bank. 83 p.

World Bank. 1980. Health Sector Policy Paper. Washington, DC. World Bank. 85 p.

World Bank. 1993. World Development Report. Investing in Health. Washington, DC. Published by Oxford University Press for the World Bank. 329 p.

World Bank. 1997. World Development Report. The State in a Changing World. Washington, DC. Published by Oxford University Press for the World Bank. 265 p.

World Bank. 1998. World Development Indicators. Washington, DC. World Bank. 388 p.

World Health Forum. 1995. The rise of international cooperation in health. World Health Forum 16:388–393.

World Health Forum. 1996. Ethics and health in a changing world. World Health Forum 17:150–155.

World Health Organization. 1958. The First Ten Years of the World Health Organization. Geneva. World Health Organization. 538 p.

World Health Organization. 1969. Statistics of Health Services and Their Activities. Technical Report Series 429. 36 p.

World Health Organization. 1976a. Reference Material for Health Auxiliaries and Their Teachers. Geneva. World Health Organization Offset Publication No. 28. 59 p in English; additional 38 p in French.World Health Organization.

World Health Organization. 1976b. Twenty-Ninth World Health Assembly, Geneva 3–21 May 1976. Part I. Resolutions and Decisions. Annexes. World Health Organization Official Records No. 233. 115 p.

World Health Organization. 1980. The Global Eradication of Smallpox. Final Report of the Global Commission for the Certification of Smallpox Eradication. Geneva. World Health Organization. 30 p.

World Health Organization. 1990. The New Emergency Health Kit. Geneva. WHO. Publication WHO/DAP/90.1.

World Health Organization. 1993. International Statistical Classification of Diseases and Related Health Problems. Tenth Revision. Volume 2. Geneva. World Health Organization.

World Health Organization. 1994. Strengthening of Health Services. WHO's Response to the Changing Needs of Countries. Publication WHO/SHS94.2.

World Health Organization. Division of Diarrhoeal and Respiratory Disease Control.1995. Integrated management of the sick child. Bulletin of the World Health Organization 73:735–740.

World Health Organization. 1996. Revised 1990 Estimates of Maternal Mortality: A New Approach by WHO and UNICEF. Publication WHO/FRH/MSM/96.11.

World Health Organization. 1997a. Care in Normal Birth: A Practical Guide. Publication WHO/FRH/MSM/96.24.

World Health Organization. 1997b. Health and Environment in Sustainable Development. Five Years After the Earth Summit. Geneva. Publication WHO/EHG/97.8. 243 p.

World Health Organization. 1998. World Health Report. Geneva. WHO obtainable from ⟨http://www.who.int/1998/whr-en.htm⟩.

World Resources 1998–99. 1998. Published for the World Resources Institute, the United Nations Environment Programme, the United Nations Development Programme, and the World Bank. New York. Oxford University Press. 369 p.

Xu W. 1995. Flourishing health work in China. Social Science and Medicine 41:1043–1045.

Yang P, Lin V and Lawson J. 1991. Health policy reform in the People's Republic of China. International Journal of Health Services 21:481–491.

Yekutiel P. 1980. Eradication of Infectious Diseases. Basel. S. Karger. 164 p.

Yergin D and Stanislaw J. 1998. The Commanding Heights. The Battle Between Government and the Marketplace That Is Remaking the Modern World. New York, Simon and Schuster.

Young ME. 1989. Impact of the rural reform on financing of rural health services in China. Health Policy 11:27–42.

Younger E. 1987. Safer motherhood. International Health News 8(Suppl. 10):1–4.

Zhang K, Liu M and Li D. 1996. Health care delivery system and major health issues in China. Medical Journal of Australia 165:638–640.

Zheng X and Hillier S. 1995. The reforms of the Chinese health care system: county level changes: the Jiangxi Study. Social Science and Medicine 41:1057–1064.

Zhu N, Ling Z, Shen J, Lane JM and Hu S. 1989. Factors associated with the decline of the Cooperative Medical System and barefoot doctors in rural China. Bulletin of the World Health Organization 67:431–441.

Zimmerman MR. 1993. The paleopathology of the cardiovascular system. Texas Heart Institute Journal 20:252–257.

Zukin P. 1987. Handbook for the Planning and Managerial Process for Health Development at the State and Local Government Area Levels in Nigeria. Nigerian National Ministry of Health. Directorate of National Health Planning and Research. 91 p.

Index